S0-ABC-438

Ophthalmic Surgery Complications

Prevention and Management

Ophthalmic Surgery Complications

Prevention and Management

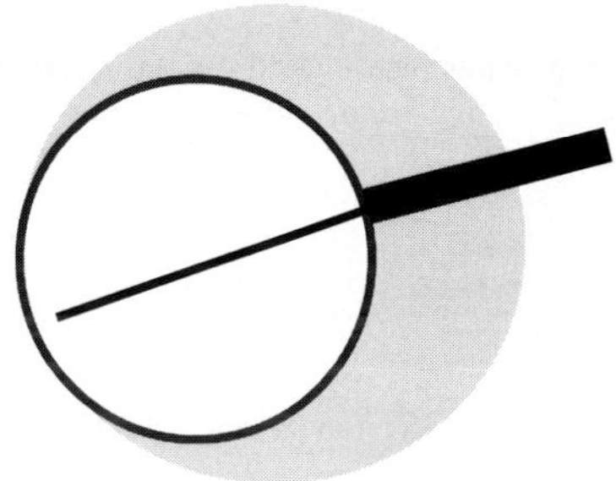

EDITED BY

Judie F. Charlton, MD
Associate Professor
Department of Ophthalmology
Residency Program Director
Robert C. Byrd Health Sciences Center
of West Virginia University
Morgantown, West Virginia

George W. Weinstein, MD
Professor and Jane McDermott Shott Chairman
Department of Ophthalmology
Director, University Eye Center
Robert C. Byrd Health Sciences Center
of West Virginia University
Morgantown, West Virginia

With 28 contributors

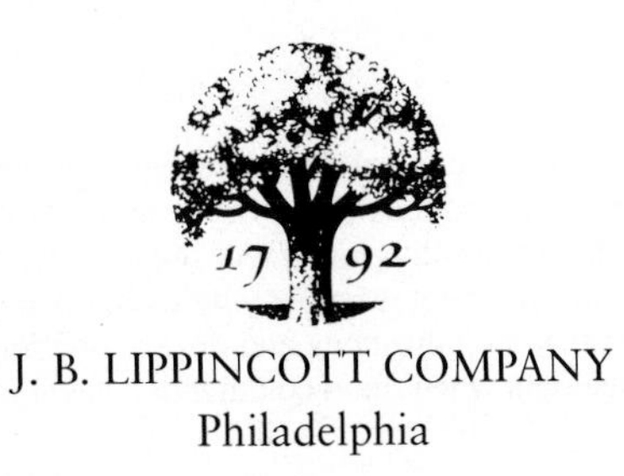

J. B. LIPPINCOTT COMPANY
Philadelphia

Assistant Editor: *Eileen Wolfberg*
Project Editor: *Jody E. Gould*
Production Manager: *Caren Erlichman*
Production Coordinator: *David Yurkovich*
Designer: *Doug Smock*
Indexer: *Ann Cassar*
Compositor: *Bi-Comp, Inc.*
Printer/Binder: *Quebecor/Kingsport*
Color Insert Printer: *Wadsworth Publishing Company*

6 5 4 3 2 1

Library of Congress Cataloging-in-Publication Data

Ophthalmic surgery complications: prevention and management/edited by Judie F. Charlton, George W. Weinstein; with 28 contributors. p. cm.
Includes bibliographical references and index.
ISBN 0-397-51295-3
1. Eye—Surgery—Complications. I. Charlton, Judie F.
II. Weinstein, George W.
[DNLM: 1. Eye—surgery. 2. Eye Diseases—surgery.
3. Postoperative Complications—prevention & control.
4. Intraoperative Complications—prevention & control. WW 168 06144 1995]
RE80.06525 1995
617.7'1—dc20
DNLM/DLC
for Library of Congress 94-26149
CIP

∞ This paper meets the requirements of ANSI/NISO Z39.48-1992 (permanence of paper).

The authors and publisher have exerted every effort to ensure that drug selection and dosage set forth in this text are in accord with current recommendations and practice at the time of publication. However, in view of ongoing research, changes in government regulations, and the constant flow of information relating to drug therapy and drug reactions, the reader is urged to check the package insert for each drug for any change in indications and dosage and for added warnings and precautions. This is particularly important when the recommended agent is a new or infrequently employed drug.

During the course of one's professional development, one is fortunate to encounter a mentor who teaches much more than ophthalmology. The lessons in diplomacy, fairness, and leading by example endure much longer than the ever changing face of medical science. This book is therefore dedicated to my mentor, friend, and coeditor, Dr. George W. Weinstein.

JUDIE F. CHARLTON, MD

CONTRIBUTORS

William H. Benson, MD
Assistant Professor of Ophthalmology
Medical College of Virginia
Richmond, Virginia

Jerome W. Bettman, Sr., MD
Emeritus Clinical Professor
Stanford University
University of California, San Francisco
Emeritus Chairman
California Pacific Eye Department
San Francisco, California

Judie F. Charlton, MD
Associate Professor
Department of Ophthalmology
Residency Program Director
Robert C. Byrd Health Sciences Center of West Virginia University
Morgantown, West Virginia

Thomas G. Chu, MD, PhD
Department of Ophthalmology
University of California at Davis
Sacramento, California

Ranjit S. Dhaliwal, MD, FRCSC
Department of Ophthalmology
Queen's University Faculty of Medicine
Kingston, Ontario, Canada

D. Michael Elnicki, MD
Assistant Professor of Medicine
West Virginia University School of Medicine
Morgantown, West Virginia

Leonard Ferenz, PhD
Bioethics Program
Department of Philosophy
University of North Carolina
Charlotte, North Carolina

Robert R. Hobson
Department of Ophthalmology
Robert C. Byrd Health Sciences Center of West Virginia University
Morgantown, West Virginia

Milton Kahn, MD
Department of Ophthalmology
Lenox Hill Hospital
New York, New York

Jonathan Kay, MD
Clinical Associate Professor of Anesthesiology and Internal Medicine
Medical College of Wisconsin
Department of Anesthesiology
St. Luke's Medical Center
Milwaukee, Wisconsin

Marilyn C. Kay, MD
Clinical Associate Professor of Ophthalmology
Medical College of Wisconsin
Department of Ophthalmology
Milwaukee, Wisconsin

Jeffrey M. Lehmer, MD
Visiting Assistant Professor
University of California, Los Angeles
Sanford and Erna Schulhofer Fellow
Department of Ophthalmology
Jules Stein Eye Institute
Los Angeles, California

Hilel Lewis, MD
Chairman, Division of Ophthalmology
Director, Cleveland Clinic Eye Institute
Cleveland, Ohio

Marc F. Lieberman, MD
Associate Clinical Professor
Department of Ophthalmology
University of California, San Francisco
Co-Director, Glaucoma Service
California Pacific Medical Center
San Francisco, California

Marian S. Macsai, MD
Department of Ophthalmology
Robert C. Byrd Health Sciences Center of West Virginia University
Morgantown, West Virginia

Nick Mamalis, MD
Associate Professor of Ophthalmology
Moran Eye Center
University of Utah Health Sciences Center
Salt Lake City, Utah

Vince Manopoli
President
Medricon, Incorporated
Hamden, Connecticut

Travis A. Meredith, MD
Clinical Professor of Ophthalmology
St. Louis University School of Medicine
St. Louis, Missouri

Dale R. Meyer, MD
Assistant Professor of Ophthalmology
Director, Oculoplastic and Orbital Surgery Service
Albany Medical College
Albany Medical Center
Albany, New York

Michelle Michael, COT, NCLC
University Eye Center
West Virginia University
Morgantown, West Virginia

Ngoc Nguyen, MD
Foundation for Glaucoma Research
San Francisco, California

Stephen A. Obstbaum, MD
Professor and Chairman
Department of Ophthalmology
Lenox Hill Hospital
New York, New York

David S. Rho, MD
Department of Ophthalmology
Lenox Hill Hospital
New York, New York

Kathleen Rose, RN
Education Coordinator
Bascom Palmer Eye Institute
Miami, Florida

Terry L. Schwartz, MD
Department of Ophthalmology
Robert C. Byrd Health Sciences Center of West Virginia University
Morgantown, West Virginia

Richard F. Spaide, MD
Clinical Assistant Professor in Ophthalmology
New York Medical College
St. Vincent's Hospital and Medical Center of New York
New York, New York

Rick Walters
Medricon, Incorporated
Hamden, Connecticut

Donna Jo Wheeler, LPN
Department of Ophthalmology
Robert C. Byrd Health Sciences Center of West Virginia University
Morgantown, West Virginia

PREFACE

Most of the currently available texts on ophthalmic surgery complications focus on recognition and management of intraoperative complications. Our goal is to expand this approach to include the prevention of complications, delayed postoperative complications, and recognition of the team approach in providing ophthalmic care. Unexpected events in surgery do not always need to lead to untoward results if the problems are approached correctly. Perhaps the best basis for definition of an untoward result is the patient's perception of the surgical outcome. Several variables affect a patient's perception of care, and the role of the billing clerks, technical support staff, and legal counsel can have an impact far beyond that of the physician. Management of surgical complications extends well beyond surgical technical expertise, and we hope that this text encompasses the full realm.

Judie F. Charlton, MD
George W. Weinstein, MD

ACKNOWLEDGMENTS

For every sense of accomplishment that goes with compiling a text, there are moments of frustration. We therefore acknowledge our families, colleagues, and coworkers for their support, understanding, and hard work on our behalf. We also acknowledge the support of Stuart Freeman and Eileen Wolfberg and thank them for extending this opportunity to us.

CONTENTS

Ophthalmic Surgery Complications

Prevention and Management

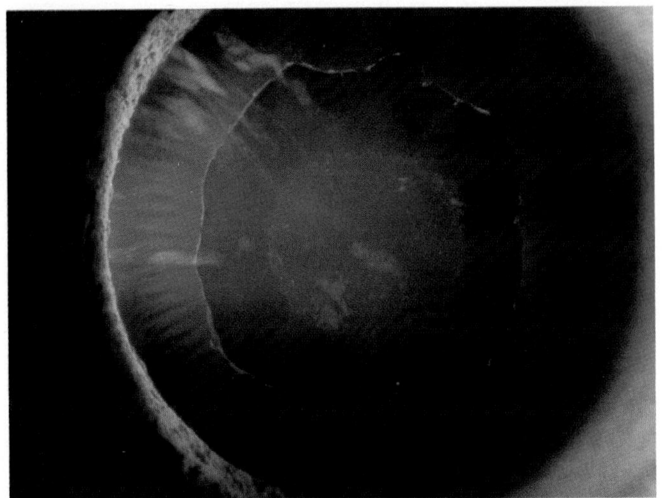

Color Figure 1-4. Pseudoexfoliation syndrome may predispose to zonular weakening and lens subluxation during surgical manipulation.

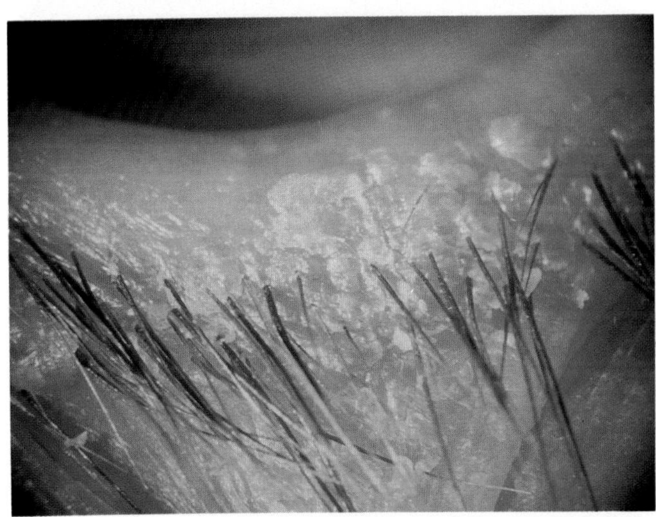

Color Figure 1-5. Severe seborrheic blepharitis should be recognized and treated before any ocular surgery is performed.

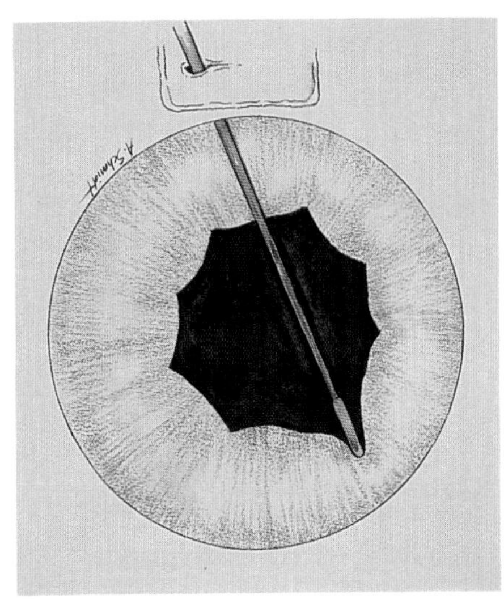

Color Figure 8-1. Illustration demonstrating Fine's technique for pupil widening, in which the iris is stretched, creating minor iris sphincter tears in multiple locations. (Courtesy of Howard Fine, MD)

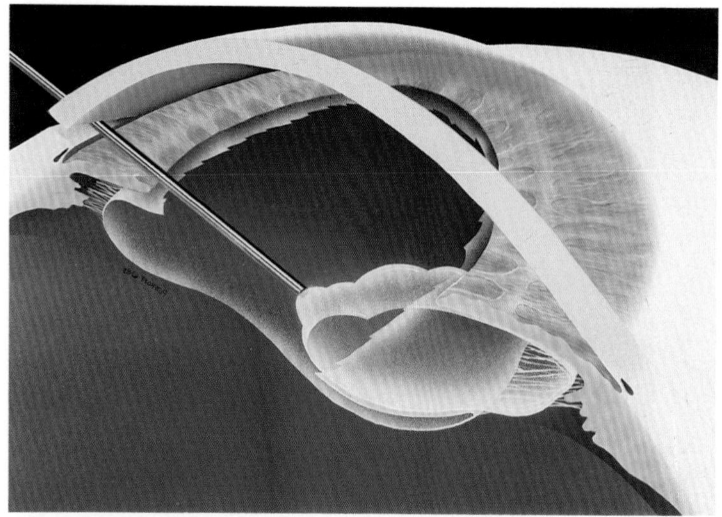

Color Figure 8-4. Illustration demonstrating the use of viscoelastic agent to widen the ciliary sulcus in preparation for implantation of the intraocular lens (IOL) within the ciliary sulcus.

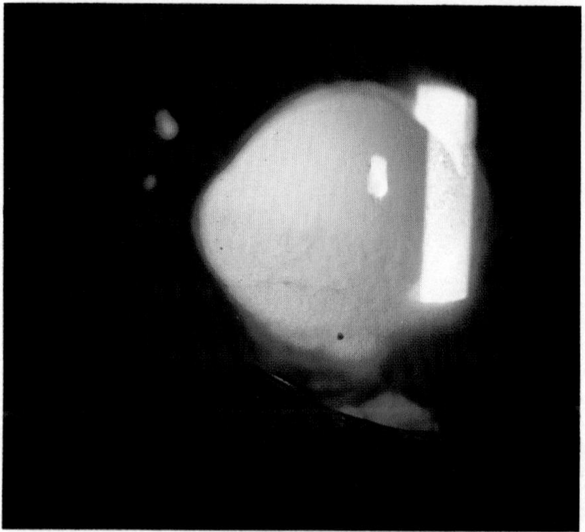

Color Figure 8-5. Slit-lamp photograph of a patient with epithelial downgrowth. Retroillumination demonstrates the retrocorneal membrane spreading from the superior cornea.

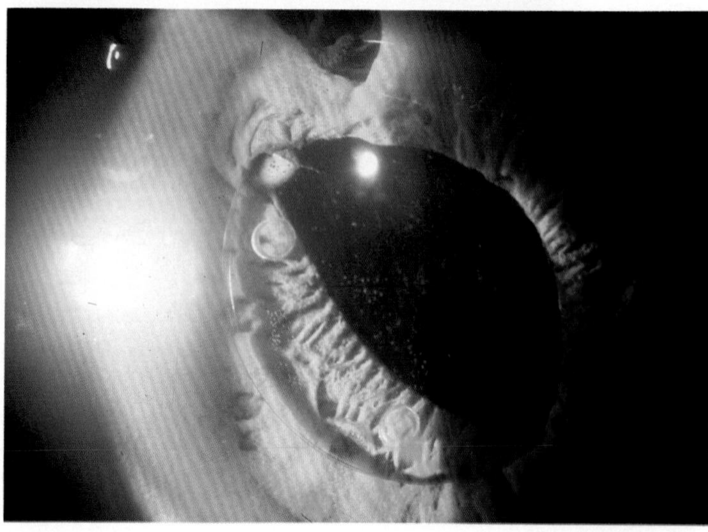

Color Figure 8-6. Slit-lamp photograph demonstrating a case of pupil capture in which a significant portion of the IOL optic is seen anterior to the iris.

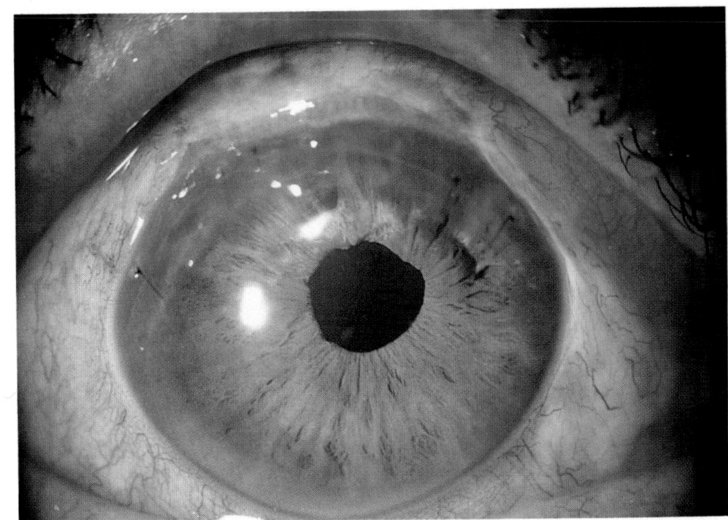

Color Figure 8-7. Slit-lamp photograph of the right eye demonstrating a case of iris tuck, in which the midstromal iris has become adherent to the intraocular lens (IOL) optic superonasally. This has not resulted in any clinically apparent dislocation of the IOL. This patient had undergone a procedure involving a corneal trephine incision for glaucoma 30 years before cataract extraction.

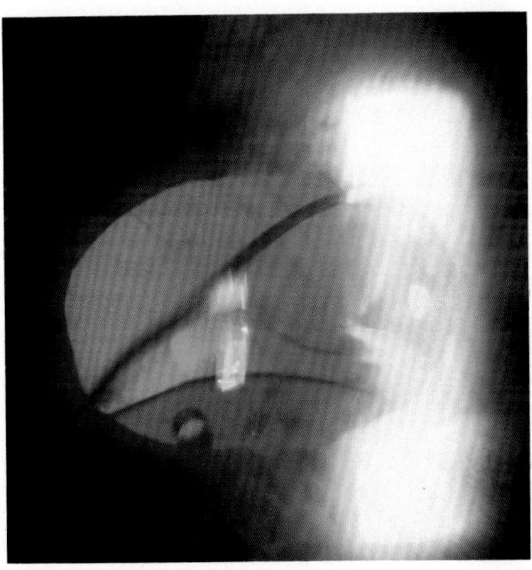

Color Figure 8-8. Slit-lamp photograph demonstrating a severe case of inferior dislocation of the IOL, so that only a small portion of the optic is visible through the pupil (ie, sunset syndrome).

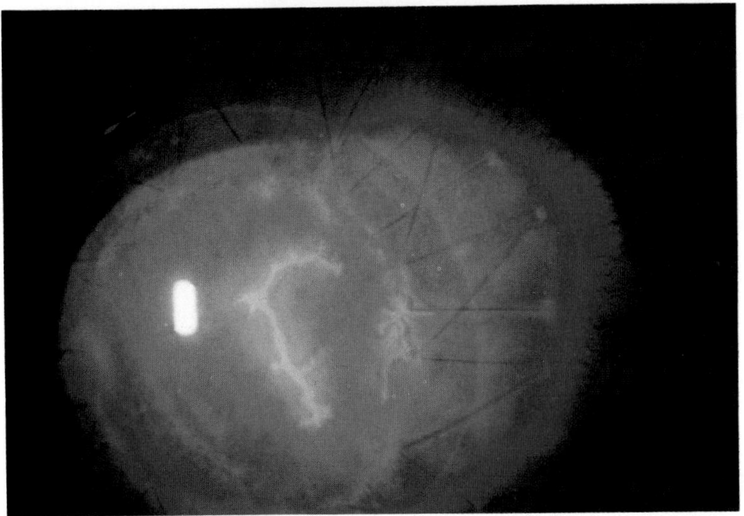

Color Figure 9-7. Fluorescein staining demonstrates classic dendritic lesion resulting from recurrent herpes simplex viral keratitis in a corneal graft. Treatment includes rapid institution of intensive topical antiviral agents. When the dendrite involves the visual axis, débridement is frequently recommended.

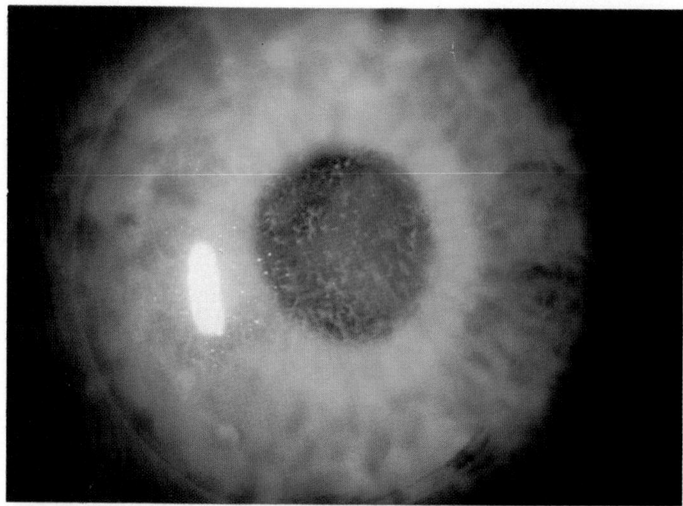

Color Figure 9-8. Recurrence of Reis-Bücklers corneal dystrophy in a penetrating keratoplasty 8 years after the initial surgery. A honeycomb-like subepithelial pattern may be seen covering the entire surface of the corneal graft.

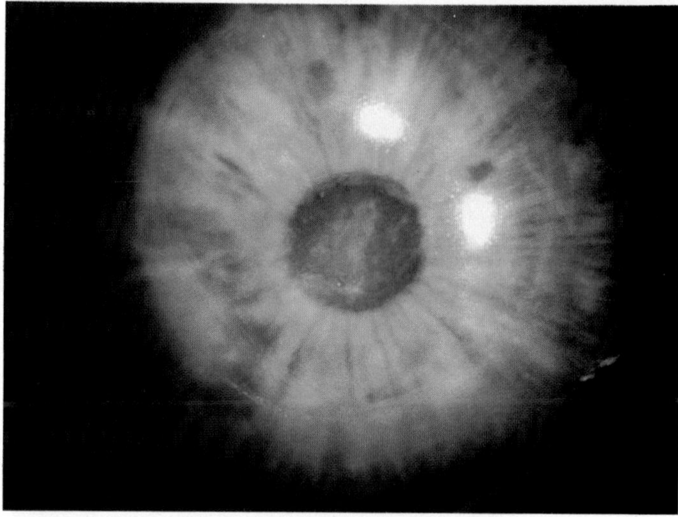

Color Figure 9-9. Recurrent lattice corneal dystrophy in a penetrating keratoplasty 6 years after the original surgery. The recurrent lattice dystrophy results in an irregular epithelial surface, which is prone to recurrent corneal erosions, as seen here. Methods of treatment have included lamellar keratectomy, excimer laser phototherapeutic keratectomy, and penetrating keratoplasty.

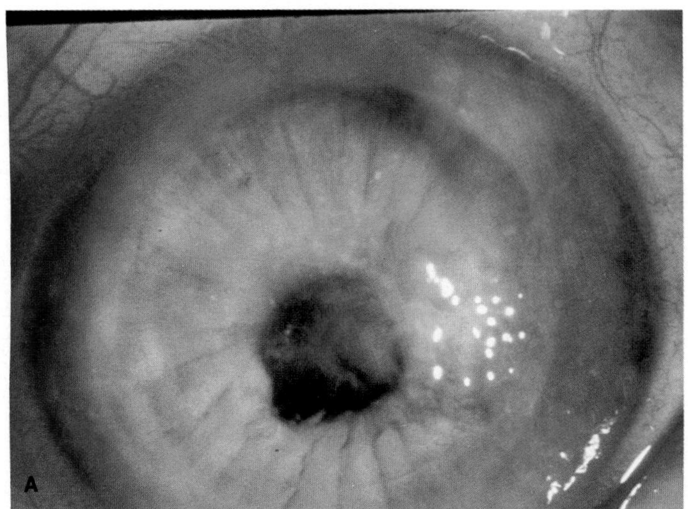

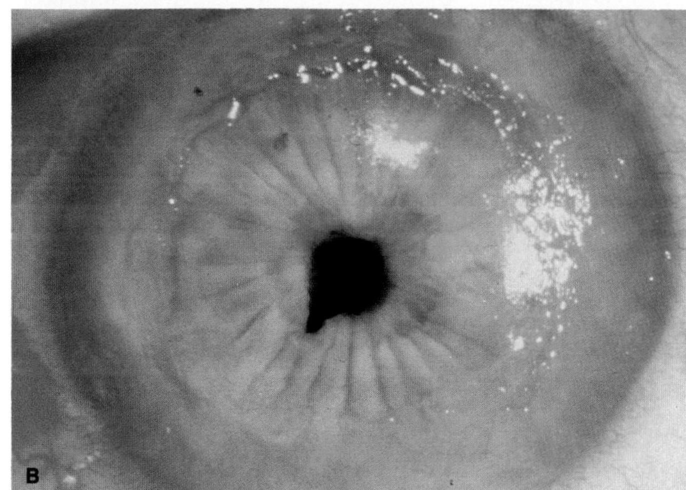

Color Figure 9-15. (**A**) Recurrent lattice corneal dystrophy 6 years after penetrating keratoplasty. (**B**) The same patient immediately after excimer laser phototherapeutic keratectomy. Note the clearing of the visual axis and the smoothing of the central corneal graft that have transpired. The patient's vision improved from the 20/200 level to 20/25 after phototherapeutic keratectomy.

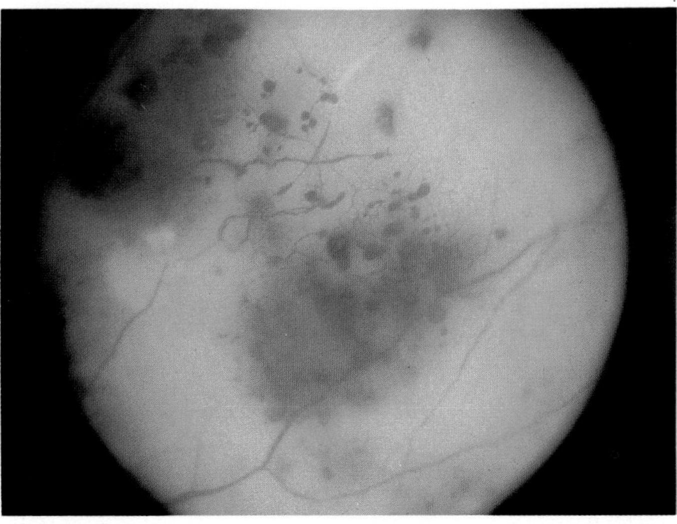

Color Figure 11-9. Fundus photograph of the characteristic telangiectatic retinal vessels seen in Coats disease with an underlying exudative retinal detachment.

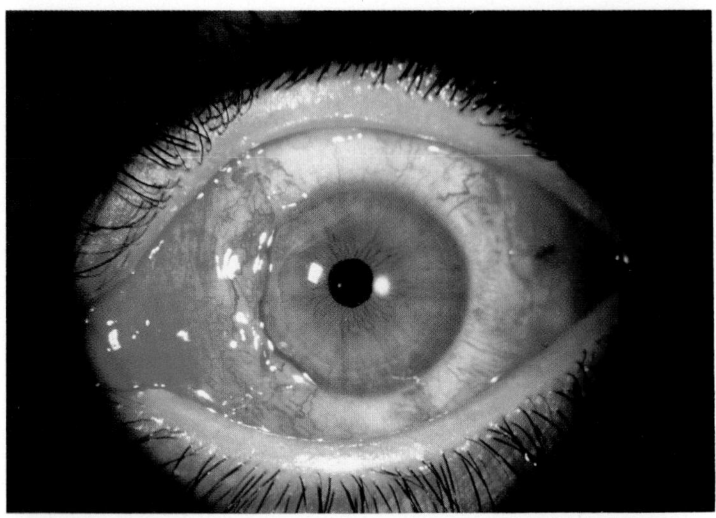

Color Figure 12-4. Dell at inferonasal limbus after large medial rectus resection. Note edematous conjunctiva with override of the cornea.

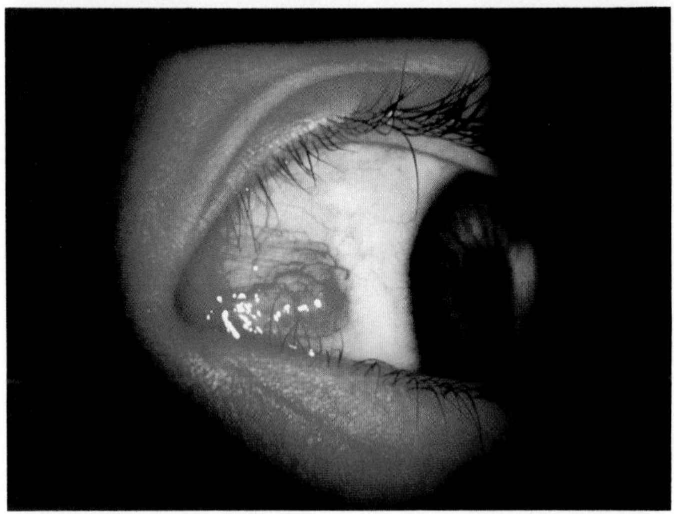

Color Figure 12-5. Hyperemia and granuloma over site of muscle insertion.

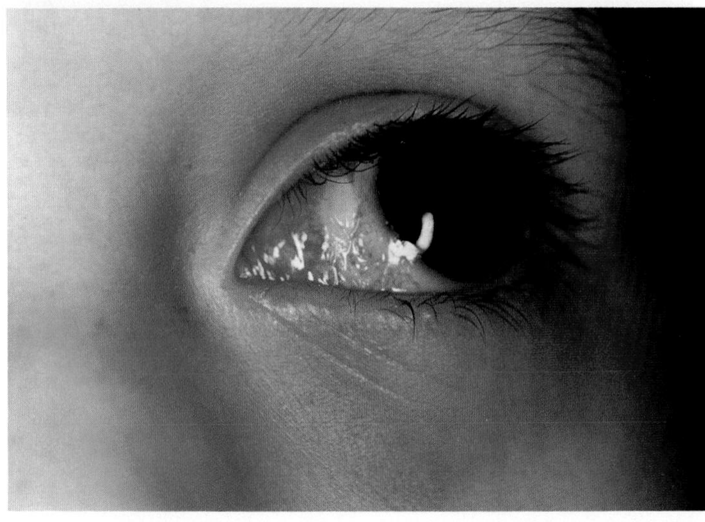

Color Figure 12-7. Tenon capsule prolapsed from conjunctival incision.

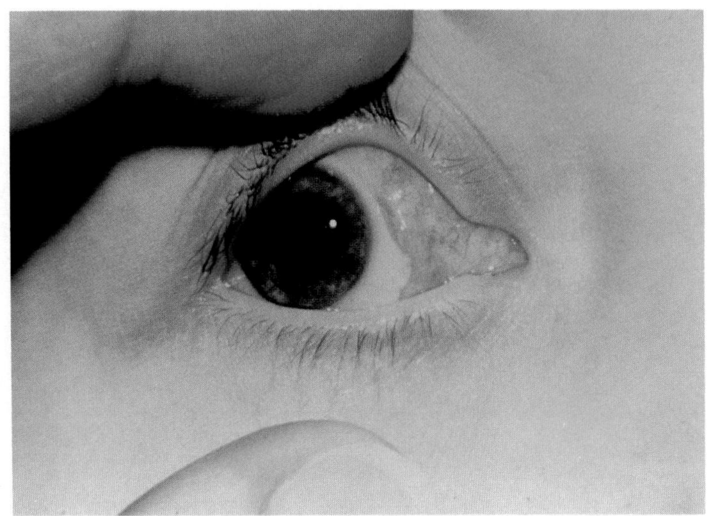

Color Figure 12-8. Prolapsed fat following surgery. (Courtesy of Linda M. Christmann, MD)

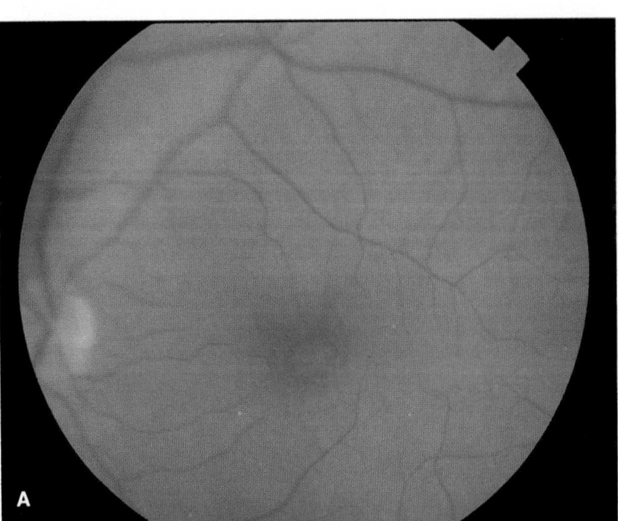

Color Figure 15-1. (**A**) Photograph of cystoid macular edema (CME), demonstrating foveal cysts.

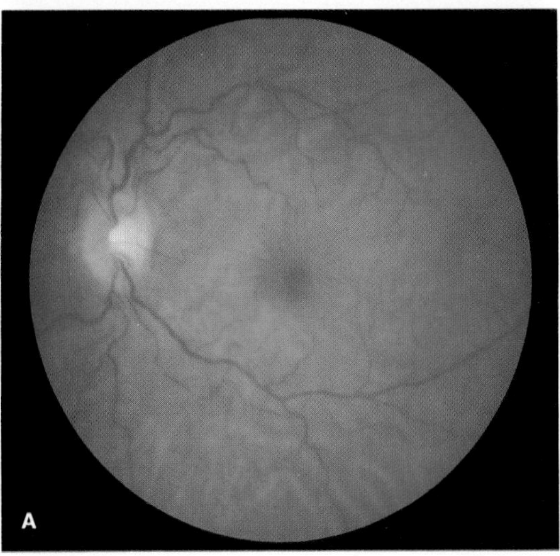

Color Figure 15-2. (**A**) Photograph of a patient with a shallow retinal detachment. The fine radiating retinal folds in the macula simulate CME.

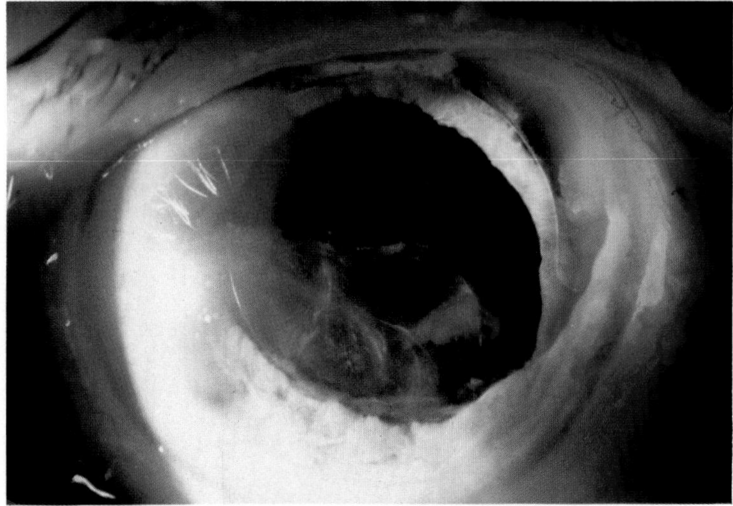

Color Figure 17-1. An 89-year-old woman with an ocular history of chronic glaucoma. She underwent uncomplicated cataract extraction, anterior chamber intraocular lens placement, and trabeculectomy. On the second postoperative day, she was awakened from sleep by severe eye pain. Notice the shallowed anterior chamber and forward displacement of the vitreous and anterior chamber lens.

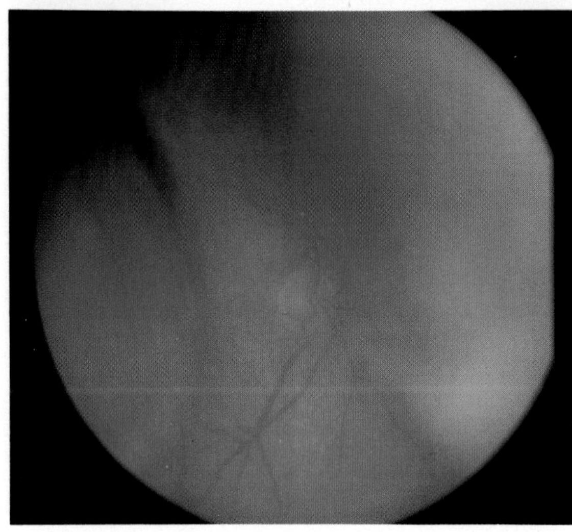

Color Figure 17-2. Same patient as in Figure 17-1. Notice the large, darkly colored, dome-shaped elevations arising from the peripheral retina and extending toward the optic nerve.

Ophthalmic Surgery Complications: Prevention and Management,
edited by Judie F. Charlton and George W. Weinstein.
J. B. Lippincott Company, Philadelphia © 1995.

1

William H. Benson

The Eye Examination

The text of this chapter focuses on the preoperative examination for those patients undergoing ophthalmic surgery. The ocular examination represents an opportunity for the ophthalmologist to obtain a proper diagnosis using specific aspects of the patient's history, physical findings, and testing parameters. The history may provide the physician with a subjective report of any functional impairment. The testing parameters and physical findings allow an objective determination of actual visual impairment.

Visual acuity and intraocular pressure represent the "vital signs" of ophthalmology. The patient's vision is the single most important parameter that must be evaluated during the ocular examination. If the patient's visual acuity is less than 20/20, the physician should account for each line of visual loss with the specific underlying disease responsible for that amount of visual dysfunction.

THE EXAMINATION PROCEDURE

The ocular examination should begin with a measurement of the patient's level of visual function. It should be assessed by both a careful history and visual testing. The history should offer an estimation of functional impairment of vision, and visual testing should measure the degree of actual visual impairment. Functional impairment of vision refers to the patient's status regarding the ability of the patient to perform everyday activities. Impairment of visual function refers to the patient's status measured in terms of the results of objective visual testing. The examination should determine whether the amount of objective visual impairment is in proportion to subjective functional impairment, and whether the underlying pathologic processes that contribute to the visual impairment have been recognized.

Snellen visual acuity is the most widely used index of visual function. It measures the patient's resolution ability for objects of uniform high contrast in a darkened room. It does not assess the eye's ability to recognize low-contrast patterns. Visual acuity may be influenced immediately after manipulating the corneal epithelium with applanation tonometry or by bleaching the retina with ophthalmoscopy. Therefore, the patient's visual acuity should be measured before any other aspect of the ocular examination is performed.

ASSESSMENT OF VISUAL FUNCTION

Other techniques for measuring visual function include contrast sensitivity and glare testing. Contrast sensitivity is a measure of the degree of contrast required to perceive a test object of a specified size. It evaluates the patient's ability to detect subtle variations of shading by presenting objects that are varied in contrast, luminance, and spatial frequency. Patients' contrast sensitivity is determined by the lowest contrast with which they are able to identify an object. The simplest device used to test contrast sensitivity employs eye charts similar to those used for testing Snellen visual acuity. Like Snellen testing, contrast sensitivity testing does not differentiate among the various reasons for a patient's visual impairment.

Glare testing attempts to determine the degree of visual impairment caused by various opacities of the media in well-lighted conditions. Glare testing attempts to simulate the symptom of glare caused by the scattering of light entering the eye and provide a measurement of the degree of resultant visual impairment. Glare disability is determined by comparing the patient's visual acuity with and without the presence of a light source directed at the eye.

As with Snellen acuity and contrast sensitivity testing, glare testing results are not specific to the underlying pathologic process causing visual dysfunction. One significant deficiency with glare testing is the lack of established standard equipment, method of administration, and scoring of the test—all of which contribute to its limited usefulness regarding the evaluation of functional disability resulting from glare.

Physical examination of the eye should follow the measurement of visual acuity. The examination should identify any ocular conditions that could account for the amount of visual impairment determined by visual acuity testing. The physical examination should include retinoscopy and refraction, evaluation of motility, pupillary function, tonometry, slit-lamp examination, and dilated fundus ophthalmoscopy.

The physical examination should begin with retinoscopy and refraction to determine whether a refractive error is present to account for any visual impairment. The retinoscope allows the physician to determine the refractive error of an eye objectively. It may be useful to determine other causes of visual impairment, such as irregular corneal astigmatism and opacities of the lens. Irregular astigmatism may be suspected with a "scissors" type of light reflex on streaking, and opacities of the cataract can be identified using retroillumination through a dilated pupil.

Manifest refraction provides a subjective determination of the refractive error of an eye. It is necessary to determine the refractive error of both eyes for those patients undergoing cataract extraction to avoid significant anisometropia after intraocular lens implantation. If a patient exhibits a unilateral cataract with high axial myopia or hyperopia in both eyes, it may be necessary to adjust the intraocular lens power to provide a balanced amount of ametropia between both eyes, thus avoiding postoperative visual problems, such as image disparity in a dissatisfied patient.

The motility examination should determine whether conjugate versions are present in all fields of gaze or whether there is a strabismic misalignment of the visual axes. Assessment of ocular alignment is generally performed with four basic types of ocular alignment tests. They include corneal light reflex tests, cover tests, dissimilar image tests, and dissimilar target tests. The tests most often used are the various cover tests that include the cover-uncover test, the alternate cover test, and the simultaneous prism-cover test.

The cover-uncover test is the main method to differentiate a phoria from a tropia. The alternate cover test (prism and cover test) measures the total deviation, both latent and manifest, but does not separate the amount of phoria from the amount of tropia. The simultaneous prism-cover test is helpful in measuring the actual manifest deviation detected by the alternate cover test. The test is performed by placing a cover before the fixating eye at the same time the prism is placed in front of the deviating eye. Longer prism powers are used until there is no shift observed in the deviated eye.

Adult patients with monocular vision loss frequently develop an exodeviation called sensory exotropia. Suppression of visual sensation in that eye from reaching consciousness prevents diplopia for the patient who may exhibit an exodeviation during the preoperative examination. The prospect for developing diplopia after surgical rehabilitation of vision in that eye should be considered by the physician and explained to the patient before surgery. If the visual result after surgery is excellent, prism therapy or surgical muscle realignment can often resolve the diplopia. However, if visual improvement after surgery remains several Snellen lines less than the best eye, diplopia may occur without a substantial improvement using spectacle prisms or muscle surgery, if the level of vision in that eye does not allow binocular fixation.

Evaluation of pupillary function should precede the administration of any pharmacologic agents that may alter the function. The physician should note all topical and systemic medications in the patient's record that may influence pupillary size and function. Pupillary shape and activity should be assessed. Observation with the slit lamp should identify whether any physical abnormalities, such as synechiae, sphincter rupture, or iris atrophy are present. A direct light source should be swung from one eye to the other and back to determine whether there is a relative afferent pupillary defect in either eye.

The presence of a relative afferent pupillary defect requires further evaluation to determine the location and origin of any occult ipsilateral optic nerve or tract lesions. It is important to recognize the lesion as a potential cause of visual impairment before dilation. Otherwise, it may go undetected until a postoperative evaluation recognizes the optic nerve or tract lesion as the reason for visual impairment.

The slit-lamp examination should precede any physical contact with the ocular surface. It should identify any abnormalities or opacities of the media of the ocular surface, anterior segment, or anterior vitreous that could account for visual impairment present at the time of the examination. It should precede tonometry so that any abnormality of the corneal epithelial surface can be considered as a significant finding. If tonometry is performed before slit-lamp examination, tonometry tip contact with the ocular surface may cause disruption of the corneal epithelium, and can alter or become confused with other separate clinical signs present during the examination. That alteration of clinical signs may lead to misdiagnosis and possible mismanagement of that problem before surgery.

Ocular surface abnormalities that may contribute to visual impairment include tear film deficiency, epithelial keratopathy, and irregular astigmatism. Clinical signs of a tear deficiency state may include a reduced tear meniscus, accumulation of mucus strands in the tear film, or punctate staining of the conjunctival or corneal epithelium with fluorescein or rose bengal stains (Fig. 1-1). Reduced basal tear production may be confirmed using Schirmer filter paper strips following the application of topical anesthesia.

Another cause of epithelial keratopathy is exposure of the ocular surface from lagophthalmos. The physician should carefully assess the patient's blinking pattern at the slit-lamp using the cobalt blue filter under low illumination after the application of fluorescein. Incomplete closure of the eyelids during involuntary blinking may lead to chronic exposure keratopathy over the inferior corneal surface. Patients should be made aware of the condition and urged to completely close and blink their eyes on a voluntary basis more frequently to avoid further problems. Patients with diabetes mellitus, previous herpetic keratitis, or long-standing rigid contact lens wear may exhibit reduced corneal sensation or signs of epithelial keratopathy from an underlying neurotrophic state. Corneal sensation to touch is provided by the nasociliary branch of the fifth cranial nerve. The level of corneal sensation can be tested subjectively by lightly touching the corneal surface with the end of a piece of dental floss and grading the patient's response as normal, reduced, or absent. Patients with preexisting epithelial keratopathy may exhibit further breakdown of the corneal surface from exposure or manipulation at the time of surgery. This can lead to persistent epithelial defects that may cause postoperative visual loss from superficial stromal scarring, sterile corneal stromal melting from topical steroid use, or infectious microbial keratitis. The physician should take all measures to treat any preexisting surface epithelial keratopathy before surgery by properly identifying the underlying cause at the time of the preoperative examination.

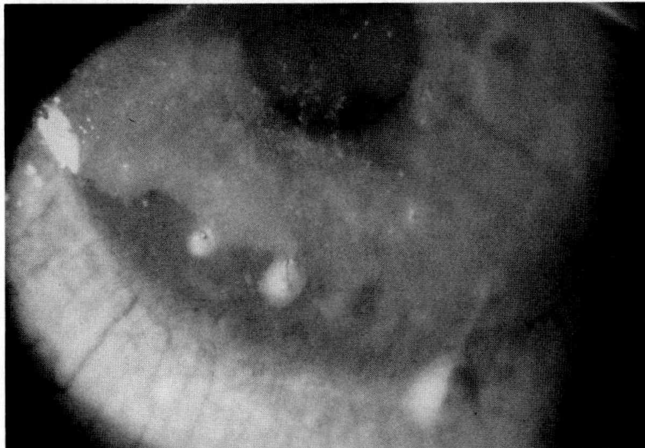

Figure 1-1. Filamentary and punctate epithelial keratopathy in a patient with keratoconjunctivitis sicca.

Another corneal surface abnormality that may contribute to visual impairment at the time of the preoperative examination is irregular corneal astigmatism from an irregular corneal curvature. Observation of distorted mires over the visual axis on qualitative keratometry or keratoscopy may suggest the presence of an irregular surface contour. Computer corneal topographic analysis can provide a quantitative and qualitative measurement of the corneal curvature at various points over the entire surface. Patients with previously unrecognized early keratoconus, or some other cause of corneal ectasia or thinning from previous inflammation and scarring may be properly diagnosed with a corneal topographic system. The diagnosis of irregular astigmatism as a cause of visual impairment can be made by refracting the patient after placing a rigid contact lens on the cornea. If improvement of vision with a rigid contact lens is obtained, the amount of improvement determines the contribution of irregular astigmatism as a source of visual impairment.

The health status of the corneal endothelium is important to determine before any intraocular surgery. The primary function of the endothelium is to maintain corneal deturgescence and preserve corneal transparency. The physician can assess the health of the endothelium by measuring corneal thickness and visualizing the posterior corneal layer under high magnification. The posterior corneal layer should be carefully examined under high slit-lamp magnification for signs of endothelial cell dysfunction, such as central guttae, folds in Descemet membrane, or increased corneal stromal thickness (Figs. 1-2 and 1-3). Increased corneal thickness can imply increased hydration from impaired endothelial cell function. Corneal thickness can be measured by optical pachometry, ultrasonic pachometry, or specular microscopy. All three methods allow accurate and repeatable measurements by one observer. However, only ultrasonic pachometry provides accurate readings by multiple observers and carries the advantage of ease of use compared with the other two methods.

Specular photographic microscopy can be used to record the corneal endothelial cell density and to evaluate endothelial cell morphology. A cell density of 2000 to 3000 cells/mm^2 with a 60% to 75% proportion of hexagonal cell morphology are indicative of a normal healthy cornea. Cell counts below normal imply some impairment of endothelial function that may not withstand the stresses of intraocular surgery. Some investigators have suggested that specular microscopy can be used to predict the response of the endothelium to cataract surgery. However, the relation between preoperative specular microscopy and surgical outcome has not been adequately determined, thus precluding its use in the routine preoperative evaluation of patients for cataract surgery. Although the slit-lamp examination provides most of the necessary information regarding the health of the endothelial cell layer, specular microscopy may be of value for those patients with a borderline corneal health status from previous intraocular surgery, inflammation, or Fuchs endothelial dystrophy.

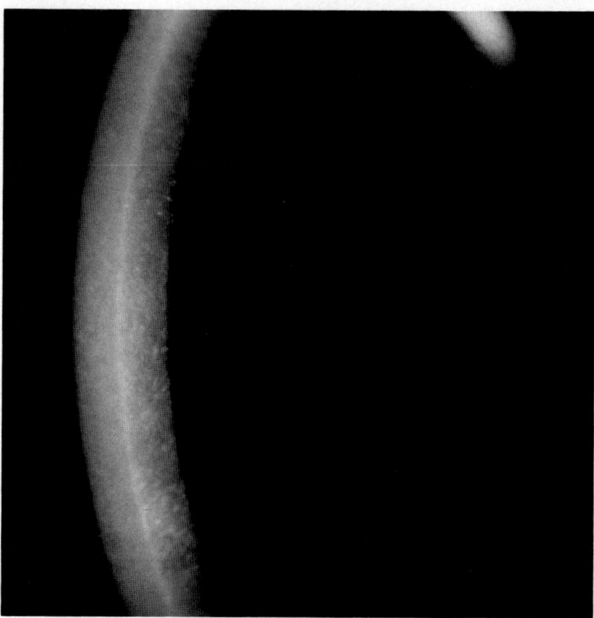

Figure 1-3. Beaten-metal appearance of the posterior corneal layer is evident with slit-lamp biomicroscopy.

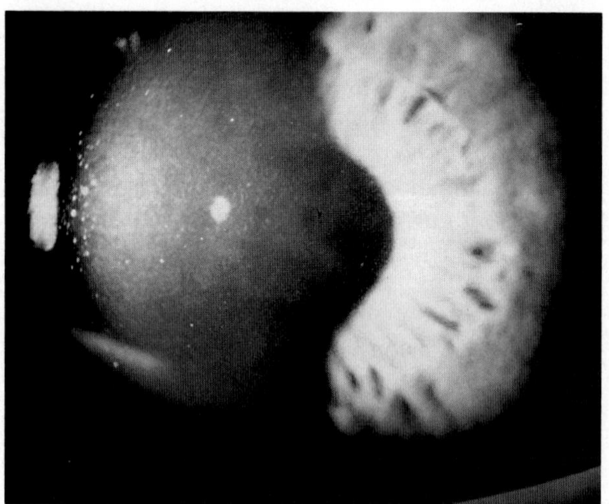

Figure 1-2. Diffuse endothelial guttae over the visual axis are seen in a patient with Fuchs endothelial dystrophy using diffuse illumination.

Further findings to note on slit-lamp examination are iris abnormalities that suggest a disorganized anterior segment from previous surgery, phacodonesis from zonular rupture, or conditions that suggest zonular weakness, such as pseudoexfoliation syndrome or previous long-standing iridocyclitis (Fig. 1-4).

MEASUREMENT OF INTRAOCULAR PRESSURE

Intraocular pressure (IOP) should be measured before any planned intraocular surgery. IOP constitutes the second "vital sign" of the eye. The presence of ocular hypotony or elevated IOP warrants further evaluation before surgery to determine its origin and avoid intraoperative complications. For those patients exhibiting an elevated IOP or hypotony, gonioscopy is essential to determine the proper diagnosis. Gonioscopy should be performed on all patients with

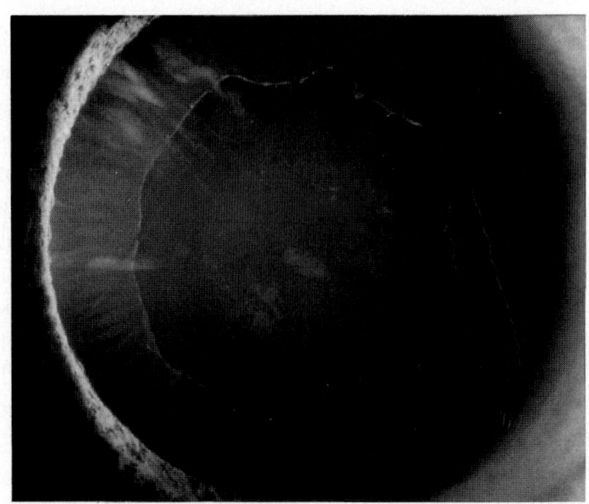

Figure 1-4. Pseudoexfoliation syndrome may predispose to zonular weakening and lens subluxation during surgical manipulation. (See color plate after page xvi.)

known glaucoma, ocular hypertension, ocular hypotony, or those with suspected disorganization of the anterior chamber angle structures. The most common type of instrument used to examine the angle structures employs a mirrored indirect system, such as the Goldmann or Zeiss lens. These lenses are placed on the corneal surface and used in conjunction with the slit lamp to provide magnification and illumination.

During gonioscopy, the physician should examine the angle in an orderly manner to identify important landmarks, such as Schwalbe line, trabecular meshwork, and scleral spur. Special attention should be given toward recognizing abnormalities, such as spindle-shaped pigmentation on the posterior corneal surface, anterior displacement or thickening of Schwalbe line, increased pigmentation, peripheral anterior synechiae, inflammatory or neovascular membranes over the trabecular meshwork, or the presence of a cyclodialysis cleft.

Various opacities of the ocular media may be recognized during the examination to account for some degree of visual impairment. Opacities of the cornea may arise from bullous keratopathy or stromal scarring over the visual axis, pigment stippling or pupillary membranes on the anterior lens capsule from previous inflammation, opacities of the cataract of the crystalline lens, opacities of the vitreous from congenital vascular remnants, vitreous hemorrhage, inflammatory debris, condensed vitreous from previous vitreous detachment, or the presence of an epiretinal membrane. For those opacities of the media that preclude an adequate view of the peripheral retina, macula, and optic nerve, B-scan ultrasonography of the eye is indicated to rule out a disorganized posterior segment or the presence of an intraocular mass lesion. In addition to qualitative B-scan ultrasonography to evaluate the anatomy of the posterior segment, it may be useful to obtain a quantitative A-scan determination of the axial length. For those patients with a long ocular axial length significantly beyond the normal range, inadvertent puncture of the globe may occur while performing retrobulbar anesthesia if the physician is not aware of the presence of a posterior staphyloma or long axial length. This may occur for those eyes in which a dense opacity of the media precludes direct visualization of the fundus by ophthalmoscopy before surgery.

Various disorders of the retina may cause a significant visual impairment out of proportion to the clinical findings noted on ophthalmoscopy. Eyes that have had previous intraocular surgery, long-standing inflammatory eye disease, or retinal vascular disease may exhibit visual loss from occult cystoid macular edema. Cystoid macular edema is a condition of fluid accumulation within the macular region in a cystic pattern centered around the fovea. If the amount of fluid accumulation is severe, the macular edema may be recognizable with contact lens slit-lamp biomicroscopy. If the amount of fluid accumulation is occult, it may only be recognized with fundus fluorescein angiography. On fluorescein angiography, fluorescein leaks from the parafoveal capillaries and accumulates in a petalloid pattern around the fovea to confirm this diagnosis.

Other causes of visual loss from macular disorders are focal areas of capillary nonperfusion from previous retinal vascular disease. These changes are visible angiographically and may be better seen with angiography than with ophthalmoscopy in many patients. These changes may be responsible for visual loss in patients who exhibit minimal diabetic retinopathy. This type of condition has been described as "dry" diabetic maculopathy, in which capillary perfusion in the perifoveolar region is poor, with resultant ischemic damage and poor visual acuity.

Impairment of optic nerve function may be present to account for visual loss noted during the preoperative examination. If a neurologic basis for visual impairment is suspected, additional testing of visual function beyond that routinely performed for a preoperative examination may be useful to establish the proper diagnosis.

Impairment of color vision, particularly red desaturation, may be noted in patients with anterior visual pathway disease through the optic nerve. Decreased visual acuity with normal color vision argues strongly against optic nerve disease. Specialized color plates, such as Handy-Rand-Rittler and Ishihara, provide a gross and nonspecific estimation of color vision. The Farnsworth-Munsell D-15 and D-100 hue comparison tests allow more accurate evaluation of color vision by requiring the patient to place pastel-colored caps in a regular sequence. Color comparison of a red object between both eyes is less standardized but may be useful in screening for subjective red desaturation, which may be suggestive of an acquired dyschromatopsia.

TESTS

Visual field testing provides specific information for many causes of visual loss along the visual pathway between the retina and the occipital cortex. Either automated static or manual kinetic perimetry can be performed. Threshold automated perimetry on the central 30 degrees using the Humphrey 30-2 or Octopus 32 program can provide a reliable indication of visual field loss from glaucoma, or retinal or neurologic disease.

Further evaluation of visual dysfunction may be performed using visual electrophysiology testing. These are the objective tests of visual potential in which the response to visual stimuli is measured electronically. The visual evoked potential (VEP) or visual evoked response provides information regarding the integrity of the entire visual pathway, but is largely a measure of macular and optic nerve visual function. The electroretinogram (ERG) provides information about a variety of diseases. A normal VEP and a normal ERG provide good evidence of an intact visual pathway between the retinal and occipital cortex. The electrooculogram reflects metabolic changes in the retinal pigment epithelium and retina. As a test of retinal function, the electrooculographic response usually parallels the electroretinographic response, with a few specific exceptions.

The history and physical examination should provide sufficient valid information concerning whether cataract is the source of functional and visual impairment in most individuals. However, tests of potential vision are available to determine whether patients with impaired vision have a potential for improved vision after cataract surgery. These tests offer the physician additional information to determine whether the significant cause of their visual impairment is cataract rather than other types of diseases.

Both subjective and objective tests of visual potential are available. The objective tests are those electrophysiologic tests previously discussed, which include electroretinography and VEP. They are generally more expensive than subjective tests because of the cost of equipment and the expertise to interpret them. Patients are usually referred to teaching institutions to obtain them because they are not available in most private physicians' offices.

Subjective tests include the potential acuity meter, suprathreshold pinhole device, Maddox rod, laser interferometer, and various blue-field entoptic image devices. Most of these tests can predict postoperative outcome reasonably accurately in eyes with a preoperative visual acuity greater than 20/200 and media clarity that allows ophthalmoscopic confirmation of a normal posterior retina and optic nerve. These tests also appear to be of value to determine the contribution of cataract to visual impairment in those individuals with either clinically detectable or occult macular or optic nerve disease, and a visible posterior pole on examination.

Potential vision tests usually do not provide an accurate estimate of visual outcome after uncomplicated cataract surgery for eyes with opaque media and a preoperative vision of 20/200 or worse. Their role appears to serve as reassurance to the physician for those patients with a cataract in which they are uncertain whether other disease processes, such as a mild to moderate atrophic macular degeneration, might limit the postoperative visual outcome.

Prevention of ocular surface infection and endophthalmitis after intraocular surgery can be accomplished with careful preoperative screening and treatment of preexisting infectious conditions. Patients should be carefully screened for the presence of chronic blepharitis, silent dacryocystitis, conjunctivitis, or keratitis (Fig. 1-5). Those patients should not be subjected to elective surgery until the disease process has been adequately treated. Patients should be questioned for epiphora, mattering or sticking of the eyelids on awakening in the morning. Direct pressure should be applied to the lacrimal sac to elicit reflux material in patients with possible occult or silent dacryocystitis. Before surgery, appropriate cultures should be obtained from the eyelid margins, conjunctival surface, or of the lacrimal sac reflux material to

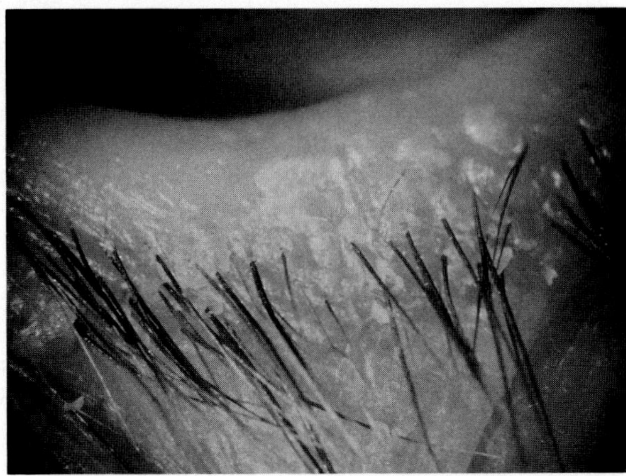

Figure 1-5. Severe seborrheic blepharitis should be recognized and treated before any ocular surgery is performed. (See color plate after page xvi.)

establish whether a heavy growth of bacteria is present on or within these tissues. Antibiotic sensitivities should be obtained so that appropriate therapeutic measures may be instituted before intraocular surgery. If the history and clinical examination indicates normal-appearing eyelid margins, conjunctival surface, and lacrimal drainage system, no further intervention is necessary before surgery. However, should these clinical entities be overlooked or ignored, those patients may pose a greater risk for postoperative infectious microbial endophthalmitis.

Patients who exhibit an elevated intraocular pressure should be appropriately treated before intraocular surgery on that eye. Those patients represent an increased risk for intraoperative expulsive choroidal effusion after decompression of the globe at the time of wound construction. Patients with an elevated intraocular pressure during the preoperative examination may exhibit further elevation of the intraocular pressure postoperatively if appropriate therapeutic measures are not instituted before surgery.

For those patients with a history of inflammatory eye disease, the physician should take all measures to determine the origin and take therapeutic measures to treat any active uveitis present at the time of the preoperative examination. These patients are at increased risk for complications both during and after intraocular surgery. Eyes that present with intraocular inflammation at the time of surgery may experience additional intraocular problems, such as hemorrhage and increased inflammation at the time of surgery. Intraoperative complications, such as hemorrhage from the conjunctiva, scleral wound, or iris vessels, can interfere with visualization of the anterior chamber structures during the procedure. Intraoperative bleeding can lead to postoperative hyphema, cellular accumulation on the intraocular lens surface, elevated intraocular pressure, and possible corneal blood staining. Preexisting inflammation or increased inflammation from iris manipulation may lead to the formation of fibrinous membranes over the lens, iris, and angle structures intraoperatively and postoperatively. These may cause reduced vision, posterior synechiae, peripheral anterior synechiae, and possible pupillary block or angle-closure glaucoma if they persist postoperatively.

The less intraocular inflammation that is present at the time of surgery, the less the chance for significant intraoperative and postoperative complications, and the better the prognosis for a good visual or functional outcome. It is recommended that eyes with active uveitis be treated with high-dose corticosteroids preoperatively. The route of administration should depend on the type, location, and severity of inflammation. However, elective surgery should be delayed as long as possible to avoid those possible complications and a poor surgical outcome. For those patients with chronic uveitis, such as sarcoidosis and juvenile rheumatoid arthritis, a cyclitic membrane extending from the ciliary body over the posterior surface of the lens may be present. This may be visualized directly with ultrasonography. Confirmation of its existence is helpful to plan the surgical procedure so that excision of the membrane with a limited anterior vitrectomy can be considered to avoid a poor visual result or eventual ciliary body detachment.

At the conclusion of the preoperative examination, several goals should be met that help achieve a successful operative procedure with the expected visual or functional result. The examination should be able to account for each line of visual loss with the specific disease responsible for that amount of impairment as well as an estimation of visual potential after surgical rehabilitation. The physician should have identified any preexisting anatomic abnormalities or disease processes that could predispose to possible intraoperative or postoperative complications. The physician should consider the pertinent clinical findings of the examination to formulate any alternative approaches or surgical modifications before surgery to reduce the risk for complications. A treatment plan should be instituted before surgery to resolve any preexisting disease processes that could otherwise carry a risk for surgical or postoperative complications. A careful, complete, and thoughtful surgical approach within the physician's realm of capability can prepare the physician to manage or prevent any complication that may be encountered during surgery appropriately. With careful preoperative planning, based on the findings of the preoperative examination, the physician can minimize risk, and maximize the clinical judgment and surgical skills necessary to achieve the desired surgical outcome.

Acknowledgment

The preparation of this chapter was supported in part by a grant from Research to Prevent Blindness, Inc.

Bibliography

Basic and Clinical Science Course, Section 5. Neuro-ophthalmology, 1992–1993. San Francisco, American Academy of Ophthalmology, 1992:18–36.

Basic and Clinical Science Course, Section 8. Glaucoma, lens, and anterior segment trauma, 1990–1991. San Francisco, American Academy of Ophthalmology, 1990:31–58.

Bates AK, Cheng H. Bullous keratopathy: a study of endothelial cell morphology in patients undergoing cataract surgery. Br J Ophthalmol 1988;72:409–412.

Berkow JW, Orth DH, Kelly JS. Fluorescein angiography: technique and interpretation. Ophthalmology Monographs 1991;5:42–48, 82–85.

Cataract Management Guideline Panel. Management of functional impairment due to cataract in adults (guideline report no. 4; AHCPR publication no. 93-0541). Rockville, MD, U.S. Department of Health and Human Services, Public Health Service, Agency for Health Care Policy and Research, August 1993.

Dubey AK, Masani PH, Schroff AP. Quantitative assessment of conventional macular functions in cases of cataract. Indian J Ophthalmol 1983;31(Suppl):895–897.

Elliott DB, Gilchrist J, Whitaker D. Contrast sensitivity and glare sensitivity changes with three types of cataract morphology: are these techniques necessary in a clinical evaluation of cataract? Ophthalmic Physiol Opt 1989;9:25–30.

Elliott DB, Hurst MA, Weatherill J. Comparing clinical tests of visual function in cataract with the patient's perceived visual disability. Eye 1990;4(Pt 5):712–717.

Graney MJ, Applegate WB, Miller ST, et al. A clinical index for predicting visual acuity after cataract surgery. Am J Ophthalmol 1988;105:460–465.

Graney MJ, Applegate WB, Miller ST, et al. An index for estimating probabilities of surgical success for cataract patients with retinal disease. J Gerontol 1990;45:M40–M44.

Howes SC, Caelli T, Mitchell P. Contrast sensitivity in diabetics with retinopathy and cataract. Aust J Ophthalmol 1982;10:173–178.

Koch DD. Glare and contrast sensitivity testing in cataract patients. J Cataract Refract Surg 1989;15:158–164.

Lempert P, Hopcroft M, Lempert Y. Evaluation of posterior subcapsular cataracts: with spatial contrast acuity. Ophthalmology 1987;94(Pt 2):14–18.

Levin ML. Opalescent nuclear cataract. J Cataract Refract Surg 1989;15:576–579.

Masket S. Reversal of glare disability after cataract surgery. J Cataract Refract Surg 1989;15:165–168.

Miller ST, Graney MJ, Elam JT, Applegate WB, Freeman JM. Predictions of outcomes from cataract surgery in elderly persons. Ophthalmology 1988;95:1125–1129.

Rao GN, Aquavella JV, Goldberg SH, Berk SL. Pseudophakic bullous keratopathy: relationship to preoperative corneal endothelial status. Ophthalmology 1984;91:1135–1140.

Smith RE, Nozik RA. Uveitis: a clinical approach to diagnosis and management. Baltimore, Williams & Wilkins, 1989:115–122.

Thornton SP, Gardner SK, Waring GO. Surgical instruments used in refractive keratotomy. In: Waring GO, ed. Refractive keratotomy for myopia and astigmatism. St. Louis, Mosby–Year Book, 1992:407–431.

Ticho U, Patz A. The role of capillary perfusion in the management of diabetic macular edema. Am J Ophthalmol 1973;76:880–886.

Waring GO. Posterior collagenous layer of the cornea: ultrastructural classification of abnormal collagenous tissue posterior to Descemet's membrane in 30 cases. Arch Ophthalmol 1982;100:122–134.

Ophthalmic Surgery Complications: Prevention and Management,
edited by Judie F. Charlton and George W. Weinstein.
J. B. Lippincott Company, Philadelphia © 1995.

2

D. Michael Elnicki

Medical History, Physical Examination, and Laboratory Screening Tests

Surgeons today must operate under a variety of constraints on patients with numerous medical conditions. Lengths of stay are continually shorter, and many procedures are now done on a largely outpatient basis. In many institutions, a cooperative approach to perioperative care has evolved between surgical, anesthesia, nursing, and medical services. Most institutions now offer medical consultation services, which can predict which patients are at risk for perioperative complications. Frequently these risks can be reduced by means of appropriate medical management.

The patient's primary care physician can often offer insights into overall medical fitness, having witnessed recoveries from previous operations and knowing the patient's past medical history in detail. It is important to invest this physician in the patient's perioperative course, as he or she will ultimately be responsible for the long-term care.

Although literature regarding perioperative medical morbidity specific to eye surgery is scanty, the complication rate is generally low. Mortality is quoted at 0.06% to 0.18% and is generally related to a preexisting condition.[1] Retrospective studies have shown that deaths related to ophthalmic surgery are usually caused by myocardial infarctions, pulmonary emboli, cardiac arrhythmias, and strokes.[2,3] Much of the mortality seen was in elderly patients.

With operations, as in any therapeutic endeavor, physicians must weigh benefits against possible risks and then match them with the utility an individual patient assigns to the procedure. Patients with significant medical concurrent diseases have increased perioperative risks. The task of the preoperative medical evaluation is to identify those patients with risk factors that are amenable to therapy, which will reduce the complication risk in a timely fashion.

It is important to distinguish between elective and emergent operations, when evaluating a patient's operative candidacy. Emergent surgery independently raises the risks of medical complications, regardless of the patient's health.[4] Concurrent diseases that are acceptable for a patient facing immediate loss of vision may be unacceptable in a candidate for elective cataract surgery.

Several authors have independently studied the ordering of preoperative testing, and have found that nondirected tests are not cost-effective and seldom affect outcomes.[5–7] Obtaining meaningful data depends on directing preoperative testing to problems identified by a careful history and physical examination. The approach outlined in this chapter relies on an organ system method to identify the type of medical problems that patients may encounter in the perioperative period. An annotated bibliography[8] and a complete textbook[9] are available on these topics, and use a similar system.

CARDIAC DISEASE

Much of the research on preventing postoperative complications focuses on cardiac mortality and morbidity. This emphasis is not surprising, because one third of postoperative deaths are from cardiac causes.[10] In the elderly, who make up much of the population undergoing eye surgery, cardiovascular disease is highly prevalent and the leading cause of mortality. In two series of ophthalmologic cases, 56% and 90% of the perioperative deaths were from cardiac causes.[2,3] The cardiac events to be prevented are death, myocardial infarction, pulmonary edema, and major arrhythmias. Each of the latter three events were causes of death in the preceding series. Predicting these events relies primarily on history and physical examination with a few basic tests. The applicability of more sophisticated tests remains unclear for all but the most high-risk patients.[11]

During the 1970s, Goldman and colleagues[10] developed a risk stratification system to predict postoperative cardiac problems in patients undergoing noncardiac surgery. That system has since been validated by others with only minor variations.[12,13] It divides patients into four risk groups, based on clinical characteristics that have been found to have independent predictive ability. Most of the important characteristics come from the history and the physical examination. The incidences of perioperative morbidity and mortality in the study cohort ranged from 0.7% and 0.2%, respectively, in the low-risk group to 22% and 56% in the highest (Table 2-1).

The relevant, patient-specific variables are signs of congestive heart failure on physical examination, recent myocardial infarction, arrhythmia or ventricular ectopy on preoperative electrocardiogram, age greater than 70 years, valvular aortic stenosis, and

Table 2-1
Perioperative Cardiac Risk Groups

CLASS	CARDIAC MORBIDITY	CARDIAC MORTALITY
I	0.7	0.2
II	5	2
III	11	2
IV	22	56

(Adapted from Goldman L, Caldera DL, Nussbaum SR, et al. Multifactorial index of cardiac risk in noncardiac surgical procedures. N Engl J Med 1977;297:845)

poor overall medical condition (Table 2-2). The urgency and location of the surgery are also important in the prediction system. Anesthetic type is not a predictor of perioperative cardiac events.[14]

Some factors from a patient's history, which are typically associated with developing cardiac disease, were found not to be predictive of cardiac events in the perioperative period. They include smoking, diabetes mellitus, mild or moderate hypertension, hyperlipidemia, and the presence of peripheral vascular disease. Smoking is a risk factor for pulmonary complications, but it does not independently predict cardiac ones. Patients with diabetes develop more complications overall, and myocardial infarction is the most common cause of death in this population.[11] A careful preoperative evaluation is needed to establish the absence of coexisting cardiac disease in patients with diabetes, because this problem is where the risk of cardiac events lies rather than in the diabetes per

Table 2-2
Predictors of Perioperative Cardiac Events

OBTAINED FROM	RISK FACTOR
History	Myocardial infarction within 6 mo Age > 70 y Advanced angina or heart failure
Physical examination	Jugular venous distention or S3 Aortic stenosis Arrhythmias
Laboratory results	Arterial: $Po_2 < 60$ or $Pco_2 > 50$ mmHg Venous: $K^+ < 3.0$ or $HCO_3 < 20$ mEq/L Blood urea nitrogen, > 50 or creatinine > 3.0 mg/dL Elevated SGOT
Specific operation	Emergency procedure Chest, intraperitoneal, or aortic procedure

SGOT, serum glutamic-oxaloacetic transaminase.

(Adapted from Goldman L. Cardiac risks and complications of noncardiac surgery. Ann Intern Med 1983;98:504)

se. Stable, moderate hypertension has been shown in several studies not to be an independent predictor of perioperative cardiac events.[10,12,14] Although patients with peripheral vascular disease have more complications when they undergo vascular surgery, this result has not been demonstrated in other procedures.[11]

Myocardial infarction is among the most feared postoperative complications and in many reports is the most common cause of death. Postoperative myocardial infarctions are often atypical in presentation, without complaints of chest pain. Not all patients with coronary disease are at high risk of myocardial infarction, however. Stable, New York Heart Association (NYHA) Class II angina (Table 2-3) has not been associated with an increased incidence of cardiac events.[11,15] However, patients with progressing or higher-grade angina should have elective procedures delayed until their coronary disease is evaluated and controlled.

A history of a previous myocardial infarction places a patient at increased risk postoperatively for another. The incidence of perioperative myocardial infarction in the general population is less than 1%. In the first 3 months after a myocardial infarction, the risk is 30%. The incidence declines to 15% from 3 to 6 months after the infarction and remains at about 5% thereafter.[14] One study found the odds of death before hospital discharge to be increased by a factor of 4.7 for patients undergoing surgery less than 6 months after a myocardial infarction.[16] A study that used intensive monitoring both intraoperatively and postoperatively was able to reduce the reinfarction rate to 6% in patients less than 3 months recovered from a previous myocardial infarction.[17] Patients with residual ischemia or left ventricular dysfunction are probably at increased risk for cardiac events. Exercise thallium stress testing, dipyridamole stress testing, and preoperative electrocardiographic monitoring for ischemia have all been used to stratify high-risk patients,[18–20] but their role has not yet been clearly defined.

Patients who have undergone coronary revascularization procedures (angioplasty or coronary artery bypass grafting) pose an interesting preoperative dilemma. They clearly have cardiac disease; however, in theory, it has been "corrected." Studies have, in fact, shown low rates of cardiac events in such individuals.[11] There may be a period after their cardiac operation where they are vulnerable, however. A high rate of events has been seen in patients having noncardiac surgery 1 month after their cardiac procedure.[13] Although there are not good data available on the subject, it is probably prudent to delay elective surgery for 3 months after coronary revascularization. A history of recurring anginal symptoms should be carefully elicited preoperatively, as it may signify either a restenosis of the corrected lesion or progression of disease into untreated vessels. In those patients with known coronary disease, it is important to quantify their level of angina preoperatively. A study of men with known coronary disease found a perioperative infarction rate of 4%, with a 2% incidence of cardiac deaths.[21] Those who have angina with only strenuous activity (NYHA Class II) do not require further evaluation. Patients whose angina follows minimal exertion or occurs at rest (NYHA Class III or IV) should be considered for further evaluation by stress testing or angiography before elective operations.

Preoperative electrocardiograms are sometimes read as "consistent with an old myocardial infarction" when the patient has no such history. Unless this finding is known to have existed on earlier studies, a 3-month delay in elective operations is probably prudent to remove the patient from the period of high risk for reinfarction. Also, because the infarction is likely to have been "silent," or without symptoms, an objective test of myocardial ischemia (ie, stress testing) should be considered.

Patients with coronary artery disease need to have their antianginal medications continued perioperatively with as little interruption as possible. As most of these drugs can be given parenterally, doing so should not be a problem even if the patient is unable to take oral medications. Efforts should be made to keep these patients euvolemic and to avoid periods of hypoxia in the perioperative period, so as not to jeopardize an already compromised delivery of oxygen to myocardial tissue.

Table 2-3
New York Heart Association Classification of Heart Disease

CLASS	SYMPTOMS WITH
I	Extreme levels of activity or asymptomatic
II	Strenuous activity
III	Mild activity
IV	Minimal effort or at rest

Cardiac arrhythmias are another major source of postoperative morbidity and mortality. Arrhythmias caused 20% and 33% of the deaths in the two series of eye surgery cases mentioned earlier.[2,3] It is interesting that arrhythmias on the preoperative electrocardiogram are predictive of pulmonary edema and myocardial infarction.[15] The findings should be considered as possibly indicative of underlying cardiac dysfunction and their origin investigated, if this has not previously been done. Exercise stress testing and measurement of left ventricular function by ultrasonography or nuclear cardiography are possible ways to proceed.

Atrial arrhythmias were found to be important markers for patients who subsequently developed complications.[10,12] The question often arises whether to begin therapy with digitalis on patients found to be in atrial fibrillation preoperatively. Controlling the ventricular response rate is important; however, if the rate is already controlled, the answer is unclear. Some authors recommend digitalizing those who would poorly tolerate rapid ventricular rates, such as those with valvular disease or compromised left ventricles.[15]

Premature ventricular contractions as an isolated finding, without structural heart disease, are not predictive of cardiac events.[11,14] However, there must be a high degree of certainty that the patient with frequent or complex ventricular ectopic beats does not have significant underlying heart disease. When ventricular ectopy is a new finding, secondary causes should be considered, such as electrolyte disturbances, hypoxemia, or myocardial ischemia.

Cardiac conduction defects are not predictive of perioperative cardiac complications. Bifascicular block, right bundle branch block, and left anterior hemiblock are not serious when they occur as isolated events.[11] Pacemaker placement perioperatively should be carried out for the indications that would normally be required, that is, symptomatic high-grade conduction defects.[14]

Patients already on antiarrhythmic agents should have them continued perioperatively. These patients should be asked about symptoms consistent with toxicity (such as nausea) or of poorly controlled heart rhythms (like palpitations, dizziness or syncope). Serum levels of the agents should be measured preoperatively to ensure they are therapeutic, with adjustments made accordingly. Which of the patients with arrhythmias to monitor perioperatively remains the subject of debate, but patients thought to be at high risk may benefit from 24 to 48 hours of telemetry postoperatively.[11,15]

Patients with a history of congestive heart failure are at increased risk of pulmonary edema in the postoperative setting, but their preoperative clinical condition is more important in establishing risk. Those with jugular venous distention or a third heart sound (S3) were found to be at increased risk for cardiac events in the initial cohort of Goldman and associates.[10] Patients with a history of pulmonary edema, NYHA Class III heart failure, signs of congestive heart failure on preoperative physical examination, or preoperative chest roentgenogram have subsequently been found to be at increased risk.[15] A left ventricular ejection fraction of less than 40% is thought to indicate increased perioperative risk, but the routine use of echocardiography or nuclear ventriculography to assess left ventricular function remains questionable.[11]

Patients with congestive heart failure need to have their cardiac medications continued without interruptions. Vasodilators and angiotensin-converting enzyme (ACE) inhibitors should be continued perioperatively. Diuretics should be adjusted to keep the patient as euvolemic as possible. The immediate preoperative period is not the time for aggressive diuretic therapy. Serum electrolytes need to be measured preoperatively. Postoperative pulmonary edema is seen in a biphasic distribution, the first occurring 30 minutes to 1 hour postoperatively and the second 24 to 48 hours later. Careful attention to volume status is critical in this interval for patients at risk for pulmonary edema. Methods of monitoring volume status in these patients should be discussed preoperatively, and some patients may require intracardiac pressure monitoring.

Patients with valvular heart disease often have some degree of ventricular dysfunction. For most valvular lesions, the perioperative morbidity is related to the degree of heart failure. Mitral valve disease, for example, has not been shown to predispose patients independently to postoperative complications.[11,14] Care needs to be taken that patients with valvular lesions not become hypervolemic or volume depleted perioperatively, as they will not compensate as well as other patients. Rate-controlling drugs, such as digoxin and β-blockers need to be continued without interruption, so that a tachyarrhythmia does not place undue strain on an already compromised heart. Diuretic use needs to be individualized, but the emphasis should be on sending the patient to the operating room in a euvolemic state.

Conversely, patients with aortic valvular lesions, particularly aortic stenosis, tolerate the volume shifts of surgery poorly and are susceptible to developing postoperative pulmonary edema. Aortic valvular stenosis is an independent perioperative risk factor, with mortalities after noncardiac surgery quoted up to 13%.[14] Patients with significant aortic stenosis frequently have no complaints, and the lesion is discovered on incidental physical examination. The murmur of aortic stenosis is harsh, systolic, and heard best at the right upper sternal border. It characteristically radiates to the neck, and is associated with a soft and delayed upstroke of the pulse (pulsus parvus et tardus).

A patient with these findings should have echocardiography performed before elective surgery to confirm the presence of a significant aortic valvular stenosis. The patient needs special attention perioperatively regarding fluid management and may require a Swan-Ganz catheter for monitoring of pressures. The issue of patients with valvular disease who are on long-term anticoagulation is discussed in the section on coagulation.

A preoperative electrocardiogram and chest roentgenogram are part of risk assessment. Clearly those with risks identified by history and physical examination need these tests, but their general preoperative use has been questioned. For young patients with no history or signs of cardiac problems, the yield of a preoperative electrocardiogram is exceedingly low and not cost-effective.[22] Studies of routine preoperative chest roentgenograms have similarly found little effect on patient outcomes if clinical signs were not also present.[23] Even these basic tests should be viewed as adjuncts to the history and physical examination, and should be ordered only if suspicion already exists that a patient may be at increased risk of complications. Specific tests of myocardial ischemia, and valvular or ventricular function are then used for subsequent evaluations on an individual basis. The use of some medications specific to ophthalmic surgery merit special attention in patients with coexisting heart disease. β-Blocker eye drops undergo some systemic absorption, and have caused bradycardia, hypotension, syncope, and precipitated heart failure in patients.[24] Sympathomimetic agents (such as phenylephrine) can increase heart rate and blood pressure, which theoretically could aggravate angina from an increase in myocardial oxygen demand.

HYPERTENSION

Hypertension is an extremely common disease, estimated to be present in 50 million Americans.[25] The prevalence rises with age, so that nearly one half of the U.S. population older than age 65 has elevated levels of systolic or diastolic blood pressure, defined as a diastolic pressure over 90 mmHg or a systolic pressure over 160 mmHg.[26] Thus, on a random basis alone, hypertensive patients will frequently be perioperative candidates, necessitating familiarity with their management.

Most hypertension is mild and is classified as "essential" (of unknown origin). Less than 10% of patients have "secondary" hypertension, or disease from a discernible cause. Most concern about patients' blood pressure, therefore, revolves around its effects on target organ damage. The organs where disease states are associated with hypertension are the brain, heart, kidneys, and vascular tree. This assessment is at least as important as blood pressure per se when assessing the hypertensive patient's operative candidacy.

The preoperative history needs to focus on the recent course of the hypertension, on side effects of therapy, and on concurrent diseases associated with hypertension, such as coronary artery disease, cerebral vascular disease, and renal compromise. A recent loss of blood pressure control would be of concern and should prompt investigation. Symptoms consistent with cerebral or cardiac ischemia may also warrant evaluation, depending on the urgency of the operation planned. A cerebral transient ischemic episode should be pursued as seriously as unstable angina.[27]

When measuring any patient's blood pressure, one needs to do so correctly to obtain meaningful data. Bulky garments should be removed, and the patient should have been seated for at least 10 minutes. Nicotine or caffeine should be avoided for at least 30 minutes. The blood pressure cuff should be large enough to cover two thirds of the circumference of the arm with the inflatable bladder portion. The patient's arm should be at heart level and supported. If an abnormal reading is obtained, it should be rechecked after 15 to 30 minutes. Orthostatic vital checks (blood pressure and pulse in two or more positions 1–3 minutes apart) remain the best assessment of intravascular volume status and, thus, the best screen for volume depletion.

Keeping the target organ concept in mind makes the examination of hypertensive patients straightforward. The heart should be examined for evidence of hypertrophy or failure. The lungs need to be auscultated for evidence of congestion (ie, rales). On abdominal examination, masses (such as aneurysms) are palpated and bruits auscultated. Peripheral arteries are auscultated and palpated as well. It is important to also assess the baseline neurologic examination, looking for focal defects or an abnormal mental status.

The laboratory assessment (Table 2-4) of the hypertensive patient follows the target organ concept as well and relies on a few basic screening tests. Patients receiving diuretics particularly need to have serum electrolytes assessed for hyponatremia or hypokalemia. Serum uric acid should also be measured in these patients because thiazides can raise uric acid levels, and the stress of surgery is well known to precipitate gouty attacks. Abnormalities in these tests should prompt further investigation and possibly consultation.

Early studies indicated that patients with hypertension were at greater risk for perioperative cardiac morbidity than patients without hypertension.[28,29] However, patients with extremely high blood pressure were included in the analysis. In their model to predict postoperative cardiac morbidity and mortality, Goldman and coauthors[10] found that hypertension was not an independent risk factor, a finding validated by later researchers.[12] A large, prospective study demonstrated that mild to moderate hypertension (diastolic pressure < 110 mmHg) is not an independent predictor of postoperative cardiac or renal complications.[30] Although the hypertensive patients had more perioperative fluctuations in blood pressure than others, tight blood pressure control did not lessen the incidence of hypertensive or hypotensive episodes in these patients. That is, the lability of hypertensive patients' blood pressures was not corrected by preoperative blood pressure control.

A more recent study addressed the question of predicting perioperative episodes of hypertension and hypotension. This study demonstrated, prospectively, that patients who became acutely hypertensive or hypotensive in the perioperative setting developed more postoperative cardiac and renal complications. The factors associated with these events were decreased exercise capacity, advanced age (>70 years), and low plasma volume.[31] Of note is that only the latter is amenable to treatment before an operation.

Based on these studies, most clinicians think that patients with mild to moderate hypertension are acceptable candidates for elective operations, barring concurrent diseases. Antihypertensive medications, with the exception of diuretics, should be continued perioperatively with as little interruption as possible. Rebound rises in blood pressure from the sudden discontinuation of drugs (eg, β-blockers and clonidine) need to be avoided. Diuretics are generally held 1 to 2 days preoperatively to avoid sending the patient to the operating room in a volume-depleted state. There are some special considerations relevant to hypertension in patients undergoing eye surgery. Hypertension has been associated with a higher risk of bleeding in vascular surgery of the eye[32]; in these cases, closer attention to blood pressure level may be warranted. Systemic absorption of topical ophthalmic preparations can be associated with fluctuations in blood pressure. The class of agents associated with

Table 2-4
Clinical Results of Hypertension and Their Assessment

TARGET ORGAN	ASSOCIATED DISEASE	ASSESSMENT
Brain	Stroke	H&P
Heart	Hypertrophy, failure, coronary artery disease	H&P, ECG, chest roentgenogram
Kidneys	Chronic renal failure	Serum Na, K, BUN or creatinine, and urinalysis
Vascular	Atherosclerosis, aneurysms	H&P

BUN, blood urea nitrogen; ECG, electrocardiogram; H&P, history and physical examination.

hypertensive episodes is the sympathomimetic, whereas β-adrenergic blockers (like timolol) are associated with hypotension.[33] These effects should be considered when adding such drugs to the regimens of hypertensive patients or when a cause of changes in blood pressure is being sought. Lastly, the diuretics acetazolamide and mannitol are sometimes used to decrease intraocular pressure. They can, however, precipitate hypotension or electrolyte abnormalities in patients on antihypertensive diuretics. The discontinuation of other diuretics should be considered, and volume status and electrolytes closely monitored when using acetazolamide or mannitol.

PULMONARY DISEASE

Pulmonary problems are among the most common in the postoperative setting. Pneumonia and exacerbations of chronic obstructive lung disease are two of the most serious, and either can lead to respiratory failure. Others, like pneumothoraxes and pleural effusions, are fairly rare. Even relatively minor complications like atelectasis and coughing can still impact on a patient's recovery, and the latter can be disastrous immediately after eye surgery.

Several physiologic reasons for postoperative pulmonary decompensation exist. The effects of anesthesia and postoperative analgesia (particularly narcotics) decrease the sigh and cough reflexes.[34] The result is alveolar collapse and areas of atelectasis. Intubation and pain decrease clearing of particles in the upper airway, predisposing a patient to infection, and inhalational gases can further decrease the clearing of secretions by inhibiting mucociliary transport.[35] These effects become most relevant in patients whose pulmonary status is already compromised.

There are readily identified patient characteristics associated with developing postoperative pulmonary problems (Table 2-5). One of the most obvious is smoking. In a prospective study of elective coronary bypass surgery, patients who smoked had a fourfold higher incidence of pulmonary complications compared with nonsmokers.[36] Smoking cessation for greater than 2 months was needed to maximize the benefits of quitting. This may seem like a long interval but is achievable before elective operations.

Other risks that have been identified include obesity, older age (> 70 years), and a history of chronic obstructive or restrictive lung disease. The risks associated with obesity are largely confined to those who are morbidly obese. These patients demonstrate numerous derangements in pulmonary physiology, which include decreased respiratory compliance, functional residual capacity, expiratory reserve volume, and sometimes ventilatory responsiveness.[35] Studies of surgery in patients with chronic obstructive lung disease have shown mortalities from 0% to 11%[37] and complication rates from 20% to 76%.[35]

The risk of postoperative respiratory problems varies with type of surgery and anesthesia. Thoracic and upper abdominal surgery have long been known to carry the highest risks. One study evaluated a cohort of patients with severe chronic obstructive lung disease undergoing a variety of surgical procedures. With outcomes clearly defined beforehand, the authors discovered postoperative pulmonary complications in more than one half of the patients undergoing coronary artery bypass surgery and major abdominal operations, whereas only 27% of those having other types of surgery developed similar complications.[37]

Patients' risks of pulmonary problems can be further lowered by using topical or regional anesthesia rather than general anesthesia. In the study mentioned previously, only 16% of patients receiving topical or regional anesthesia developed respiratory problems.[37] Anesthetic choice will depend on a variety of factors, but the risk of pulmonary complications should be considered in the decision process. It may be difficult to predict all those at risk by history

Table 2-5
Predictors of Increased Risk of Pulmonary Complications

History and Physical Examination
Age (> 70 y)
Smoking
Chronic obstructive lung disease
Obesity
Respiratory infection
Laboratory Data
P_{CO_2} > 45 mmHg
FEV_1 < 2 L or < 50% predicted
FVC < 50% predicted
FEV_1/FVC < 50% predicted
MVV < 50% predicted
Operation
Surgical site
Type of anesthesia

FEV_1, forced expiratory volume in 1 s; FVC, forced vital capacity; MVV, maximum ventilatory volume.

and physical examination alone. A study attempting to identify men with compromised lung function found the sensitivity and specificity of the combined history and examination to be only 51% and 64%, respectively, with positive and negative predictive values of 8% and 95%.[38] The presence of one or more known risk factors should, nevertheless, prompt the supplementation of history and physical examination by laboratory testing. Chest roentgenogram, spirometry, and arterial blood gases can all lend valuable information to assist risk assessment. The presence of a mass or infiltrate on chest roentgenogram would obviously prompt further investigation. An abnormal spirometry (see Table 2-5) can be both predictive and directive regarding further therapy (Table 2-6). Hypoxia has not been shown to be a reliable predictor of pulmonary complications, but hypercapnia ($P_{CO_2} >$ 45 mmHg) is associated with a tenuous preoperative state and postoperative problems.[34,35]

Predicting which patients are likely to develop pulmonary difficulties is a worthwhile endeavor, because viable therapeutic options exist. More than 20 years ago, investigators demonstrated that the complication rate of a high-risk group (based on the parameters mentioned earlier) could be decreased to that of a low-risk group using specifically directed therapy.[39] Since then, other investigators have validated the ability to reduce the prevalence of pulmonary complications in the postoperative setting.[40,41]

Depending on the anticipated difficulties and the operation planned, the following interventions can be selectively instituted. The respiratory service can best teach incentive spirometry preoperatively, while the patient is alert and not anesthetized. Chest physical therapy can be instituted before surgery and continued in the postoperative period. Patients' chronic pulmonary medications should be continued without interruption, and most can be given parenterally if patients are unable to take medications orally. Patients with reversible bronchospasm can be given bronchodilators. Purulent sputum production indicates a bacterial pulmonary infection, which can be treated with antibiotics perioperatively. Narcotics diminish sighing and coughing, so their use should be minimized in high-risk patients. Obese patients should be encouraged to lose weight preoperatively, as even a 10% loss can improve pulmonary status.[35]

The research on postoperative pulmonary complications has not specifically addressed ophthalmologic surgery. The risks and benefits of therapy, therefore, remain difficult to quantify. The position paper of the American College of Physicians, which addressed preoperative pulmonary function testing, stated that there were inadequate studies to base recommendations on their use for surgery involving the head and neck.[42] None of the studies mentioned earlier, for example, discussed ophthalmologic procedures.

There are some respiratory considerations specific to eye surgery. The use of β-blocker eye drops has been associated with flares of obstructive lung disease.[1] Anticholinergic drops can dry out respiratory secretions, making them more difficult to clear. This can be a significant problem for patients with chronic bronchitis. Many patients with chronic pulmonary disease need to expectorate copious secretions in the mornings. Waiting until afternoon for their operations may allow them to complete this process beforehand. Flare-ups of many pulmonary diseases involve coughing. If this could seriously complicate the planned

Table 2-6
Interventions to Prevent Pulmonary Complications

INTERVENTION	INDICATION
Bronchodilators	Wheezing (bronchospasm) Reversibly decreased FEV_1
Antibiotics	Fever, purulent sputum
Supplemental oxygen	Hypoxemia*
Chest physiotherapy	Difficulty clearing secretions
Incentive spirometry, breathing exercises, or intermittent positive-pressure breathing	Patient or procedure at risk for pulmonary complications
Smoking cessation	All patients
Early mobilization	
Minimization of narcotics	

* Patients who chronically retain carbon dioxide may decompensate if given more than 1–2 L/min of oxygen.

operation, delaying elective surgery until after the flare-up is controlled may be judicious.

ENDOCRINE PROBLEMS

Diabetes Mellitus

Diabetes mellitus occurs in about 5% of the adult population, and patients with diabetes mellitus are frequently encountered on ophthalmology services. Diabetic retinopathy remains the leading cause of blindness in Western countries.[43] Patients with diabetes have a 20 times increased relative risk of blindness over the general U.S. population and a 14% cumulative prevalence of visual impairment.[44] It has been estimated that a patient with diabetes has a greater than 50% lifetime chance of undergoing surgery, and vitrectomy and cataract extraction are two of the most common operations performed on patients with diabetes.[45]

Clinicians routinely group patients with two different diseases (types I and II diabetes mellitus) into the category of "patients with diabetes," but important pathophysiologic differences between them exist, which impact on their respective perioperative management. The most common form of diabetes is type II (formally called adult onset), which has a strong autosomal pattern of inheritance and presents later in life. These patients tend to be obese and insulin resistant. Their serum insulin levels are often increased, and type II patients are not prone to developing ketosis. The stresses of surgery, however, may cause glucose levels to rise dramatically in these patients. Patients with type I diabetes (formerly called juvenile onset) have a disease characterized by the lack of insulin production. The disease is thought to be autoimmune in nature, and the patients are generally younger at presentation and not obese. They are prone to ketosis because of their inability to increase insulin production on demand. These patients require a constantly available supply of glucose and exogenous insulin, or they will develop diabetic ketoacidosis (DKA).

The perioperative complications, to which patients with diabetes are prone, can be divided into those specific to the abnormal biochemistry characteristic of their disease and those related to damaged diabetic target organs. The former depend more on the degree of metabolic derangement present. In contrast, the latter seem to correlate more with the duration of the patient's diabetes. The biochemical defect of type I diabetes is the lack of insulin, whereas patients with type II diabetes are unable to use their insulin effectively to control blood glucose levels.

Of the biochemical complications that patients with type I diabetes encounter, DKA is the most serious, with associated mortalities up to 10%. The stress of surgery, with its associated increases in cortisol and catecholamine secretion,[46] can be enough to cause DKA in susceptible patients. DKA can occur even if usual insulin doses are maintained and can occur without dramatically elevated serum glucose levels.[47] Measurements of serum bicarbonate levels, pH, or ketones are needed for assessment of DKA in patients at risk.

The ketosis-resistant, type II patients may develop a hyperosmolar state after stressful events, such as surgery. These patients characteristically have high blood glucose levels and develop polyuria. They may become dehydrated and lapse into a hyperosmolar coma, which has been associated with mortalities up to 40%.[48]

Compromised wound healing, another non–organ-specific complication, has long been recognized to occur in patients with diabetes. Abnormal leukocyte function, tissue perfusion, and hormonal influences have all been considered as explanations. Experimental data and clinical outcomes both support controlling blood glucose perioperatively to promote wound healing and prevent infections.[49]

Over time, the abnormal metabolic state of diabetes mellitus causes damage to several target organs (Table 2-7). In addition to the eyes, organs commonly manifesting the effects of diabetes are the kidneys and nervous system. Having diabetes greatly increases a patient's risk for atherosclerosis, with its resulting damage to the heart and vascular tree.

Diabetic nephropathy is related to the length of time a patient has had diabetes and to the degree of glycemic control over that time.[50,51] Its presence may necessitate altering the doses of renally metabolized drugs. To assess the degree of nephropathy, one needs to check a urinalysis for serum electrolytes and serum creatinine. The finding of peripheral edema on physical examination may be indicative of hypoalbuminemia secondary to urinary protein loss. Albuminuria progressing to the nephrotic syndrome is a hallmark of serious diabetic renal disease.[50,51] Patients with this level of proteinuria may be particularly sensitive to the fluid status shifts associated with surgery, and they are prone to developing thromboemboli.

Table 2-7
Preoperative Evaluation of Diabetic Patients

Assess diabetic control
Recent
With previous surgery
Assess associated comorbidity
Cardiac
Coronary artery disease
Congestive heart failure
Peripheral vascular disease
Renal insufficiency
Neuropathy
Peripheral
Autonomic
Important laboratory values
Electrolytes
Serum creatinine
Urinalysis (ketones, protein)
Serum glucose and HbA_{1c}
Electrocardiogram

HbA_{1c}, hemoglobin A_{1c}.

There are numerous forms of diabetic neuropathy, and the presence of both peripheral and autonomic neuropathy should be assessed preoperatively. Nearly one half of patients with diabetes eventually develop neuropathies,[52] and the most common peripheral neuropathy is a distal polyneuropathy.[45] It is manifested by losses of deep tendon reflexes, vibratory sense, and position sense in a "stocking-glove" distribution. Patients complain of burning, aching, or numbness in the affected areas. They are at risk for skin breakdown and cutaneous ulcers[45] because of their decreased sensation.

Those patients with autonomic neuropathy often demonstrate postural blood pressure drops, without the normal rise in heart rate. Patients with autonomic neuropathy are at increased risk of myocardial infarctions, sudden death, and postoperative hypotension.[44,52] They also frequently have gastroparesis, which can cause nausea and vomiting. Patients with gastroparesis often give histories of early satiety, diarrhea, abdominal bloating and vomiting after meals. Metoclopramide, which increases gastric motility, can help these patients if they develop nausea or vomiting perioperatively.

Although diabetes has not been found to be an independent predictor of cardiac risk in several studies,[10,12] patients with diabetes are at high risk of coronary artery disease. The most common cause of perioperative mortality in surgical patients with diabetes is coronary artery disease.[44] Careful attention should be given to taking a history for symptoms suggestive of angina or congestive heart failure. The physical signs relevant to cardiac risk need to be sought as well carefully. All patients with diabetes should have a recent cardiogram and chest roentgenogram available preoperatively. A sudden loss of glycemic control in the perioperative period should always prompt a search for a myocardial infarction as the etiology, whether or not the patient has complained of chest pain.

The effects of atherosclerosis in patients with diabetes are not confined to the heart, and peripheral vascular disease in these patients is common. Because of concomitant neuropathy, patients may not complain of pain with an ischemic extremity. During the preoperative physical examination, pulses should be palpated, and each extremity examined for lesions or signs of tissue ischemia. Any abnormalities that may be noted postoperatively can then be evaluated with a baseline having been clearly established.

Diabetic control can be assessed by monitoring serial serum glucose or measuring glycosylated hemoglobin (HbA_{1c}). Home blood glucose monitoring is increasingly practical with the widespread availability of accurate glycometers that rely on fingerstick blood samples. Although difficult to perform for extended periods, frequent assessment of serum glucose levels gives the range and diurnal patterns of diabetic control. The glycosylated hemoglobin assay, in contrast, gives the average level of glucose control over the preceding 1 to 2 months. This method is not affected by acute metabolic fluctuations and cannot be falsified by patients. It is generally considered to be the most accurate index measure of glycemic control,[48] but each method yields different, valuable information.

Several studies have supported tight glycemic control as a means to prevent the long-term complications of diabetes.[53–55] These findings do not necessarily translate directly into perioperative care; however, the issues of wound healing and ketosis, mentioned previously, argue for maintaining perioperative glycemic control. In this setting, clinicians must navigate between the deleterious effects of hyperglycemia and the potential disaster of an anesthetized hypoglycemic patient.

The best method of maintaining glycemic control in the perioperative period remains unclear, so a considerable amount of individualization is required in constructing a sound perioperative diabetic regimen (Table 2-8). Preoperative glycemic control, previous perioperative problems, and the nature of the

Table 2-8
Major Principles of Diabetic Perioperative Management

Monitor blood glucose frequently
- Avoid hypoglycemia
- Avoid prolonged hyperglycemia

Importance of metabolic control
- Prevent ketosis/acidosis
- Avoid electrolyte shifts
- Avoid volume depletion

Supply enough glucose to prevent hypoglycemia and for basal energy needs (5–10 g/h)

planned procedure need to be considered. A preoperative fasting serum glucose greater than 180 or a glycosylated hemoglobin level over 10 are indicative of poor glycemic control and should prompt consideration of a continuous insulin infusion.[56] Patients undergoing longer procedures and who have a history of diabetic complications following previous operations should also be considered for insulin infusions.

Patients who have been given a hypoglycemic agent, whether insulin or an oral agent (Table 2-9), need to have a continuous supply of intravenous glucose until fully awake and eating. Which intravenous fluid is the best perioperative nutritional source remains a subject of debate, with some authors arguing for lactated Ringer solution and others for 5% to 10% dextrose in 0.45% saline.[44,57] What is probably more important is that those caring for the patient be aware of and comfortable with the solution used, and that it not be changed back and forth.

There can be no gaps in glucose monitoring between operating room, recovery room, and ward room. These arrangements should be established in advance of the procedure. Blood glucose levels should be checked on arrival in the recovery room, arrival on the ward, and every 4 to 6 hours thereafter, until the clinical situation is stable. Those patients on intravenous insulin drips will need more frequent monitoring perioperatively (every 30 minutes to 2 hours). Intravenous boluses of insulin should not be used because of the short biologic half-life (about 20 minutes) and the risk of hypoglycemia.

Most type I patients undergoing surgical procedures require constant insulin infusion. Patients who require insulin but are well controlled and undergoing relatively minor surgery may be adequately managed by giving a portion of their intermediate action (NPH or Lente) insulin subcutaneously before surgery, while they receive intravenous dextrose (Table 2-10). The safety of this approach has been demonstrated in several studies, some of which specifically included ophthalmologic procedures.[44] Diet-controlled patients with diabetes or those on oral hypoglycemic agents usually require only close postoperative glucose monitoring, with insulin coverage given if blood glucose levels rise. Although the oral agents should be withheld the day of surgery, patients receiving them need to be given a continuous glucose supply, as these agents have long active half-lives.

Adrenal Suppression

Eye disease may be a manifestation of many systemic processes. For example, patients undergoing operative procedures for iritis may have an underlying

Table 2-9
Hypoglycemic Therapy

Oral agents—need to be stopped preoperatively
Glipizide, glyburide, tolbutamide, and tolazamide all have durations of action 12–24 h. Chlorpropamide has a duration of > 36 h. All of these intervals can be dramatically prolonged in the elderly.

INSULIN PREPARATIONS	ONSET (h)	PEAK (h)	DURATION (h)	PREOPERATIVE PROCEDURES
Regular	0.3–0.7	2–4	5–8	Use sliding scale.
NPH or Lente	1–2	6–12	18–24	Hold evening dose and give ⅓–½ of AM dose
H-Ultralente	4–6	12–16	24–36	Give usual dose.

ss, sliding scale.

(Adapted from Zinman B. The physiologic replacement of insulin. N Engl J Med 1989;321:363; and Gerich JE. Oral hypoglycemic agents. N Engl J Med 1989;321:1231)

Table 2-10
Diabetic Management Regimens: Subcutaneous Insulin vs Continuous IV Insulin

Not IV boluses
Continuous IV Insulin
- NPO after dinner night before OR.
- Begin infusing solution containing D5 at 10 PM.
- Regular insulin in normal saline (0.5–1 U/h).
- Check BG after 1 h, qh in OR, then q2–4h.
- Keep BG 120–200; remember electrolytes, acidosis.

Subcutaneous Insulin
- Start D5 maintenance IV in AM (or PM before).
- Give ⅓–½ of usual AM intermediate insulin (ie, NPH or Lente).
- Monitor BG q1h in OR, arrival to RR and ward, then q4–6h.
- Cover with sliding-scale regular.

BG, blood glucose; IV, intravenous; NPH, neutral protamine Hagedorn; NPO, nothing by mouth; OR, operating room; RR, recovery room.

connective tissue disease, such as systemic lupus erythematosus. Many patients with connective tissue diseases and vasculitides are on long-term corticosteroid therapy, and have developed iatrogenic adrenal suppression. Similarly, other patients have coincidental concurrent diseases (eg, chronic obstructive lung disease) that require corticosteroids and lead to the same adrenal state. In the perioperative period, the body's usual output of corticosteroids is increased sevenfold. A hypoadrenal patient cannot meet this increased demand and may develop postoperative shock.

If a patient has recently received more than 10 mg of prednisone daily, or the equivalent dose of another adrenocorticoid preparation, for more than 1 month (or > 20 mg for longer than 1 week), the patient should be considered to be adrenally suppressed.[60,61] When there is doubt about the patient's adrenal status, an adrenocorticotropic hormone (ACTH) stimulation test can be performed. If the patient has adequate adrenal reserves, blood samples drawn 0.5 and 1 hour after the ACTH injection will show a 20 μg/dL or greater rise in serum cortisol levels from at least one of the samples.

During the preoperative evaluation, the clinician should be suspicious of patients with features characteristic of either adrenocortical excess or insufficiency. Patients who have been exposed to supraphysiologic amounts of corticosteroids for prolonged intervals develop central obesity, striae, rounded faces and fat deposits ("buffalo humps") over the cervical spine. Their skin bruises easily and develops a parchment appearance. These patients often are glucose intolerant and have hypokalemia. Hypoadrenalism, when not iatrogenic, is most commonly autoimmune in etiology. Addisonian, or hypoadrenal, patients are characterized by hyperpigmentation, weight loss, fatigue, and weakness. They often will have the associated laboratory findings of hyponatremia, hyperkalemia, and eosinophilia.

Patients with adrenal insufficiency should receive a perioperative corticosteroid "boost." For major surgery, this is done by giving 100 mg of hydrocortisone (or the equivalent) intravenously every 6 to 8 hours starting the night before surgery. The dose is then tapered to 50 mg every 6 hours after 24 hours (postoperative day 1) and then to 25 mg every 6 hours on the second postoperative day. The following day, the patient's usual corticosteroid dose can be resumed. If only a minor operation is planned, a one-day boost of 100 mg of hydrocortisone every 6 to 8 hours is adequate.[60] The side effects that should be monitored when using high-dose corticosteroids include mental status changes, hyperglycemia, or hypokalemia.

Thyroid Disease

Both hypothyroidism and hyperthyroidism have been associated with increased perioperative risks. Therefore, if either is expected clinically, elective surgery should be delayed until a patient is in a euthyroid state. Thyroid disease is most commonly seen in women and the elderly, and the elderly are less likely to demonstrate the associated physical findings commonly seen in younger patients.[62]

Clues that can be gathered on history regarding hypothyroidism include weight gain, cold intolerance, constipation, hair loss, and lethargy. On physical examination, these patients are frequently bradycardiac and hypothermic with decreased deep tendon reflexes. Their skin is characteristically dry and flaky. They may exhibit generalized alopecia and have a nonpitting pretibial edema.

Chemical confirmation of hypothyroidism is generally achieved by measuring the serum thyrotropin-stimulating hormone (TSH) level. Only rarely is a patient's hypothyroidism due to primary pituitary failure. A low serum thyroxine (T_4) level is suggestive, but it can also be a consequence of various systemic illnesses in which the patient's thyroid is normal. This condition is called the euthyroid sick syndrome.[62]

The complications seen with increased frequency in hypothyroid patients are cardiac (congestive heart failure), gastrointestinal (constipation or ileus), and psychiatric (acute confusional states). Hypothyroid patients also experience more hypotension than matched controls.[63] The congestive heart failure that these patients develop, although reversible with thyroid replacement, may respond poorly to conventional therapies.

Surgery performed on a hyperthyroid patient carries the risk of precipitating thyroid storm,[61] which is associated with significant morbidity and excess mortality. Once made euthyroid, patients who were previously hyperthyroid carry no increased perioperative risk in elective surgery.[60]

Hyperthyroid patients commonly give histories of weight loss without loss of appetite, palpitations, diarrhea, heat intolerance, nervousness, and insomnia. Again, however, elderly patients may present atypically, complaining only of fatigue and weakness, and appearing depressed.[62] This presentation is called the "apathetic hyperthyroidism" of the elderly. On physical examination, most hyperthyroid patients are tachycardiac, hyperthermic, and hyperreflexic. They often have a fine generalized tremor and may have hyperdynamic cardiac flow murmurs. Characteristic ocular findings include lid lag and exophthalmos. Many of the systemic findings of hyperthyroidism are obscured by β-adrenergic–blocking drugs.

A clinical diagnosis can be chemically confirmed by an elevated T_4 or a suppressed TSH. A free thyroxine level or free T_4 index is more reliable than a total T_4 in conditions associated with increased thyroxine binding globulin (eg, pregnancy, estrogen replacement, or liver disease).

COAGULATION

Several studies have demonstrated the uselessness of routine screening coagulation tests as a means of uncovering coagulopathies.[5,6,64] Yet, they continue to be performed on many patients. One study examined consecutive surgical patients, obtaining prothrombin time (PT), partial thromboplastin time (PTT), platelet counts, and bleeding time (BT) levels on each (at a cost of $65.70). Blinded observers divided the tests into those directed by information obtained on history and physical examination, and nondirected (or screening) tests. All the coagulopathies found were on the "directed" tests, and the authors thought that 46% of the tests could be safely omitted.[64]

Clearly, not all patients have the same bleeding risks. A healthy individual undergoing cataract surgery, for example, is not the same as a patient with cirrhosis having retinal surgery. The key when evaluating a preoperative patient regarding hemostasis is to obtain clues to risks from the history and physical examination. The nature of the procedure planned and the consequences of bleeding must be factored into the equation. Then coagulation studies can be ordered in a cost-effective and worthwhile manner.

The preoperative history needs to contain several specific questions about bleeding. Was excessive bleeding a complication of prior operations, births, or dental extractions? Did the patient require a transfusion postoperatively? The patient needs to be asked about current and recent medication usage. Warfarin (Coumadin), cytotoxic agents, aspirin, and nonsteroidal antiinflammatory agents all can affect coagulation parameters for considerable lengths of time. Questions about the existence of any concurrent illnesses, like liver and kidney disease, need to be asked. The interviewer should ask about any recent spontaneous bruising or bleeding. Inquiring about a family history of bleeding problems is important, as many coagulopathies are inherited, and some may only become clinically apparent under stresses like surgery.[65]

The emphasis of physical examination is on hematologic organs and sites of pathologic bleeding. The skin should be examined for pallor, jaundice, bruises, or petechiae. Petechiae are red, macular lesions seen on the extensor surfaces of extremities and are associated with thrombocytopenia. The presence of lymphadenopathy should raise concern. Splenomegaly and hepatomegaly are important findings, possibly indicating consumption of platelets or inadequate production of hepatic synthesized coagulation factors.

If the planned procedure carries minor consequences of bleeding, and the history and physical examination raise no questions of clotting abnormalities, no further studies are necessary.[66,67] For patients undergoing major operations but who have no history suggestive of problems, a PT, PTT, and platelet count will suffice preoperatively. When the history and physical examination have raised questions regarding a patient's hemostasis capacity or where bleeding would be a catastrophe, a BT should be added. If the patient's history is highly suspicious of a clotting problem, regardless of the operation planned, these tests should be ordered. If there are abnormalities found or doubt remains, a hematology consultation is probably in order.

Once the laboratory values are obtained, they need to be interpreted and not ignored. When clotting abnormalities are found, a complete blood count should also be checked. A hemoglobin over 10 g is preferred preoperatively to ensure the adequacy of oxygen transport, but blood volume is probably more important. Patients with chronic anemias and hemoglobins between 5 to 10 g are not at increased risk, in contrast to those with recent blood loss and decreased blood volumes.[66] Ideally, a patient should have a platelet count greater than 100,000/μL preoperatively, but for most procedures more than 50,000 will be adequate.[66] At counts less than 50,000 excessive postoperative bleeding is a potential risk, particularly if a functional defect exists. Elective surgery should be delayed until the situation is clarified. Platelet transfusions can be given if the operation is emergent, but if there is a consumptive disorder present, the effect may not be adequate for hemostasis. An unexplained, prolonged PT or a prolonged PTT, beyond the normal ranges, can be from a variety of causes, and special testing is needed to clarify them.

Patients on chronic anticoagulant therapy require special consideration. The reason they are receiving anticoagulants needs to be discussed with the primary care physician. The bleeding risks of the procedure and the expected degree of immobility afterward need to be considered. The goal is to minimize the "window" of time where the patient is not anticoagulated, without compromising hemostasis and causing bleeding complications perioperatively. To that end, it should be remembered that blood can be replaced, but an embolic event, like a stroke, can be catastrophic.

Patients with prosthetic heart valves are usually anticoagulated with warfarin. Prosthetic aortic valves carry a small risk of thrombosis during the perioperative period. These patients can have their warfarin dose held for 2 to 3 days preoperatively, allowing their PT to normalize. If rapid reversal is needed for urgent surgery, vitamin K or plasma infusions can be used. After the operation, the usual dose of warfarin can be resumed. Those patients with prosthetic mitral valves are at higher risk of thromboembolic events. Their anticoagulants should also be stopped preoperatively and a normal PT achieved. When the surgeon thinks it is safe from a wound standpoint (12–24 hours postoperatively), a heparin infusion should be started and continued until adequate anticoagulation is achieved with warfarin as indicated by the PT.[68]

As with hemostasis, patients' risk of thromboembolic events varies with their concurrent diseases and the planned procedure. Some common conditions that place patients at high risk for thromboembolic events are listed in Table 2-11. Prolonged immobilization postoperatively is itself a risk factor for thromboemboli. Prophylactic measures have been shown to be effective for high-risk procedures and patients, and they should be instituted preoperatively. Depending on the patient and the procedure, recommendations include heparin, warfarin, dextran, compression stockings, pneumatic compression boots, vena caval filters, and combinations of these measures.[69] Patients with hematocrits greater than 50% should be phlebotomized to less than 50% before elective surgery.

Those patients with a previous history of thromboembolic events should be considered at higher risk. A personal or family history of unexplained or repeated thromboses may signify a primary coagulopathy, several of which are inheritable. Proteins S and C are vitamin K–dependent, hepatically synthesized anticoagulants. Deficiencies in their production are associated with venous thromboses. The defects have an autosomal dominant inheritance pattern, and both can be acquired disorders seen in association with systemic (eg, liver) diseases.[70] Antithrombin III is also synthesized by the liver, but independently of vitamin K. Its deficiency appears as an acquired condition associated with the nephrotic syndrome, liver disease, or disseminated intravascular coagulation. The defect can also be inherited in an autosomally dominant fashion, via lack of protein production or production of a defective protein. In one series of patients with deep venous thromboses 3% were found to have this defect, and another found that one

Table 2-11
Common Conditions Associated With Increased Risks of Thromboembolic Events

Artificial heart valves
Congestive heart failure
Erythrocytosis
Estrogen therapy
Inflammatory bowel disease
Malignancies
Myeloproliferative disorders
Nephrotic syndrome
Obesity

half of those with the defect had suffered a thrombotic event.[71] Serum levels of all three of the previously mentioned proteins can be obtained if a deficiency in them is suspected.

One final acquired, hypercoagulable state deserving mention is the antiphospholipid syndrome. The antiphospholipid antibody and the lupus anticoagulant have been associated with several pathologic events including recurrent arterial and venous thromboses. Their presence may be signaled by a falsely positive syphilis test or a prolonged PTT. The role that these antibodies play in hypercoagulability, their mechanism of action, and the best treatment all remain controversial.[72]

HEPATIC DISEASE

When evaluating a patient with liver disease preoperatively, it is important to remember the multiple tasks performed by the liver and biliary tree. Hepatocytes are responsible for the synthesis of myriad proteins including clotting factors. The liver metabolizes and the biliary tree excretes a variety of drugs and toxins. The action of many pharmacologic agents can be potentiated and prolonged in patients with hepatobiliary disease. The liver is intricately involved in glucose metabolism, and patients with compromised hepatic function have decreased glycogen stores available for times of energy demand.

Patients with significant hepatic pathology are at increased risk for a variety of postoperative complications. These include encephalopathy, infections, bleeding complications, drug toxicities, acute renal failure, and electrolyte derangements.[9,73,74] These patients may develop new or worsening jaundice, or ascites postoperatively as well. If a patient has a history of hepatic problems after previous operations, associations with drugs or anesthetics used should be sought. The patients with known liver disease should also be asked about gastrointestinal bleeding, as they have a much higher incidence of this problem than the general population.

A comprehensive preoperative evaluation can help to predict which problems pertain to an individual patient and what can be done to prevent them. Generally speaking, a patient who has only a history of liver disease, such as jaundice, will do well perioperatively if the preoperative assessment of liver function is normal. This is done by the assessment of blood levels of total bilirubin, serum glutamic-oxaloacetic transaminase (SGOT) or serum glutamic-pyruvic transaminase (SGPT), alkaline phosphatase, and albumin, and assessment of PT.[73] In many patients with chronic liver disease, these values are not normal and are poorly predictive of complications. Child's classification system has been shown to have predictive value for patients undergoing surgical procedures.[73,74] It uses the presence of hyperbilirubinemia, hypoalbuminemia, malnutrition, encephalopathy, and ascites to divide patients into high-, medium-, and low-risk groups (Table 2-12).

Table 2-12
Preoperative Severity of Liver Disease

	CHILD'S CLASS		
PARAMETERS	A	B	C
Clinical			
Ascites	None	Easily controlled	Poorly controlled
Encephalopathy	None	Minimal	Moderate/severe
Nutrition	Excellent	Good	Poor
Laboratory			
Albumin (g ≠ dL)	> 3.5	3–3.5	< 3
Bilirubin (mg ≠ dL)	< 2	2–3	> 3
Perioperative mortality (for portal shunts)	0–1%	9–10%	> 50%

(Adapted from Siefkin AD, Bolt RJ. Preoperative evaluation of the patient with gastrointestinal or liver disease. Med Clin North Am 1979;63:1309; and Mullen J. Consequences of malnutrition in the surgical patient. Surg Clin North Am 1981;61:456)

On physical examination, the patient with significant hepatobiliary disease demonstrates numerous findings. Lesions seen on skin examination include scleral icterus, jaundice, palmar erythema, and spider angiomas. Men with alcoholic liver disease have gynecomastia and testicular atrophy. If the liver disease is severe enough to have caused portal hypertension (ie, has progressed to cirrhosis), patients demonstrate splenomegaly, ascites, and cutaneous venous shunting around the portal system (eg, caput medusae). The liver should be palpated for hepatomegaly, but often the most diseased livers are not enlarged. On neurologic examination, the examiner may find peripheral neuropathies, cranial nerve abnormalities, cerebellar signs, and mental status abnormalities, most of which are due to coexisting alcohol abuse or malnutrition.[74] The classic sign of hepatic encephalopathy is asterixis, a jerking tremor at the wrists or ankles on dorsiflexion. This sign is not specific for liver disease and can be seen with other metabolic encephalopathies, such as uremia.

Coagulopathies, thrombocytopenia, and anemia are all associated with chronic liver disease, regardless of etiology. An elevated PT from hepatic disease is serious and denotes diminished synthesis of hepatic coagulation factors, something temporarily reversible with vitamin K and plasma infusions. A history of abnormal bleeding, or the presence of petechiae or bruises should prompt further investigation. The PT, a platelet count, and a complete blood count should always be performed preoperatively on patients with known liver disease.

Serious liver disease seldom exists as an isolated event. In the United States, alcohol and drug abuse are strongly associated with chronic liver disease. A careful history regarding current and past substance abuse should be taken, with emphasis given to the course of previous hospitalizations and withdrawal syndromes. Serologies for infectious hepatitis (both B and C viruses) and human immunodeficiency virus should be ordered if appropriate. If there is a question of current habituation, a prophylactic regimen should be started preoperatively and continued postoperatively. Only about 5% of patients admitted for alcohol abuse develop the severest form of withdrawal, delirium tremens, but the untreated mortality for it is as high as 20%.[75] A regimen used for alcoholics is given in Table 2-13. Patients addicted to other drugs need to be individualized. Many patients with substance abuse problems are seriously malnourished. Malnourished patients are at increased risk for wound infections and other postoperative problems.[76] Nutritional needs should be assessed and supplements given (see Table 2-13). The value of delaying surgery while hyperalimentation is being given remains questionable in all but the most grossly malnourished individuals. A large, prospective study was unable to demonstrate any net benefit from preoperative hyperalimentation to any but severely malnourished patients.[77] The history and physical examination should guide the use of laboratory testing in patients with liver disease (Table 2-14). In addition to assessing hepatic function as well as hematologic and coagulation status, renal function needs to be assessed in these patients by obtaining a serum creatinine. In patients with poor nutritional status, serum magnesium and phosphate levels should be assessed and replacement given if they are low.

RENAL DISEASE

Improvements in dialysis, transplantation, and supportive techniques have lengthened and improved the quality of life for patients with chronic renal disease. They are increasingly candidates for elective procedures not related to their kidney problems. These patients merit special attention, however, as they have increased postoperative risks that parallel the degree

Table 2-13
Prophylactic Therapy for Alcoholic Patients

Delirium tremens: medium-duration benzodiazepine*
- Diazepam (Valium), 2–5 mg or chlordiazepoxide (Librium), 25–50 mg PO or IV q6h (increase for signs of withdrawal and decrease for somnolence†)

Nutrition
- Thiamine, 100 mg IV or IM qd × 3 d
- Folate, 1 mg PO or IV qd × 3 d
- Multivitamins, 1 tablet PO qd
- Magnesium and phosphate (if low)

Coagulation: prolonged PT
- Vitamin K, 10 mg SQ qd × 3 d
- Fresh frozen plasma‡

IM, intramuscularly; IV, intravenously; PO, by mouth; PT, prothrombin time; qd, every day; SQ, subcutaneously.

* This is only a prevention regimen, and doses in patients with actual delirium tremens will be *greatly increased.*

† Half-lives are prolonged in hepatic failure.

‡ If PT is still prolonged after vitamin K, use enough fresh frozen plasma to achieve a normal PT.

Table 2-14
Laboratory Evaluation in Patients With Liver Disease

Hemostasis
Hemoglobin/hematocrit
Platelet count
PT
Tests of liver damage/function
Alkaline phosphatase
SGOT or SGPT
Total bilirubin
Albumin
PT
Associated chemistries
Electrolytes
Magnesium
Phosphate

PT, prothrombin time; SGOT, serum glutamic-oxaloacetic transminase; SGPT, serum glutamic-pyruvic transaminase.

of compromise in their renal function. Complications to which they are prone include hypertensive and hypotensive episodes, electrolyte disturbances, volume overload, bleeding and clotting problems, infections, delirium, and cardiac problems.[46] Doses of renally excreted drugs need to be adjusted according to the patients' degree of renal compromise.

Patients with renal disease should always have a preoperative electrocardiogram, chest roentgenogram, and careful assessment of cardiovascular status on preoperative history and physical examination (Table 2-15). Sixty percent of deaths in patients on dialysis are from cardiovascular diseases, and cardiac disease develops in these patients at younger ages than in other individuals.[78] An elevated serum creatinine conveys increased perioperative cardiac risks and is included in the risk stratification system of Goldman and associates.[10] The specific cardiac problems that these patients develop include coronary insufficiency, arrhythmias, valvular disease, and pericarditis.

Most patients with severe renal disease have chronic anemias, to which they are compensated. They will not, however, replace operative blood losses as normal individuals do. They are at risk for upper gastrointestinal hemorrhages, which cause the deaths of 3% to 7% of patients with chronic renal failure.[79] A history of peptic disease or gastrointestinal bleeds should be inquired about preoperatively and consideration given to prophylaxis. In addition to bleeding complications, patients with protein-losing renal diseases, particularly those with the nephrotic syndrome, have an increased incidence of thromboembolic events, such as deep venous thromboses and pulmonary emboli. Studies have found incidences of thromboembolic events in nephrotic patients up to 44%.[80] Their urinary wasting of antithrombin III and abnormal platelet function are thought to play important roles, but the cause of the hypercoagulability is probably multifactorial. Plans for prevention of pulmonary emboli need to be discussed if these patients are to be immobilized postoperatively.

In addition to those with known kidney disease, many patients having eye surgery have concurrent diseases that put them at risk for compromised renal function. The two most common examples are diabetes mellitus and hypertension. Any patient with either of these problems, or other conditions known to lead to compromised renal function, should have a screening preoperative urinalysis and serum creatinine measured to assess renal function.

Acute and chronic problems that leave a patient volume depleted (such as vomiting or diarrhea) can predispose a patient to acute renal failure. Both volume and electrolytes should be corrected preoperatively. Patients with compromised renal function particularly are unable to control their volume status when physiologically stressed. Assessment of volume status is best done by measuring the patient's blood pressure and heart rate in two positions (eg, supine and sitting), waiting at least 1 minute between measurements. Hypovolemic patients will drop their blood pressures or raise their heart rates after positional changes. A difference of greater than 20 mmHg or 20 beats/min is considered significant.

Table 2-15
Preoperative Laboratory Evaluation of Renal Disease

Known renal disease
ECG
Chest roentgenogram
Urinalysis
Blood values
Complete blood count
Electrolytes
BUN/creatinine
PT, PTT, bleeding time
Suspected renal disease
Urinalysis
Serum creatinine

BUN, blood urea nitrogen; ECG, electrocardiogram; PT, prothrombin time; PTT, partial thromboplastin time.

ACUTE CONFUSIONAL STATE

Delirium or the development of an acute confusional state is a problem of increasing magnitude in our aging society. As a postoperative complication, delirium is almost uniformly seen in elderly patients. The reason for the susceptibility of the elderly to this complication is unclear. However, the elderly's aging cholinergic nervous systems, decreased rates of oxidative metabolism, and difficulties with autoimmunity have all been implicated.[81,82]

Dementia is commonly mistaken for delirium, but differentiating the two is important. Dementia is an insidious, chronic loss of intellectual function and is usually irreversible. Delirium is a sudden and global change in mental status. It is characterized by altered perceptions, hallucinations, and a fluctuating course. Although electroencephalographic studies can be suggestive of the disorder, it remains a clinical diagnosis.[83] Delirium frequently has a discernible and reversible course, but untreated has a significant mortality.

In populations undergoing emergent surgery, such as hip fracture repair, rates of delirium are high. Incidences over 50% have been reported in several studies.[84–87] Acute confusion still occurs commonly but less frequently (10%–20%) in elderly patients undergoing elective surgery.[88,89]

The development of this complication is important, because it has been linked to several unfavorable clinical outcomes. Postoperative delirium has been associated with prolonged hospital stays and various poorer functional outcomes. These patients have an increased mortality and an increased likelihood of being discharged to a nursing home.[85,86]

Predicting which patients are at risk for acute postoperative confusion is a topic receiving much attention in the medical literature. Several attempts to identify hospitalized elderly patients at risk for acute confusion have been published.[84,90–92] The variables these studies identified as independent predictors of delirium are shown in Table 2-16. Risk seems to increase with age as a continuous variable. That is, the older the patient, the more likely delirium will be a complication. Men may be more susceptible than women. Patients with an abnormal baseline mental status are more likely to become confused postoperatively. Medication with central nervous system side effects, particularly drugs with anticholinergic properties, put older patients at increased risk for delirium.

Postoperative confusion can be reduced by paying close attention to general medical care and medications used. Although multiple drug classes have been associated with the development of delirium, anticholinergic agents, sedative-hypnotic drugs, and narcotics are the most common offenders. Of particular concern regarding ophthalmic surgery patients is the use of anticholinergic eye drops (eg, atropine and scopolamine), which have been reported to cause confusion and hallucinations.[1] Regular reorientation of patients, and frequent verbal contact with patients have been effective in preventing confusional episodes[84] and can be started preoperatively.

When faced with a confused patient, the first point to establish is whether this is a new problem. Then, one must consider treatable conditions (Table 2-17) including drug withdrawal or overdose, metabolic

Table 2-16
Prospectively Identified Variables Associated With the Development of Delirium

SOURCE	PATIENTS	PREDICTORS OF DELIRIUM
Inouye et al (1993)	General medical age > 70 y	Visual impairment, severe illness, cognitive impairment, high blood urea nitrogen/creatinine ratio
Schor et al (1992)	General medical age > 80 yr, age > 65 y	Cognitive impairment, fracture, infection, male gender, neuroleptic or narcotic use
Williams-Russo et al (1992)	Elective knee replacement	Increased age, male gender, alcohol use
Williams et al (1985)	Hip fracture Age > 60 y	Increased age, cognitive impairment, prior activity level

Table 2-17
Initial Studies for Patients With Delirium

Serum electrolytes (particularly Na^+)
Blood urea nitrogen/creatinine
Serum glucose
Complete blood count
Po_2
pH
Electrocardiogram
Chest x-ray

disturbances, hypoxemia, shock, infections, anemia, myocardial infarction, and stroke. Any of these medical problems can have acute confusion as the presenting symptom in elderly patients. Exacerbations of the patient's known, chronic conditions (such as obstructive lung disease or congestive heart failure) should always be considered when evaluating delirious patients.

References

1. Adler AG. Perioperative management of the ophthalmology patient. Med Clin North Am 1987;71:561.
2. Duncalf D, Gartner S, Carol B. Mortality in association with ophthalmic surgery. Am J Ophthalmol 1970;69: 610.
3. Petruscak J, Smith B, Breslin P. Mortality related to ophthalmological surgery. Arch Ophthalmol 1973;89: 106.
4. Djokvic JL, Hedley-White J. Prediction of outcome of surgery and anesthesia in patients over 80. JAMA 1979;242:2301.
5. Kaplan EB, Sheiner LB, Boeckmann AJ, et al. The usefulness of preoperative laboratory screening. JAMA 1985;253:3576.
6. Turnbull JM, Buck C. The value of preoperative screening investigations in otherwise healthy individuals. Arch Intern Med 1987;147:1101.
7. Nar BJ, Hansen TR, Warner MA. Preoperative laboratory screening in healthy Mayo patients: cost effective elimination of tests and unchanged outcomes. Mayo Clin Proc 1991;66:155.
8. Caputo GM, Gross R. Medical consultation on surgical services: an annotated bibliography. Ann Intern Med 1993;188:290.
9. Kammerer WS, Gross RJ. Medical consultation. In: The internist on surgical, obstetric, and psychiatric services, ed 2. Baltimore, Williams & Wilkins, 1990.
10. Goldman L, Caldera DL, Nussbaum SR, et al. Multifactorial index of cardiac risk in noncardiac surgical procedures. N Engl J Med 1977;297:845.
11. Mangano DT. Perioperative cardiac morbidity. Anesthesiology 1990;72:153.
12. Detsky AS, Abrams HB, McLaughlin JR. Predicting cardiac complications in patients undergoing non-cardiac surgery. J Gen Intern Med 1986;1:211.
13. Michel LA, Jamart J, Bradpiece, HA, et al. Predictor of risk on noncardiac patients after cardiac operations. J Thorac Cardiovasc Surg 1990;100:595.
14. Weitz HH, Goldman L. Noncardiac surgery in the patient with heart disease. Med Clin North Am 1987;71:413.
15. Goldman L. Cardiac risks and complications of noncardiac surgery. Ann Intern Med 1983;98:504.
16. Browner WS, Li J, Mangano DT. In-hospital and long-term mortality in male veterans following noncardiac surgery. JAMA 1992;268:228.
17. Rao TK, Jacobs KH, El-Etr AA. Reinfarction rate following anesthesia in patients with myocardial infarction. Anesthesiology 1983;59:499.
18. Raby KE, Goldman L, Creager MA, et al. Correlation between preoperative ischemia and major events after peripheral vascular surgery. N Engl J Med 1989; 321:1296.
19. Coley CM, Field TS, Abraham SA, et al. Usefulness of dipyridamole-thallium scanning for preoperative evaluation of cardiac risk for nonvascular surgery. Am J Cardiol 1992;69:1280.
20. Carliner NH, Fisher ML, Plotnick GD, et al. Routine exercise testing in patients undergoing major noncardiac surgery. Am J Cardiol 1985;56:51.
21. Ashton CM, Peterson NJ, Wray NP, et al. The incidence of perioperative myocardial infarction in men undergoing noncardiac surgery. Ann Intern Med 1993;118:504.
22. Goldberger AL, O'Konski M. Utility of the routine electrocardiogram before surgery and on general hospital admission. Ann Intern Med 1986;105:552.
23. Tape TG, Mushlin AI. How useful are routine chest x-rays of preoperative patients at risk for postoperative chest disease? J Gen Intern Med 1988;3:15.
24. Adler AG, McElwain GE, Merli GJ, et al. Systemic effects of eye drops. Arch Intern Med 1982;142:2293.
25. Joint National Committee on Detection, Evaluation and Treatment of High Blood Pressure. The fifth report of the Joint National Committee on Detection, Evaluation and Treatment of High Blood Pressure (JNC V). Arch Intern Med 1993;153:154.
26. Elnicki M, Kotchen T. Hypertension: patient evaluation, indications for treatment. Geriatrics 1993;48:47.
27. Merli GJ, Bell RD. Preoperative management of the surgical patient with neurologic disease. Med Clin North Am 1987;71:511.

28. Prys-Roberts C, Meloche R, Foex P. Studies of anesthesia in relation to hypertension: I. Cardiovascular responses of treated and untreated patients. Br J Anesth 1971;43:122.
29. Prys-Roberts C, Foex P, Greene LT, et al. Studies of anesthesia in relation to hypertension: IV. Br J Anesth 1972;44:335.
30. Goldman L, Caldera DL. Risks of general anesthesia and elective operation in the hypertensive patient. Anesthesiology 1979;50:285.
31. Charlson ME, MacKenzie CR, Gold JP, et al. Preoperative characteristics predicting intraoperative hypotension and hypertension among hypertensives and diabetics undergoing noncardiac surgery. Ann Surg 1990;212:66.
32. Adler AG. Perioperative management of the ophthalmology patient. Med Clin North Am 1987;71:561.
33. Adler AG, McElwain GE, Merli GJ, et al. Systemic effects of eye drops. Arch Intern Med 1982;142:2293.
34. Jackson MV. Preoperative pulmonary evaluation. Arch Intern Med 1988;148:2120.
35. Mohr DN, Jett JR. Preoperative evaluation of pulmonary risk factors. J Gen Intern Med 1988;3:277.
36. Warner MA, Offord KP, Warner ME, et al. Role of preoperative cessation of smoking and other factors in postoperative pulmonary complications: a blinded prospective study of coronary artery bypass patients. Mayo Clin Proc 1989;64:609.
37. Kroenke K, Lawrence VA, Teroux JF, et al. Operative risk in patients with severe obstructive pulmonary disease. Arch Intern Med 1992;152:967.
38. Mannino DM, Etzel RA, Flanders D. Do the medical history and physical examination predict low lung function? Arch Intern Med 1993;153:1892.
39. Stein M, Cassara EL. Preoperative pulmonary evaluation and therapy for surgery patients. JAMA 1970;211:787.
40. Celli BR, Rodriguez KS, Snider GL. A controlled trial of intermittent positive pressure breathing, incentive spirometry, and deep breathing exercises in preventing pulmonary complications after abdominal surgery. Am Rev Respir Dis 1984;130:12.
41. Roukema JA, Carol EJ, Prins JG. The prevention of pulmonary complications after abdominal surgery in patients with noncompromised pulmonary status. Arch Surg 1988;123:30.
42. American College of Physicians. Preoperative pulmonary function testing. (Position Paper) Ann Intern Med 1990;112,793.
43. Merimee TJ. Diabetic retinopathy: a synthesis of perspectives. N Engl J Med 1990;322:978.
44. Hirsch IB, McGill JB, Cryer PE, et al. Perioperative management of surgical patients with diabetes mellitus. Anesthesiology 1991;74:346.
45. Nathan DM. Long-term complications of diabetes mellitus. N Engl J Med 1993;328:1676.
46. Werb MR, Zinman B, Teasdale SJ, et al. Hormonal and metabolic responses during coronary artery bypass surgery: role of infused glucose. J Clin Endocrinol Metab 1989;69:1010.
47. Foster DW, McGarry JD. The metabolic derangements and treatment of diabetic ketoacidosis. N Engl J Med 1983;309:159.
48. Reynolds C. Management of the diabetic surgical patient. Postgrad Med 1985;77:265.
49. Goodson WH, Hunt TK. Wound healing and the diabetic patient. Surg Gynecol Obstet 1979;149:600.
50. Reddi AS, Camerini-Davalos RA. Diabetic nephropathy: an update. Arch Intern Med 1990;150:31.
51. Selby JV, Fitzsimmons SC, Newman JM, et al. The natural history and epidemiology of diabetic nephropathy: implications for prevention and control. JAMA 1990;263:1954.
52. Harati Y. Diabetic peripheral neuropathies. Ann Intern Med 1987;107:545.
53. Reichard P, Nilsson BY, Rosenquist U. The effect of long-term intensified insulin treatment on the development of microvascular complications of diabetes mellitus. N Engl J Med 1993;329:304.
54. Chase HP, Jackson WE, Hoops SL, et al. Glucose control and the renal and retinal complications of insulin-dependent diabetes. JAMA 1989;261:1155.
55. The Diabetes Control and Complications Trial Research Group. The effect of intensive treatment of diabetes on the development and progression of long-term complications in insulin-dependent diabetes mellitus. N Engl J Med 1993;329:977.
56. Gavin LA. Management of diabetes mellitus during surgery. West J Med 1989;151:525.
57. Degoute CS, Ray MJ, Manchon M, et al. Intraoperative glucose infusion and blood lactate: endocrine and metabolic relationships during abdominal aortic surgery. Anesthesiology 1989;71:355.
58. Zinman B. The physiologic replacement of insulin. N Engl J Med 1989;321:363.
59. Gerich JE. Oral hypoglycemic agents. N Engl J Med 1989;321:1231.
60. McGlynn TJ, Simons RJ. Endocrine disorders. In: Kammerer WS, Gross RJ, eds. Medical consultation: the internist on surgical, obstetric, and psychiatric services, ed 2. Baltimore, Williams & Wilkins, 1990:275.
61. Houston MC, Ratcliff DG, Hays JT, et al. Preoperative medical consultation and evaluation of surgical risk. South Med J 1987;80:1385.
62. Gregerman RI. Thyroid diseases. In: Hazzard WR, Andres R, Bierman EL, Blass JP, eds. Principles of geriatric medicine and gerontology, ed 2. New York, McGraw-Hill, 1990:719.
63. Ladenson PW, Levin AA, Ridgway EC, et al. Complications of surgery in hypothyroid patients. Am J Med 1984;77:261.
64. Rohrer MJ, Michelotti MC, Nahrwold DL. A prospective

evaluation of the efficacy of preoperative coagulation testing. Ann Surg 1988;208:554.
65. Hoyer LW, Tuddenham EG. Excessive bleeding caused by defective coagulation. In: Lichtman MA, ed., Hematology for practitioners. Boston, Little, Brown, 1978:297.
66. Fellin F, Murphy S. Hematologic problems in the preoperative patient. Med Clin North Am 1987;71:477.
67. Rapaport SI. Preoperative hemostatic evaluation: which tests, if any? Blood 1983;61:229.
68. Elliot DL, Tolle SW, Linz DH. Preparing the medically compromised patient for surgery. Postgrad Med 1985;77:269.
69. Gaasch WH. Diagnosis, treatment, and prevention of pulmonary embolism. JAMA 1992;268:1727.
70. Rick ME. Protein C and protein S: vitamin K-dependent inhibitors of blood coagulation. JAMA 1990; 263:701.
71. Nachman RL, Silverstein R. Hypercoagulable states. Ann Intern Med 1993;119:819.
72. Lockshin MD. Antiphospholipid antibody syndrome. JAMA 1992;268:1451.
73. Siefkin AD, Bolt RJ. Preoperative evaluation of the patient with gastrointestinal or liver disease. Med Clin North Am 1979;63:1309.
74. Charness ME, Simon RP, Greenberg DA. Ethanol and the nervous system. N Engl J Med 1989;321:442.
75. Turner RC, Lichstein PR, Peden JC. Alcohol withdrawal syndromes. J Gen Intern Med 1989;4:432.
76. Mullen J. Consequences of malnutrition in the surgical patient. Surg Clin North Am 1981;61:456.
77. The Veterans Affairs Total Parenteral Nutrition Cooperative Study Group. Perioperative total parenteral nutrition in surgical patients. N Engl J Med 1992;325:525.
78. Becker RC. Cardiovascular disease in patients with chronic renal failure. Cleveland Clin J Med 1988; 55:521.
79. Boyle JM, Johnston B. Acute upper gastrointestinal hemorrhage in patients with chronic renal disease. Am J Med 1983;75:409.
80. Llach F. Thromboembolic complications in nephrotic syndrome. Postgrad Med 1984;76:111.
81. Francis J. Delirium in older patients. J Am Geriatr Soc 1992;40:829.
82. Lipowski Z. Delirium in the elderly patient. N Engl J Med 1989;320:578.
83. Francis J, Kapoor W. Delirium in hospitalized elderly. J Gen Intern Med 1990;5:65.
84. Williams MA, Campbell EB, Raynor WJ, et al. Reducing acute confusional states in elderly patients with hip fractures. Res Nurs Health 1985;8:329.
85. Gustafson Y, Berggren D, Brannstrom B, et al. Acute confusional states in elderly patients treated for femoral neck fracture. J Am Geriatr Soc 1988;36:525.
86. Berggren D, Gustafson Y, Eriksson B, et al. Postoperative confusion after anesthesia in elderly patients with femoral neck fractures. Anesth Analg 1987;66:497.
87. Gustafson Y, Brannstrom B, Berggren D, et al. A geriatric-anesthesiologic program to reduce acute confusional states in elderly patients treated for femoral neck fractures. J Am Geriatr Soc 1991;39:655.
88. Hole A, Terjessen T, Breivik H. Epidural versus general anesthesia for total hip arthroplasty in elderly patients. Acta Anaesth Scand 1980;24:279.
89. Millar HR. Psychiatric morbidity in elderly surgical patients. Br J Psychiatry 1981;138:17.
90. Inouye SK, Viscoli CM, Horwitz RI, Hurst LD, Tinetti ME. A predictive model for delirium in hospitalized elderly medical patients based on admission characteristics. Ann Intern Med 1993;119:474.
91. Schor JD, Levkoff SE, Lipsitz LA, et al. Risk factors for delirium in hospitalized elderly. JAMA 1992;267:827.
92. Williams-Russo P, Urquhart BL, Sharrock NE, Charlson ME. Post-operative delirium: predictors and prognosis in elderly orthopedic patients. J Am Geriatr Soc 1992;40:759.

Ophthalmic Surgery Complications: Prevention and Management,
edited by Judie F. Charlton and George W. Weinstein.
J. B. Lippincott Company, Philadelphia © 1995.

3

Jerome W. Bettman, Sr.

Informed Consent

THE CONTINUING PROCESS OF INFORMED CONSENT

The best prophylactic of medicolegal claims is good rapport. The most important aspect of good rapport is communication, and communication is the essence of informed consent.

Proper informed consent is not a one-time event that occurs before an operation or a medical procedure; rather, it is a continuing process. This process may start before the ophthalmologist sees the patient. If the ophthalmologist is on a television program or in an advertisement, what is said or written may be part of the informative process. This is also true of advice given over the telephone or in the office by the office personnel.

If ophthalmologists continue to inform patients during the entire period of care and if they take patients into their confidence in the decision-making process, it is extremely unlikely that patients will sue. Conversely, what causes patients to sue? Usually an unpleasant surprise makes patients angry, and these patients are likely to seek an attorney.

HOW TO INFORM AND DOCUMENT

It is especially important that patients be fully informed before an operation or major medical procedure. How and when should this be done?

It is wise to use a carefully written, printed form. Most forms contain appropriate information about the procedure: the complications and the alternatives as well as a statement that not every complication can be addressed. The courts have decided that not every unusual complication need be addressed. The material should be written in a layperson's language and should include the possibility of loss of vision or loss of the eyeball. The latter is a possibility in almost every surgical procedure in or around the globe. If the patient accepts the peril of loss of vision or the eye, it might be assumed that the patient would have accepted lesser perils, although the latter should be addressed. The form should be signed by the patient, dated, and witnessed.

Having a patient read and sign such a form is insufficient. It is essential that the patient understands what is in the form. It is mandatory that surgeons themselves discuss the problem with the patient and ask questions about the material in the form so that one is assured that the patient does understand.

Such a form should be given to the patient in advance of the day of operation. The patient should take it home, read it at leisure, and discuss it with family if desired. The patient who is given a form on the day of surgery may correctly say that the decision had been made before receiving the form or that signing of the form was a perfunctory event, such as signing a form before admission to the hospital. The latter is frequently not read, and the signing of that form is mandatory before one is admitted to the hospital. This is different from signing an "informed consent" form, a copy of which the patient should receive.

SIGNIFICANCE OF THE DOCUMENTED FORM

If a suit comes to trial, the signed consent form may be valuable in defense, but this situation is not always true. I was an expert witness in two illustrative suits.

Both were based on informed consent before refractive keratomy procedures, the suits were against the same surgeon, and the same consent form was used. The consent form was a good one: it covered all the important complications and the alternatives. In one suit, there was a defense verdict because the judge said that the form had been signed by the patient, and it included a statement that the patient understood the form.

During the suit in the other case, it was stated that the patient only received the form just before the operation, that the patient had already decided to have the procedure done because of the surgeon's television appearance and a brochure that had been mailed, and that the patient did not understand the significance of the form or its content. This resulted in a verdict for the plaintiff. The conclusion must be that the printed consent form may be important in the defense, but it cannot be relied on.

Some surgeons use a taped message or videotape to inform the patient. This is acceptable as a part of the process, but it does not absolve the surgeon from personally explaining some aspects, asking the patient if the material is understood, and asking questions of the patient to ensure that it is understood.

Some surgeons tape the conversation with the patient during the informing process. This is acceptable provided it is done carefully and according to a protocol. With a large practice, however, there can be a problem of storage and expense.

The truly important aspect is what is in the patient's head, not what is printed on a form. One should always remember that well-informed patients rarely sue.

Giving documentation of the information to the patient is essential. The reason for the emphasis on the documentation of informed consent is that patients frequently do not recall what was said by the physician, especially if the risk is one of potential loss of vision or of the eye. This has been demonstrated in three controlled series of cases, one in the ophthalmic literature,[1] one in thoracic surgery,[2] and one in plastic surgery.[3] The essential message is the same in each, as discussed subsequently.

Ophthalmologists who have a claim against them should be aware of these three publications. They document that patients frequently do not recall being told about many complications, especially those that are a significant threat to vision or to the eyeball.

Priluck and colleagues[1] did a prospective study on 100 patients undergoing a primary scleral buckling procedure for rhegmatogenous retinal detachment. Before surgery, each patient was given a detailed 15- to 20-minute discussion by one of the authors following a standard protocol. Two to 11 days later in the postoperative period, standard questions were asked according to protocol to determine what the patients did remember. Ninety-seven percent of the patients stated that they had a satisfactory preoperative discussion, but 54% of the patients who gave inadequate responses denied the subject had ever been discussed preoperatively. Only 23% of the patients recalled that hemorrhage or infection could possibly occur intraoperatively or postoperatively, and only 3% were aware that either of these complications could essentially destroy the eye.

The other two studies, one by Robinson and Merav[2] and the other by Lieb and associates,[3] produced similar results. The former was conducted on a series of patients with open heart surgery, and questions asked 4 to 6 months postoperatively showed a retention rate of only 29% for primary recall. The study in plastic surgery showed a retention rate of 35%.

The patients in these studies had no reason to be untruthful; they actually did not recall most complications that had been discussed. It is to be expected that patients who have entered a malpractice claim will frequently and honestly deny that certain essential facts were not discussed even though they were. It is of obvious importance to be able to refer to documentation of these items in claims in which lack of informed consent is a factor.

THREE METHODS OF DOCUMENTATION

There are three methods of documentation. The seriousness of the patient's condition guides one in selecting a particular method. For a relatively minor case, it is sufficient for the ophthalmologist to write by hand on the patient's record: "The procedure, the complications, including systemic hazards, the alternatives, and anesthetic risks were explained to the patient, and the patient appeared to understand." This notation should be dated and signed, and, if desired, it can be witnessed. The statement must be in the physician's own handwriting, however, because of the fact that depositions and trials frequently take place years after the event. At that time, neither the patient nor the physician remembers what was said, if anything, but the statement was written at the time; it is inferred that the statement was actually made because the physician took the time to record it.

The second method of documentation, that of using a printed form, was discussed earlier. The third method may be used rarely, when the usual consent forms are insufficient, in which case it is wise to use a printed consent form as well. An example of such a case involves a patient who has a neovascular membrane that has encroached to within one third of the disc diameter of the fovea, although the visual acuity is 20/20. Laser photocoagulation is essential to prevent the loss of all central vision, but, if done, the acuity after such treatment will probably be reduced to approximately 20/50, even though the therapy has been applied with great caution. In this situation, it might be wise to proceed as follows:

1. Explain the situation thoroughly with emphasis on the indications and complications.
2. Ask for feedback to be sure the patient understands.
3. Clarify any points as indicated.
4. Have the patient write what is understood in the patient's own handwriting.
5. Have the patient correct any misunderstandings, and date and sign this notation.

This documentation cannot be denied because it is written in the patient's own handwriting.

In elective procedures, the need for fully informing the patient is much greater. This is especially true in plastic surgery, or in operations using drugs or devices not approved by the Food and Drug Administration. In my experience, the surgeon compares the postoperative result with the preoperative status and may be pleased, but the patient tends to compare the postoperative result with the normal side and may be unhappy. In such instances, documentation with preoperative and postoperative photographs is invaluable.

WHEN THE INFORMATION DOES NOT HAVE TO BE GIVEN

There are three circumstances in which the information leading to consent does not have to be given.

1. Patients should first be told that there are significant hazards involved, including the possibility of loss of sight, eye, or life, and then asked if they wish to know more about them. If they say, "no," this fact should be recorded in the record in the doctor's handwriting, dated, signed by patients, and witnessed. No further disclosure is then required. However, if there is an unusual risk of which patients should be aware, they should be told anyway. Patients who have a retinal detachment in one eye and lattice degeneration and a cataract in the other eye should be made aware of the hazard of retinal detachment before the cataract is removed, even if they have indicated that they do not wish to hear about the risks.
2. Some patients are totally unable to tolerate hearing about risks, or cannot comprehend the information, because of psychiatric problems. This difficulty should be confirmed by a psychiatrist and the information regarding risks should be given to relatives.
3. Some cases are true emergencies, in which there is no time to discuss consent. These situations are rare in ophthalmology.

One must also understand that the patient has the right to withdraw consent, either verbally or in writing, at any time.

An additional caveat is that consent should be obtained for what is to be done, and any additional procedures should not be done without additional consent. As an example, if consent is obtained for a strabismus operation, one might be tempted to cut off a superficial lid growth while the patient is under anesthesia. If any complication related to the removal of the growth occurs, the surgeon could be liable.

INFORMING A PATIENT THAT A COMPLICATION HAS OCCURRED

If a complication occurs after a procedure, it is essential that the surgeon be aware of how to inform the patient. The following guidelines should be observed.

After a complication has occurred, it is in the surgeon's best interest as well as the patient's to tell the patient what happened. The surgeon should be honest and not try to obscure the fact that a complication did occur. It is hoped that during the process of informing the patient before surgery, the patient was made aware of the fact that no outcome can be guaranteed. After a problem has arisen, the surgeon must inform the patient that the problem with his or her eye is within that group of complications of which the patient was informed preoperatively.

The most difficult medicolegal cases to defend are those in which the surgeon was not forthright with the patient or in which the surgeon did not seem sympathetic or particularly concerned. Patients are likely to show graceful acceptance of even the most difficult situations if they have been treated with kindness and sympathy. Again, it is essential that patients are properly informed at every stage of the procedure, from the time they are first seen through the postoperative period. If this has not been the case, surprised, angry patients are likely to seek an attorney.

Surgeons should tell patients immediately that they regret any complications and that they will do everything in their power to help. They should also reassure patients that they will do their best to provide the best possible care in dealing with the surgical results.

The patient may ask, "How did these complications occur?" It does little good to blame the patient or oneself; even when the patient might have been at fault, this explanation is usually not accepted. It is more satisfactory to blame the eye by saying, "It proved to be a difficult eye." This statement is probably correct or the complication would not have occurred.

The surgeon should suggest consultations before the patient becomes uneasy about the complication. There are two reasons for this: (1) Consultation tends to give the patient more confidence, and (2) the surgeon can choose a competent consultant. The surgeon should tell the patient about various ophthalmologists' skills, training, and experience, and hence who can be most helpful to both the patient and surgeon. A complex situation may be made much more complicated by a deficient consultant.

If the complication is less serious, it is nevertheless essential to tell that to the patient honestly. It is also critical to assess the significance of the complication and what future problems, if any, may occur. Surgeons must always be sympathetic and assure patients that they are available to provide any necessary help in the future.

One should always adhere to the following principles:

1. Be certain that proper information is imparted to the patient in a manner that is clearly understood, so that the patient can give meaningful consent to surgery. This is essential.
2. Discuss the complication and its effects honestly. Never obfuscate the situation.
3. Be sympathetic and kind.
4. Reassure the patient that the best care is being provided.
5. Suggest consultants, whom the patient might wish to see.

References

1. Priluck et al. What patients recall of the preoperative discussion after retinal detachment surgery. Am J Ophthalmol 1979;87:620.
2. Robinson G, Mirav A. Informed consent: recall by patients tested postoperatively. Ann Thorac Surg 1976;22:209.
3. Leeb D, et al. Observations on the myth of informed consent. Plastic Reconstructive Surg 1976;58:280.

Ophthalmic Surgery Complications: Prevention and Management,
edited by Judie F. Charlton and George W. Weinstein.
J. B. Lippincott Company, Philadelphia © 1995.

4

Michelle Michael
Judie F. Charlton

The Role of the Ophthalmic Technician

Comprehensive eye care can best be provided by a team of professionals who work and communicate well together. All persons involved, including physicians, optometrists, technicians, nurses, scheduling clerks, and receptionists, must have a clear understanding of their respective roles in the office, clinical, or surgical setting, and of their responsibility to the patient. When a patient undergoes eye surgery, this teamwork is especially important. The ophthalmic technician can support the ophthalmologist's efforts to provide high-quality surgical care by establishing a rapport with the patient, coordinating the patient's office visits, performing important screening and diagnostic testing, and guiding the patient through the steps in preparing for and recovering from surgery. A technician who carries out these diverse responsibilities effectively contributes to a successful surgical outcome and to the management of complications, should they occur.

ESTABLISHING A RAPPORT WITH THE PATIENT

A patient's attitude toward the ophthalmologist can be as important as the ophthalmologist's medical and surgical expertise in ensuring a successful outcome to ophthalmic surgery. A patient who trusts the ophthalmologist and is convinced of the ophthalmologist's knowledge and concern for the patient is more likely to be realistic and cooperative throughout the preoperative and postoperative periods. Such a patient is better prepared to understand and comply with postoperative care instructions and to be satisfied with the surgical results. In the event of surgical complications, patients with good attitudes toward their care providers are more likely to cope with the complications effectively and less likely to be litigious. The patient's attitude depends a great deal on the professionalism and courtesy of everyone the patient encounters in the ophthalmologist's practice.

A telephone call is usually the first contact the patient makes with the ophthalmologist's practice. Patients' calls need to be handled in a manner that inspires confidence in the office and protects the physician from unnecessary interruptions. Calls are generally answered by the receptionist and then referred to the ophthalmic technician if screening and triage are necessary. The technician should be warm and courteous, helping the patient to feel at ease while maintaining an attitude of professionalism.

The patient's first office visit is as important as the first telephone call in establishing a rapport with the patient. Even calling the patient into the examination room should be handled with courtesy and sensitivity to the patient's needs. To call the patient, one walks into the reception area and calls the patient's name. Yelling a name from a door is not professional and shows a lack of interest on the part of the technician. The patient's full name should be called in a clear, friendly tone of voice that expresses hospitality.

As the patient responds, the technician makes a quick physical assessment. A patient using a walker or in a wheelchair should be offered assistance. As the patient approaches, the technician should make eye contact and introduce himself or herself, remembering that the patient may have impaired hearing or vision. Patients are addressed as "Mr." or "Ms." and the last name. Calling patients by their first name is unprofessional unless one is given permission to do so. If the patient is visually impaired, the technician offers his or her arm to escort the patient to a room, giving specific directions (eg, "Let's go down the hall and then turn to our right through a doorway"). These instructions put the patient at ease and allow some autonomy.

After acquaintance with the patient is established, the technician can offer him or her a business card listing the technician's name and the name, address, and telephone number of the physician or clinic. Not only is this gesture a nice marketing device, but it also makes this encounter more personal for the patient and ensures that the patient will leave the office with this information handy. Another simple way to personalize the office is for all staff members to wear name tags. The needs of the patient's family members must be accommodated as well. If a member of the family prefers to come with the patient to the examination room, and the patient does not object, the technician makes sure that the person is made comfortable. The examination is explained to the family member as well as to the patient. Some family members prefer not to come into the examination room, or the patient prefers to see the physician alone. If a family member remains in the reception area, that person should be kept updated as to how long the examination will take, particularly if special testing is needed. This courtesy helps avoid undue worry for the person waiting. It is beneficial to have brochures or newsletters containing information on office hours, insurance, emergency numbers, and new medical developments in the reception area for patients and their families to read while waiting.

Once the visit is completed, the patient is escorted back to the reception area, and to waiting family members if present.

SCREENING BY THE TECHNICIAN

History

The patient's medical history and reason for the current visit are the first and most important items of information for the technician to obtain. A history is the story of a patient's medical complaint. The physician uses the history recorded by the technician to understand and evaluate the patient's current eye problem. A thorough history may disclose information that could help prevent surgical complications, such as a family history of anesthetic reaction.

There are two types of patients who enter an ophthalmologist's office: those who desire a routine eye examination and those with symptoms of an ocular disorder. It is sometimes impossible to distinguish between the two on the basis of history. Thus, it is important to question the patient with the expectation of finding some ocular disease. If the history is simply recorded as "no complaints" or "routine examination," third-party payers may deny coverage of the examination even though real ocular disease exists.

The history should be subdivided to maintain organization and protocol. Subdivisions may include the chief complaint, systemic medical problems, current ocular and systemic medications, allergies, and family history. Every physician has a unique preferred method. The technician must have a clear understanding of the physician's preferred format.

The technician determines the answer to the following question: Who referred the patient to the office? (That is, was it an ophthalmologist, a family physician, an optometrist, friends or relatives, or did the patient come on his or her own initiative?) Knowing the referral source is important so that the physician can send follow-up letters to referring physicians to keep the lines of communication open in the medical community. The following related questions are also important: Why does the patient think that he or she was referred? Why did the patient come to this office? The answers to these questions provide much helpful information. It is important to distinguish between the patient who is there to obtain a second opinion regarding cataract surgery and the patient who just wants a preliminary examination. The next documentation is the patient's age and occupation.

The patient's chief complaint is the most important information that the technician can elicit for the physician. The chief complaint constitutes the headline of an ophthalmic story. In a sentence or two the technician writes the primary reason the patient has come to the ophthalmologist. It is best to use language as close as possible to the patient's own words. The questions should be direct, simple, and straightforward. The question "How do your eyes trouble you?" is a good place to start. After the chief complaint is recorded, the patient is questioned in more detail about primary symptoms. One should try to pinpoint specific complaints and symptoms, date of onset, and duration of course.

Once the chief complaint is established, the patient is asked about previous eye history. Information regarding past eye surgery is recorded, along with the dates operations were performed and listings of previous eye medications and eye problems. Knowledge of family history of eye disease can be most helpful, especially in familial diseases such as myopia, strabismus, and glaucoma. However, one must remember that a negative family history does not exclude genetic problems such as retinitis pigmentosa. Many patients do not know the ocular status of relatives or prefer not to discuss family problems.

Medical history and general health, past and present, are also discussed. Common diseases such as diabetes, hypertension, cardiac disorders, and arthritis should be mentioned. One should obtain information about any systemic medications that the patient may be taking. Often, the patient does not know the name of the medication but may say, for example, "red pill" or "green tablet." In these cases, the patient can be asked why he or she takes the medication. Most patients are aware of the general nature of their medications.

If a patient is unsure about medications, it is helpful to ask the patient to write the names and doses of all his or her medications before the next visit, and place the list in a wallet or purse for handy reference. In addition to helping complete records, this list makes medical information accessible to care givers in the event of an emergency. Compiling the list also trains patients to be more aware of their medications.

An important part of a patient's medical history is a record of known allergies. The technician asks the patient about allergic responses to the following types of substances:

1. Contactants (cosmetics and tapes)
2. Drugs (internal or applied topically)
3. Inhalants (dust and pollen)
4. Ingestants (foods)
5. Injectants (tetanus antiserum)

The importance of a given symptom is difficult to determine based on information obtained in the history. Technicians should refrain from trying to interpret the symptoms that patients report, and should confine their role to gathering the information systematically, and recording it as clearly and completely as possible. Interpretation is the domain of the physician, who combines all the findings from the history, physical examination, and laboratory testing to determine a final diagnosis and treatment plan for each patient.

Assessment of Visual Acuity

One of the most common tests a technician is asked to perform is assessment of visual acuity. Accurate preoperative and postoperative visual acuity measurements are especially important in evaluating a patient who has had a surgical complication. Visual acuity is measured by determining the smallest character that the patient can clearly distinguish, both close up and at a distance. The most common tool used in the United States to measure visual acuity is the Snellen chart. A Snellen chart consists of letters carefully designed to subtend a 5-minute angle to the eye at a specified distance. Twenty feet or 6 m is considered standard for measuring distance vision, and 13 in. is standard for measuring close-up (near) vision. The charts are calibrated to these distances.

Initially, the patient's distance vision is checked while the patient is wearing his or her current glasses or contact lenses. The patient stands 20 ft from the Snellen chart. Each eye is checked independently, with an occluder placed over the eye that is not being measured. The occluder should not exert any pressure on the eye. The patient is asked to read the smallest line on the chart that is clear. Near vision should also be checked, especially if the patient has any complaints or is approaching the age that presbyopia is likely to occur. The same procedure is followed, except that the patient holds a card with the Snellen chart on it 13 in. from the eyes.

In general, corrected visual acuity is more valuable information for the ophthalmologist than uncorrected visual acuity. Instances when uncorrected visual acuity is important include performing a disability determination, qualifying an individual for certain types of employment (firefighter or professional driver), and evaluating a patient after a surgical procedure that was likely to change the patient's refraction, such as cataract surgery.

After acuity with correction is determined, a pinhole device is placed over the patient's eye (still with correction). The patient is asked to pick one hole and look through this. Then the patient is asked, "Does this make it brighter or darker? Can you read any further on the chart?" The pinhole eliminates peripheral rays of light, improves contrast, and generally improves vision to almost normal if the vision loss is caused by a refractive error. The pinhole test is used to differentiate whether vision loss is due to refractive error or disease of the eye. Vision loss caused by eye disease does not improve during the pinhole test. Thus, pinhole testing gives the examiner an idea of potential acuity. Also, the patient may find it encouraging to see how a change in glasses prescription would improve his or her vision.

Although the Snellen chart is the only visual acuity assessment tool discussed at length in this chapter, other options are available for patients with special needs. Patients who cannot read are usually tested with the *E*-game, a variation of the Snellen chart that uses capital letter *E*s pointing left, right, up, and down. Patients are asked to point in the direction the *E* is turned.

When measuring visual acuity in preschoolers, first try the Snellen letters or numbers. If the child does not know letters or numbers, try the *E*-game, then Allen pictures. Allen pictures are standardized images of objects recognizable by most young children including ducks, telephones, hands, and cars. The images are designed to subtend an angle of 5 minutes with the eye as are the Snellen letters. If the child is too small to identify Allen pictures, Teller cards are a good option. Teller cards are special cards made with black-and-white contrast lines on one half with homogenous gray on the other half. Children who cannot speak respond to Teller cards by looking at the striped side if they can distinguish the lines, or by ignoring them if the lines are too fine to distinguish from the gray side. Teller cards are available commercially and provide reliable visual acuity assessment in preverbal children.

What happens when the patient cannot read the largest letter on the chart? The technician holds fingers before the patient's eye in good light, and the vision is recorded as the farthest distance at which the patient can count the fingers. Visual acuity is charted as "counting fingers at 3 ft" ("CF 3ft"). If the patient cannot distinguish fingers, the examiner should wave a hand in front of the patient's eye. If hand movements are perceived by the patient, this is charted as "hand movements at 2 ft" ("HM 2ft"). If the patient cannot detect hand motion, the room is darkened, and a bright test light is shone into the patient's eye from four quadrants. The patient is asked to point in the direction of the light. If the patient can accurately point to the light, vision is recorded as "light perception ('LP') with direction." If the patient is unable to distinguish direction but can detect light, "LP without direction" is recorded. If the patient is unable to detect indirect light turned all the way up, vision is recorded as "no light perception" ("NLP"). Care should be taken not to hold the light source too close to the patient, because the patient may respond to heat from the light rather than to the light itself.

Refraction

The next step for the technician is to determine the patient's best glasses prescription. The patient's current glasses correction is measured and recorded. A manual lensometer or an automated lensometer may be used. It is helpful to record the type of instrument used in the chart.

There are two types of refractometric methods: objective and subjective. Objective methods have the advantage of obtaining measurements without requiring the patient to give answers and are performed with streak retinoscopy or with an automated refractor. The disadvantages of these methods are that they require a moderate-sized pupil and that information cannot be relied on to provide sufficient data for a final prescription. Conversely, subjective methods can be performed with small pupils, and they provide more precise and reliable data.

The retinoscope is the most useful instrument for the refractionist, and retinoscopy is the chief objective method of determining refractive error. There are two types of retinoscope, spot and streak, with the Copeland Streak (Copeland Optic, Chicago, Ill) being the most popular. One must remember to use 66 cm working distance, and, when converting to diopters, to subtract 1.50 D from the final sphere.

Subjective refractometry employs the Phoropter (American Optical, Warner Lambert Co. Tech Inc., Buffalo, NY) or trial frames and loose lenses. Information regarding retinoscopy and autorefraction and the current glasses prescription are entered in the Phoropter. It is best to fog the patient's vision before starting the refraction by beginning with +2.00 D over the patient's current spectacle correction. The technician notes the patient's clinical responses to changes of spherical and astigmatic lenses while having the patient read progressively smaller letters.

Two tools are used for determining axis and power of correct cylinder: the astigmatic dial or clock, and the cross cylinder. With the astigmatic dial or clock, the patient is located 20 ft from the chart and asked to select the blackest line on the chart. The astigmatic dial resembles a sunburst with outgoing radial lines. Astigmatism is corrected when two principal axes are equally dark.

The cross cylinder is the most popular method of refraction. A cross cylinder is a lens consisting of two cylinders of equal power but opposite designation, one plus and the other minus. Their axes are 90 degrees apart. In most cross cylinders, the red mark indicates the minus power, and the white mark indicates the plus power. The entire lens is mounted on a ring either attached to the Phoropter or loose on a handle. The cross cylinder is used to determine both the axis and the power of the cylinder.

There are four basic steps to a good refraction.

1. Start with sphere.
2. Work on cylinder (cross cylinder).
3. Define axis (cross cylinder).
4. Refine sphere. (For every 0.50-D cylinder added, subtract 0.25-D sphere.)

When the best possible refraction is obtained, the technician should record the best visual acuity obtained with this refraction.

Refractometry is an art that requires patience and much practice. In addition to knowing optics, the technician must be able to elicit consistent responses from the patient. While refractometry is a useful skill for a technician to develop, only licensed practitioners (ophthalmologists and optometrists) may prescribe the refraction. Opticians may dispense the refraction, but they are not licensed to prescribe.

Evaluation of Pupil

The pupil can be evaluated with a simple pen light. A normal pupil reacts not only to light but also to accommodation. Accommodation occurs when one looks at near objects. All pupils that react to light also react to accommodation. There are, however, some uncommon neurologic disorders in which the pupils react to accommodation but not to light. The technician must be able to assess the pupil's ability to react to light.

The patient is seated in a dim room and asked to look at a distant object. The technician brings the light from the side and shines it directly into the pupil. A normal pupillary response is constriction. To check consensual light reflex, the technician brings the light to one eye while watching the fellow eye. The unilluminated eye should constrict. A swinging flashlight compares direct and consensual reflexes of the same eye. The technician brings a bright light to one eye and watches the response. It is helpful to note whether the pupils react briskly or sluggishly. Then, the technician swings the light over to the patient's other eye and notes the constrictive reflex.

In a normal reaction, miosis happens bilaterally as the light swings back and forth. If the optic nerve senses less light, the impaired eye shows paradoxical dilation. This condition is called an *afferent pupillary defect (APD),* or *Marcus Gunn pupil* (Fig. 4-1). An APD may be relative or absolute. A relative APD reacts to direct light stimulus but constricts further when the light is swung to the other eye. The severity of the APD can be rated +1 to +4, with +4 being the larger defect.

When charting pupillary response, the technician should record the size of the pupil in both dilated and constricted phases. The shape of the pupil is normally round and regular. Some irregularities in shape are from congenital abnormalities, inflammation of the iris, trauma, or surgical intervention (Fig. 4-2). The pupils should be equal in size and react equally to both direct and consensual light stimulation as well as near stimuli. This information should be recorded in the chart as follows:

Pupil (Describe characteristics, eg, "round and reactive.")
+ or − APD (If an APD is present, note which eye is abnormal, and grade the amount of the defect, eg, +3 APD OS.)
Reaction response time (Grade as +1 to +4 (with +4 being brisk and +1 being sluggish.)

Assessment of pupillary function is an important part of both the preoperative and postoperative ophthalmic assessment. If an APD is noted, surgical intervention may not be indicated in some cases. Noting an APD preoperatively may help explain less than optimal postsurgical results. An APD noted postoperatively for the first time may alter the course of postoperative care. Accurate assessment of the pupils is especially important in the event of surgical complications. Pupils should never be pharmacologically dilated until after an accurate assessment is obtained.

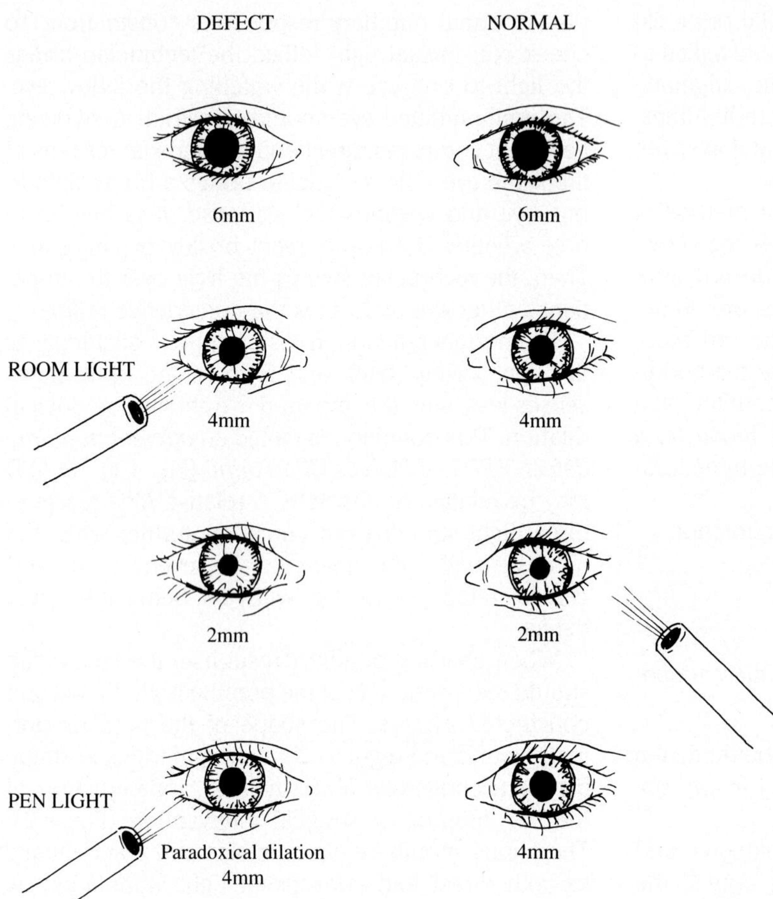

Figure 4-1. Relative afferent pupillary defect (Marcus Gunn pupil), right eye.

Evaluation of Extraocular Motility

Extraocular motility may be evaluated by measuring corneal light reflex. Two common methods are the Hirschberg test and the Krimsky method. The Hirschberg test is the most popular. With this test, 1 mm of decentered corneal light reflection corresponds to 7 degrees or 15 prism diopter of ocular deviation. The Krimsky method is a more refined test; it uses prisms placed before the fixating eye to center corneal reflection in the deviated eye. The technician should have the patient look in primary and all eight cardinal positions of gaze to detect any weakness of extraocular muscles. The technician should also note if diplopia or pain is present in any of the eight positions of gaze. Ocular motility is especially important in evaluating complications as a result of retinal detachment, orbital, or strabismus procedures.

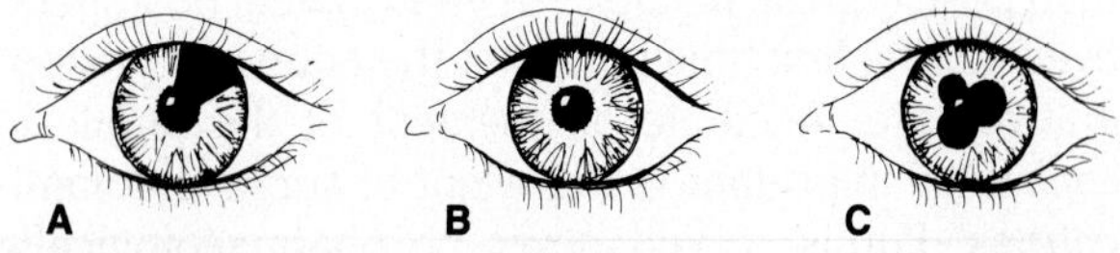

A B C

Figure 4-2. Pupil abnormalities: sector iridectomy (**A**), peripheral iridectomy (**B**), and irregular pupil from posterior synechiae (**C**).

Ending the Screening

Depending on how the office is structured, some ophthalmologists ask the technician to continue the screening examination by performing tonometry. Possible tonometry methods include applanation, pneumotonometry, Tonopen, (Oculab, Inc., Glendale, CA) and noncontact. A technician who is familiar with corneal structure and anatomy might also do a slit-lamp screening examination. Other ophthalmologists prefer that the technician end the screening examination after measuring motility. They do not want tonometry performed before their examination because any type of corneal contact may disturb the clarity of the cornea. Also, the extra light exposure from a preliminary slit-lamp examination may make it difficult for the ophthalmologist to check or reproduce the refraction if any question arises.

At whatever point the technician ends the screening, he or she should always sign the chart note, because it is a legal document. Technicians should be trained in proper charting methods and some medicolegal issues. The technician should leave proper space for the physician's examination and notes. Some physicians prefer that the technician use a screening sheet first.

ASSISTING WITH THE OPHTHALMIC EXAMINATION

When a clinic is running smoothly, and the technician does not have patients waiting to be screened, most physicians prefer that the technician accompany them into the examination room. The technician can assist the physician in many facets of the ocular examination. One of the most important ways the technician can assist the physician is to complete the examination record by writing on the chart as the physician dictates the notes. The technician might also be asked to instill dilating drops or perform additional tasks, such as intraocular lens calculations, photography, visual field testing, or contact lens insertion or removal. At the end of the examination, the technician should be available to escort the patient back to the waiting room. This is especially important if the patient's eyes have been dilated, because the patient's vision may still be blurred.

ARRANGING SURGERY

One of the most important contributions a technician can make to a patient's care is to coordinate the procedures necessary for a patient to have surgery. The technician must be familiar with the appropriate preoperative testing and evaluation, the documentation required, and the appropriate follow-up care needed after surgery. Surgical patients must feel confident that their cases are being handled competently from the time they decide to have surgery to the time of their final surgical outcomes. Although arrangements vary according to office and physician preferences, several steps need to be taken before surgery can be performed. These steps include informed consent to surgery, scheduling of surgery, preoperative testing and consultation, verification of billing and reimbursement procedures, and patient education.

Informed Consent

Once the ophthalmologist and the patient have agreed to proceed with the surgery, the technician should obtain the correct consent form for the physician to review with the patient, and the technician should be available to witness the patient's signature. Because patients sometimes ask the technician questions about their surgery, the technician should be knowledgeable regarding the surgical procedure but should always leave to the physician the matter of obtaining informed consent. Some offices have successfully used videotapes to standardize how surgical procedures are explained to patients. Nevertheless, videotapes are not interactive, and patients must be given ample opportunity to address their questions with the physician. A patient who is aware of possible complications is better able to make an informed decision to have the surgery and will be better prepared to cope with complications, should they occur.

Scheduling Operation and Preoperative Testing

Medicare mandates that most ophthalmic procedures be performed on an outpatient basis. If a patient's health makes hospital admission necessary, prior authorization from the patient's third-party payer must be obtained. There are three types of admission to the hospital.

1. *Emergency admission.* Serious ocular calamity—immediate surgery required because of nature of condition (eg, intraocular foreign body, lacerated globe).
2. *Urgent admission.* Problem that needs attention within the next day or so (uncontrolled glaucoma, orbital tumor, or dislocated lens).
3. *Elective admission.* An ocular disorder that is chronic and that will not deteriorate because of delay in admission.

Third-party payers often request explanation of why hospital admission is necessary. Parameters such as the need for intravenous or intramuscular medications, or frequent monitoring of vital signs, often justify the admission. If an unexpected complication occurs, the need for hospitalization is not anticipated. In this case, the patient should be admitted, and the patient's insurance carrier should be contacted as soon as reasonably possible.

Outpatient surgery has many advantages, including patient acceptance, cost-effectiveness, and improved control of operating room scheduling. Although the steps to scheduling outpatient surgery vary according to the policies and preferences of individual units and physicians, a sequence of events do need to occur for scheduling to proceed smoothly. Furthermore, it is important to have a centralized schedule (written or computerized) with checks and balances for all procedures and tests that need to be scheduled for each patient. Otherwise, small but important tasks that must be completed before surgery can be easily overlooked.

The first step is to request time in the operating room. Next, plans for preoperative testing and physical examination are arranged with the patient. If possible, the operation is scheduled, informed consent is obtained, and ophthalmic preoperative testing is performed the same day the patient is signed up for surgery. This not only saves the patient a trip back to the office, but also makes the patient feel that he or she is receiving organized and professional health care. Calculations for intraocular lens implants must be performed in advance so that a lens of correct power may be ordered and delivered in a timely manner.

The technician should schedule the surgery at a time that is convenient for the patient and the physician. The duration of each operative procedure, and the number of cases the surgeon can perform and follow postoperatively each week, should be considered. When possible, all preoperative tests and consultations are scheduled on the same day. The patient receives an explanation of the amount of time the preoperative history and physical examination as well as tests (blood, electrocardiogram, chest x-ray study) will take, and an attempt is made to schedule these at the patient's convenience. If the patient has had any testing done recently, copies of the results are requested to avoid unnecessary duplication.

History and Physical Examination

A history and physical examination can be performed in one of two ways. A preprinted history and physical form can be given to the patient to take to his or her local family physician to complete. A letter of explanation should accompany the examination form, informing the other physician of when the surgery is scheduled, what type of surgery is planned, the type of anesthesia planned, and guidelines regarding specific screening tests the ophthalmologist would like to have performed. Providing the physician who is to perform the history and physical examination with a form helps ensure that he or she will not misunderstand what is needed. Otherwise, the physician may merely write "cleared for surgery" on a prescription pad rather than sending the information in a form suitable for incorporation into the medical record. It may be advisable to have the patient hand carry the completed documentation to the surgical unit on the day of the operation to prevent its being lost in the mail.

The other method is to perform the history and physical examination at the ophthalmologist's office. The examination can be performed by the ophthalmologist, a resident in training, a colleague, or a physician assistant working under the direction of a physician. Blood may need to be drawn in the office, or laboratory tests may need to be scheduled. All testing should be prearranged with the local laboratory or hospital to avoid any scheduling errors with the patient.

Anesthesia Consultation

The patient may need an anesthesia preoperative consultation. General anesthesia is used for all children's surgery, most strabismus procedures, enucleations, and removal of orbital tumors. Local anesthesia is preferred for adults undergoing other types of procedures, such as surgery for cataracts or glaucoma. It may be advisable to have an anesthesiologist or nurse anesthetist present during the operation to monitor vital signs and administer intravenous sedatives. Such an arrangement may be termed *monitored anesthesia care.* Having an anesthesiologist present is especially helpful in the event that a complication occurs. A complication often lengthens the surgical time, and properly rendered anesthetic agents can keep the patient comfortable and lying still for the extra time needed.

Whenever monitored anesthesia care is administered, the anesthesia service must evaluate the patient before surgery. This is usually done the morning of the outpatient procedure, but the anesthesia service may prefer to have a preoperative consultation with the patient a few days before the operation, especially if the patient has multiple medical problems, or if general anesthesia is planned.

Local anesthesia may be administered topically or by infiltration. There are four primary methods of administering infiltrative local ocular anesthesia:

1. Facial nerve block, which stops the patient from blinking
2. Retrobulbar anesthesia
3. Direct subconjunctival infiltration
4. Peribulbar anesthesia

Nursing Assessment

The patient may also need to be scheduled for a nursing assessment at the outpatient surgery facility. A nurse or nurse practitioner reviews the patient's medications and tells the patient what to bring to the facility, what time to arrive the morning of surgery, what the time of discharge is likely to be, and what experiences the patient can expect during his or her stay on the unit.

Verifying Billing and Reimbursement Procedures

When scheduling a patient for surgery, it is appropriate to discuss surgical fees, insurance, and payment options. It is best to discuss these issues in advance, not only to facilitate payment to the office, but also to help the patient plan for any expenses for which he or she may be directly responsible. The technician or person responsible for scheduling should meet with the patient in a private, quiet room, and should take time to discuss these issues before setting the date for surgery.

The insurance carrier should be consulted to see if prior authorization is required from a third-party payer. Some insurance carriers require additional information and documentation, such as a second opinion, a required level of visual acuity before cataract surgery, visual field testing and documentation, or photography. If this information is not obtained before surgery, it may be difficult to resubmit claims and obtain reimbursement from the insurance carriers.

Patient Education and Orientation

The technician should also provide the patient with information about the procedure and how to prepare for surgery. A thorough understanding of what to expect may help alleviate the patient's fears. Some patients learn better by oral instruction, some by printed information, and some by visual direction. Consequently, the technician should talk with the patient to decide which method is best for that individual. If space allows, the office might include a patient education room, which would contain pamphlets, literature, and a television for viewing educational videotapes about the procedure to be performed. The more knowledgeable the patient is, the more realistic he or she will be about expected surgical results and possible complications.

The patient should be informed in advance of the need to wear a patch overnight after the operation. Also, the appointment schedule for the next few weeks should be explained. The patient will not be able to drive home after the operation and may also need to arrange transportation for some time afterward. Patients do not like to learn of postoperative limitations on physical activity. Discussing in advance the patient's responsibilities during the postoperative period greatly increases the patient's compliance and thus reduces the risk of postoperative complications.

The office should have maps printed and information on where to park, nearby hotels and their rates (some hotels give discounts for patient referrals), where to call for emergencies, what time to arrive on the day of surgery, and any other practical issues concerning patients and their families.

Telephoning the Patient

Telephoning the patient the day before surgery to see if there are any last-minute questions or concerns is always a good idea and assures the patient that members of the office staff are organized and caring. Although a call from the surgeon is preferred, a call from the technician is useful to verify times and procedures.

Patients should also be telephoned the evening after the surgery. This call is usually made by the nursing staff or the technician. If possible, the caller should be someone that the patient has met in the office or operating room.

Discharging the Patient

A patient should be discharged the day of surgery only if there is a competent adult to provide transportation home. If the patient has good sight in the unpatched eye, it is usually not necessary that someone stay with the patient overnight. Someone should be available, however, for the patient to call should he or she have a problem. The name of this person should be recorded on the chart.

The patient and the caregiver should be given thorough instructions before leaving the ambulatory surgery facility. If the patient was sedated, these instructions should be given both verbally and in writing, as the patient's memory may be temporarily impaired. Written instructions should be presented in large, bold type.

POSTOPERATIVE CARE

First Postoperative Visit

The first postoperative visit is an important event for the patient. The technician should remember that although postoperative visits are a daily routine for the clinic staff, the patient's first postoperative visit is a one-time occurrence for him or her, and the patient is likely to be apprehensive about the surgical outcome.

When walking the patient back to the examination room, the technician should ask in a pleasant tone of voice how the patient's evening went. When in the confidential setting of the examination room, he or she should ask whether the patient had any pain or nausea. The technician should also ask how the patient feels today and whether the patient has any discomfort or questions.

Once the patient is comfortably seated, the eye bandage is gently removed. Not only is the patient's face tender, but the patch often has a tendency to stick to lids and lashes. Next, the external eyelid and the facial skin to which the tape adheres are gently cleaned. Sterile saline or another suitable irrigating solution is used on a clean gauze pad. Tissues have a tendency to stick to the face where tape has been. This simple act of cleansing helps the patient feel refreshed and cared for.

The next step is to check the patient's vision. This is best done by checking for hand motion or counting fingers vision first. If the technician starts with the eye chart first and the patient does not immediately see it, the patient is likely to be discouraged and unhappy with the surgical results. Also, visual acuity is checked with a pinhole test to verify whether vision does indeed improve with each postoperative visit. It is normal for many patients to have hand motion vision on the first postoperative visit and still go on to develop excellent vision.

Postoperative Instructions

Postoperative instructions can easily be given by the technician, which saves time and allows the rapport that the technician has already established with the patient to come into effect. A compassionate, knowledgeable technician contributes greatly to the welfare of surgical patients. The patient is given both oral and written instructions. For most intraocular procedures, instructions should explain the need to wear a shield at night until the patient is further instructed and to wear glasses during the day to protect the eye. The technician should make sure that the patient understands that the old glasses prescription may not work well after surgery. In fact, the patient may see better without glasses. The patient is informed that looking through a lens that is no longer correct will not damage the eye, and the importance of wearing the glasses for protection is emphasized.

The technician should discuss the level of activity allowed (eg, the patient should not bend over at the waist, strain, or lift anything heavier than 10 lb). If the patient experiences nausea, excessive straining with bowel movements, or extreme coughing, he or she should notify the ophthalmologist.

Medications should be discussed with both the patient and a family member or caregiver. Discussion should include each type of medication, the dosage, and techniques for administration. Some patients benefit from marking the number of times per day a medication should be given on the bottom of the bottle itself, or making an X, which means, "Shake this one." Patients and caregivers are shown how to instill drops and ointment so that container contamination and ocular injury are avoided (Fig. 4-3).

For patients who live alone and are uncomfortable with instilling the drops directly into their eyes, an alternative technique may be taught. The patient may recline back and close his or her eye. The drop should be instilled at the inside corner of the eye. When the eye is opened with the patient still reclined, the drop will run into the eye. Although this technique

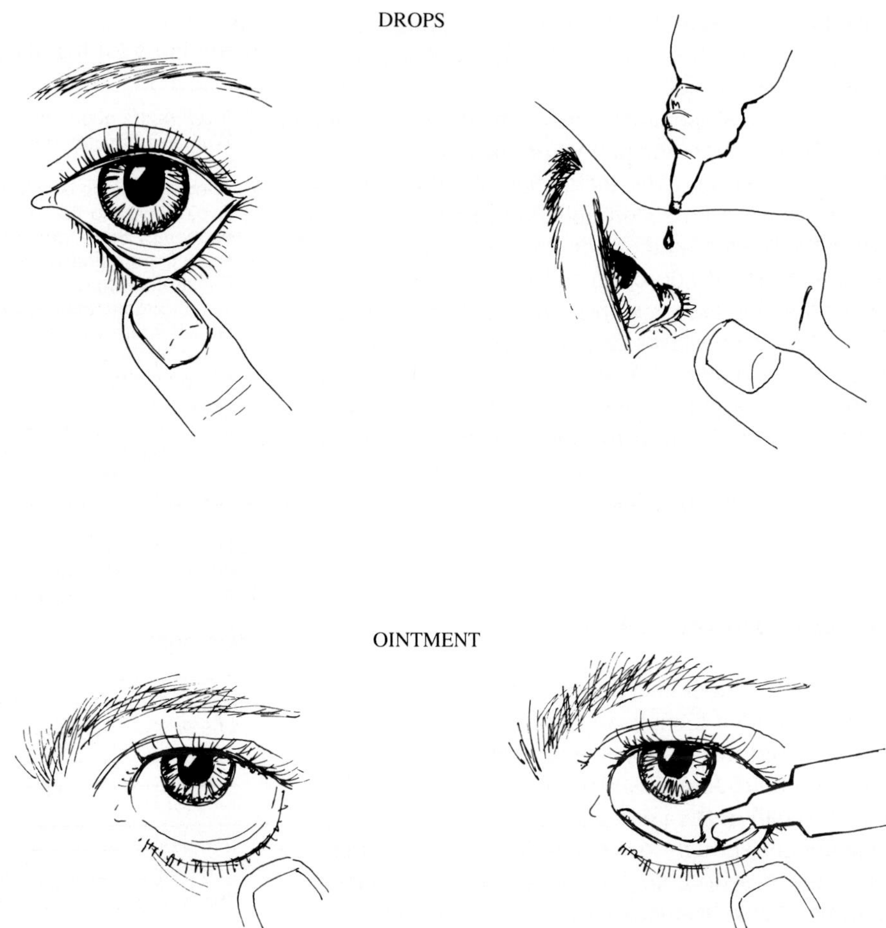

Figure 4-3. Instillation of drops and ointment.

is not as good as direct instillation, it is better than missing the dose. Certain drops may cause systemic side effects; for example, timolol may decrease heart rate. To decrease systemic absorption and at the same time enhance ocular penetration, punctal occlusion is helpful. Punctal occlusion is performed by putting pressure at the inside corner of the eye with a clean finger immediately after instillation of the drop. Closing the eye for 3 to 5 minutes after drop instillation also helps.

The technician shows the patient and caregiver how to clean the eye. Cleaning should be done with a clean gauze pad or tissue, and some type of nonpreserved sterile irrigating solution. Tap water will do in most cases. The patient should be taught not to rub the eye but to dab at it instead. If continuous patching is necessary, the technician shows the caregiver how to do this and has the caregiver patch the patient's eye there in the office. Two eye pads are best: one folded over and a second placed on top, with approximately four to six pieces of tape firmly adhering. Taping is always performed diagonally from forehead to cheek, away from the hairline and mouth to allow normal eating and facial movements. The technician emphasizes to the patient that using drops correctly and listening to the physician's orders make a difference in the surgical outcome.

Subsequent Postoperative Visits

The key to providing effective postoperative care is knowing the patterns of the physician's practice. With today's advances in cataract surgery, including one-stitch and no-stitch surgery, stabilized keratometry readings and refraction are achieved much earlier than before. Awareness of the physician's preferences saves time for everyone concerned, because the technician can perform the appropriate tests without being asked and does not waste time on unnecessary procedures. For example, keratometry readings at the 1-week postoperative visit may be considered unnecessary by the physician.

On these postoperative screenings, the technician should help instruct the patient on the continued use of eye medications. The technician should find out whether refills are needed and should have the prescriptions written and ready for the physician to check and sign if appropriate. The physician is provided, when necessary, with a tapering drop schedule (Table 4-1). These tasks can all be performed before the physician enters the room, thus saving time for the physician and the patient. It is also important to remind the physician to tell the patient when he or she may resume normal activities. This matter is often overlooked by the physician.

Table 4-1.
Instructions for Instilling Eye Drops*

1. Instill medications into the lower lid.
2. Wait 3–5 minutes between medications if more than one is used.
3. Keeping the top of the dropper or tube clean is essential. Avoid touching the top of the dropper or tube to anything, especially the fingers or any part of the eye.
4. Store the medication at room temperature; refrigerate only if instructed to do so.
5. Use the medication only in the eye for which it is ordered.
6. Do not share your medication with anyone.
7. Use only the ophthalmic medication that your physician has prescribed.
8. Never use eye drops that have changed color.
9. Do not transfer the medication from one bottle to another.
10. When using both eye drops and eye ointment, administer the drops first.
11. Always follow the directions on your prescription label and the instructions given to you by your physician.
12. Do not skip doses, and never use the medication more often or longer than prescribed.
13. Keep eye medication out of the reach of children.

Medications

1. ________________________right eye/left eye
One drop________Times a day until________; then
One drop________Times a day until________; then
One drop________Times a day until________; then
________________________________.

2. ________________________right eye/left eye
One drop________Times a day until________; then
One drop________Times a day until________; then
One drop________Times a day until________; then
________________________________.

3. ________________________right eye/left eye
One drop________Times a day until________; then
One drop________Times a day until________; then
One drop________Times a day until________; then
________________________________.

*If refills are needed, please call the Eye Center at (304) 598-4820. We will need the name of your medication, the dosage, and the telephone number of the pharmacy where the medication will be picked up.

Answering Patient Calls

Calls from postoperative patients should be directed immediately to a technician or physician; the receptionist should not simply take a message or put the patient on hold. Almost any problem that prompts the patient to call in the immediate postoperative period is significant enough to warrant the surgeon's attention. Patients who complain of any of the following should be brought immediately into the office: pain, bulging eye, decrease in vision, flashes or floaters, or purulent discharge. These complaints need immediate attention. Minor complaints that occur further into the postoperative period may be communicated to the physician at his or her convenience, and the technician may be asked to call the patient back. For example, if a patient complains of a mildly scratchy eye 6 weeks postoperatively, the surgeon might recommend that the patient use artificial tears as needed.

Telephone calls should always be documented in the patient's chart and in a telephone log if available. If the technician talks to the patient on behalf of the physician, this fact should be documented in the chart along with the date, time, and a synopsis of the conversation, with the entry signed by the technician. This protocol is important for legal reasons.

The technician can be a great asset to the physician in total-quality patient care. A knowledgeable technician with good communication skills and a strong rapport with patients can make a significant contribution to preventing and managing surgical complications.

Bibliography

Jackson-Williams B. Ophthalmic surgical assisting. In: Willoughby CO, ed. Ophthalmic technical skills series, ed 2. Thorofare, NJ, Slack, 1993.

Milder B, Rubin M. The fine art of prescribing glasses. Gainesville, FL, Triad Scientific, 1978.

Stamper RL. Ophthalmic medical assisting: an independent study course. San Francisco, American Academy of Ophthalmology, 1991.

Stein H, Slatt B, Stein R. The ophthalmic assistant: fundamentals and clinical practice. St. Louis, CV Mosby, 1988.

Ophthalmic Surgery Complications: Prevention and Management,
edited by Judie F. Charlton and George W. Weinstein.
J. B. Lippincott Company, Philadelphia © 1995.

5

Vince Manopoli
Rick Walters

The Role of the Billing Clerk

In the past several years, the complexity of insurance reporting has increased significantly. This increased complexity has been brought about by the need to translate increasingly complicated surgical procedures into precise procedure codes according to *Physicians' Current Procedural Terminology, Fourth Edition* (commonly CPT or CPT-4), and diagnosis codes according to the *International Classification of Diseases, 9th Revision, Clinical Modification* (commonly ICD-9 or ICD-9-CM), as well as to comply with more intricate insurance submissions and payment requirements. These factors are keenly felt by the billing clerk, especially when he or she submits claims for complex surgical procedures, complications following surgery, and conditions with multiple diagnoses.

Although the traditional function of the billing clerk has remained the same (ie, to submit claims in a manner that will be easily accepted by the insurer and result in maximum payment to the provider), the level of expertise required to do this has increased. This factor has made the role of the billing clerk increasingly important to medical practices. Payment depends on understanding the complexities of insurer billing requirements and keeping abreast of changes, because coding systems, as well as policies of Medicare and other payers, are updated annually.

This chapter provides several key concepts used in billing for complex ocular surgery, and for complications following surgery, that remain applicable despite the changes that may occur in specific policies. It also provides practical examples of the policies of insurers and of their effects on reimbursement for surgical procedures. For reference, discussion includes correct CPT-4 procedure coding and ICD-9 diagnosis coding for many ocular surgery situations that can involve complications.

PATIENTS LIKELY TO HAVE COMPLICATED CODING

The effective billing clerk must be alert to patients who have had complications previously, who are likely to develop complications, or whose cases involve complex management options. These patients often have multiple conditions or diagnoses and often have suffered from a catastrophic event.

A common mistake of many practices is to assume that the billing clerk has easy access to the patient's complete medical history, which, in fact, is rarely the case. Thus, unless the clerk has easy access to the medical record *and* the physician, the surgery dictation (or operative notes) should clearly outline underlying conditions. The clerk who tries to rely on the immediate facts at hand, such as the patient's age, may be misled to erroneous coding of the situation (eg, using the diagnostic term *congenital* for a child when the condition or disorder is actually not congenital).

The following list includes examples of problematic diagnoses common in ophthalmology that often entail complications and potential coding problems. The billing clerk should double-check for complications as well as the proposed coding on the claim when the following diagnoses arise:

Congenital/Infantile Ophthalmic Defects (743 series)

Retinopathy of prematurity (362.21)

Congenital cataracts (743.33)

Aniridia (743.45)

Simple buphthalmos (743.21)

Diagnoses Suggesting Reoperations That May Affect Selection of CPT-4 Coding

History of malignant neoplasm, eye (V10.84)

Old retinal detachments (361.07)

Recurrent pterygium (372.45)

Recurrent iridocyclitis (364.02)

Recurrent corneal erosion (371.42)

Prolapse of iris (364.8)

Accident Victims

Fall stairs/steps (E880)

Fight/brawl (trauma) (E960.0)

Fall from chair/bed (E884.2)

Foreign body, magnetic (360.50–360.59)

Foreign body, nonmagnetic (360.60–360.69)

Occurrences During Surgery That Affect Coding

Vitreous prolapse (379.26)

Subluxation of lens (379.32)

Posterior dislocation of lens (379.34)

Occurrences After Surgery That May Affect Coding

Hyphema (364.41)

Acute endophthalmitis (360.01)

Ocular fistula causing hypotony (360.32)

Expulsive choroidal hemorrhage (362.62)

Subluxation of IOL (996.53)

By remembering the diagnoses of patients most likely to have complicated claims, and by attempting early identification of those cases needing close monitoring, physicians can treat patients carefully and efficiently, focusing their energies on diagnoses where close monitoring has the highest potential for return. The best method is to develop a list of problematic patient types and conditions that are most likely for each physician's practice. The physician should communicate to staff the specific procedure and diagnosis codes to use as well as any other requirements necessary for appropriately documenting these patient conditions.

ICD-9 DIAGNOSIS CODING

In medical claims submissions, ICD-9 diagnosis coding is increasingly important. As insurers look to reduce expenses and claims processing costs, they increasingly rely on coverage determinations based on diagnosis codes. All too often, the staff members of a clinical practice focuse all attention on procedural coding and forget the language of medical necessity, the ICD-9 diagnosis coding. Complex coding depends heavily on appropriate, specific ICD-9 diagnosis coding, because additional services made necessary by surgical complications are most often the subject of review and scrutiny. Careful diagnosis coding can result in higher payments for multiple surgical procedures as well as increased coverage of ancillary services.

The codes and descriptions in ICD-9-CM, Volume One, are divided into chapters representing 17 primary areas of disease processes. It also includes two additional supplemental chapters: one for "V" codes and the other for "E" codes. Each chapter represents an organ system; thus, most ophthalmology codes are found in one location (360.0–379.99). Furthermore, each chapter is organized into *major categories*, designated by three digit codes. For example:

361
Retinal detachments and defects

For purposes of reporting specificity, categories are often broken into *subcategories*, which are designated by the fourth digit (the first digit to the right of the decimal). These fourth-digit codes are termed *subcategory codes*, for example:

361.0
Retinal detachment with retinal defect

Finally, the fifth digit or *subclassification codes* are often used to give maximum specificity and clarification. Based on the preceding example, the fifth-digit subclassifications are as follows:

361.00
Retinal detachment with retinal defect, unspecified

361.01
Recent detachment, partial, with single defect

361.02
Recent detachment, partial, with multiple defect

361.03
Recent detachment, partial, with giant tear

. . . . . .

. . . . . .

361.06
Old detachment, partial

361.07
Old detachment, total or subtotal

Reimbursement often depends on the level of coding specificity. That is, if fourth- or fifth-digit codes apply to the diagnosis code, physicians need to report them; otherwise, they may be denied payment. The major problem most billing clerks face is that physicians have been trained to give general, not specific, diagnoses. The best solution is to redo office paperwork, including encounter forms, internal fee slips, and computer lists, to eliminate all codes that are not the most specific available. Using "nonspecific" codes is tempting, but it can lead to reduced payment and denials.

Special symbols (such as the lozenge), punctuation (such as parentheses), and conventions (such as italicized codes) are included in ICD-9-CM to assist with one's understanding of codes and their appropriate use. The use of these formats is often ignored by the novice coder, and inevitably codes are misused or incorrectly ordered.

Punctuation

[ ] *Brackets*

Brackets are used at times in ICD-9 definitions to enclose synonyms, alternative wordings, or explanatory phrases. These are often used in dictation or medical records and are extremely helpful. For example:

365.0
Borderline glaucoma [glaucoma suspect]

377.14
Glaucomatous atrophy [cupping] of optic disc

365.61
Glaucoma associated with pupillary block
Use additional code for associated disorder, such as:
seclusion of pupil iris bombé (364.74)

: *Colon*

Colons are used after an incomplete term that needs one or more of the modifiers. The modifiers are listed in alphabetic order and make it assignable to a given category. For example:

364.04
Secondary iridocyclitis, noninfectious
Aqueous:
cells
fibrin
flare

{ } *Braces*

Braces are used to enclose a series of terms, each of which is modified by the statement appearing at the right of the brace, and may not be used for other indications. For example:

364.53
Pigmentary iris degeneration

Acquired heterochromia Pigment dispersion syndrome Translucency	} of iris

One can better understand how the preceding symbols are used in ICD-9-CM by taking the time to locate instances where they appear in the physician's ophthalmology code section.

Conventions

Two important conventions are used in ICD-9-CM. First, **bold type** is used for all codes and titles in ICD-9-CM, Volume One. Second, *italic type* is used to list background disease processes. *Codes printed in italic type are not to be listed as the patient's primary diagnosis.* However, they may be used as a secondary diagnosis. For example, the following should never be used as the primary reason for treating a patient:

365.41
Glaucoma associated with chamber angle anomalies

Because it clearly states in ICD-9-CM,

> *Code also associated disorder, as:*
> Axenfeld's anomaly (743.44)
> Reiger's anomaly or syndrome (743.44)

Thus, both the manifestation of the condition and its underlying cause need to be listed. The tabular list provides help by giving references to underlying conditions. These appear with the note "Code also underlying disease." Codes that list this note are also in italic type. The most common example in ophthalmology is diabetic retinopathy. For example:

362.0
Diabetic retinopathy
Code also diabetes (250.5)

362.01
Background diabetic retinopathy
Diabetic retinal microaneurysm
Diabetic retinopathy NOS

362.02
Proliferative diabetic retinopathy

To report services related to a patient suffering from diabetic retinopathy, the service listed on the claim form would be linked to both ICD-9 codes (eg, 250.5 and 362.01).

NEC and NOS Abbreviations

Users of ICD-9-CM will be familiar with the two abbreviations, NEC (*N*ot *E*lsewhere *C*lassified) and NOS (*N*ot *O*therwise *S*pecified). Each has a specific meaning and importance to coding and reimbursement.

The abbreviation NEC has two distinct uses in ICD-9-CM. First, it may be used by coders who do not have enough information available to determine which specific diagnosis code should be used in situations where ICD-9-CM provides specific diagnoses. For example, the physician may be treating a patient for cytomegalovirus retinitis, but the specific vector may not be known. A review of the ICD-9-CM Index shows that codes are based on whether the disease was transmitted or congenital.

Cytomegalovirus Inclusion Disease (078.5)

Congenital Cytomegalovirus Disease (771.1)

The abbreviation NOS appears throughout the tabular list and is used to denote "unspecified" codes. Codes with NOS as part of their definition may be used when the coder does not have enough information to select a more definitive diagnosis. Suppose the physician has determined that the patient has open-angle glaucoma; furthermore, no other information that would help categorize the disease is currently available. In such a situation, the physician would look first in the index as discussed earlier:

Glaucoma

. . .

. . .

Open-angle glaucoma, unspecified (365.1)

Primary open-angle glaucoma (365.11)

. . .

. . .

. . .

Note that the subheading "open-angle glaucoma" that precedes the specific diagnoses refers one to the NOS codes. By reviewing code 365.1 in the tabular list, one finds the following:

365.1
Open-angle glaucoma, unspecified

Wide-angle glaucoma NOS

When submitting NOS or "unspecified" ICD-9-CM codes, it is helpful to explain the disease more fully, so that the payer can make a determination in the physician's or patient's favor. A simple written statement may suffice, or if the patient's problem is unusual or complex, a note may be in order. *In ophthalmology, there is usually enough information available to be specific. Physicians should be conscientious about selecting coding with the fifth digit.*

"Includes:"

The ICD-9 listings for ophthamology diagnoses rarely use the "Includes:" nomenclature, but alternative descriptions are often listed. For example:

368.41
Scotoma involving central area
Scotoma:
Central
Centrocecal
Paracentral

The following code illustrates the use of the "Includes:" nomenclature:

055
Measles
Includes:
Morbilli
Rubeola

The problems of patients suffering from either type of measles could be coded using listings from the 055 series.

"Excludes:"

The ICD-9 term "Excludes:" is always surrounded by a box so that it will be more easily noted. Physicians need to be aware of conditions that are excluded from groups of codes. An example of an "Excludes" note follows:

364
Other disorder of iris and ciliary body

Prolapse of iris NOS
Excludes:
prolapse of iris in recent wound (871.1)

Thus, if a patient has experienced prolapse resulting from a wound, codes from the 364.8 group should not be reported, and 871.1 should be used instead.

Publishers of ICD-9-CM may use their own symbols for special purposes, such as noting new or changed codes, highlighting that fifth-digit codes apply, and so forth. One should review the definitions of publisher-specific symbols that may appear in the ICD-9-CM text.

Five Steps to Better ICD Coding

Coding with ICD-9-CM can be made easier by following five steps:

1. *Locate the code.* Locating codes in ICD-9-CM does not have to be as difficult a task as it may appear.

   Identify the main terms in the physician's diagnosis statement. For example, if the physician has written the patient's diagnosis as, "The patient has a partial retinal detachment, OD," one would take note of the terms "retinal," and "detachment." With the terms noted, one would look first in the ICD-9-CM Index.

   Locate the main term in the Volume Two Index. In the ICD-9-CM Index, terms are listed by condition or problem, not by anatomic area or site. Using the preceding example, one would look under the term "detachment." The following appears under "detachment" in the ICD-9-CM Index:

   Detachment: (cartilage), (cervix), (choroid), (knee), (ligament), (placenta), (retina), (vitreous humor)

   Check any notes appearing after the main term. In the instance just given, there are several notes describing recent and old detachments that are helpful when one needs to determine whether the detachment should be reported as recent or old.
2. *Code to the highest level of certainty.*
3. *Code only the reason for the visit or encounter.*
4. *Reference each service with the diagnosis that is the reason for the service.*
5. *Never use "rule out," "probable," "suspected," or "questionable" conditions as you would a confirmed diagnosis.* Use codes selected from Chapter 16, "Symptoms, Signs and Ill-Defined Conditions" in these cases, as discussed below.

"Symptoms, Signs and Ill-Defined Conditions"

The ICD-9-CM provides codes that the physician can use until a more definitive diagnosis is reached. These codes can be found in Chapter 16 of ICD-9-CM under the title "Symptoms, Signs and Ill-Defined Conditions." In this section, one finds codes for conditions ranging from convulsion to cachexia. Of greater use to ophthalmologists are the 368 series codes, "Visual Disturbances," and code 379.9, "Unspecified Disorders," which include the following:

Sudden vision loss (368.10)
Visual discomfort (368.13)
Visual distortion (368.15)
Visual field defects (368.41–47)
Color vision deficiencies (368.5)
Pain in or around eye (379.91)
Redness or discharge of eye (379.93)
Blurred vision (NOS) (368.8)
Swelling on mass of eye (379.92)

"V" Codes

Many physicians and staff are afraid to report "V" codes because they know that in many cases the patient's insurance policy does not cover services associated with them. Although a physician may be well-meaning, this problem is really the patient's concern, not the physician's. Patients purchase specific coverage when they buy health insurance, and many carriers today do not cover adult "well visits." Thus, it is the patient's responsibility to pay for noncovered services, and in these cases, accurate reporting usually leaves the physician no choice but to use the "V" codes. Thus, the physician should not feel guilty about reporting "V" codes when it is appropriate to do so. Some useful "V" codes are listed in the following:

V10.84
History of neoplasm of other sites, eye

V42.5
Corneal transplant

V43.0
Globe replacement

V43.1
Pseudophakia (lens replacement)

V45.6
States following surgery of eye and adnexa
[Excludes 379.31, V43.0 and V43.1]

V52.2
Artificial eye

V59.5
Donor cornea

V72.0
Examination of eyes and vision

"E" Codes

The "E" codes are supplementary and used to describe external causes of injuries and poisonings. *"E" codes are never reported by themselves and should be added only when they affect coverage.* Physicians rarely use "E" codes, because most third-party payers do not use these codes as a basis for making payment determinations. The most common application for "E" codes is Worker's Compensation, in which their use can ease claims processing. These codes make follow-up easier because they convey why the patient received the service. Some common ophthalmology examples follow:

E880
Fall stairs/steps

E960.0
Fight/brawl (trauma)

E884.2
Fall from chair/bed

Also listed in the "E" code section are drug codes. These codes are used to report that the patient's condition was induced by use of a specific drug, or that the patient is suffering from the toxic effect of a specific drug. These codes are likely to be submitted with a diagnostic test procedure and with another primary ophthalmic diagnosis, such as:

366.45
Drug-induced cataract

365.3
Corticosteroid-induced glaucoma

362.55
Toxic maculopathy

These codes are then followed by the appropriate "E" code for the drug being taken by the patient, as given in the "E" code definitions or in the Table of Drugs and Chemicals in Volume I. Examples are as follows:

E931.4
Plaquenil

E933.1
Prednisone

E955.3
Pilocarpine

E942.2
Antiarteriosclerotic drugs (Lovastatin, Mevacor)

E932.0
Systemic steroids

SURGERY BILLING RELEVANT TO COMPLEX CASES

Surgery complications require detailed coding on claims submissions, which is generally done by (1) affixing CPT modifiers that precisely describe the surgical situation to the CPT code for the procedure, (2) carefully ordering procedures on the submission, and (3) knowing when a lesser procedure is considered part of a major procedure—and thus when its payment is included in the major procedure payment.

The CPT guidelines specifying when modifiers are to be used in describing surgical situations were largely standardized for Medicare in 1992, and few local modifiers continue to be used. At the same time, however, it became necessary to use modifiers for several services that did not previously require them. Fortunately, Medicare and most other payers all use CPT coding, so that practices no longer have to keep track of multiple coding systems.

The effective billing clerk must have a good understanding of CPT modifiers that apply to special situations and of when they are to be used. A poor comprehension of these modifiers lowers reimbursement, considerably increases the time spent trying to straighten out billing problems, and delays payment. The major modifiers that arise with ophthalmic surgery complications and that must be used as indicated whenever applicable are discussed in the following sections. We have also indicated the Medicare payment guidelines for these situations to aid in defining their use. Also, for purposes of definition, we consider the phrase "same physician" to mean any physician who is employed within a financial entity (eg, group practice).

Unlisted Procedure or Service Codes

Unlisted Procedure or Service Codes are defined as follows in CPT: "It is recognized that there may be services or procedures performed by physicians that are not found in CPT. Therefore, a number of specific code numbers have been designated for reporting unlisted procedures. When an unlisted procedure number is used, the service or procedure should be described." Each of these unlisted procedural code numbers (with the appropriate accompanying topical entry) relates to a specific section of the book and is presented in the guidelines given in that section.

GUIDELINES FOR USE

1. Use the Unlisted Procedure code from the topical section of CPT that is the most specific for the procedure (eg, unlisted procedure of the anterior segment); it must be accompanied by a special report.
2. Do not use an unlisted code as a "shortcut" when the correct code is not immediately apparent. Note that use of the Unlisted Procedure codes (those CPT codes ending in -99) always result in a time-consuming review of the claim.
3. Always double-check that a more appropriate CPT code is not available. Note that in many cases in which claims are submitted using Unlisted Procedure codes, a more appropriate and specific CPT code is actually available and should be used instead.
4. If you determine that an appropriate, specific CPT code is not available, double-check with the insurer to which the claim will be submitted for any specific instructions for billing that procedure. In many cases, doing so verifies that the insurer will accept the particular unlisted code for that procedure.

Multiple Procedure Modifier (-51)

The specific guideline in CPT for the Multiple Procedure modifier (-51) is as follows: "When multiple procedures are performed on the same day or at the same session, the major procedure or service may be reported as listed. The secondary additional, or lesser procedure(s) or service(s) may be identified by adding the modifier '-51' to the secondary procedure or service code(s). . . . This modifier may be used to report multiple medical procedures performed at the same session, as well as a combination of medical and surgical procedures, or several surgical procedures performed at the same operative session."

GUIDELINES FOR USE

1. Use this modifier to clarify that a multiple surgery situation exists, and to indicate the secondary services or procedures.
2. Attach the modifier to the *secondary* procedure and to subsequent procedures beyond that; do *not* attach the modifier to the major procedure of the operative session.
3. Omit the -51 modifier when a particularly complicated situation requires two more essential modifiers (Assistant Surgeon [-80] and Related Procedure [-78]), because the claims reviewer should be able to discern that it was a multiple surgery by the date of service.
4. Under Medicare, procedures should be submitted in descending order of Medicare Fee Schedule Amount, regardless of whether Medicare is the primary or the secondary payer. Because one may not have accurate payment amounts for other payers, ordering is done either according to Medicare rule or in descending order of fees.
5. Medicare and most other payers reduce payment as follows:
   First procedure: 100%
   Second procedure: 50%
   Third through fifth procedures: 25%
   Subsequent beyond five: 25%
6. Surgical coders should check all procedures on the Uniform Physician Billing Rules (see later)

before submitting multiple procedures to guard against "unbundling" of services.

Within ophthalmology, the use of the multiple surgery modifier is most common in cases of trauma and plastic surgery, although increasingly, more complex anterior segment cases are being performed and should be submitted as multiple surgeries. Common multiple ophthalmology procedures along with their cause include the following:

Extracapsular cataract removal with insertion of intraocular lens prosthesis followed by vitrectomy:

66984
Extra cap. cataract removal with IOL
Diagnosis: 366.16

67010-51
Vitrectomy, mechanical partial
Diagnosis: 379.26

Remove and replace IOL performed with Pseudophakic Penetrating Keratoplasty

66986
Remove and replace IOL
Diagnosis: 996.53

65755-51
Penetrating keratoplasty in pseudophakia
Diagnosis: 371.57

67010
Vitrectomy, mechanical partial
Diagnosis: 379.26

Note: The procedural order depends on the individual payer's rules.

Uniform Physician Billing Requirements

The Uniform Physician Billing Requirements (UPBRs) give guidelines concerning mandatory bundling of surgery procedures that would otherwise be considered multiple surgeries. Column 1 represents the major procedure codes for which payment may be made. Column 2 procedures are considered component parts of the Column 1 procedures for which separate payment may not be made. Billing the secondary procedures in addition is considered "unbundling," which is contrary to the UPBR reporting regulations, and is a Medicare violation.

The UPBR guidelines apply to Medicare surgery services performed in all settings. The UPBRs do not apply to all insurers but are a good guide for coders. If indeed the codes appear on the listing, there is most likely a definition overlap in the codes being submitted; in this event, one should be sure to check the operative report carefully. All physicians should review the listing of their common multiple procedures, and surgical coders should check all procedures on the UPBR before billing. Lastly, all multiple surgery payments must be monitored to ensure they are correct; one should be aware that multiple surgery claims have a high incidence of payment errors under Medicare and other payers.

Unusual Procedural Services (-22) and Reduced Procedural Services (-52)

The specific guideline in CPT for the Unusual Procedural Services modifier (-22) is as follows: "When the service(s) provided are greater than that usually required for the listed procedure, it may be identified by adding modifier '-22' to the usual procedure number. . . . A report may also be appropriate."

GUIDELINES FOR USE

1. Be aware that Medicare and other payers infrequently augment payment for procedures submitted with the -22 modifier; thus, do not rely on this regularly to report services.
2. Determine whether another coding approach is available that can accurately represent the full service (ie, a multiple surgery).
3. Medicare reviews submissions with the -22 modifier on a case-by-case basis. In those exceptional cases in which payment for the service is increased, it is generally about 15% to 20% above the usual payment for the procedure.

The specific guideline in CPT for the -52 Reduced Services Modifier is as follows: "Under certain circumstances a service or procedure is partially reduced or eliminated at the physician's election. Under these circumstances the service provided can be identified by its usual procedure number and the addition of the modifier '-52,' signifying that the service is reduced. This provides a means of reporting reduced services without disturbing the identification of the basic service." Its most common use is for reporting aborted surgery, for which rules vary by carrier. Because this situation requires insurers to make independent payment determinations, the physician should monitor payment.

Cosurgeon Situations

The CPT definition of the Two Surgeons (Cosurgeons) modifier (-62) follows: "Under certain circumstances the skills of two surgeons (usually with different skills) may be required in the management of a specific surgical procedure. Under such circumstances, the separate services may be identified by adding the modifier '-62' to the procedure number used by each surgeon for reporting his services."

The -62 modifier is used for complex surgical procedures, including those for which management of surgical complications is essential; in ophthalmology, the modifier is used most often in trauma cases. Situations of "team surgery" generally do not occur in ophthalmology. Most situations that at first might appear to be team surgery can be more accurately reported as multiple surgery with cosurgeons (more than two surgeons may be involved in each surgical procedure). Also, Medicare and other insurers generally define "different skills" of surgeons to refer to different medical specialties (ie, ophthalmic surgeons, plastic surgeons, and neurosurgeons).

Most insurers pay for surgical procedures performed by cosurgeons at 150% of the usual payment amount, with each surgeon receiving one half (75% of the combined payment amount). The issue that this generally raises is that if the "cosurgeons" perform operations with widely differing payment rates, the surgeon receiving the greater fee will have his or her payment reduced. For cases in which both surgeons are ophthalmologists or only one procedure is involved, one surgeon should bill as an assistant surgeon rather than as a cosurgeon.

Assistant Surgeon Situations

The CPT definition of the Assistant Surgeon modifier is as follows: "Surgical assistant services may be identified by adding the modifier '-80' to the usual procedure number(s)." Note that this is the appropriate modifier for surgical assistant services in the nonteaching hospital setting.

The CPT definition of the modifier for Assistant Surgeon When Qualified Resident is not Available (-82) is as follows: "The unavailability . . . the usual procedure code number(s)." Note that this is the appropriate modifier for surgical assistant services in the teaching hospital setting. Since Medicare pays for graduate medical education, a resident must not be available in any case in which one submits for the assist at surgery.

Because complex ophthalmic surgery is likely to require the use of assistant surgeons, a coder should remember several common problems: (1) Both surgeon and assistant surgeon must use the same codes. (This problem is common with nongroup practices.) (2) Assistants are usually paid between 16% and 25% of the surgeon's payment for the full surgery procedure. (3) Insurers are increasingly not covering surgical assistants; in fact, as of 1993, Medicare no longer covers assistants at cataract surgery with intraocular lens (IOL) implant.

Subsequent Surgery Situations (-76/-77/-78/-79)

There are two modifiers intended for situations in which the initial procedure was unsuccessful and must be repeated, including the -76 modifier, Repeat Procedure by the Same Physician, and the -77 modifier, Repeat Procedure by Another Physician. These modifiers are not often used, because other billing methods, including the use of the reduced services modifier (-52) and careful application of the carrier's global surgery rules, are generally used instead.

The modifier for Return to the Operating Room for a Related Procedure (-78) is relatively new and is used moderately in ophthalmology. The CPT definition follows: "Return to the operating room for a Related Procedure during the Postoperative Period: The physician may need to indicate that another procedure was performed during the postoperative period of the initial procedure. When this subsequent procedure is related to the first, and requires the use of the operating room, it may be reported by adding the modifier '-78' to the related procedure."

The -78 modifier can be used with any insurer that has established a postoperative period. The diagnosis code for the primary procedure is used again for the return operation (although the return procedure may include other diagnoses).

Under Medicare, surgical procedures performed during the postoperative period of the initial major surgical procedure are defined as "related to" when they have lesser relative value units (RVUs). This means that according to Medicare, procedures are considered to be related if a procedure of lesser value follows one of greater value. This rule is not based on any medical facts or judgment, but instead is an administrative method of defining "related to." In general, procedures that are considered "related to" (-78) are paid at a reduced rate, typically 50%. Some insurers other than Medicare are considering application of this rule, but their policies are still in the formative stages.

Some examples of procedures that would be considered related to each other under the Medicare rules are as follows:

YAG capsulotomy (66821-78) following ECCE w/IOL (66984)

Retinal laser for proliferative retinopathy (67228) followed by retinal focal laser for maculopathy (67210-78)

Primary glaucoma filter (66170) followed by revision of filter (revision operative wound) (66250-78)

The -79 modifier (Unrelated Procedure or Service by the Same Physician During the Postoperative Period) is fairly common in ophthalmology. One major reason is that patients often have surgery on a second eye within the postoperative period of the first. The CPT definition is as follows: "The physician may need to indicate that the performance of a procedure or service during the postoperative period was unrelated to the original procedure. This circumstance may be reported by using the '-79' modifier."

This modifier is used to indicate that the performance of a procedure or service during a postoperative period was unrelated to the original procedure. The diagnosis coding for the second procedure may be different from the coding for the first, but it need not be so. Consistent with the -78 modifier, Medicare has chosen to define procedures "unrelated to" as those having greater RVUs than the original procedure. Also, in the case of ocular surgery, the use of the "-LT" and "-RT" modifiers for left and right eye designation is necessary along with the -79 modifier, because procedures on the second eye are considered "unrelated" by definition.

Some common example of "Unrelated Procedures" are as follows:

Repair detachment w/buckle (67107) followed by repair detachment w/vitrectomy (67108-79)

Pan-retinal laser for proliferative retinopathy (67228-79) following focal laser for maculopathy (67210)

YAG in right eye (66821-79-RT) following ECCE w/IOL in left eye (66984-LT)

Postoperative Periods

All visits with the primary surgeon during a designated period following surgery are included in payment for one global surgical package. This rule does not apply, however, if the visit is for a problem unrelated to the diagnosis for which the surgery was performed or is for an added course of treatment other than normal recovery from the surgery. Each insurer or governmental agency sets its own postoperative period. These periods vary from 0 to 180 days and are usually procedure-specific, although many health maintenance organizations use a set amount for all surgery (eg, 42 days).

Most insurers expect that all services provided by the surgeon for postoperative complications (eg, removing stitches or servicing infected wounds) are included in the global package if they do not require additional trips to the operating room. For office visit services, reimbursement is made for diagnoses that are unrelated to the original condition (the -24 modifier attached to the visit code). Also, most insurers cover medically indicated diagnostic tests (92020-92287) performed during the postoperative period.

Often, poor diagnostic coding results in the nonpayment of visits provided in the postoperative period. Two examples are (1) a patient with open-angle glaucoma (365.15) requiring an examination 60 days after cataract surgery (66984, 365.15) and (2) a patient suffering from sudden vision loss resulting from retinal detachment (368.10, 362.10) after a filtering procedure (66170). The latter case would be unrelated, whereas the former may be related, depending on several factors including the patient's previous history and postoperative course.

CPT CODES REPRESENTING COMPLICATIONS

There are several CPT-4 codes directly representing ophthalmology complications and reoperations. These codes are fairly straightforward, that is, they represent the reoperation.

65125
Modification of ocular implant

65150
Reinsertion of ocular implant

65175
Removal of ocular implant

65920
Removal of implanted material (anterior segment)

66185
Revision of aqueous shunt to extraocular reservoir

66250
Revision/repair of operative wound

66825
Repositioning of IOL, requiring incision

66986
Exchange of IOL

67112
Repair retinal detachment, previously operated upon

67115
Release encircling material

67120
Removal of implanted material, anterior segment, extraocular

67121
Removal of implanted material, anterior segment, intraocular

67909
Reduction overcorrection of ptosis

The following are exceptions in which the procedure code represents an "add-on" service and is reported with another surgical procedure to represent the difficulty of reoperating:

67331
Strabismus surgery—patient with previous eye surgery or injury that did not involve the extraocular muscles

67331
Strabismus surgery on patient with scarring of extraocular muscle (eg, prior ocular surgery, strabismus or retinal detachment surgery) or restrictive myopathy surgery (eg, dysthyroid ophthalmopathy)

67343
Release of extensive scar tissue without detaching extraocular muscle

Four Rules for Better Coding

Because accuracy of coding directly affects reimbursement and coverage, diligence in all cases is in the best interest of a medical practice. Because most claims are uneventful, the 80/20 rule can often be applied to ophthalmic coding—that is, 20% of claims generate 80% of the work and problems. Therefore, the following set of rules can serve to guide the physician's efforts:

1. Focus on those patients whose diagnoses make them most likely to have complicated claims or cases; in this way, your energies will be concentrated on cases with the highest potential return.
2. Use ICD-9 codes in a way that clearly conveys the patient's condition and the reason for services. Doing so increases the chances of appropriate payment determination and assists in detecting services that were provided and not clearly documented.
3. Be sure to use surgery modifiers whenever appropriate, especially the -51 modifier for multiple surgeries and the -78 and -79 modifiers in the postoperative period; remember to use them in conjunction with the "UPBR" bundling guidelines and rules for correct ordering of multiple surgeries.
4. Become familiar with the CPT-4 codes, which commonly represent services associated with complication and reoperations, but remember that each patient responds differently to treatment, and thus you may need to consider coding combinations that are uncommon.

Use of these rules and familiarity with CPT-4, ICD-9, and medical payment policy should improve one's management of the coding of complex patient cases and should ultimately speed payment of claims.

Ophthalmic Surgery Complications: Prevention and Management,
edited by Judie F. Charlton and George W. Weinstein.
J. B. Lippincott Company, Philadelphia © 1995.

6

Kathleen Rose

The Perioperative Role of the Nurse

PERIOPERATIVE NURSING IN THE 1990s

From the 1800s to the present, the role of the nurse in the operating room has been in a state of evolution. Originally, the nurse accompanied the patient from the ward, assisted during the surgical procedure, and attended to the care of the same patient through recovery and discharge. An era of specialization saw the nurse become more technically oriented in the role of scrub nurse. Then, the Association of Operating Room Nurses (AORN), with input from the American Nurses Association (ANA) redirected efforts of the professional nurse in the operating room to concentrate on patient-centered activities, providing the foundation for the "Standards of Practice: O.R. as a Basis for Safe and Effective Clinical Practice." The AORN first described *perioperative* nursing to its membership in 1978, expanding the nurse's scope of practice to include the preoperative, intraoperative, and postoperative phase of the surgical experience. This expanded role at times brings nurses back to their beginnings in the operating room. Certain aspects of care and responsibilities have always been present: the roles of coordinator, caregiver, patient advocate, and educator. Thus, the nurse is in the position to provide continuity and to meet the individual needs of patients experiencing the surgical process.

In times of health care reform, the need for nurses to expand and develop their scope of knowledge and experiences has been even greater. The mastery of skills and knowledge of procedures in various phases of the patient's surgical experience is imperative for nurses to maintain high standards of care and to meet the increasing health care demands of a cost-conscious society.

As in any situation involving multiple players, teamwork is the name of the game. Only with all players working together and communicating can the goal be scored. The nurse is in the unique position to function as the quarterback and lead the team to a successful outcome by supplying the tools, ensuring that they are used properly, and supporting the participants. Each member of the team, including the patient, family or friends, clerk, physician, technician, and nurse, plays an important role in ensuring that the patient has a positive outcome. The price of complications in the perioperative arena is paid in financial, physical, and emotional terms for those involved. As outpatient care proliferates and cost-effective services are demanded, the prevention of complications becomes an increasing priority.

Professional Nursing Practice

The public continues to become more conscious of the health care industry as it has a growing financial impact on daily life. The public's expectations of health care providers and quality care is based on perceptions of those things important to their physical and psychological comfort. Most often, patients relate quality with sensitivity to their needs or respect for them as individuals. They really are not able to assess the professional competence of staff members. Knowledge of the Patient's Bill of Rights and

Responsibilities is a good guide for meeting the patient's perceptions of quality:[1]

- Each patient should be treated as an individual, not a disease.
- Privacy needs should be considered when conversing to or about the patient; discussions should take place where they cannot be overheard by other patients in the surgical area.
- The patient should be involved in decisions about planning and implementing his or her care.
- The concerns of the patient should be addressed, not ignored or dismissed. It may only be a matter of reassuring the patient, but if a topic is mentioned, it is of importance.
- Above all, communication is vital: the patient is kept informed, because waiting in the dark is frustrating and conveys an uncaring message.

Dissatisfaction with the care received often preoccupies the patient to the point that the experience increases stress, pain, and inability to listen and then comply with discharge instructions adequately. The ideal nurse in the perioperative setting lives up to the scout motto of being prepared, is assertive, and is ready to serve as the patient's advocate in situations that demand quick, competent decision making. Attention to standards developed by the ANA, the AORN, and the Joint Commission for the Accreditation of Healthcare Organizations (JCAHO) ensures good preparation and patient advocacy.

The JCAHO has placed new emphasis on staff orientation, education, and competency. The ANA has defined nursing practice as the diagnosis and treatment of human responses to actual or potential health problems and has established the nursing process as the systematic approach to professional nursing practice. Use of the nursing process for each phase of the perioperative experience—through assessment, development of a nursing diagnosis, comprehensive planning, implementation of the plan, and evaluation of the patient's progress in meeting the outcomes expected—provides the benchmark for the delivery of high standards in nursing care.[2]

Documentation of the nursing process should be accurate, brief, and complete, making the use of well-developed flow sheets and preprinted forms a practical option.

Environment

Patients also look at the environment to which they are introduced. Cleanliness, attractive decor, low noise levels, and good maintenance of equipment add to patient confidence and satisfaction. Good housekeeping and temperature control help in the prevention of postoperative complications, such as endophthalmitis, which is frequently attributed to introduction of particles during the procedure.

Universal Precautions mandate the use of appropriate cleaning solutions for equipment and surfaces after use. The Occupational Safety and Health Administration requires the use of Universal Precautions throughout the health care environment. All patients are therefore treated as if potentially infectious, with no need for specific isolation procedures for those patients known to have human immunodeficiency virus (HIV) infection, acquired immunodeficiency syndrome (AIDS), or hepatitis B. In fact, it is those patients who have not been diagnosed with such infections that should cause concern for health care workers. The use of protective barriers is indicated in the surgical setting; face shields should be used where there is potential for splashing of body fluids to the face.[3]

Health care workers are advised to be aware of their HIV status. When a health care worker tests positive for the HIV virus, he or she is advised to voluntarily consult with the state board or with a panel of experts convened to confidentially determine what changes in practice may be indicated for the individual. Professionals with exudative lesions or weeping dermatitis are also advised to refrain from all direct patient care and handling of patient care equipment until it is evaluated.[4]

PERIOPERATIVE NURSING PROCESS

Provision of optimal care for the ophthalmic patient requires specific nursing skills and knowledge that allow the nurse to assess the surgical site, observe for complications, and anticipate and act quickly in emergencies. The nurse needs the ability to make decisions based on knowledge of ophthalmic anatomy and physiology, medications, ophthalmic conditions, and medical interventions. With these tools, the nurse can answer patient questions as well as anticipate and prevent complications.

Preoperative Phase

Since the introduction of diagnosis-related groups, most ophthalmic surgery is performed on an outpatient or emergency basis, giving physicians a lot of ground to cover in a short period. It is tempting to skip over the details of patient education to focus only on the technical aspects of the surgical procedure, complete the mounds of documentation needed, and move on to the next patient because health care providers do not have the time to sit and talk. Nurses need to adapt their thinking and act on the aspects of care where they can develop their roles during the process of health care reform. Patient assessment and patient education are two major areas in which nurses can use their skills to affect the patient outcome.

Patient Education

Patient and family expectations and attitudes throughout the surgical experience have a great impact on their ability to cooperate, understand, and meet the continuing care needs of the patient. It cannot be said enough,"Discharge planning begins before the time of admission." Deliberate, planned education is needed to ensure that educational needs are met in what is usually a short time in a fast-paced setting. Ideally, patient education is started in the physician's office, where special needs can be identified and provided for in a timely manner.

The initial patient contact is frequently made by clerical personnel or someone other than the nurse. These people should have good interpersonal and interviewing skills. They should be well versed in explaining anticipated routines to the patient and prepared to refer appropriate questions to a designated nurse. Interviewers who have detailed information available relating to the patient they are calling and who are able to answer the patient's questions present a picture of organized and efficient personnel who are providing future care. Instructions presented in an unhurried, caring conversation set the tone for patients to trust in and cooperate with the health care providers they and their families encounter during the surgical experience. Basic components of preadmission instructions anticipate the questions that the patient may forget to ask until the conversation is over include the following:

- Expected arrival time
- Transportation, directions, and parking arrangements
- Insurance cards or referral forms needed
- Proper clothing (eg, sunglasses and hat)
- Medications to bring (eg, ophthalmic, insulin, or systemic)
- Money or credit cards for prescriptions
- Local telephone contact for the day of surgery
- Items or people not to bring (eg, valuables or children)
- A responsible adult to accompany the patient on discharge and help in continuing care needs
- Special needs of concern to the patient
- Policies or procedures unique to the institution (eg, smoking restrictions, need for parents to be available)
- When to eliminate food and liquids before surgery

Assessment

Assessment of the patient begins with initial contact. The nurse must be aware of the patient's emotional condition, physical limitations, self-care capabilities, and decision-making capacity. Many patients undergoing ophthalmic procedures are elderly and have an array of medical conditions that may be exacerbated with surgical intervention. A printed form is helpful to document assessment information uniformly so that it is easily used by the entire health care team (Fig. 6-1). The assessment provides the groundwork for the rest of the nursing process. The nurse may use data collected by others when assessing the patient, including current medications, the last dose of those medications, coping mechanisms, and pain relief methods previously effective. Although an ocular examination has been done previously by the physician, the nurse should perform a gross external examination, looking for signs of inflammation (eg, redness or drainage) that may warrant rescheduling an elective procedure to avoid potential postoperative infections. A systems review, including breath sounds and baseline vital signs, should be completed the morning of surgery to alert the physician of any potential problems. After the patient's current and previous health status is assessed, a nursing diagnosis can be determined and a plan of care developed to assist the patient in achieving the highest level of self-care possible with appropriate support provided.

(Text continues on p. 64.)

NURSING ADMISSION INTERVIEW

A. Preadmission Visit: _____ yes _____ no Mode of admission ____________________

Date ________ Blood pressure __________ Pulse __________ Height __________

Time ________ Temperature __________ Respiration ________ Weight __________

Pre-admission or local phone number ______________________________

R.N. Signature ______________________________

B. History

Principal language: ________ interpreter ______ information source: patient ____ other ______

Reason for admission ______________________________

- Ocular History ______________________________
- Diabetes ______________________________
- Other: ______________________________
- Transfusions ______________________________
- Immunizations:
  - a. last tetanus: ______________
  - b. childhood up to date ____ yes ____ no

ALLERGIES: ______________________________

Current Medication and Route	Dose	Frequency	Day of Admission: date/time of last dose

Figure 6-1. Nursing admission interview form to document assessment of patients. (**A**) Preadmission data and history. (**B**) Systems assessment and day-of-admission data.

A

NURSING ADMISSION INTERVIEW

Systems Assessment Instructions: Check if applicable. *indicates description in progress note.

1. OPHTHALMIC:
- __ functional vision
- __ blind OD OS
- __ prosthesis OD OS
- __ red sclera OD OS
- __ drainage OD OS
- __ pain OD OS
- __ lid edema OD OS
- __ ________
- __ ________

2. ENT:
- __ normal hearing
- __ hard of hearing AD AS
- __ pain AD AS
- __ tinnitus AD AS
- __ vertigo
- __ nasal discharge
- __ sinus pain
- __ ________
- __ ________

3. NEUROLOGIC:
- __ alert
- __ oriented
- __ confused
- __ disoriented
- __ lethargic
- __ dysphagia
- __ memory deficit
- __ paresthesia
- __ paresis
- __ syncope
- __ tremors

____
____

4. CARDIOVASCULAR:
heart rhythm: __ regular __ irregular
- __ edema: ________
- __ varicose veins: ________

____
____

5. RESPIRATORY:
- __ normal breathing
- __ cough: ________
- __ dyspnea

____
____

6. SKIN:
- __ warm __ cool __ moist __ dry
- __ pale __ flushed __ cyanotic
- __ rash: ________
- __ lacerations: ________
- __ ecchymosis: ________
- __ decubit: ________

____
____

- __ IV: type: ________
  date inserted: ________
  skin condition: ________

____

7. GI: diet: ________
- __ nausea
- __ diarrhea
- __ constipation
- __ laxative of choice: ________
- __ ostomy: ________

____

8. GUI/GYN:
- __ no complaints of urinary distress
- __ pain __ burning __ dysuric
- __ catheter inserted on: ________

____
____

- __ dialysis: access: ________
  skin condition: ________

____
____

- __ menstruating __ pregnant
- __ l.m.p. ________

____

9. MUSCULOSKELETAL:
- __ ambulates well __ unsteady gait
- __ cane __ walker used to ambulate
- __ joint pain: ________
- __ contractures: ________
- __ amputation: ________
- __ prosthesis: ________
- __ weakness: ________

____
____

10. PSYCHOSOCIAL:

occupation: ________
smoker/amt: ________
alcohol/amt.: ________
drugs/type: ________
sleep aids: ________
sleep pattern:

____

coping mechanisms for pain/anxiety:

____
____

Living will: __ yes __ no
Health care surrogate: __ yes __ no
If yes,
name: ________
Organ donor: __ yes __ no

Comments: ________

____
____
____
____

Special needs & concerns: ________

____

R.N. Signature ________ Date ________ Time ________

C. Day of Admission

Date ________
Time admitted ________
Admitted via ________

Orientation to Environment:
- __ telephone
- __ nurse call light/TV
- __ electric bed
- __ side rail policy
- __ side rail release signed
- __ bath room/emergency light
- __ shower
- __ smoking policy
- __ recliner

Blood pressure ________
Temperature ________
Pulse ________
Respiration ________
Breath sounds: __ clear __ rales __ ronchi __ wheeze

Height ________
Weight ________

- __ Physical assessment unchanged since preadmission.
- __ Change in physical assessment. *

Disposition of valuables:
- __ given to: ________
- __ safe __ no valuables

Disposition of medications:
- __ given to: ________
- __ home
- __ medicine closet
- __ Instructed not to self-medicate

Prosthetics/Aids brought to BPEI:
- __ cane
- __ wheelchair __ walker
- __ glasses __ contact lens
- __ dentures: __ upper __ lower
- __ hearing aid: __ AD __ AS

Comments: ________

R.N. Signature ________

*see progress notes Revised on: ________

B

Patient and family education must be documented, including the assessment of learning needs, establishment of current knowledge base, and determination of patient expectations. Simple questions as shown in the patient education section of the flow sheet in Figure 6-2 can be used.

Discharge planning needs should also be identified at this time, such as determination of alterations needed in the home environment to provide safety during the postoperative period when vision and depth perception may be affected. Alterations might include removing throw rugs, providing sleeping arrangements on the ground floor to avoid stairs, rearranging the play areas for small children in the family so that toys will not be laying around, and changing to soft-light bulbs so that halls and rooms provide adequate light while minimizing glare. A key factor in preventing complications after discharge is the patients' ability to care for themselves and comply with the instructions given. Few insurance companies provide payment for home health services after ophthalmic surgery. A supporting adult should be included in assessment and planning of care as well as the home care instructions. The nurse should focus on making the patient feel confident to go home by providing the information and instructions needed, promoting a sense of well-being, and reinforcing patients' abilities rather than limitations during their interactions.

Planning

Confirmation that a responsible adult will be present to accompany the patient home may necessitate a telephone call to verify estimated arrival time of the companion. Some facilities have policies to cancel surgery or use only local anesthesia if assisted transportation cannot be confirmed.

The perioperative plan of nursing care should be based on department standards of care and further individualized for the patient based on assessment information. Arrangements for continuing-care needs identified during the admission interview should be handled at this point. An example of such a standardized form can be seen in Figure 6-3.

Planning during the preoperative phase includes verifying the informed consent obtained by the physician, reinforcing information, and clarifying misunderstandings. The consent should be written in language the patient can understand. The physician needs to be notified if patients cannot verbalize the nature of the procedure or why they are there or if they have misgivings about their decision.

Implementation

Implementation of the patient and family teaching plan should anticipate routines and focus on postoperative expectations. Information previously explained may need to be reinforced (in the doctor's office, some patients tend to stop listening after they hear the word *surgery*). When a separate preadmission visit is made to the facility, allowing the patient to meet the surgical staff and view the surgical suite may be beneficial. The patient should be instructed to expect some pain and to inform the nurse so that relief may be obtained. Knowledge of discharge criteria provides a purpose for postoperative routines and involves the patient in the process.

Attention to details is an important part of preparing the patient for surgery. A preoperative checklist (see Fig. 6-2) is often used to ensure that routines are completed:

- Written consent has been attained.
- Laboratory reports have been received and assessed.
- The patient has not ingested food or liquids, as directed.
- The prescribed preoperative medication has been administered.
- Intravenous medication has been initiated per protocol.
- Recent vital signs have been documented.
- Eye makeup has been removed.

Positive identification of the eye to be operated on should be confirmed with the patient and may even be marked with a dot or marker before going into the surgical suite. The patient should void before any sedative is administered; otherwise, involuntary voiding may later embarrass the patient and pose a safety risk when he or she attempts to ambulate while under the influence of medication.

Evaluation

Evaluation during the preoperative phase includes verification of patient preparation. A note documenting the patient's status is necessary throughout each

(*Text continues on p. 68.*)

PATIENT CARE FLOW SHEET

PATIENT EDUCATION

Assessment

1. Patient has ability to learn: yes ____ no ____ if no, why? ____________
1. Patient is ready to learn: yes ____ no ____ if no, why? ____________
3. Other responsible adult is available to share in learning? yes ____ no ____
4. Patient had understanding of problem/condition: yes ____ no ____
5. Further information requested: ____________
6. Special learning needs: ____________
7. Comments: ____________

R.N. Signature ____________ Date ____________

Implementation

Method:
- A. Verbal
- B. Demonstration
- C. Written material
- D. Audio/visual

Evaluation:
1. Learning continues, reinforcement needed.
2. Learning objective met
3. Family/s.o. particpated in learning.

Teaching Content (Date, Key, & Initial)

Patient should be able to:	Initiated	Reinforced	Comments
1. Verbalize a basic understanding of problem.			
2. Describe pre-operative routine.			
3. Use aseptic technique to administer drops/ointment			
4. Use correct procedure for dressing change			
5. State names, doses, action side effects and food/ drug interactions of discharge medications			
6. Other:			

Pre-Operative Data

(Check appropriate line when completed)

____ CBC
____ P-6
____ U/A
____ EKG
____ X-RAY
____ A-SCAN
____ ____________
____ ____________

____ Surgical consent
____ General consent
____ History & physical
____ Medical clearance
____ ID band in place
____ Vital signs recorded
____ Voided
____ Keyplate on chart

____ Contacts removed
____ Glasses removed
____ Make-up removed
____ Nail polish removed
____ Dentures removed
____ Hearing aid ____ AS ____ AD
____ Jewelry removed: ____________

Last po intake ____________
Post S.A.N.: VS ____________
BS ____________

CAUSE FOR DELAY ____ NO DELAY

____ Consent
____ Orders
____ Medical clearance
____ Late pt. arrival
____ Lab tests
____ O.R.
____ Unit staff
____ Other ____________

Time to O.R. ____________ via ____________ accompanied by ____________

Comments: ____________

R.N. Signature ____________ Date ____________

Figure 6-2. Preoperative portion of patient care flow sheet.

OPHTHALMIC NURSING CARE PLAN

___ Patient and/or significant other ______________________ are involved in planning care.
___ Patient is child age ___. Parent or significant other ______________________ participated in planning care.

Instructions: Date (month/day) appropriate items as initiated/reassessed/evaluated
Reassess plan each shift. Sign at end of page 2.

Nursing Diagnosis	Expected Outcomes	Interventions	Evaluations
___ *Altered Visual Acuity* indicate OD OS OU related to: ___ blindness ___ cataract ___ enucleation ___ external ___ glaucoma ___ infection ___ muscle surgery ___ optic nerve disease ___ retinal detachment ___ trauma ___ tumor ___ vitrectomy ______	Patient will be able to perform ADL ___ without assistance ___ with assistance of SO at time of discharge. Safe environment will be provided to patient during hospital stay.	___ Provide safe and unobstructed walkway. ___ Instruct patient to call for assistance as needed. ___ Blind care. ___ Instruct and monitor position compliance: ______ ___ Ambulate post op. ___ Teach sighted guide technique. ___ Keep side rails up. ___ Provide crib for child under 6 years. ___ Make referrals. ___ Isolation precautions.	Patient is able to perform ADL ___ without assistance ___ with assistance of significant other. ___ Patient is free of injury during hospitalization. ___ Referral made to: ______
___ ***Nausea, vomiting, pain, discomfort*** related to: ___ increased IOP ___ infection ___ surgery ___ other	Nausea/vomiting will be controlled. Pain/discomfort will be relieved or minimized.	___ Instruct patient to verbalize discomfort. ___ Utilize patient's usual coping mechanism to minimize discomfort, as appropriate. ___ Instruct patient to report effectiveness of intervention. ___ Check IOP if pain or discomfort persists.	___ Patient tolerates oral intake without nausea. ___ Patient states no pain since surgery. ___ Patient is free of pain, discomfort at discharge. ___ Pain/discomfort is controlled by:
___ ***Altered mental status*** related to: ___ age ___ bilateral patch ___ loss ___ sleep deprivation ___ other: ______	Anxiety will be minimized during hospital stay.	___ Provide opportunity for patient to verbalize fears, anxiety. ___ Organize nursing activities to allow maximum rest between care. ___ Solicit input from significant other/family. ___ Make appropriate referrals.	___ Patient anxiety was minimized during hospital stay. ______ ___ Referral made to: ______

Figure 6-3. Ophthalmic nursing care plan.

OPHTHALMIC NURSING CARE PLAN

Date (month/day) appropriate items as initiated/reassessed/evaluated. Sign at end of this page.

Nursing Diagnosis	Expected Outcomes	Interventions	Evaluations
— ***Knowledge deficit*** related to: — disease — surgical procedure — special procedure	Patient/significant other will state understanding of disease process, treatment modality and alternatives.	— Insure that explanation is given. — Provide instructional aids: ______	— Patient or significant other states he received adequate information to make informed decision. — More information needed. See progress note.
— ***Self care deficit*** related to care after discharge.	Patient/significant other will: 1. verbalize understanding of discharge instructions; 2. administer eye drops using aseptic technique; 3. administer eye drops without causing injury to affected eye; 4. identify potential hazards related to eye safety at home/work/play.	— Explain discharge instructions to patient and significant other. — Demonstrate aseptic eye drop application. Give information about medication, use and complications. — Provide practice time for return demonstration. — Assist patient/SO to evaluate home environment to identify hazards to eye safety.	— Patient/SO verbalizes understanding of discharge instructions. — Demonstrates aseptic application of eye drops. — Applies eye drops without injury to affected eye. — Identifies hazards to eye safety related to activities and age. — Verbalizes intent to use protective shield/glasses. — Verbalizes ability to manage continued care needs after discharge.
— ______	Condition will be monitored during hospital stay:		— Condition unchanged during hospital stay. — Condition requires further follow up.
— ______			

Date	7 - 3 R.N. Signature/Initials	3 - 11 R.N. Signature/Initials	11 - 7 R.N. Signature/Initials

Figure 6-3. Continued

phase of the perioperative process. Information about the patient and care needs that is to be relayed to different members of the health care team should be documented in a consistent place in the medical record. Medications requested by a medical consultant for intraoperative administration, monitoring of blood glucose levels, and the patient's intolerance of lying flat are examples of information that should be communicated.

Intraoperative Phase

Nursing care in the operating room requires specific knowledge of ophthalmic anatomy and physiology, aseptic technique, the nursing process, surgical procedures, and legal implications of surgery. The AORN requires that the circulating nurse be a registered nurse (RN) at all times.[5]

The nurse needs to be competent in assembling, using, and troubleshooting equipment to prevent disruption during the procedure. He or she should be prepared to respond to patient's fears with calm confidence and efficiency. As in all other areas of nursing practice, comprehensive documentation gives a clear picture of the patient and the interventions implemented (Fig. 6-4).

Assessment

Patient assessment is one of the major functions of nurses during the intraoperative phase of the surgical process. Positive identification of the patient, the surgical site, and allergies are to be confirmed. The patient's level of anxiety should be assessed in relation to the time and amount of preoperative medication administered. After the retrobulbar injection, the nurse must monitor the patient for potential reactions, including hypotension, convulsions, or respiratory arrest. After the nerve block is administered, a pressure-reducing device may be used on the eye, such as a mercury balloon (this device requires observation for reflex bradycardia, tissue damage to the ear from poor placement, or corneal abrasions).

Planning

To ensure familiarity with institutional procedures and to demonstrate competency, nurses assisting with surgical procedures should complete a thorough orientation period before assuming their responsibilities. Documented hands-on in-service training should be completed before any new equipment is used.

Assembling equipment before the administration of anesthesia allows the nurse to anticipate and resolve problems before surgery begins. For example, the vitrectomy handpiece should be attached to the appropriate tubing, and the power console, suction device, lighting, and recording equipment should be tested. Scrub nurses ensure that equipment within the sterile field is functional, that the microscope is set up, and that the light bulb on the scope is working. They are responsible for the availability and care of the surgical instruments that may be needed. All instruments should be checked for sterility, broken tips, sharpness, stiffness, and general integrity before the procedure begins. A sponge, needle, and instrument count is completed according to individual policies. Nurses must understand the sequence of events for the specific procedure scheduled.

Consistency in both nursing staff and surgeons can produce optimal teamwork when the scrub nurse can become so familiar with the surgeon's routine that each step or response to unusual events can be anticipated. Up-to-date files listing individual surgeon preferences and routines are helpful for staff and orientation of new personnel.

Implementation

Use of an intravenous line and monitoring equipment is usually initiated in a holding area if not begun previously. One of the most important nursing roles during the intraoperative phase is that of the circulating nurse; he or she brings the other team members together, coordinates the care, and acts as the patient advocate. By orienting the patient to the operating room environment, explaining basic equipment and anticipated routines, introducing personnel, and reassuring the patient during the procedure, patient anxiety can be diminished. The circulator reviews all information about the patient's status, communicating relevant changes to other team members. Surgical site preparation and patient positioning and draping, are also the responsibilities of the circulating nurse.

NOISE REDUCTION. Noisy activity should be minimized once the patient enters the operating room. Because most ophthalmic surgery is performed while the patient is awake, conversation can be heard, so only topics of immediate concern should be discussed while the surgery is proceeding. Messages for personnel involved in the procedure should be taken at another location. To avoid frightening the patient, words used in the operating room must be chosen carefully. The use of *trim* as opposed to *cut* and the avoidance of words with negative implications (*oops, uh-oh*) are prime examples. In the event of complications, voices should be controlled and events should proceed quickly but quietly. If the patient becomes restless during the procedure or wakes suddenly, touching his or her hand under the drape may help calm and reorient him or her. The circulator should talk calmly to the patient. If a rapport has been developed earlier, the patient will be reassured by a known voice, whereas several different voices can be confusing.

POSITIONING. Patient comfort during the procedure promotes compliance and a positive attitude. The patient is placed in a supine position with the head just at the edge of the table. The head should be secured with the patient looking directly up so that the head is neither rotated nor tilted. The wrist rest should be secured perpendicularly 2.5 cm below the lateral canthus. The area under body surfaces should be padded. A pillow, blanket, or towel under body spaces may provide additional comfort or support when placed under the knees of a patient with low-back pain or arthritis. A safety belt should be placed above the knees and the wrist gently secured to the table.[6]

SITE PREPARATION. With clean, gloved hands, the nurse dips a cotton-tipped applicator into a weak 5% solution of povidone-iodine (*not* scrub solution), separates the eyelids, and cleans the base of the lashes and lid margins, allowing a few drops of the solution to enter the cul-de-sac. pHisoHex should be used if the patient is allergic to iodine. Care should be taken to ensure that it does not enter the cul-de-sac.

A folded 4 × 4-in. pad is dipped into the preparation solution, with any excess squeezed out. Beginning at the margins of the closed lid, the lid is gently cleaned in a circular motion that moves out to the boundaries of the nose, forehead, and cheek. This step is repeated three times, with the pad changed each time the outer boundary of the site is reached; a used pad is never returned to the preparation site.

Using an irrigating bulb, the globe and cul-de-sac are thoroughly irrigated with normal saline solution. Solution left can cause sloughing of the corneal epithelium, which would degrade the view through the cornea, making intraocular structures difficult to visualize during the procedure.

The eye and cheek are painted with preparation solution a final time. Excess solution is immediately removed by patting the area with dry 4 × 4-in. pads, finishing at the ear. The ear is checked to ensure that solution has not pooled there and that the area is completely dry before draping.

DRAPING. Various materials and methods are used for draping the head. Applying the sterile drape is a cooperative effort. The drape should be handled as little as possible, and gloved hands should not touch the patient's skin during draping. The circulating nurse positions the patient's head so that the scrub nurse can place the end of the drape under the head. Disposable adhesive plastic drapes stick firmly to the eyelid and seal the area around the lids. A large drape is positioned over the torso. One should avoid reaching across the unsterile field to drape the opposite side.

STERILE TECHNIQUE. The importance of maintaining sterile technique during the operative procedure cannot be overemphasized. The circulator finds tact and assertiveness skills helpful when identifying and correcting a break in sterile technique by any member of the surgical team. A gown or glove contaminated when bumped into the microscope or when instruments are introduced into the surgical field should be replaced immediately.

Any products brought into the sterile field should be carefully verified. Identification labels should be placed on syringes of medication or solution containers before they are passed to the surgeon. Inappropriate introduction of antibiotics or steroids into the eye can result in irreversible damage to the cornea. Use of color-coded labels for frequently used medications provides added safety. Whenever there is any question about contents of a container, it should be discarded and fresh solution obtained. The scrub nurse should verify the power of intraocular lenses and handle them only with forceps before they are passed to the surgeon.

CARE AND HANDLING OF SPECIMENS. The JCAHO recommends that all potentially diagnostic tissue removed from a patient be examined by a pathologist. Related policies and procedures should be in writing for each institution. Containers should be

(*Text continues on p. 72.*)

PERIOPERATIVE RECORD

DATE: **TIME ARRIVED:** **B/P** **PULSE**

HOLDING AREA PATIENT IDENTIFICATION:	LIMITATIONS:	PROCEDURE/LOCATION	CONSENTS	____ % SaO_2 (RA)
☐ VERBAL ☐ ALERT	☐ NONE	OD OS OU	☐ OPERATIVE	☐ LAB DATA
☐ CHART ☐ ORIENTED	☐ AUDITORY	AD AS AU	☐ GENERAL	☐ EKG
☐ ARM BAND ☐ DISORIENTED	☐ VISUAL	OTHER ________	OTHER:	☐ MED. CLEARANCE
☐ STAMP PLATE ☐ DROWSY	☐ MOBILITY	VERIFICATION	☐ 2ND OPINION	☐ LASH TRIM
	☐ LANGUAGE	☐ VERBAL ☐ OP CONSENT		☐ MERCURY BAG

HOLDING AREA COMMENTS:	I.V. START:	I.V. DISCONTINUE:
ALLERGIES: ☐ NKA LIST:	SOL. #1:	#1 INFUSED:
	SITE: ANGIO:	CONDITION: SITE: ANGIO:
	BY: @ a.m. p.m.	BY: @ a.m. p.m.
	SOL. #2:	#2 INFUSED:
	SITE: ANGIO:	CONDITION: SITE: ANGIO:
H.A. R.N.	BY: @ a.m. p.m.	BY: @ a.m. p.m.

OPERATING ROOM CIRCULATOR CHECK LIST

			ALLERGIES: ☐ NKA
☐ VERBAL	☐ ALERT	☐ CONSENT SIGNED	LIST:
☐ CHART	☐ ORIENTED	OD OS OU	
☐ ARM BAND	☐ DISORIENTED	AD AS AU	
☐ STAMP PLATE	☐ DROWSY	OTHER:	

ANESTHESIA	OR #	IC #	OR/ANES IN	OR START	OR STOP	OR/ANES OUT
GEN. ☐ LOC/SED. ☐ LOCAL ☐			A.M. P.M.	A.M. P.M.	A.M. P.M.	A.M. P.M.

PRE-OP DIAGNOSIS

POST-OP DIAGNOSIS

OPERATIVE PROCEDURE

SURGEON LAST NAME	ASSISTANT SURGEON #1 LAST NAME
ASSISTANT SURGEON #2 LAST NAME	ASSISTANT SURGEON #3 LAST NAME

ANESTHESIOLOGIST FIRST NAME LAST NAME	NURSE ANESTHETIST FIRST NAME LAST NAME
RELIEF FIRST NAME LAST NAME	RELIEF FIRST NAME LAST NAME

CIRCULATING RN FIRST NAME LAST NAME		SCRUB NURSE FIRST NAME LAST NAME	
RELIEF #1 FIRST NAME LAST NAME	IN / OUT	RELIEF #1 FIRST NAME LAST NAME	IN / OUT
RELIEF #2 FIRST NAME LAST NAME	IN / OUT	RELIEF #2 FIRST NAME LAST NAME	IN / OUT

Figure 6-4. Perioperative record.

POSITION FOR SURGERY	OPERATIVE SITE PREPARATION				PREP
☐ SUPINE ☐ RT LAT ☐ LT LAT		PREPPED	COVERED	TAPED	☐ BETADINE SOLUTION
☐ HEAD POSITION PER M.D.	OD				☐ BETADINE SCRUB
☐ ARMS POSITIONED BY______	OS				☐ PHISOHEX
☐ SAFETY STRAP	OU				☐ OTHER:
☐ SIDERAILS UP	AD				
☐ OTHER	AS				
	AU				

EQUIPMENT	UNIT #	EQUIPMENT	UNIT #	LASER ☐ NA	#	PULSE / WATT	BOVIE ☐ NA
☐ NA		CATARACT		ARGON		/	#
VITRECTOMY		STAT VISC					PACEMAKER YES☐ NO☐
FRAGMENTOR		DRILL/SAW		INDIRECT		/	GR. PAD SITE
AIR PUMP		BLANKET/COVER		DIODE		/	BY: R.N.
LIGHT SOURCE		OTHER:		OTHER:			SKIN PRE-OP
CRYO							SKIN POST-OP
M.P.C.							

CIRCULATING NURSES COMMENTS:

____

____

____

____

____

____

____

____

____

____

PATIENT OUTCOME STANDARDS MET YES ☐ NO ☐

DISCHARGED TO: ☐ RECOVERY ☐ ROOM

SIGNATURE R.N.

SPECIMENS ☐ NA
☐ TISSUE
☐ F.S.
☐ MICRO
☐ FOREIGN BODY
☐ OTHER

LOCAL CASES ☐ NA	URINARY CATHETER ☐ NA
EKG LEADS APPLIED ☐YES ☐NO	☐ ON ARRIVAL
PULSE OXIMETER APPLIED ☐YES ☐NO	☐ IN OR @ BY
VITAL SIGNS PRE-OP: B/P ______ P______ R ______	SIZE TYPE ☐ LEFT IN ☐ REMOVED @
VITAL SIGNS POST-OP: B/P ______ P______ R ______	AMOUNT CC

SPONGE COUNTS	COUNTED IN	FIRST	FINAL	SIGNATURE NA ☐
LAPS				
RAYTEC				
NEEDLES				
BLADES				
OTHER				INSTRUMENTS YES ☐ NO ☐

PROSTHESIS ☐ NONE

Figure 6-4. Continued

labeled with the name of the preservative within *before* being placed in the operating room. Mistakes in identifying solutions can have life-threatening consequences. The usual tissue preservative is 10% formalin; however, it is important to have the correct solution for each type of specimen. Foreign-body samples should be sent without preservatives. Safety precautions and monitoring routines must be observed when handling hazardous chemicals such as formalin. Staff handling the solution must be regularly educated about procedures to follow in the event of a spill. Special spill kits should be readily available.

Tissue removed by the surgeon is passed to the scrub nurse and then placed into the labeled container held by the circulator for proper handling. If not given directly to the circulator, specimens should be kept moist in a sterile container and not placed on a gauze pad, where they can be easily overlooked. The circulator should confirm the description and source of the specimen with the surgeon when receiving the container.

Each tissue sample is to be sent for pathologic analysis in a separately labeled container. Containers and lids should be labeled with the patient's keyplate. Additional information should be written on the attached laboratory request, including the following:

- Specimen description and source location (eg, "right upper lid")
- Examination requested
- Name of the surgeon
- Time and date obtained

A system for tracking each specimen should be in place. A log listing the patient's name, each specimen obtained, the date obtained, the time and date sent, and where it was sent and by whom should be maintained. Specimens for frozen section are examined immediately by the pathologist. A report of findings should be given directly to the surgeon, either verbally or in writing, without being relayed by the circulator.

Preparedness for Complications

Knowledge of the potential complications of ophthalmic procedures allows the nurse to anticipate the supplies needed and to reassure the patient in case a different course of action is required. The circulating nurse needs to obtain medications, know the location of equipment, and how to set it up and use it quickly. The scrub nurse must act quickly, anticipating the needs of the surgeon and having sutures and instruments readily available.[7]

Nurse as First Assistant

The RN first assistant has the knowledge and skills of both the scrub and the circulating nurses, with additional education and experience in those skills needed to assist the surgeon during the operative procedure. He or she practices under the direction of the surgeon but does not function in a dual role as scrub nurse during the procedure. Each institution must establish a credentialing process, ensuring competence for nurses functioning in this extended role. Some functions unique to the role of RN first assistant include the following:[8]

- Use of microsurgical instruments
- Tissue handling
- Exposure of the surgical site
- Retraction
- Suturing
- Provision of hemostasis

Successful management of complications is enhanced by a confident, skillful first assistant able to use good judgment in stressful situations. Table 6-1 provides examples of a first assistant's nursing interventions for selected ocular complications. Most of these interventions involve the use of manual dexterity, which is a learned skill, and experience is needed to improve techniques and control hand movements. General guidelines to be observed by the first assistant include the following:

1. Tremors can be minimized by keeping elbows at the sides of the body and resting the hands on the patient's brow or cheek. One should avoid putting pressure on the face or orbit, which can cause intraocular contents to extrude.
2. When using instruments, it is easier to look around the microscope and bring them into the light of the microscope than to peer through the microscope. Care must be taken not to drop instruments or pass things directly over the patient's eye. Corneal surfaces must be kept wet with balanced salt solution. Proper irrigation allows for better visualization and smaller light reflex. The first assistant should work out a system not to obscure the surgeon's view. All actions should be performed with care and in an unhurried manner, concentrating on the task

Table 6-1
Ocular Complications

EVENT	POTENTIAL NURSING RESPONSE
Allergic reaction	Preparation of benadryl or epinephrine
Corneal burns	Equipment maintenance/in-service training
Vitreous loss	Vitreous cutter/vitreous tray
Expulsive hemorrhage	Keratoprosthesis/quick preparation of suture
Orbital hemorrhage	Cautery/pressure dressing
Retrobulbar hemorrhage	Canthotomy scissors
Hypotony	Balanced salt solution reform chamber
Choroidal hemorrhage	Draining electrode
Dislocated lens nucleus	Vitreous cutter
Intraocular pressure	Tonometer/surgery
Iris prolapse	Surgical repair
Flat anterior chamber	Healon
Wrong eye/wrong intraocular lens	Consent/incident report
Loss of vision	Counseling/patient education
Infection/endophthalmitis	Antibiotic therapy

at hand and eliminating the potential for complications.

Intravenous Conscious Sedation

Perioperative nurses also deliver sedation and monitor patients receiving intravenous sedation during the surgical procedure. Patient acuity often creates challenges for nurses during minor procedures. Stringent guidelines, policies and procedures, and parameters for the monitoring of patients receiving intravenous conscious sedation should be in place before a nurse undertakes the responsibility. The AORN has issued a statement of recommended practices for nurses monitoring patients receiving intravenous conscious sedation, which will help in developing institutional practices.[9]

Only nurses without other circulating, scrubbing, or monitoring responsibilities should monitor patients under intravenous conscious sedation, and such patients should be limited to those with predictable outcomes. The nurse taking on this responsibility must have considerable experience, advanced skills, and an extensive knowledge base; these areas of expertise should be defined by the institution. A knowledge of anesthetic agents, their physiologic effects, and potential patient response is minimal. Management of potential complications, such as airway management and emergency situations, should be included in competency validation. Other policy statements to be defined include the following:

- Types of patients the nurse can monitor
- Types of surgical procedures appropriate
- Medications that the nurse can administer
- Maximum dosages that the nurse can administer
- Skills of the nurse that validate competence
- Policies stating equipment required in the room
- Need for an airway management expert on site
- Requirement for a physician to be in attendance
- Written identification of minimal monitoring parameters
- Written discharge criteria for the patient

Evaluation

The circulating nurse assesses the patient as a whole being before the patient leaves the operating room. Speaking to the patient aids in orientation and provides reassurance that he or she is progressing as expected to the next phase of the surgical experience. The nurse's assessment of the patient's status is documented on the perioperative record. The circulator should also confirm with the surgeon the procedure that was performed before documenting it on the record. Additional documentation of charges for medications, equipment, and supplies used should be reviewed for accuracy. The report should be given to the nurse who is continuing to care for the patient either in the postanesthesia care unit (PACU) or other recovery area. Communication of unusual events during the procedure, special equipment needed during the postanesthesia phase, and a summary of the patient's status should be reported.

Postanesthesia Phase

Even with excellent preoperative education, the experience of waking up with the treated eye patched and shielded is startling. Because of the possibility of poor vision in the eye that did not undergo surgery, patients often awaken frightened and hostile. Familiar voices, a calm atmosphere, and a comforting touch can help the patient adjust to unfamiliar surroundings.

Assessment

The anesthesiologist or nurse anesthetist should give the nurse caring for the patient in the postanesthesia period a thorough report about the drugs administered and the patient's reactions to them. The patient is monitored until the effects of anesthesia have worn off. Figure 6-5 is an example of a postoperative documentation form. Airway patency and optimal breathing are the first priority. Breath sounds are checked with a stethoscope; blood pressure, pulse, temperature, and cardiac rhythm are also assessed and documented.

When assessing the level of consciousness and orientation, it should be noted whether the patient is conversing, whether the speech is clear, whether the patient wakes to gentle stimulation by calling his or her name, and so forth. The color and temperature of skin, ability to move extremities, and presence of peripheral pulses should also be noted. Initial assessment provides the baseline for further reassessment by others. Additional observations include the following:

- Fluid intake and output
- Comfort level and need for aggressive management
- Dressing and surgical site
- Presence, color, and amount of drainage
- Security of dressing and shield
- Specific observations related to the surgery
- Adjustable sutures intact
- Increasing swelling at the site
- Specific observations related to preoperative medical status
- Changes in cardiac rhythm
- Glucose level in diabetics
- Suspected aspiration if the patient has respiratory difficulty or is wheezing

Planning

Preparation for life-threatening complications is essential. A good preoperative screening process makes the occurrence of respiratory or cardiac arrest a rare situation in an ophthalmic setting but can give a false sense of security. Drills, mock codes, familiarity with crash carts, emergency procedures, and up-to-date supplies ready for use are of utmost importance. Personnel monitoring patients in the PACU should be competent in current advanced cardiac life support and knowledgeable of treatment algorithms. Respiratory or cardiac arrest is rarely seen without some warning. The nurse should monitor the patient's vital signs and be alert to subtle changes that give clues to an impending arrest situation:

- Changes in skin or poor capillary refill
- Changes in blood pressure
- Changes in heart rate
- Changes in respiratory pattern
- Chest pain with vagus nerve action
- Restlessness and apprehension
- Arrhythmias or blocks should be observed for progression
- Slowly rising or decreasing Po_2

Implementation

The family and, when ready, the patient should be informed of any complications in a timely manner. The physician frequently talks to them about unexpected or unmet outcomes in the PACU. The nurse should be present to provide reassurance for the patient and to support the physician. Reinforcing information and allowing the patient and family to express their feelings are helpful.

In the event of postoperative hypertension, nonpathologic factors should be ruled out (eg, pain or emotional distress, the catecholamine release that comes with waking up, a full bladder, hypoxemia). Close monitoring and medical intervention should be initiated quickly.

The Agency for Health Care Policy and Research has published national guidelines for pain management in both adults and children. The multidisciplinary panel that developed these guidelines recognized that traditional practices are inadequate for relieving pain and that nurses and physicians may need to reassess their attitudes and prejudices about pain management. Pain should be assessed every 2 hours during the first postoperative day. Effective pain management should begin preoperatively through education of the patient about expectations, use of intensity scales, and consideration of the patient's wishes. The panel recommended that pharmacologic management of moderate postoperative pain begin with nonsteroidal antiinflammatory drugs. Moderately severe to severe pain should be treated initially with an opioid analgesic.

Based on the type of anesthesia used, initial con-

PATIENT CARE FLOW SHEET

POST - OPERATIVE PERIOD

Initial Assessment

Time of return from O.R.: ____________ via _____ accompanied by ________________

Mental status: alert _____ drowsy _____ lethargic _____ oriented _____ disoriented _____

Skin: warm _____ dry _____ moist _____ cool _____ / Color ____________

Moving all extremities: yes _____ no * _____

IV infusing: yes _____ no _____

Operative site: ____________________ Dressing: ____________________

Placed in post-op position (____________________) & instructions given: yes _____ no * _____

Vital signs: B/P _______ T _____ P _____ R _____

Comments: ____

____

R.N. Signature ________________________________ Date ____________

Reassessment

Ambulation:

alone _____ with assistance _____ tolerated well _____ other* ____________ Time: ____________

Operative site: ____________________ Dressing ____________________ Time: ____________

Intake: Tolerated p.o. fluids: yes _____ no _____ nausea _____ Time: ____________

Tolerated solid food: yes _____ no _____ nausea _____ Time: ____________

Output: Voided: q.s. _____ without difficulty _____ other * _____ Time: ____________

Vomited: amount _____ description ____________________

Medication given: ____________________ Time: ____________

Relief obtained: yes _____ no * _____ Time: ____________

Comfort: Pain: _____ Location: __________ Intensity __________

Medication given: ____________________ IM / SC site _______ Time: ____________

Relief obtained: yes _____ no * _____ Time: ____________

Vital Signs:

B/P _____ T _____ P _____ R _____ Time ____________

B/P _____ T _____ P _____ R _____ Time ____________

Comments: ____

____

R.N. Signature ________________________________ Date/Time: ____________

R.N. Signature ________________________________ Date/Time: ____________

Discharge Data

Status: Comfort ____________________________

Dressing ____________________________

Mobility ____________________________

Systemic condition monitored since admission & unchanged: yes _____ no * _____

Escorted from the unit by ____________________ , ambulatory ___ w/c ___ stretcher ___

Transportation by ____________________ to ____________ with ____________

Time of discharge ____________________

Phone # after discharge ____________________

Comments: ____

____

____

R.N. Signature ________________________________ Date ____________

* See Progress Notes

Figure 6-5. Postoperative portion of patient care flow sheet.

siderations should be reassessed, and progress toward meeting discharge criteria should be evaluated at frequently defined intervals. Discharge criteria need to be defined in writing for each facility and should allow for clinical judgment without compromising patient safety. Various tools, such as the Robertson and Aldrette scoring guides, can be used, but good nursing assessment is still crucial. Each patient should be seen by an anesthesiologist before discharge if general anesthesia was administered. All assessments, interventions, and patient responses to interventions must be documented. Any alterations in facility protocol should be documented, including rationale, specific circumstances involved, and follow-up planned.

Some of the most frequent complications resulting in extended stay in a hospital or observation unit include persistence of premedication, unrelieved pain, and persistent nausea and vomiting. Factors contributing to nausea and vomiting include pain, narcotic use, sudden movement or position changes, hypotension, obesity resulting from a decreased rate of gastric emptying, and the site of the surgical procedure (as in strabismus).

Patients should not be discharged home until established criteria are met:

- Adequacy of respiratory function
- Temperature and other vital signs within normal range
- Acceptable level of orientation
- Ability to ambulate
- Ability to tolerate fluids
- Ability to void

The patient who has not met the discharge criteria but who insists on leaving should sign an Against Medical Advice discharge form. Bearing in mind the needs of the patient and the patient's rights while maintaining a professional attitude should prevent this situation from becoming a personal battle of wills. Attempts should be made to find what is causing the alteration in the plan previously discussed with the patient and what can be done to alleviate any dissatisfaction. When it has been determined that the patient is ready to leave, all the same instructions are to be provided as for a planned discharge in addition to considerations for the patient's safety. Patient outbursts of anger or hostility should not be taken personally.

Patient and Family Education

Patient and family education focuses on assisting patients to meet their self-care needs. Inform family members of their role. Instructions must be in the language understood by the patient and should be both verbal and written. A copy of the written instructions in both the patient's language and in English becomes part of the medical record. Education postoperatively is built on instruction previously initiated. Timing, relevance, and the amount of information presented affect the learning process. Safety and prevention of complications are of prime concern at this time. Care of the dressing and surgical site, infection control, signs and symptoms requiring attention, a telephone number to call in an emergency, and the follow-up appointment should be included (see Fig. 6-6). Instructions for medications to be taken at home, including the name, dose, and time, should be written. A demonstration and return demonstration of the procedure for instilling eye drops and ointments may be indicated. Any alterations in the routine for systemic conditions should be discussed with the patient, including any indications for follow-up with the physician. Thorough education requires evaluation of what was learned and how behavior has changed. The nurse must ascertain a patient's understanding of the instructions and document that understanding. Patients are often asked to sign a statement that they understand the instructions.

Evaluation

When reviewing the plan of care before discharge, the nurse should evaluate the patient's progress toward meeting the expected outcomes previously established. Alternative plans and follow-up arrangements should be verified. Many organizations have the nurse telephone the patient within 48 hours of discharge. This follow-up call can be incorporated into the quality assessment and improvement program. Patient response to the call is generally positive, and it allows the nurse to discuss the patient's general condition, any problems that he or she encountered during the surgical visit or postoperatively, and the effectiveness of pain management, as well as to answer any questions about home care. The benefits of this call go beyond ensuring quality patient care: the contact encourages the patient to trust and seek future health care from the same providers and facilities.

DISCHARGE INSTRUCTIONS

Diagnosis: ______________________ Procedure: ______________________

DIET:
- ☐ Resume your diet
- ☐ Special instructions ______________________

ACTIVITY:
- ☐ Rest in bed today
- ☐ Resume normal activity
- ☒ Avoid strenuous activity
- ☐ Do not lift more than 5 pounds
- ☐ Maintain special position: ______________________
- ☐ Do not sleep on operated side
- ☐ Sleep with your head slightly elevated
- ☐ Do not bend below your waist

EYE CARE:
- ☐ Wear shield at all times
- ☐ Wear shield when sleeping
- ☐ Do not use pad or shield
- ☒ Do not rub your eye
- ☒ Avoid dusty, dirty places
- ☒ Observe safety precautions to avoid bumping your head
- ☒ Use a fresh tissue each time you touch your eye
- ☐ Wear pad and shield until you see your doctor
- ☐ Change the pad when it becomes moist
- ☐ Wear glasses when awake for safety
- ☒ Keep water out of your eye
- ☒ Avoid straining with bowel movements
- ☒ Cleanse eyelids with a clean cloth, rayon ball, or tissue, and clean water
- ☒ Take care not to contaminate the medicine dropper or tip by touching it to your eye

- ☒ WASH YOUR HANDS BEFORE AND AFTER TOUCHING YOUR EYE AND INSTILLING MEDICATIONS.
- ☒ CALL YOUR DOCTOR IF YOU HAVE INCREASED PAIN, SWELLING, REDNESS, BLEEDING, DRAINING, FLASHING LIGHTS, FLOATERS, QUESTIONS OR CONCERNS.

- ☒ CALL YOUR DOCTOR **IMMEDIATELY** IF YOU HAVE A SUDDEN DECREASE IN VISION FROM THE LEVEL IT WAS AT DISCHARGE.
- ☐ OTHER: ______________________

MEDICATIONS: ______________________

____

____

____

- ☐ Continue your usual medications, as directed by your medical doctor
- ☐ Bring your **eye medications** to your doctor's office
- ☐ Do not use eye medications until you see your doctor, and receive additional instructions.

FOLLOW-UP: Appointment: Doctor ______________ Phone # ______________
Location ______________________
Date ______________ Time ______________

•IF YOU HAVE ANY PROBLEMS OR QUESTIONS CALL YOUR DOCTOR OR EYE CLINIC

- ☐ Copies of laboratory tests given, to take to your private medical doctor
- ☐ See your private medical doctor for follow-up regarding ______________________
- ☐ Other: ______________________

Printed Instructions Given:
- ☐ How to use prescribed medication
- ☐ Medication instruction sheet
- ☐ Physician's instruction sheet
- ☐ Other: ______________________

I/WE HAVE RECEIVED AND UNDERSTAND THESE INSTRUCTIONS.

____
Patient (other/relationship)

Instructions given by: ______________________
(nurse)

Date ______________ Time ______________

Figure 6-6. Discharge instructions for the patient and family.

MEETING THE NEEDS OF SPECIFIC PATIENT POPULATIONS

Children

As a result of congenital anomalies and trauma, children are seen in the ophthalmic setting at all developmental stages. Their perceptions of hospitalization are frequently based on fear of the unknown. A staff knowledgeable about the care of children and a flexible program geared to various developmental age groups should produce a positive response to the experience and ensure the cooperation of the child and parent. Assessment of the child's emotional readiness and the family dynamics is the starting point when preparing the child for surgery. The fear or guilt of a parent is often relayed to the child. Children usually understand more than they verbalize. Speaking directly to the child in addition to the parents helps build rapport. Good preoperative preparation sets the stage for a smooth recovery.

Pediatric surgery requires significant modifications in the perioperative routines. A preoperative tour of the surgical suite allowing both the child and a parent to change into surgical scrubs can go a long way in alleviating anxiety in both parties. Meeting the staff who will care for the child the day of surgery and trying on a surgical mask or touching the blood pressure cuff or other appropriate equipment can produce surprising, intelligent questions from the child.

Specific videos, toys, puppets, or demonstrations should be developed for giving instruction to various developmental age groups. Activities that encourage a more positive experience for the child should be built into the system. A ride to the operating room in a wagon or toy car may reduce fears. The child should be allowed to pick a flavoring to apply inside the anesthesia mask and to bring a favorite toy into the operating room. Whenever possible, parents should be permitted to accompany the child into the holding area to help relieve anxiety. They should be the last people the child sees before surgery and the first ones he or she sees when waking up in the recovery area, where they can hold and support the child.

Popsicles and juices can be given in the PACU to speed recovery. Aggressive treatment of nausea, vomiting, and pain should be given priority. An increasing trend using desflurane intraoperatively has been helpful in avoiding postoperative nausea and vomiting, decreasing recovery time, eliminating admissions, and controlling costs. Children under general anesthesia for ocular muscle surgery should be monitored closely for bradycardia and hypotension caused by the oculocardiac reflex.[10]

It is important to remember that children are not small adults. Their anatomy and physiology are different. The pediatric airway has a smaller diameter with high resistance to flow. The use of cold mist in the recovery room helps to increase the airway diameter. The trachea lacks firm cartilage support, resulting in airway collapse if the neck is hyperextended. The use of diaphragmatic breathing impedes air movement when the child's movement is restricted. Pressure on the diaphragm results in reflux and potential aspiration. Therefore, postoperatively the best position for a child is on the right side or a semi-Fowler position. Sudden changes in assessment parameters have intense results; children do not have the reserves to fall back on and can experience respiratory arrest brought on by fatigue. The nurse must be able to recognize decompensation in a child. A good baseline assessment preoperatively helps to determine who is at risk for postoperative respiratory complications. Assessment parameters include behavior, color, respiratory rate, breathing pattern, breath sounds, and heart rate. Knowledge of the normal ranges for vital signs in various age groups is essential when caring for children. Respiratory arrest in children is most often secondary to hypoxemia from respiratory depression. Hypoxemia results in decreased heart rate exacerbating to asystole, which is difficult to reverse. Because of their small cardiac mass, fibrillation is uncommon in children. Postoperative monitoring should indicate immediate interventions when there are changes in the baseline parameters focusing on the airway. Appropriately sized resuscitation equipment, medication dosages, and dosage charts must be available wherever pediatric care is provided. In the event of an arrest situation in a child, airway management is the key to successful resuscitation.[11,12]

Postintubation croup may be seen 1 to 3 hours after extubation. It is most common in the 1- to 4-year age group and is characterized by hoarseness, croupy cough, stridor, restlessness, and edema. After treatment with epinephrine and corticosteroids, children should be observed for at least 2 hours in the surgical center; if they remain stable, they can be sent home with consideration given to their age, severity of the episode, reliability of the parents, and availability of support measures, such as a humidifier and emergency systems in the home.[12] As with most nursing situations, the key to providing optimal pediatric care is *assess, monitor,* and *anticipate.*

Discharge instructions should be given to the child as well as the parents. Even young children can take an active role in complying with the instructions if they assume responsibility. Directions to leave a patch in place and avoid running or sports have more impact when given by health care personnel and reinforced by the parents.

Elderly Patients

The visually impaired elderly often bring with them at least one other chronic health condition or disability. As with other groups of patients, the whole person must be addressed. Assessment must deal with the physical, psychological, functional, and social aspects of the person preparing for surgery. Physiologic changes associated with the aging process vary among individuals, both in timing and in the specific body systems involved. Many people are self-sufficient and mentally astute in their 90s, whereas others in their 60s have become "old," displaying deteriorated physical and cognitive functioning. Visual impairment at a time when other diminished physical capabilities become apparent (unsteady gait, decreased hand strength, and difficulty hearing) presents new hazards and difficulties in daily living. Those caring for older adults need to present a positive awareness of their circumstances, abilities, and limitations.

Although adaptations in routine are easily understood when caring for children, increased awareness of the unique needs of the elderly must be encouraged so that health care providers tailor programs and facilities for them. A positive attitude toward and respect for the elderly can promote effective communication and rapport, thereby influencing their emotional response and surgical outcome. A strong sense of independence may prevent older persons from asking for assistance, or fear of bothering friends and neighbors may cause patients to ignore instructions to have another responsible adult accompany them on discharge. The nurse should confirm the discharge arrangements during the admission interview on the day of surgery.

As the patient's advocate, the nurse validates the patient's competency and understanding of the informed consent. An initial assessment should include accurate height and weight information, which is needed for proper medication and anesthetic dosages. Baseline assessment parameters also need to be documented. Blood pressure and temperature norms may be altered because of vascular considerations, and comparison of lung sounds is especially important postoperatively. Assessment of risk factors leading to injury should not be overlooked when planning perioperative care and home care, including steadiness of gait, propensity for confusion, and level of independence.

Surgery should be scheduled early in the day to maintain a routine pattern for those who rise early; early discharge to a familiar environment should be encouraged, avoiding the "sundown effect" seen in those prone to confusion late in the day. Patients' intraoperative attention to sensory perception is significant. Loud noises in a strange environment may cause disorientation or confusion. Encourage patients to wear hearing aids and dentures into the operating room to promote communication. Provide reassurance and reinforce instructions in a calming voice because short-term memory is diminished in some elderly patients. Reassess positioning during the surgical procedure to prevent circulatory impairment.

Postoperative assessment parameters should be adjusted to the norms of the individual. Core temperature is often lower in the elderly, making a temperature of 99°F an elevation. Respiratory problems related to weakened compensatory mechanisms are the leading complications seen in the elderly and should be monitored closely. Wheezing that may be indicative of pulmonary edema or bibasilar rales suggestive of congestive heart failure should prompt immediate intervention. Fluid overload and voiding may also be a concern. Postoperative confusion may be avoided by providing some time reference, early contact with family, monitoring of Sao_2 levels, and intervention as indicated to prevent hypoxemia. If confusion does occur, look for possible causes, such as hyponatremia or pain.

Discharge planning and instructions are a high priority in the care of the elderly. The physiologic changes of aging make the older person more susceptible to adverse drug reactions. Medications to be taken after discharge should be reviewed with the patient and reinforced with the family. Instructions about the dose, frequency, and special storage should be given. Careful explanation of medication side effects and ophthalmic symptoms that indicate a need to call the physician is warranted because some people confuse these responses with consequences of aging.

Surgery may compound or increase awareness of the usual visual changes associated with aging that have occurred so gradually they were not noticed previously. Increased light sensitivity, recovery from glare, and altered depth perception are a few of the changes. Adaptations to the home environment that may be needed to promote safety and prevent falls or injury should be discussed. Maintenance of independence and adjustment to the activities of daily living are often related to the support and attitude of others. The patient and family should be advised to remove obstacles such as small stools, glass coffee tables, wastebaskets, or area rugs from halls and pathways, and to add decals or stained glass ornaments to sliding glass doors. Glare can be minimized by positioning tablecloths or heavy matte surfaces under lamps. Stairs and ramps should have handrails on both sides. Contrasting color surfaces add depth and prevent accidents. Adding color to fixture surfaces in an all-white bathroom makes edges more visible. Colored tape should be placed on white pot handles, and white dishes should not be used on a white tablecloth. Whenever possible, instructions for older patients should be provided in large print. Time should be taken to review instructions in an unhurried manner and to provide realistic expectations for older patients and their families.

Patients With Diabetes

Diabetes mellitus is one of the major causes of visual impairment, manifested most commonly as blurred vision, cataracts, glaucoma, and retinopathy. Diabetic retinopathy is a progressive disease that requires regular visits to the ophthalmologist. The patient with diabetes is therefore a frequent candidate for surgical intervention. The intrinsic side effects of diabetes, such as diminished ability for wound healing, present greater potential for complications and need for aggressive interventions in this patient population. The development of abnormal new blood vessels in proliferative diabetic retinopathy may cause scar tissue, resulting in a traction retinal detachment or vitreous hemorrhage that requires laser therapy or a vitrectomy. Although laser therapy may be successful in stabilizing retinopathy, the cauterization may damage healthy tissue and consequently reduce night and peripheral vision. As vision becomes increasingly impaired, many patients with diabetes respond with depression or anger. Their physical condition may be compounded by neglect of their usual diet, medication, exercise, and self-care routines. Fluctuations in blood sugar levels can cause blurred vision as well as additional emotional response.

Controlling the blood sugar level is the single most important safeguard against the complications of diabetic retinopathy. Facility protocols should arrange for a physician to be available and prepared to manage the needs of the patient with diabetes during the surgical experience. The nurse should obtain a detailed history of hypoglycemic and hyperglycemic experiences from the patient. This should include past responses to changes in activity, illness, and early signs of reactions.

Stress, infection, and anesthesia alter the patient's insulin requirements. Fundamental decisions regarding the patient's insulin regimen must be planned and discussed with the patient before the day of surgery. Various methods may be used, ranging from withholding the usual insulin dosage the day of surgery and giving regular insulin coverage throughout the day based on blood sugars to administration of an insulin drip. Monitoring and responding to alterations in the blood sugar level on the day of surgery are major nursing responsibilities. Administration of intravenous fluids containing dextrose should not be a major concern for most patients with diabetes. Five percent dextrose in water provides only 20 calories per 100 mL. The small increase in blood sugar that it may cause is easily controlled. However, studies have shown significant rise in blood sugar as a result of lactated Ringer solution. Many physicians order acetazolamide (Diamox) postoperatively, so it should be noted that it is one of several medications that may increase blood sugar levels. Whatever regimen is prescribed for the patient with diabetes, the nurse must stay alert to signs of both hypoglycemia and hyperglycemia. Liquids with concentrated sugar content should be readily available, such as honey, fruit juice, and regular soft drinks. Fifty percent dextrose should be administered to any diabetic patient with altered consciousness. An intravenous access may be indicated for a longer length of time, until the patient is able to void and tolerate oral intake.[13]

Having diabetes is an emotionally difficult experience in itself; adding the stress of surgery and dealing with unfamiliar situations may be more than the patient can handle. The nurse caring for the patient with diabetes should consider and understand individual experiences.

SUMMARY

Ophthalmology offers nurses many challenges for the future. They need to leave behind attitudes protecting territories and traditional roles. Nurses demonstrating knowledge and expertise are in the ideal position to be innovators in the changing health care system, providing new avenues to meet patient needs. Nurses can function in many roles in multiple settings, caring for the whole person.

References

1. Messner R. What patients really want from their nurses. AJN 1993;23:38–41.
2. American Nurses Association. Standards of clinical nursing practice. Washington, DC, American Nurses Association, 1991.
3. Centers for Disease Control. Update: universal precautions for prevention of transmission of human immunodeficiency virus, hepatitis B virus, and other bloodborne pathogens in healthcare settings. MMWR 1988;37:377–382.
4. Florida Department of Health and Rehabilitative Services. Florida recommended guidelines on health care workers infected with HIV and/or HBV. Tallahassee, HRS State Health Office, AIDS Program, 1992.
5. Association of Operating Room Nurses. Standards and recommended practices. Denver, Association of Operating Room Nurses, 1993:19.
6. Yamada S, et al. An eye on comfort: positioning a patient for ophthalmic surgery. J Ophthal Nurs Technol 1993;12:75–78.
7. Fairchild S. Perioperative nursing: principles and practice. Boston, Jones & Bartlett, 1993:345–347.
8. Rothrock J. The RN first assistant, ed 2. Philadelphia, JB Lippincott, 1993.
9. Association of Operating Room Nurses. Recommended practices: monitoring the patient receiving IV conscious sedation. AORN J 1993;57:978–983.
10. Eustis HS, Eiswirth CC, Smith DR. Vagal responses to adjustable sutures in strabismus correction. Am J Ophthalmol 1992;114:307–310.
11. Emergency Cardiac Care Committee and Subcommittees, American Heart Association. Guidelines for cardiopulmonary resuscitation and emergency cardiac care. VI. Pediatric advanced life support. JAMA 1992;268:2262–2274.
12. Gildea J. Crisis plan for pediatric codes. AJN 1986;568.
13. Lorber D, Tibaldi J. Care of the hospitalized patient with diabetes. Pract Diabetol 1987;6:16–17.

Bibliography

Agency for Health Care Policy and Research. Acute pain management in infants, children, and adolescents: operative and medical procedures. Rockville, MD, Public Health Service, US Department of Health and Human Services, 1992.

Agency for Health Care Policy and Research. Clinical practice guidelines for acute pain management: operative or medical procedures and trauma. Rockville, MD, Public Health Service, US Department of Health and Human Services, 1992.

Boyd-Monk H, Steinmetz C. Nursing care of the eye. Norwalk, CT, Appleton & Lange, 1987.

Burden B. Ambulatory surgical nursing. Philadelphia, WB Saunders, 1993.

Daniels N. HIV-infected professionals, patient rights, and the "switching dilemma." JAMA 1992;267:1368–1371.

Garrett G. A new lease of life: nursing care of elderly surgical patients. Prof Nurse 1992;81:15–8.

Goldblum K. Knowledge deficit in the ophthalmic surgical patient. Nurs Clin North Am 1992;27:715–724.

Ivey DF. Local anesthesia: implications for the perioperative nurse. AORN J 1987;45:682–689.

Kitz D, et al. Discharging outpatients: factors nurses consider to determine readiness. AORN J 1988;48:87.

Kwitko M, Weinstock F. Geriatric ophthalmology. Orlando, Grune & Stratton, 1985.

Litwack K. Managing postanesthetic emergencies. Nursing 91 1991;49–55.

Mackowiak L, McCarthy R. Managing diabetes on "sick-days." AJN 1989:950–951.

Meeker MH, Rothcock JC. Alexander's care of the patient in surgery, ed 9. St. Louis, Mosby–Year Book, 1991.

Miner DG. Anesthesia: the perioperative nurses role. Todays OR Nurse 1990;12:24–29.

Murphy M, DeBack V. Today's nursing leaders: creating the vision. Nurs Admin Q 1991;16:15–21.

Newbold P. Improve customers' perception of quality: communicate value. Trustee 1987:18–19.

Peplau, H. Interpersonal relationships in nursing. New York, Springer Publishing, 1991.

Puta DF. Nurse-physician collaboration toward quality. J Qual Assur 1989;3:11–18.

Ruehl C. Nursing care of the cataract patient. Nurs Clin North Am 1992;27:732–743.

Schremp P. Nursing management of the choroidal hemorrhage patient. Ophthal Nurs Forum 1986;2:4.

Smith S. Diabetic retinopathy. Nurs Clin North Am 1992;27:750–759.

Summers S, Ebbert D. Ambulatory surgical nursing: a nursing diagnosis approach. Philadelphia, JB Lippincott, 1992.

Thomson-Keith E. Care of the ophthalmology patient. Denver, Association of Operating Room Nurses, 1986.

Vaughan D, Asbury T, Tabbara K. General ophthalmology. Norwalk, CT, Appleton & Lange, 1989.

Watson D, James D. Intravenous conscious sedation: implications of monitoring patients receiving local anesthesia. AORN J 1990;51:1512–1522.

Watson ME, Fine IH. The first assistant's role in managing phacoemulsification complications. J Ophthal Nurs Technol 1991;10:172–186.

Zander K. Nursing case management: strategic management of cost and quality outcomes. J Nurs Admin 1988;18:23–30.

Ophthalmic Surgery Complications: Prevention and Management,
edited by Judie F. Charlton and George W. Weinstein.
J. B. Lippincott Company, Philadelphia © 1995.

7

Marilyn C. Kay
Jonathan Kay

Complications of Anesthesia for Ocular Surgery

CANCELLATION OF ADULT OCULAR SURGERY

Economic and social considerations have led to the conversion of most ophthalmic surgical procedures from an inpatient setting to an outpatient setting. Preoperative assessment occurs in the surgeon's office and by telephone evaluation from the anesthesiologist or his or her surrogate. Cancellation of the surgery deprives the patient of a timely operation, disrupts the operating room schedule, disrupts the surgeon's schedule, and may be avoidable. Most last-minute "medical" cancellations can be avoided if preoperative screening is appropriate from both the history and laboratory standpoints. Preoperative medication errors can be avoided if certain guidelines are followed.

An accurate current medical history must be obtained. The patient must be questioned about chronic conditions or the medications for their treatment. Hypertension, cardiovascular disease, and diabetes mellitus should be controlled and stable to avoid perioperative complications of anesthesia, whether regional or general anesthesia is planned. The use of a standardized questionnaire to detect changes in the patient's recent health may help the surgeon determine whether a visit with the patient's internist will result in better health before surgery (Table 7-1).[1,2] For example, recent shortness of breath, recent onset of ankle swelling, or a change in the patient's diabetic medication requirements must be addressed in advance of any elective surgery.

The increase in frequency of malignant hyperthermia in patients with strabismus makes this entity of particular interest to ophthalmologists.[3] Other factors in the history that may heighten the suspicion of such a medical condition include muscle cramps or abdominal cramping with caffeine use.[3] The history of death under anesthesia of a healthy young person in a patient's family raises the specter of malignant hyperthermia. The original records, if available, must be reviewed by an anesthesiologist, and the written reports of any muscle biopsy results should be obtained. Other reasons for an unexpected perioperative demise, such as sepsis, thyroid storm, or neuroleptic malignant syndrome, must be ruled out. Simply proceeding with a "malignant hyperthermia–safe" anesthetic is tempting but labels the patient, and perhaps his or her progeny, as susceptible to malignant hyperthermia, perhaps unnecessarily. The ready availability of dantrolene has reduced the mortality of malignant hyperthermia to less than 10%.[4]

Preoperative Laboratory Tests

Patients older than 60 to 70 years of age need a complete blood count (CBC), electrolyte panel, blood urea nitrogen or creatinine measurement, chest roentgenogram, and electrocardiogram (ECG). Electrolyte levels, especially the potassium determination, are particularly important in any patient on digoxin or diuretic therapy. If they are too low or too high, arrhythmias or heart problems may develop during surgery.[5] A high glucose level must be detected and controlled because the hyperglycemic brain is more prone to ischemic damage than a euglycemic one, should blood pressure drop during the opera-

Table 7-1
Preoperative Questions to Be Answered by the Patient

What prescription medications do you take?
What medications do you buy over the counter?
Do you or anyone in your family have bleeding problems?
Have you recently had chills, fever, or a cold?
Do you have muscle cramps?
Do you have stomach cramps from drinks containing caffeine?
Do you get up at night more than once to urinate?
Do you have heart trouble?
Do you have skipped heartbeats?
Do you have chest pain?
Do you take blood thinners, or aspirin or other arthritis medication?
Do you smoke?
Are you pregnant?
Do you cough? Do you have to sleep on several pillows to breathe?
Do you have seizures?
Do you have allergies to local anesthetics?
Do you or does anyone in your family get high fevers from anesthesia?
Is there a history of sickle cell trait or anemia in your family?

tion.[6] The age of 40 to 60 years is a gray area; a relatively healthy person may need only a CBC and ECG. Conversely, a smoker receiving diuretics and digoxin would need all the same laboratory investigations as a 70-year-old. In healthy patients under 40 to 50 years of age, little laboratory testing is required; again, exceptions exist if the patient is on chronic diuretic therapy or has a history of chronic illness. Otherwise, a CBC may be the only test needed for elective, relatively superficial surgery, such as most ophthalmic surgery (Table 7-2).[7–9]

An abnormal or suspicious spot on a chest roentgenogram rarely poses a significant threat to the patient undergoing anesthesia for eye surgery. However, this abnormality must be discussed with the patient at the time it is recognized. If an abnormality such as a new lesion, which may represent malignancy, is discovered on a chest roentgenogram, the risk–benefit ratio of delaying the exact diagnosis of the chest lesion versus delaying the desired elective eye surgery must be discussed with the patient and his or her family and personal physician.

The discovery of previously undiagnosed diabetes mellitus the day of ocular surgery represents a significant threat because if any unexpected neurologic event occurs perioperatively, the prognosis worsens in the presence of hyperglycemia.[6,10] Recommendations for management of hypokalemia have changed because of studies that show no danger from hypokalemia in the absence of cardiomegaly, cardiac arrhythmia, digoxin therapy, or known cardiovascular ischemia.[11,12] Hyperkalemia in an otherwise asymptomatic individual may be due to hemolysis of the blood sample. The most common cause of true hyperkalemia is drug therapy, not more exotic or

Table 7-2
Screening Studies That Should Be Performed Preoperatively for Asymptomatic Adults Undergoing Ocular Surgery*

AGE (y)	MALE	FEMALE
Under 40	None	Hemoglobin or hematocrit Urine pregnancy test
40–59	ECG BUN or creatinine Glucose	Hemoglobin or hematocrit ECG BUN or creatinine Glucose Possible urine pregnancy test
Over 60	Hemoglobin or hematocrit ECG BUN or creatinine Glucose Chest roentgenogram	Same as for male

BUN, blood urea nitrogen; ECG, electrocardiagram.

*In addition, any patients on diuretics must have serum potassium determined. Any patient with cardiac or pulmonary disease, or recent upper respiratory infection or a patient with a smoking history who is over 40 should have a chest roentgenogram.

dangerous causes such as Addison disease or uremia.[13]

Abnormalities in the ECG must be carefully evaluated despite the relatively stress-free nature of most elective ocular surgery. The consideration in elective situations is whether the patient is in as good a condition as possible for the procedure. Common abnormalities that may pose problems and lead to delay in surgery include new-onset atrial fibrillation, ST-T segment changes on the ECG signifying ischemia, evidence of new myocardial infarction, and premature ventricular contractions. New atrial fibrillation may be benign or may be a marker of significant ischemic disease, including myocardial infarction. Chronic lung disease, pulmonary emboli, or congestive heart failure can also be the cause of new-onset atrial fibrillation. Appropriate consultation and medical work-up is required when there is a finding of new atrial fibrillation.

ST-T segment changes on ECG signify ischemia, and the first order of business would be to compare these with old ECGs if available. Stable changes in an asymptomatic patient are less ominous than brand new changes in a patient with episodic chest discomfort. Similarly, the exact age of a myocardial infarction is medically important. The incidence of reinfarction decreases to a risk of 5%, 6 months after the original myocardial infarction.[14–16]

Although more than five premature ventricular contractions per minute is associated with an increased perioperative morbidity, premature ventricular contractions must be considered in the context of the patient's history. Are potassium and magnesium levels normal? Are there symptoms of ischemia? Is there cardiomegaly on a chest roentgenogram? Premature ventricular contractions can occur in the setting of substance abuse, such as alcohol, caffeine, or cocaine use. Considerable judgment must be used in the decision to proceed in such circumstances with elective surgery.[17]

Medications to Be Continued the Day of Surgery

There is always a question as to what medications the patient should continue right up through the morning of surgery and what medications the patient should discontinue. The following is a guideline for commonly prescribed medications.

Patients should generally continue taking antihypertensive agents up to the time of surgery to avoid rebound hypertensive crises with the associated myocardial compromise that may occur. Such medications include transcutaneous clonidine, oral β-blockers, calcium-channel blockers, and angiotensin-converting enzyme inhibitors. These medications can be taken with a sip of water the day of surgery despite the nothing-by-mouth (NPO) status of the patient.[18]

Digoxin can be withheld if the patient tends to be bradycardic and if the intended anesthetic technique and surgical procedure might induce further bradycardia. For example, a patient scheduled to undergo strabismus surgery who has a resting heart rate of 45 beats/min should not take the digoxin the morning of surgery. However, a patient who is receiving digoxin to help control ventricular heart rate response to atrial fibrillation should receive the normal dose of digoxin the morning of surgery. However, it is easier for the anesthesiologist to slow the patient's heart rate down with additional doses of digoxin during the procedure than to speed it up. If the patient's digoxin level is too high and the heart rate too low, the placement of a temporary pacemaker may be required.

The patient's routine antiseizure medications should be administered the morning of surgery with a sip of water, because stress and particularly general anesthesia can provoke seizures in those patients who are susceptible.[19]

The patient who has taken corticosteroids for more than 1 month within the 6 months to 1 year before the surgery traditionally is covered with the equivalent of 300 mg of hydrocortisone. One hundred milligrams is administered intravenously (IV) at the start of the case, an additional 100 mg is given IV at the end of the procedure, and another 100 mg is given IV 6 hours after the end of the procedure. However, investigators have suggested lower doses, in the range of 25 to 30 mg IV, for procedures associated with minimal physiologic stress.[20]

The automated glucose measuring devices now available to patients have made the management of diabetes easier. For short procedures, a "no insulin, no glucose" policy works well with close monitoring of the blood glucose perioperatively. In addition, during the procedure, intravenous solutions without dextrose, such as normal saline, are given. After the procedure, the patient receives a portion of his or her usual insulin after demonstrating successful calorie intake (usually one half to two thirds of the usual daily dose of insulin). For longer procedures (2 hours or more), insulin should be given as an infusion of at least 4 U/h of regular insulin with close glucose monitoring every 30 minutes. Alternatively, for longer procedures or for patients who tend to have higher blood glucose levels, a quarter to a half of the patient's long-acting insulin is given at the end of the procedure, and blood glucose level is measured every 30 minutes. If the glucose is over 200 mg/dL, an insulin drip is added.[20] An anesthesiologist and internist may necessarily be involved to help manage blood glucose levels in the recovery area in patients with diabetes, such as those described earlier.

Although thyroid medications have a long half-life, they should be continued on the day of surgery.[21]

Medications to Be Omitted on the Day of Surgery

Oral antihyperglycemics should be omitted the day of surgery because of their long duration of action, which could lead to hypoglycemia late in the day if the patient's caloric intake has not risen on schedule after surgery has been completed.

Diuretics also should be omitted the day of surgery. A patient having a local procedure may become uncomfortable from the full bladder caused by taking the dose of diuretic before coming to the operating room. Because of the preoperative fasting required by most anesthesiologists, a patient under general anesthesia may be unacceptably hypotensive as the result of a diuretic and having had inadequate fluid intake before the induction of anesthesia.

Administration of drugs that interfere with platelet function, such as aspirin or the nonsteroidal antiinflammatory agents (ibuprofen, indocin, naproxen, and sulindac), should be discontinued for the duration of one platelet life-span, at least 7 days. Similarly, warfarin therapy should be discontinued until the prothrombin time has returned to normal unless the patient has an artificial heart valve. In the case of an artificial heart valve, especially a mitral valve, warfarin sodium is discontinued until the prothrombin time reaches 15 seconds. Heparin therapy then is started and infused until 2 hours preoperatively.[22] Heparin and warfarin administration is restarted after 12 to 24 hours of normal hemostasis postoperatively. An internist must be involved in management of patients with heart valve disorders to determine the appropriate level of anticoagulation drugs.

Another drug that some have recommended stopping before surgery is nicotinic acid because it can cause an exaggerated hypotensive response in patients that take such a vasodilator.[23] This vasodilation occurs during general anesthesia.

Monoamine oxidase inhibitors, although not as popular as they once were for treatment of depression, are still in use. To avoid the exaggerated hypertensive response to indirect-acting, systemically released vasopressors that occurs during general anesthesia especially, administration of these medications should be stopped for 2 to 3 weeks before anticipated elective surgery.[24]

CANCELLATION OF PEDIATRIC OCULAR SURGERY

Is a CBC or any other laboratory screening necessary in a child undergoing elective eye surgery? There is no evidence that abnormalities on a CBC impact on the choice of management of anesthesia in asymptomatic children.[25] A family history of sickle trait or sickle disease is significant because some aspects of anesthetic management that change in such patients. Other laboratory work, such as bleeding time or routine urinalysis, is unnecessary in the healthy child and serves only to traumatize the youngster in his or her interaction with medical personnel.[25]

There are certain issues in pediatric patients that should be addressed to avoid cancellation of pediatric ocular surgery at the last minute. The question always arises in performing surgery on children as to when to proceed with the child who apparently has an upper respiratory infection. There is a great deal of difference between a healthy child with allergic rhinitis who "always looks like this" according to the parents and the child with a temperature higher than 38°C with a sore throat, malaise, and anorexia. Making the parents aware of the dangers of proceeding with general anesthesia in the patient with an upper respiratory infection usually is sufficient to temper their disappointment at having to delay the elective procedure. The ophthalmologic follow-up of a sick child when the elective surgery is carried out is unpleasant under the best of circumstances, because the patient will feel worse than usual postoperatively. The presence of fever postoperatively is difficult to interpret. The presence of nasal discharge may endanger the results of the surgery should the infective discharge enter the ocular area. We recommend that part of the preoperative teaching of the parents should include discussion of the symptoms of an upper respiratory infection so that a trip to the hospital, only to determine that the child is too sick to proceed with surgery, can be avoided.

How long should a child be on NPO status before receiving an anesthetic? The preoperative fast is uncomfortable for adults and children alike and somewhat risky for children less than 2 years of age. Young children and infants may become dehydrated and hypoglycemic easily if kept on NPO status for longer than 4 to 6 hours. The purpose of preoperative fasting is to reduce particulate matter in the stomach and lower the gastric fluid volume and acidity should aspiration of the stomach contents occur. Allowing clear liquids as late as 2 hours before surgery does not adversely affect the volume or pH of gastric contents, and it makes the experience for the patient more comfortable.[18,26,27]

PREVENTION OF COMPLICATIONS OF LOCAL ANESTHESIA

History of Allergy

The patient reporting an allergy to all of the "caines" has frequently had an intravascular injection of epinephrine, a vasovagal attack, or even a panic attack rather than a true allergic reaction. True allergic reactions occur, but are extremely rare, being less than 1% of local anesthetic reactions.[28,29] A careful history is critical in making the correct diagnosis. Sweating, tachycardia ("My heart was pounding"), headache, and hypertension all suggest intravascular injection of epinephrine. Conversely, an overdose of local anesthetic produces tinnitus, a bad taste in the mouth, and central nervous system changes such as confusion, slurred speech, or respiratory arrest. The hallmarks of a true allergic reaction to a "caine" include wheezing, urticaria, and respiratory distress.

True allergy to local anesthetics is more likely with the ester derivatives such as procaine, tetracaine, chloroprocaine, and benzocaine.[29] Confounding the issue of allergies to local anesthesia is the allergic response that may occur to the preservative paraben, which is widely used in multidose vials of local anesthetics and is also found in cosmetics, foods, and as a preservative for other medications.[30] Skin testing in advance of the day of a prospective operation by appropriate personnel with adequate monitoring and resuscitation equipment nearby is desirable in patients suspected of an allergy to local anesthetics.[31] If the patient demonstrates an ester allergy, xylocaine, bupivacaine, or mepivacaine should be used as an alternative local anesthetic.

Local anesthetic injection into the retrobulbar space can lead to an accidental perforation of the globe or retrobulbar hematoma.[32–34] It is not the purpose of this discussion to address basic techniques in giving local anesthetic injections. The reader is directed to basic texts in ocular surgery for discussion of the techniques for retrobulbar injection, peribulbar injection, van Lint block, and Nadbath block for facial akinesia. A disturbing complication of anesthetic injection into the retrobulbar space, respiratory arrest, is one with which the reader should be acquainted. Case reports of apnea, respiratory arrest, and cranial nerve palsies in the eye being injected and on the opposite side from the retrobulbar injection began to surface in the anesthesia and ophthalmology literature in the early 1980s.[35–37] Anatomic studies of the position of the retrobulbar needle in relation to the optic nerve when the adducted and supraadducted position of the eye is used during injection showed that it was possible to inject into the subdural space with a standard Atkinson-type needle.[38–40] The cases of respiratory arrest or cranial nerve palsies in association with respiratory difficulties represent actual brain-stem anesthesia from injection of the anesthetic agent into the subdural space, with subsequent dissection into the circulating cerebrospinal fluid and the occurrence of depression of the reticular formation and dysfunction of cranial nerves in the involved area. One way to avoid such complications involves changing the traditional positioning of the eye during the retrobulbar anesthetic injection so that the nerve is rotated away from the track of the needle rather than moving the eye so that the nerve is directly in the way of the needle as occurs in the typically adducted and supraadducted position.[40–42]

If the eye is kept in its primary position looking straight ahead, the retrobulbar optic nerve moves more medially and coils loosely in the orbit out of the way of an advancing retrobulbar needle. Likewise, using less sharp, nondisposable retrobulbar needles that are short (less than 1.25 in.) lessens the chance of perforating the optic nerve sheath, which would result in injection into the subarachnoid space.[42] Although the concentration of the anesthetic has been implicated as the source of the respiratory arrest in one series, it is more likely that a larger volume, and therefore a larger total dose of anesthetic in that volume, was delivered to the brain stem through an advertent subdural injection.[43]

Should apnea or respiratory arrest or cranial neuropathies occur subsequent to a retrobulbar injection, it is imperative that the patient be supported with mechanical ventilation, including intubation if necessary, to keep him or her adequately oxygenated. Fortunately, apnea seldom lasts more than 30 to 50 minutes, but during that time, it is important that the patient be stabilized by medical personnel experienced in such situations. Less serious respiratory complications may be treated successfully by an oral airway and ventilatory assistance with a mask. Often, if the patient recovers from the respiratory event, surgery can proceed without sequelae.

The peribulbar technique for anesthesia of the eye during ocular surgery was devised partly to avoid the complications mentioned from retrobulbar injections. To our knowledge, respiratory arrest has not been reported secondary to peribulbar injections, but retrobulbar hematomas or perforation of the eye can still occur.[33]

Respiratory distress and dysphagia can occur from the Nadbath block, an injection of the stylomastoid foramen, which is used to provide facial akinesia.[44,45]

The complications occur when, in the process of injecting the anesthetic agent in the area of the facial nerve as it exits the stylomastoid foramen, the anesthetic agent is injected more deeply and bathes cranial nerves IX, X, and XI as they exit the jugular foramen (Fig. 7-1). This leads to paralysis of these nerves, and the patient becomes dysphagic, coughs, has a hoarse voice, and develops stridor or severe respiratory insufficiency. This complication tends to occur in thin individuals where it is easier to bury the needle deeply because there is little subcutaneous fat in the area. Management of the respiratory distress requires suctioning of the pharynx, repositioning the patient on his or her side, and supplementing inspired gases with oxygen by nasal cannula or even intubation of the trachea.

Precautions suggested to decrease the chance of respiratory distress after a Nadbath block include using a short hypodermic needle and advancing this needle only partway into the area to be injected to avoid delivery of the anesthetic agent deeper than the stylomastoid foramen. Use of a small volume of solution (less than 3 mL) also helps avoid this complication.[45]

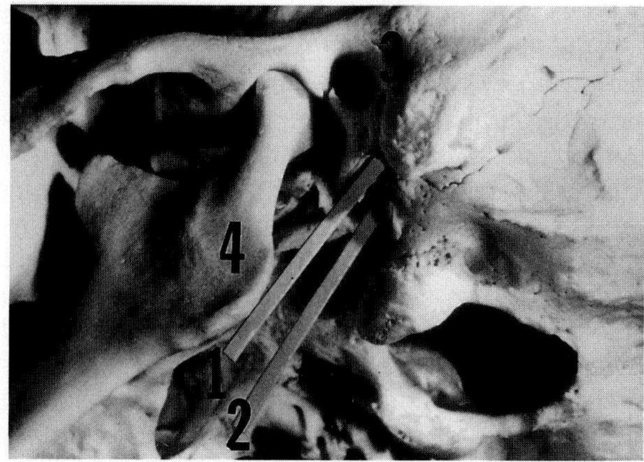

Figure 7-1. Note stylomastoid foramen (1), jugular foramen (2), Int. auditory meatus (3), and left mandible (4) on skull in right lateral decubitus position.

Systemic Toxicity From Local Anesthetics

Anesthetic toxicity can occur when a high concentration per milliliter of local anesthetic agent is given.[28] For example, it is the custom in some centers to use 4% xylocaine for a peribulbar injection. If the peribulbar injection is not successful the first time, there may be a temptation on the part of the surgeon or anesthesiologist to reinject the area. It does not take a large volume of 4% xylocaine to reach the toxic xylocaine dose where central nervous system dysfunction and cardiac depression can occur.[28] The total volume of 4% xylocaine that can safely be given to a 70-kg patient, for example, is limited to 7.5 mL. Likewise, a smaller individual would be able to tolerate no more than 5 mL of 4% xylocaine in the peribulbar area or other area for injection.

Complications From Sedation

Respiratory Arrest With Intravenous Sedation

Respiratory arrest after intravenous sedation can occur with any of the agents commonly used. Small increments given IV have a larger safety margin than one large increment that depresses the patient's respiratory apparatus to the level that intubation is required. For example, titrated increments of midazolam, 0.5 mg every 1 to 2 minutes; propofol, increments of 10 mg IV; or pentothal, increments of

25 mg IV are useful and avoid the problems with overdosage, such as respiratory difficulties, confusion, or lack of patient cooperation that can jeopardize the upcoming surgery. If respiratory arrest occurs with IV midazolam, flumazenil is available for reversal in the dosage of 0.1 to 0.2 mg IV. However, flumazenil is associated with the occurrence of seizures in patients, most often in those who are habituated to benzodiazepines. Propofol can be "reversed" by turning off the IV drip and supporting the patient with oxygen or assisted ventilation if necessary. Likewise, if there is an overdosage of barbiturate, the patient must be supported with assisted ventilation or intubation until he or she becomes responsive.

Preoperative Sedation in Children

It is difficult to avoid traumatizing a child in the process of sedating him or her. An optimal anesthetic is one that the child does not recall. Giving the child some preoperative sedation that will not delay discharge to home is preferred. In a child who can take juice in a cup, oral midazolam, 0.4 to 0.75 mg/kg in 5 mL of juice or cherry acetaminophen syrup 30 minutes before the anticipated surgery, leads to a relaxed, cheerful child who has no memory of the holding area or the operating room.

Rectal methohexital, 20 to 30 mg/kg, or midazolam, 0.3 mg/kg, can be given by rectal catheter about 1 hour before surgery. When the child reaches the expected level of calmness, the drug remaining in the rectum can be withdrawn by aspiration of the small catheter.[46]

PREVENTION OF COMPLICATIONS OF GENERAL ANESTHESIA

Malignant Hyperthermia

Malignant hyperthermia* is a hypermetabolic disorder of skeletal muscle characterized by intracellular hypercalcemia. This intracellular derangement results in acidosis, membrane destruction, and ultimately death if not treated. Malignant hyperthermia presents clinically as an elevation of expired carbon dioxide, "inappropriate" tachycardia, increased muscle tone, peripheral skin mottling, cyanosis, and sweating. Because of the extraordinary use of oxygen, the blood on the surgical field becomes extremely dark. The use of succinylcholine during intubation accelerates this syndrome. All of the inhalational agents have been implicated as triggering agents for malignant hyperthermia.[47]

As mentioned in the section on preoperative screening, a high level of suspicion and a careful history help the clinician anticipate the need for treatment.

Because stress may trigger the reaction, anxiolytic agents such as opioids, benzodiazepines, barbiturates, antihistamines, and anticholinergics are recommended preoperatively.

Intravenous dantrolene sodium, 2.5 mg/kg, should be administered to a patient waiting in the holding area 30 minutes before the anticipated surgery (when there is a documented prior episode of malignant hyperthermia). Further dantrolene administration after the surgery is not recommended in such a patient, but the patient must be observed for 4 to 6 hours.[47] In other malignant hyperthermia–susceptible patients, the use of a "safe" anesthetic and a safe machine, with vigilance for any heart rate or carbon dioxide elevation is sufficient. A safe anesthesia machine is prepared by draining or removing the vaporizer, changing the tubing, changing the carbon dioxide absorbent, and flowing oxygen at 10 L/min for 20 minutes through the machine.[47]

Local anesthesia with either ester or amide anesthetics is safe. IV propofol is considered safe. Nitrous oxide is a "weak" triggering agent.[47] Should an acute malignant hyperthermia crisis be recognized during the case, it is imperative to stop the surgery and administration of all inhalational agents, discontinuing the use of succinylcholine, if applicable. The patient is hyperventilated with 100% oxygen, and the dantrolene is mixed as soon as possible. The patient is packed with external ice packs; gastric, rectal, and wound (if applicable) ice lavage is carried out as well. In extreme cases, iced peritoneal lavage and even cardiopulmonary bypass has been used to aggressively cool the patient who triggers a malignant hyperthermia attack. Urine output must be measured by Foley catheter because of the risk of myoglobinuric acute renal failure. Complications of exces-

**The telephone number for the Malignant Hyperthermia Hotline is 209-634-4917.*

sive bleeding must be watched for as disseminated intravascular coagulation is a risk.

The most common side effects of dantrolene sodium are nausea, weakness, and phlebitis.

Nausea and Vomiting

Pediatric patients experiencing nausea and vomiting in the recovery area can receive 0.075 mg/kg of droperidol IV.[46] There is no evidence that a dose of droperidol prolongs recovery from strabismus surgery.[48] The adult dosage is 0.625 to 1.25 mg IV push of droperidol.[46] Alternative strategies for nausea and vomiting control include the use of metoclopramide 100 μg/kg IV in children and 10 to 15 mg IV in adults.[46]

Ondansetron has also been shown to lower the incidence of gastric distress postoperatively in the pediatric outpatient population (adult dose, 4 to 8 mg IV push; pediatric dose, 0.15 mg/kg IV push).[49]

Excess Sedation

The use of "balanced" general anesthesia in which small amounts of several different types of medications are titrated to avoid the side effects of large doses of any one type has been effective in reducing prolonged anesthesia.

Neuromuscular blocking agents of short duration (12 minutes for mivacurium) and intermediate duration (30 minutes for atracurium and vecuronium) administered with an infusion pump allow the anesthesiologist to fine-tune the degree of neuromuscular blockade during balanced anesthesia. This fine-tuning avoids having the surgery end before the neuromuscular blocking agents can be reversed.

The shorter-acting narcotics, such as sufentanil, have potencies up to a 1000 times that of morphine. Alfentanil has an offset that is so rapid that it is frequently used as a continuous infusion in shorter ocular cases. These agents help provide short-term stability of hemodynamics during intense stimulation without the cost of prolonged excessive sedation. Their use immediately before intubation as part of an anesthetic induction has become virtually universal.

MANAGEMENT OF COMPLICATIONS OF LOCAL ANESTHESIA

Seizures

Seizure secondary to the intraarterial injection of local anesthetic agent into the ophthalmic artery can occur from retrograde flow of the anesthetic into the cerebral circulation.[50] Most such seizures are short-lived. As little as 1.8 mL of 2% lidocaine has been reported to produce such a seizure. Such seizures are instantaneous with injection and should be supported with airway maintenance and blood pressure support.[51]

Restlessness

The causes of restlessness during regional anesthetic should be sought rather than simply sedating the patient. Elderly patients who are deaf are extremely challenging when they are covered by the operating room drapes. Placing a stethoscope in the patient's ears may allow him or her to communicate with the anesthesiologist speaking into the stethoscope head. Common problems are the need to void, discomfort on the operating table (a small amount of narcotic IV is indicated), and feeling smothered (turn up the airflow under the drape or place a cool towel on the patient's exposed arm for diversion). Low-dose propofol at 5 to 20 μg/kg/min has been effective in reducing restlessness, but the dangers of oversedation must be recognized.

Nausea and Vomiting

Additional caveats regarding control of nausea and vomiting are that because metoclopramide may cause a dystonic reaction, it is recommended that the first dose be given under the supervision of a physician in the recovery area. Both metoclopramide and ondansetron do not cause sedation as droperidol does.

Urinary Retention

Urinary retention is caused by the anticholinergic challenge of some drugs such as droperidol and atropine combined with a rapid IV fluid bolus that can distend the patient's bladder, especially men with prostatism. Urinary retention is a common cause for restlessness in the recovery room and should be treated by placement of a Foley catheter.

Blood Glucose and Electrolyte Management

All diabetics should have their blood glucose levels checked before and after the surgical procedure. Small doses of regular insulin may be required to bring their glucose levels below 200 mg/L postoperatively, and this requires the input of the anesthesiologist or an internal medicine physician.

Hypokalemia below 3.5 mg/L must be treated.

Coughing

If the patient begins to cough either during the surgical procedure or in the recovery room, lidocaine, 1 mg/kg IV, may be effective in decreasing the cough. Extubating the patient "deeply" during general anesthesia or the use of a laryngeal mask airway during general anesthesia may prevent coughing from laryngeal irritation.

Hypertension

Postoperative hypertension can occur from three causes: noxious stimuli, adverse physiology in the patient, and medications. Noxious stimuli include pain, anxiety, a full bladder, and the presence of an endotracheal tube. Removing the stimulus works better than the medical therapy of the hypertension.

Adverse physiologic conditions that predispose to hypertension include hypercarbia, hypoxemia, hypoglycemia, congestive heart failure or pulmonary edema, and increased intracranial pressure. The treatment is clear once the diagnosis of the abnormal physiology is made. Medications, or their absence, can cause postoperative hypertension. The patient may be due for a dose of medication or may have missed a scheduled dose the morning of surgery. Sympathomimetic agents used for the treatment of asthma during the case may also cause postoperative hypertension. Medications used for the treatment of postoperative hypertension are given, in consideration of the patient's heart rate and whether he or she already has bronchospastic disease or cardiac disease. Carefully titrated doses of IV labetalol, apresoline, and verapamil are commonly used. These agents must be given under the supervision of the anesthesiologist or internist.

Eye Pain

Eye pain in same-day adult surgical patients may be treated by either intramuscular or IV ketorolac, at the dose of 30 to 60 mg, or with small carefully titrated doses of fentanyl, 25 to 50 μg IV. Longer-acting narcotics like morphine or demerol may delay the patient's discharge because of excessive sedation.[52]

References

1. Berger, JJ. The patient for outpatient surgery. Problems in Anesthesia 1991;5:613.
2. Roizen MF. Pre-operative evaluation. In: Miller RD, ed. Anesthesia, ed 3. New York, Churchill Livingstone, 1990:743.
3. Durbin CG. Malignant hyperthermia syndrome: identification and management. In: Berry FA, ed. Anesthetic management of difficult and routine pediatric patients. New York, Churchill Livingstone, 1990:399.
4. Miller JD, Lee C. Muscle diseases. In: Katz J, Benumof JL, Kadic LB, eds. Anesthesia and uncommon diseases. Philadelphia, WB Saunders, 1990:626.
5. White PF. Pre-operative evaluation and premedication of ambulatory surgery patients. Refresher Courses in Anesthesiology 1991;19:219.
6. Pulsinelli WA. Increased damage after ischemic stroke in patients with hyperglycemia with or without established diabetes mellitus. Am J Med 1983;74:540.
7. Kaplan EB, Sheimer LB, Boeckmann AJ. The usefulness of pre-operative laboratory screening. JAMA 1985;253:3576.
8. Neelan M, Roizen MF. Laboratory testing. Probl Anesth 1991;5:575.
9. Warner MA, Shields SE, Chute CG. Major morbidity and mortality within one month of ambulatory surgery and anesthesia. JAMA 1993; 270:1437.
10. Longstreth WT, Inui TS. High blood glucose level on hospital admission and poor neurological recovery after cardiac arrest. Ann Neurol 1984;15:59.
11. Vitez TS, Soperle LE, Wong KC. Chronic hypokalemia and intraoperative dysrhythmias. Anesthesiology 1985;63:130.

12. Hirsch IA, Thomlinson DL, Slogoff S. The overstated risk of pre-operative hypokalemia. Anesth Analg 1988; 67:131.
13. Rimmer JM, Horn JF, Gennari FJ. Hyperkalemia as a complication of drug therapy. Arch Intern Med 1987;147:867.
14. Tarhan S, Moffitt CA, Taylor WF, Guilani E. Myocardial infarction after general anesthesia. JAMA 1972; 220:1451.
15. Steers PA, Tinker JH, Tarhan S. Myocardial reinfarction after anesthesia and surgery. JAMA 1978; 239:2566.
16. Rao TLK, Jacobs KH, El-Etr AA. Reinfarction following anesthesia in patients with myocardial infarction. Anesthesiology 1983;59:499.
17. Ross AF, Tinker JH. Cardiovascular disease. In: Brown D, ed. Risk and outcome in anesthesia. Philadelphia, JB Lippincott, 1992:39.
18. Stoelting RK. NPO and aspiration pneumonitis: changing perspectives. Refresher Course in Anesthesiology. 1993;21:41.
19. Stoelting RK, Dierdorf SF, McCammon RL. Diseases of the nervous system. In: Stoelting RK, ed. Anesthesia and co-existing disease, ed 2. New York, Churchill Livingstone, 1987:335.
20. Kay J. Endocrine disorders. In: Cheng EY, Kay J, eds. Anesthesia and the medically compromised patient. Philadelphia, JB Lippincott, 1990:362.
21. Roizen MF. Diseases of the endocrine system. In: Katz J, Benumof JL, Kadis LB, eds. Anesthesia and uncommon diseases. Philadelphia, WB Saunders, 1990:260.
22. Florete OG, Gallagher TJ. Cardiac disease: congestive heart failure, coronary artery disease, and valvular disease. In: Cheng EY, Kay J, eds. Anesthesia and the medically compromised patient. Philadelphia, JB Lippincott, 1990:2.
23. Roizen MF. Anesthetic implications of concurrent disease. In: Miller RD, ed. Anesthesia, ed 3. New York, Churchill Livingstone, 1990:874.
24. El Ganzouri AR, Ivankovich AD, Braverman B, McCarthy R. Monoamine oxidase inhibitors: should they be discontinued pre-operatively? Anesth Analg 1985;64:592.
25. Mulroy JJ, Lynn AM. The medical evaluation of pediatric patients. Semin Anesth 1992;11:200.
26. Schreiner MS, Triebwasser A, Keon TP. Ingestion of liquids compared with pre-operative fasting in pediatric outpatients. Anesthesiology 1990;72:593.
27. Bready LL, Solomon DE. Preparation for surgery. Probl Anesth 1991;5:386.
28. Sobol WM, McCrary JA. Ocular anesthetic properties and adverse reactions. Int Ophthalmol Clin 1989; 29:195.
29. Aldrete JA, Johnson DA. Evaluation of intracutaneous testing for investigation of allergy to local anesthetic agents. Anesth Analg 1970;49:173.
30. McLeskey CH. Allergic reaction to an amide local anesthetic. Br J Anesth 1981;53:1105.
31. Arora S, Aldrete JA. Investigation of possible allergy to local anesthetic drugs. Anesthesiol Rev 1976:13.
32. Grizzaid WS, Kirk NM, Pavan PR, Antworth MV, Hammer ME, Roseman RL. Perforating ocular injuries caused by anesthesia personnel. Ophthalmology 1991;98:1011.
33. Hay A, Flynn HW, Hoffman JI, Rivera AH. Needle penetration of the globe during retrobulbar and peribulbar injection. Ophthalmology 1991;98:1017.
34. Edge KR, Nicoll JMV. Retrobulbar hemorrhage after 12,500 retrobulbar blocks. Anesth Analg 1993; 76:1019.
35. Rosenblatt RM, May DM, Barsoumian K. Cardiopulmonary arrest after retrobulbar block. Am J Ophthalmol 1980;90:425.
36. Myers EF. Brainstem anesthesia after retrobulbar block. Arch Ophthalmol 1985;103:1278.
37. Beltraneva HP, Vega MJ, Garcia JJ, Blakenship GB. Complications of retrobulbar marcaine injection. J Clin Neuro Ophthalmol 1982;2:159.
38. Unsold R, Stanley JA, DeGroot J. The CT-topography of retrobulbar anesthesia. Albrecht von Graefes Arch Klin Ophthalmol 1981;217:125.
39. Drysdale DB. Experimental subdural retrobulbar injection of anesthetic. Ann Ophthalmol 1984;16:716.
40. Smiddy WE, Michels RG, Kumar AJ. Magnetic resonance imaging of retrobulbar changes in optic nerve position with eye movement. Am J Ophthalmol 1989;107:82.
41. Morgan CM, Schatz H, Vine AK, et al. Ocular complications associated with retrobulbar injections. Ophthalmology 1988;95:660.
42. Katser DA, Drews RC, Rose BT. An anatomic study of retrobulbar needle path length. Ophthalmology 1989;96:1221.
43. Wittpenn JR, Rapoza P, Sternberg P, Kuwaskemia A, Saklad J, Patz A. Respiratory arrest following retrobulbar anesthesia. Ophthalmology 1986;93:867.
44. Wilson CA, Ruiz RS. Respiratory obstruction following the Nadbath block facial nerve block. Arch Ophthalmol 1985;103:454.
45. Koenig SB, Snyder RW, Kay J. Respiratory distress after a Nadbath block. Ophthalmology 1988;95:1285.
46. Morrison JE, Lockhart CH. Pre-operative fasting and medication in children. Anesth Clin North Am 1991;9:731.
47. Rosenberg H, Fletcher J, Seitman D. Pharmacogenetics. In: Barash PG, Cullen BF, Stoelting RK, eds. Clinical anesthesia, ed 2. Philadelphia, JB Lippincott, 1992:589.

48. Lerman J, Eustis S, Smith DR. Effect of droperidol pretreatment of post-anesthetic vomiting in children undergoing strabismus surgery. Anesthesiology 1986; 65:322.
49. Lawhorn CD, Brown RE, Schmitz ML, et al. Prevention of post-operative vomiting in pediatric outpatient strabismus surgery. Anesthesiology 1993;79:A1196.
50. Aldrete JA, Roma-Sales F, Arora S. Inadvertent arterial blood flow as a pathway for central nervous system toxic responses following injection of local anesthetics. Anesth Analg 1978;57:428.
51. Meyers EF, Ramierz RC, Boniu KI. Grand mal seizures after retrobulbar block. Arch Ophthalmol 1978; 96:847.
52. Hammonds WD, Donnigan D. Clinical use of ketorolac tromethamine. Probl Anesth 1993;7:268.

Ophthalmic Surgery Complications: Prevention and Management,
edited by Judie F. Charlton and George W. Weinstein.
J. B. Lippincott Company, Philadelphia © 1995.

David S. Rho
Milton Kahn
Stephen A. Obstbaum

8

Complications of Cataract Surgery

Cataract surgery is one of the most successful surgical procedures performed in medicine. As in any discipline, however, complications can and do occur. This chapter provides an approach to the prevention, diagnosis, and management of many complications associated with cataract surgery, focusing particularly on those accompanying phacoemulsification.

PREOPERATIVE EVALUATION

The preoperative assessment of a patient with an operable cataract is important in planning the surgical procedure. The information obtained from a comprehensive ophthalmic examination of the patient with a cataract may prevent or minimize the occurrence of untoward situations during the surgical procedure. The patient's past medical and ophthalmic history, use of topical and systemic medications, family history of medical disease, and allergic history are essential elements of the preoperative evaluation.

Several specific aspects of the comprehensive examination are particularly germane in preparation for cataract/intraocular lens (IOL) surgery. The condition of the scleral tissue often determines the type of surgical incision. Patients with rheumatoid arthritis, for example, may have thinned sclera as a consequence of scleromalacia. This condition could influence the ophthalmologist to select an alternative incision site or to perform a corneal incision.

Clarity and health of the cornea are essential elements to assess preoperatively for technical modifications ensuring excellent visibility during surgery and preservation of endothelial health after surgery. In addition, the determination of whether to perform a cataract/IOL procedure alone or in combination with a penetrating keratoplasty is generally made preoperatively and discussed with the patient.

The effect of pupil dilation can be assessed at this time as well. A pupil that dilates widely usually facilitates cataract surgery. Pupils that do not dilate adequately require intraoperative iris surgery or the use of devices that can stretch the pupil sufficiently to ensure uncomplicated surgery.[1,2]

Anterior chamber depth is assessed to determine the ease of the surgical procedure. Anatomically shallow anterior chambers are often associated with anteriorly inserted iris roots that may cause iris prolapse during surgery. In addition, asymmetric anterior chamber depths may indicate zonular laxity of the crystalline lens.

The appearance of the crystalline lens and the characteristics of the cataract are important to note during the examination. The extent of cataract formation and density of the lens as reflected in the degree of brunescence might influence the strategy for removing the cataract. The skill and experience of the ophthalmologist often dictate the surgical approach. Iridodonesis, phacodonesis, and asymmetry of anterior chamber depth are signs of loose zonules and suggest formulation of a preoperative plan for cataract surgery. These findings are more frequently observed in eyes with exfoliation syndrome.

In eyes in which a surgeon has performed vitrectomy, and in eyes with loosened zonules, an excessively deep anterior chamber may develop with phacoemulsification. Identification of these eyes and appropriate chart notation can permit modifications in technique that normalize surgery.

PREOPERATIVE COMPLICATIONS

Corneal Abrasion

Visualization of intraocular structures is a key element in successful intraocular surgery. Preservation of corneal clarity is, therefore, a desirable goal for surgery. Disruption of the corneal epithelium limits clear visibility. Care should be taken to ensure corneal clarity during presurgical preparations, including povidone-iodine (Betadine) preparation, drape placement, and lid speculum insertion.

Retrobulbar Hemorrhage

Recent trends in topical anesthesia for cataract surgery notwithstanding, orbital hemorrhage can be associated with retrobulbar injection and less commonly with peribulbar injection.

The earliest signs of retrobulbar hemorrhage include a tense, immobile globe that gives firm resistance to retropulsion, taut eyelids, diffuse subconjunctival hemorrhage, and, at times, ecchymosis of the lids. Direct or indirect ophthalmoscopy should be performed to assess the status of the central retinal artery. The goal of treatment of this condition is to maintain patency of the central retinal artery by reducing the pressure head against it.

Management includes the use of topical β-blockers and intravenous carbonic anhydrase inhibitors or hyperosmotics. A lateral canthotomy can be performed if the lids are tense and the globe protuberant. If the intraocular pressure is not sufficiently lowered by the preceding techniques, anterior chamber paracentesis may be performed. Any sources of active bleeding should be attended to, with direct orbital pressure applied to facilitate hemostasis. The decision to terminate the procedure or to continue with surgery depends on the ability to reverse the findings mentioned earlier, and to create a relatively normal state. If this result is readily accomplished, surgery can continue.[3] If, however, the orbit remains full, the globe cannot be retropulsed, and the lids are taut, it is prudent to postpone the surgery until later.

Globe Trauma

Perforation of the globe, although rare, may occur during retrobulbar anesthesia.[4] Sudden softening of the eye and collapse of the posterior chamber are the hallmarks of this occurrence. Myopic eyes with a longer axial length are more susceptible to this injury during peribulbar or retrobulbar anesthesia. In this instance, the surgery should be stopped, and the patient should be referred to a vitreoretinal specialist for further evaluation and management.

INTRAOPERATIVE COMPLICATIONS

Orbital Adnexa

Inadvertent trauma to the eyelids, superior rectus, and levator occur infrequently perioperatively or intraoperatively. Injury may include hemorrhage, neurapraxia, or direct tissue damage. Bridal suture placement has been implicated as a potential cause of damage to the superior rectus or to the closely apposed levator complex, which may result in postoperative ptosis.

Conjunctiva and Episclera

The conjunctiva and episclera are relatively forgiving structures. Significant manipulation and surgical injury to these tissues are tolerated both functionally and cosmetically because they regenerate rapidly after surgery. Significant distortion of anatomy and scarring will, however, prove important if concomitant or future glaucoma-filtering procedures are planned.

Cornea

Descemet Membrane Detachment

Detachment of Descemet membrane may occur during the insertion of any instrument into the anterior chamber, especially large instruments, such as the phacoemulsification or irrigating–aspirating (I–A) tips. The occurrence of Descemet membrane detachment is greater with a relatively shallow anterior chamber, because there is less space between the cornea and iris.

This complication may be avoided by the careful insertion of instruments into the anterior chamber, with all instruments directed posteriorly through the corneoscleral incision, avoiding the corneal endothelium and Descemet membrane. The phacoemulsification or I–A tips should be in irrigation-only mode during instrument insertion, and the phacoemulsification tip is usually introduced with the bevel down. Injection of a viscoelastic material increases the space between the cornea and iris, facilitating the atraumatic entry of instruments. If persistent restriction of instrument movement is observed after successful insertion of the instrument into the eye, the incision should be enlarged to prevent obstruction of flow into the anterior chamber.

Descemet membrane detachment may also occur during IOL insertion. It is important to recognize that the internal aperture of the wound may differ significantly from the length of the external opening. Less commonly, if a partial detachment of Descemet membrane occurs and is unnoticed by the surgeon, it may be accidentally or mistakenly engaged as a cortical remnant, and the detachment may extend. Descemet detachment has occurred as a consequence of a clear corneal incision and subsequent instrumentation through the incision.

If a relatively small Descemet membrane detachment occurs, repair is not generally necessary. The corneal stroma usually remains clear overlying the detachment, and visibility is not compromised. If a significant portion of Descemet membrane becomes detached, the detached portion can be reposited to its normal anatomic position by the injection of either viscoelastic material or air central to the detachment. Inadvertent injection of the viscoelastic material between Descemet membrane and the corneal stroma prevents reappositioning of these two layers and may actually extend the Descemet detachment. A second instrument introduced through a paracentesis incision can also be used to assist in repositioning a localized Descemet detachment. However, direct contact with the corneal endothelium should be avoided if possible. A large Descemet membrane detachment can be repositioned by suturing it to the stroma.

Endothelial Trauma

Trauma to the corneal endothelium usually occurs from either direct contact by an instrument or from nuclear fragments that are liberated during phacoemulsification. In both instances, some degree of protection to injury of the endothelium is afforded by the use of viscoelastic materials that coat or bind to the endothelium, and create space in the anterior segment. Trauma secondary to nuclear fragments created during phacoemulsification is also less likely with the capsulorhexis and in situ phacoemulsification techniques.

Anterior Chamber Hyphema

Intraocular blood can limit both intraoperative visualization and postoperative visual acuity. Other potential complications of blood in the anterior chamber include premature miosis intraoperatively; delayed or incomplete miosis at the end of surgery; and an increased risk of corectopia, pupillary capture, IOL decentration, and posterior capsule opacification postoperatively. Finally, intraocular hemorrhage increases the severity and duration of the postoperative inflammatory response.

Although the issue is somewhat controversial, preoperative discontinuation of aspirin and anticoagulants is appropriate for eyes in which a conventional incision is contemplated. In instances in which anticoagulants cannot be discontinued, a corneal incision can be performed. In addition, an attempt should be made to avoid temporal, posterior, or deep incisions because the blood vessels encountered in these locations tend to be larger in caliber.

Conjunctival and episcleral bleeding is minimized by cauterizing vessels before entering the anterior chamber. Active bleeding sites on the conjunctiva or episclera may be treated by direct pressure, clamping with forceps, cautery, or topical epinephrine. If bleeding is noted after passing a needle during suturing, hemostasis can sometimes be achieved simply by tying the suture.

An important cause of hyphema is an iridodialysis. The bleeding tends to be brisk because the major iris circle comprises blood vessels near the iris root that are large in caliber. An iridodialysis usually occurs when the iris is inadvertently engaged by an instrument or IOL being passed into the anterior chamber. This result is more likely to occur when the chamber is shallow or if there is increased posterior pressure.

Bleeding from the iris or angle is managed by irrigating the blood from the eye with balanced saline or depressing the posterior lip of the corneoscleral incision. Other adjuncts to hemostasis in iris bleeding include intraocular epinephrine irrigation, and air or viscoelastic agent injection in an attempt to tamponade an obvious intraocular source of bleeding. The infusion bottle height may also be raised to help tamponade the bleeding. Direct cauterization of vessels can be attempted if all the previously cited measures fail.

Iris

During the preoperative evaluation, the surgeon determines the suitability of the patient for phacoemulsification or extracapsular cataract extraction (ECCE), considering the nature of nuclear hardness, related ocular conditions, and the relative ease and completeness of pupil dilatation. Various techniques to widen the pupil are available to facilitate phacoemulsification. These include radial sphincterotomy, multiple sphincterotomies, sector iridectomy, or the use of devices to widen the pupillary aperture, such as iris retractors[1,2] (Fig. 8-1).

A major concern occurring during phacoemulsification is iris prolapse. This situation usually occurs with a wound that is placed near the iris root and can be avoided if the entry into the anterior chamber is made somewhat corneal. Once iris prolapse occurs, it is recurrent during the procedure and may be troublesome. It is often wise to suture this incision and make another one to complete the phacoemulsification. In those instances in which iris prolapse has occurred, the wound construction is often inadequate to permit a sutureless, self-sealing closure. The corneoscleral wound should be closed with deeply placed sutures to minimize the risk of iris incarceration postoperatively. The peripheral iris tissue can be swept toward the pupil to ensure that no tissue is incarcerated in the wound.

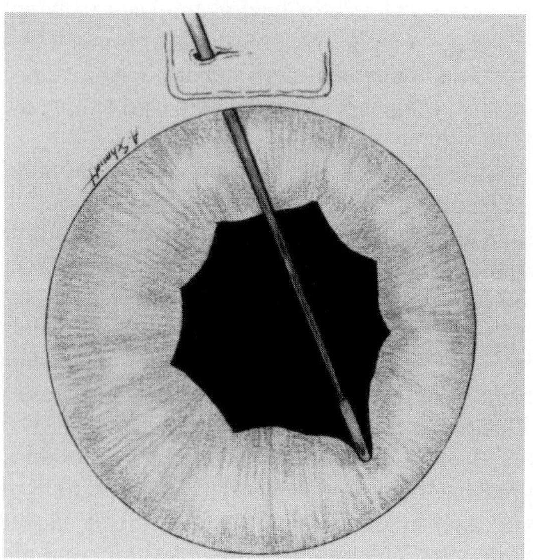

Figure 8-1. Illustration demonstrating Fine's technique for pupil widening, in which the iris is stretched, creating minor iris sphincter tears in multiple locations. (Courtesy of Howard Fine, MD) (See color plate after page xvi.)

Sphincter tears may occur during ECCE nucleus expression. In planned ECCE, if the pupil does not dilate adequately before nucleus expression, some form of pupil widening can be performed.

Iris trauma may result in depigmentation and flaccidity of the iris, predisposing to the development of iris incarceration, corectopia, and peripheral anterior synechiae formation. The iris retraction syndrome also develops as a consequence of these circumstances. Cystoid macular edema may occur as a late complication of iris trauma.

Several measures may minimize inadvertent iris trauma. Preoperative administration of a cyclooxygenase inhibitor maintains pupil dilatation, as does nonpreserved epinephrine delivered through the infusion bottle. A viscoelastic agent maximizes the space between the iris and the cornea, and widens the pupil. The anterior chamber is entered in irrigation mode to push the iris posteriorly and facilitate entry of the phacoemulsification tip. The phacoemulsification tip may be introduced bevel down initially to avoid engaging the iris. The bevel may then be rotated up, after advancing the tip so that it is within the center of the pupil.

Lens

Extension of Anterior Capsulotomy Radial Tear

The conventional can-opener anterior capsulotomy consists of multiple small radial tears. During other portions of the extracapsular procedure, nucleus removal, and irrigation and aspiration, these small tears can extend to the lens equator and, at times, even extend to the posterior capsule. Similar events can also occur with the so-called envelope technique. Other factors contributing to the development of radial tears include insufficient corneoscleral wound length and an anterior capsulotomy opening that is too small, each of which may cause greater resistance to nucleus expression during ECCE; significant posterior pressure; and high pressure of the I–A bottle.

CAPSULORHEXIS. Capsulorhexis is a method of creating a smooth-edged, continuous tear capsulotomy that obviates many of the problems arising with the can-opener type of anterior capsulotomy.

Capsulorhexis is easier to perform with a stretched anterior capsule and deepened anterior chamber. The use of a viscoelastic material is advocated to maintain chamber depth, although Blumenthal has alternatively suggested the use of an anterior chamber maintainer with constant flow.[2a] In an anterior chamber of appropriate depth, a carefully performed capsulorhexis can be successfully performed in a predictable manner. If the capsulorhexis tear begins to move peripherally, it frequently reflects a shallowing of the anterior chamber and an increase in posterior pressure. Once this problem is recognized, one can stop the capsulorhexis, refill the anterior chamber with viscoelastic material, and then attempt to continue the capsulotomy. If an anterior capsular tear extends radially and is too peripheral to be recovered, repeated efforts to redirect the tear circumferentially may cause further peripheral extension of the tear. There are two options to manage this situation. One can return to the origin of the capsulorhexis to create a second continuous circumferential tear in the opposite direction as the original tear. A small tangential cut with Vannas scissors is often helpful to start the second tear (Fig. 8-2). A second alternative is to use the multiple-puncture, can-opener technique to connect the remaining unconnected portions of the capsulotomy. Should this latter option be used, however, nuclear cracking should not be performed because a risk of extending a capsular tear to the equator exists.

A capsulorhexis that is too small compromises the ease of nucleus removal and makes aspiration of the superior cortex more difficult. These potential problems with a small capsulorhexis may be alleviated by enlarging the capsulorhexis. The technique for expanding the size of the capsulorhexis is similar to that described as the first option earlier. For ECCE, a cystotome or Vannas scissors may be used to create relaxing radial incisions at the 2- and 10-o'clock positions, acknowledging that these incisions may themselves extend peripherally during nucleus expression.

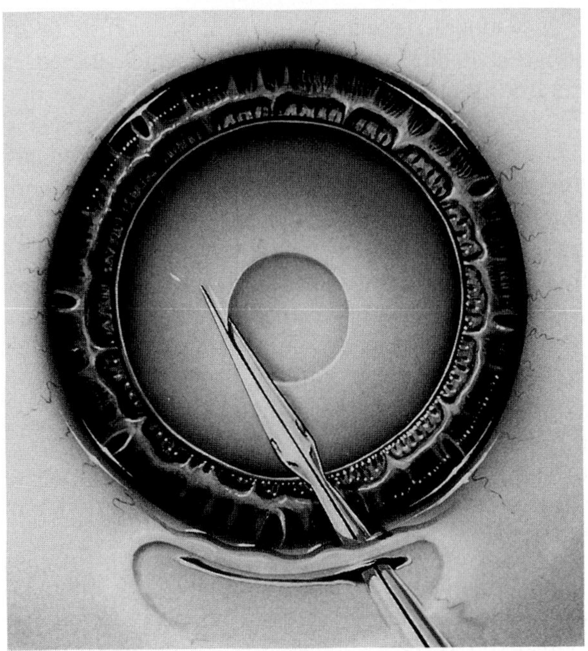

Figure 8-2. Illustration demonstrating the use of Vannas scissors to create a new tear in a capsulorhexis that is thought to be too small. This same technique may be used to create a second tear in patients in whom control of the initial capsulorhexis has been lost and cannot be recovered. (Courtesy of Howard Gimbel, MD)

Posterior Capsular Tear

A tear in the posterior capsule may occur during various stages of cataract surgery. Posterior capsular tear and vitreous loss increase the risk of postoperative sequelae, including the development of cystoid macular edema and retinal detachment. However, with appropriate recognition and proper surgical management, a posterior chamber IOL (either in the ciliary sulcus or in the capsular bag) can be implanted, and a good surgical outcome can be anticipated.

In several conditions, posterior capsular tears develop more frequently: brunescent cataract, Morgagnian cataract, and cataracts in younger patients. Brunescent cataracts are characterized by harder nuclei and may be associated with weakened zonules.

Morgagnian cataracts are characterized by a liquefied cortex and a dense nucleus that is situated in the inferior portion of the capsular bag. During the capsulotomy, the liquefied cortex escapes after the initial anterior capsular puncture, causing a generalized laxity of the lens and making it more difficult to complete the capsulotomy. The escaping liquefied cortex obscures a clear view of the capsule and also allows the posterior capsule to move anteriorly. Zonular weakness is also a common finding that further complicates the capsulotomy and may eventuate in a posterior capsule tear.

In younger patients, the lens cortex tends to be adherent to the posterior capsule, which increases the risk for an inadvertent posterior capsule tear during cortical cleanup. In addition, decreased scleral rigidity occurs in younger patients as well as a greater tendency for scleral collapse and secondary anterior chamber shallowing. Greater elastic and intrinsic intralenticular forces exist at the site of zonular attachment, not only increasing the chance for posterior capsule tear but also making the management of a posterior capsule tear more difficult.

MANAGEMENT. In general, management of posterior capsular tears depends on the period during the surgery when the rent or tear is noted, presence of vitreous in the anterior chamber, and experience of the surgeon.

Posterior Capsule Tears During ECCE. Although it is unlikely for capsular rupture to occur before nucleus expression, if a posterior capsule tear is noted before nucleus removal, steps should be taken to remove the nucleus atraumatically from the eye without widening the posterior capsular defect. Nuclear material is poorly tolerated in the vitreous cavity and may be associated with an intense inflammatory reaction and ultimately a retinal detachment.

Either a Sheets glide or a high-viscosity viscoelastic material can be used to cover the posterior capsule tear, both to protect the posterior capsule from additional trauma, and to prevent the loss of nuclear or cortical material into the vitreous. A second instrument can help direct the nucleus or nuclear fragments away from the posterior capsule tear. An anterior vitrectomy should then be performed, meticulously removing all formed vitreous from the corneoscleral wound and anterior chamber.

Posterior Capsule Tears During Phacoemulsification. If a tear in the posterior capsule is encountered during phacoemulsification, the decision to continue phacoemulsification of the nucleus or convert to an ECCE depends on the skill and experience of the surgeon. If one elects to convert to ECCE, the nucleus fragments can be removed with a lens loop. Alternatively, if the surgeon decides to continue with phacoemulsification, use of a viscoelastic agent to tamponade a small rent or insertion of a Sheets glide to block a larger one often permits successful completion of phacoemulsification. Another management option includes the conversion of a linear posterior capsule tear into a continuous round capsulorhexis. A second instrument may be used either to direct nuclear remnants away from the posterior capsule tear or block the posterior capsule rent physically to prevent the loss of nuclear material into the posterior chamber.

Low emulsification power, low fluid flow, low vacuum, and a lowered bottle height are used after a posterior capsule tear to minimize the risk of nucleus fragment loss posteriorly, posterior capsule movement, anterior chamber shallowing, and vitreous hydration and subsequent prolapse.

Loss of Nucleus Into the Vitreous Cavity. Loss of the lens nucleus into the vitreous is relatively rare but requires prompt attention (Fig. 8-3). Management depends on the surgeon's experience with vitreoretinal techniques. For surgeons who do not usually perform vitreoretinal surgery, we recommend thoroughly clearing the anterior segment of residual nuclear and cortical material, as well as vitreous, while maintaining as much of the anterior and posterior capsules as possible. A posterior chamber IOL can be implanted at this time. The wound is closed appropriately and the patient referred to a vitreoretinal surgeon for pars plana nucleus removal. In those instances in which the surgeon is adept with vitreoretinal surgery, the nucleus can be removed by means of a pars plana or combined approach at the time of the primary surgery.

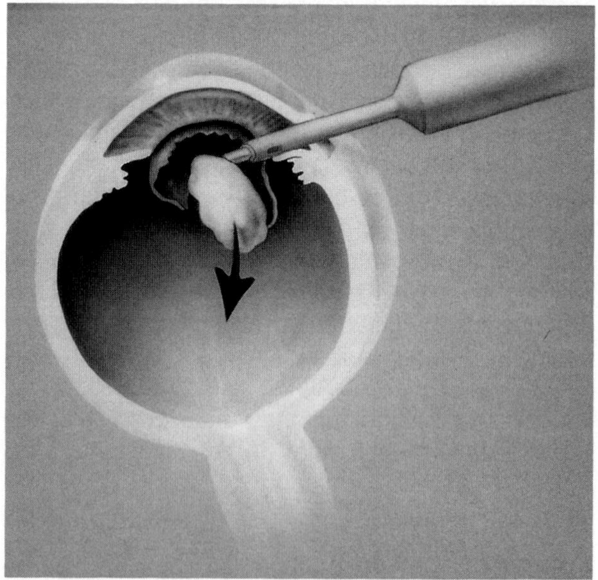

Figure 8-3. Illustration demonstrating loss of the nucleus into the vitreous cavity during phacoemulsification as a result of a rupture of the posterior capsule. (Courtesy of George Weinstein, MD)

Posterior Capsule Tears During Cortical Cleanup. When a posterior capsule tear occurs during cortical cleanup, the surgeon should weigh the potential risks in pursuing residual cortex and causing additional trauma to the posterior capsule and zonules. In most cases, leaving cortex behind is well tolerated, and it often resorbs over time.[5]

If the capsular bag is particularly tenuous, and only a small amount of cortex is present, we recommend foregoing extensive cortical cleanup. If further cleanup is necessary, one should minimize stress to the capsular bag, removing only as much cortex as can be easily aspirated, without further manipulation of the capsular bag.

Cortical material remote from the posterior capsular tear should be removed first. Any movement of the I–A tip and cortical stripping should be directed toward the rent to prevent extension of the tear or propagation of a zonular dialysis in the vicinity of the tear.

Low infusion and aspiration rates should be used to minimize fluid flux within the eye, which may create convection forces directed at the posterior capsule and extend a posterior capsule tear; this approach also minimizes anterior chamber shallowing, vitreous hydration, and prolapse. Extreme caution is exercised in the area of the posterior capsular tear, and the surgeon should consider leaving cortical material if it appears to be present at or adjacent to a portion of the posterior capsule that is clearly absent or where zonular integrity is in question.

Because irrigation can hydrate the vitreous and widen a posterior capsular tear, the "dry" cortical cleanup technique should be considered. A viscoelastic material is injected into the anterior chamber and then aspiration is performed, either manually or with the automated aspiration handpiece with the irrigation port disconnected. Alternatively, aspiration may be performed with the simultaneous low infusion of saline or viscoelastic agent through a second site.

Zonular Dialysis

Preoperative evaluation may reveal several clues that zonular integrity is compromised, most important of which are phacodonesis and iridodonesis. Weakened or absent zonules cause lens and iris tremulousness with eye movements. Visible vitreous strands in the anterior chamber also indicate imperfect zonular integrity in the anterior chamber. Less subtle signs are the edge of the lens visible within the pupil, indicative of a greater degree of zonular dialysis sufficient to cause lens subluxation. Unequal chamber depths are also indicative of lens luxation.

Among the risk factors associated with zonular dialysis are Marfan syndrome, homocysteinuria, Weill-Marchesani syndrome, microspherophakia, and pseudoexfoliation syndrome.

Some degree of zonular disruption is a frequent occurrence during ECCE. Wilson and colleagues[6] studied the zonular integrity of 27 postmortem eyes, 20 of which had undergone ECCE. All the zonules associated with at least one major ciliary process were found to be disinserted in 45% of the eyes that had undergone ECCE, and 25% of eyes had all of the zonules associated with 5 to 14 adjacent ciliary processes disrupted. Zonular disruption is likely to occur during ECCE, but disruption is clinically apparent in only a small percentage of the cases.

Skuta and associates[7] reported five cases in which ECCE had been performed in patients with known pseudoexfoliation syndrome. All five patients developed zonular rupture intraoperatively, three with complete zonular rupture and the remaining two patients with partial zonular rupture—despite large pupillary apertures created by sector iridectomies or complete radial sphincterotomies. It is notable that despite extensive zonular dialyses, the anterior hyaloid face remained intact in all five patients, thus suggesting that zonular dialysis, even if complete, is not always associated with vitreous loss. At many different points during cataract extraction, a zonular dialysis can occur.

During capsulorhexis or a can-opener capsulotomy, a radial tear may extend peripherally to the lens equator, with subsequent zonular dialysis. If this occurs, care should be taken to avoid subsequent aspiration of the torn portion of the anterior lens capsule during the remainder of the case.

Zonular dialysis may occur during hydrodissection, or viscodissection and delineation of the lens nucleus, when a bolus of fluid may extravasate through a preexisting site of weakness in the equatorial lens capsule. This problem may also occur during nucleus rocking or expression during ECCE, nucleus cracking in cases of phacoemulsification, and irrigation and aspiration if a shard of lens capsule is inadvertently aspirated. Finally, zonular dialysis may occur during IOL insertion, when the entire capsular bag is placed under stress.

Once zonular dialysis has occurred, the principles for management are similar to that for a posterior capsule tear. Phacoemulsification and cortical irrigation and aspiration should be performed under low power and flow rates. Any intraocular manipulation should be initiated away from the site of zonular dialysis but with the forces directed toward the zonular dialysis to prevent further extension of the dialysis.

IOL Insertion After Posterior Capsular Tear

After cortical cleanup and, if necessary, anterior vitrectomy, one must decide where the intraocular lens should be placed. The anterior and posterior lens capsules should be clearly visualized and their structural integrity assessed.

In a case in which a small tear has occurred in the central posterior capsule but has not extended toward the periphery (ie, zonular integrity is intact), then the IOL may be placed directly within the capsular bag.

Similarly, if a tear has extended to the periphery but fewer than 5 clock hours of zonular integrity are absent, one may still consider IOL placement in the capsular bag. In this case, the posterior capsular bag should be inflated with viscoelastic material, taking care not to inject too much, and the haptics placed as far away from the tear as possible to avoid extending the tear. Once the IOL has been placed into the capsular bag, it should not be rotated because this approach can also extend the tear and increase the risk of losing IOL into the vitreous.

For most instances in which any tear has occurred in the posterior capsule, an IOL with a relatively large optic without holes should be selected. This choice is appropriate given the increased likelihood for subsequent IOL decentration secondary to either asymmetric posterior capsule contraction after posterior capsule tears or decreased zonular integrity in the case of zonular dialysis.

If a posterior capsule tear is large, has peripheral extensions, or if the extent of the posterior capsule tear is poorly visualized, then the anterior lens capsule should be assessed for the suitability for IOL placement in the ciliary sulcus. The IOL power for ciliary sulcus placement should be decreased by 0.5 diopter from the original calculations based on placement of the IOL in the posterior capsule bag.[8]

Viscoelastic material should be injected just under the iris to collapse the capsular bag (Fig. 8-4). As with capsular bag IOL insertion, the IOL should be inserted to minimize stress on the intact remaining zonules, with the haptics oriented away from areas of zonulysis.

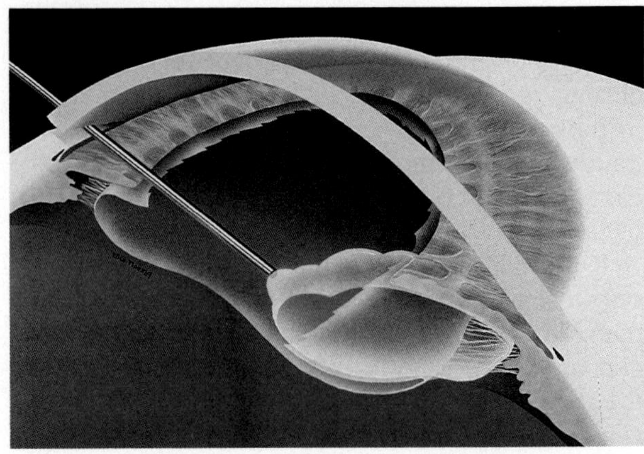

Figure 8-4. Illustration demonstrating the use of viscoelastic agent to widen the ciliary sulcus in preparation for implantation of the intraocular lens (IOL) within the ciliary sulcus. (See color plate after page xvi.)

Once the IOL has been placed in the ciliary sulcus, one can test IOL fixation and centration by gently displacing the IOL optic toward its haptics and observing for spontaneous recentering (the so-called bounce-back test).[9] If the IOL does not spontaneously recenter, the IOL should be rotated to a different axis.

If after rotation the IOL remains poorly fixated or centered, one must consider either a scleral-fixation IOL or an anterior chamber IOL. Alternatively, one may consider suturing only one of the haptics, provided that the zonules 180 degrees away from the sutured haptic are intact.

If significant defects of both the anterior and posterior lens capsules are observed, an IOL should be placed in the anterior chamber. The IOL power should be decreased 1.5 to 2.0 D from the original calculations based on IOL placement in the posterior chamber.

If the patient has known corneal endothelial disease or low endothelial cell counts, or significant preexisting damage to angle structures, an anterior chamber lens would be less desirable, and one may consider scleral fixation of the IOL.

Management of Residual Viscoelastic

At the conclusion of surgery in which a posterior capsule tear has occurred, an important decision arises regarding any viscoelastic agent that had been injected into the eye intraoperatively. Any attempt at removal of viscoelastic material risks the creation of intraocular pressure flux.

One option is to leave the viscoelastic agent in the eye at the end of surgery, expecting a transient 10- to

30-mmHg intraocular pressure elevation for the first 24 to 48 hours postoperatively. The pressure rise may be managed with topical β-blockers and oral carbonic anhydrase inhibitors, but the viscoelastic material eventually absorbs spontaneously regardless of medical therapy.

If the patient has a known history of glaucoma or optic neuropathy, whereby intraocular pressure elevation may be more poorly tolerated, one may elect to remove the viscoelastic material at the end of surgery. Viscoelastic materials are most effectively removed with the I–A unit, although some lower-molecular-weight agents can be removed manually, with a syringe and simultaneous injection of saline.

Vitreous Loss

Measures to prevent vitreous loss include limiting posterior pressure and avoiding sudden changes in anterior chamber volume by controlled nucleus expression during ECCE, the use of low phacoemulsification power, and low I–A rates during cortical cleanup. Jaffe and associates[10] reported a 3% incidence of vitreous loss, however, even by experienced surgeons.

Guzek and colleagues[11] reported that the only significant risk factor for the occurrence of both zonular breaks and vitreous loss was insufficient pupil dilatation preoperatively. In their study of 1000 ECCE cases, they reported a 2.8% incidence of vitreous loss in patients with pupils larger than 6 mm compared with an incidence of 5.9% in patients with pupils smaller than 6 mm. They also confirmed the generally accepted fact that zonular breaks, although not necessarily vitreous loss, occurred more commonly with pseudoexfoliation syndrome. They did not find high myopia, advanced cataract, glaucoma, advanced age, or diabetes mellitus to be risk factors for capsular breaks, zonular breaks, or vitreous loss.

If vitreous loss is suspected, a thorough assessment of the surgical wound and anterior chamber should be performed for the presence of cortical vitreous. A dry cellulose sponge may be placed at the scleral incision, which, if gently pulled, demonstrates a spinbarkeit effect; viscous strands adhere to the sponge if vitreous is present at the wound. One may also see distortion of the pupil if vitreous is present in the anterior chamber when the preceding procedure is performed. Alternatively, a spatula may be gently swept over the pupil and reveals pupillary movement if vitreous is present in the anterior chamber.

If vitreous is found at the surgical wound or in the anterior chamber, then a vitrectomy should be performed using an automated vitrector. The goal is the complete removal of vitreous from both the surgical wound and the anterior chamber. The guillotine action of the vitrector, with brief intervals of alternating aspiration and cutting, ensures a minimal amount of net tractional forces imparted to the vitreous. Signs that the anterior chamber is clearing of vitreous include the restoration of a round pupil, settling of a previously drawn-up pupil posteriorly, and an increase in the ease of aspiration through the vitrectomy port.

If an automated vitrector is not available, then manual vitrectomy should be performed. The cellulose sponge should be placed as far into the wound as possible to ensure that it is free of formed vitreous; however, it should be displaced a minimal distance from the wound before cutting it flush with the scleral surface to avoid traction on the retina. Manual vitrectomy should be performed until the surgical wound is found to be completely free of vitreous.

Complications of vitreous loss include vitreous incarceration, with the potential for impaired wound healing, epithelial or fibrous downgrowth, corneal stromal edema secondary to vitreocorneal touch, iritis, glaucoma, vitreous hemorrhage, cystoid macular edema, retinal detachment, and proliferative vitreoretinopathy.

Retina

Intraoperative retinal complications are relatively few. Photic maculopathy has become more common with the greater light intensity capability of modern operating microscopes. The key factor in the development of photic maculopathy is the intraoperative surgical time.[12] Once the cataractous lens, which acts as a natural light filter, is removed, one should attempt to minimize potential damage to the retina. This goal is accomplished by the use of a light filter in all aspects of the surgery that do not require precise intraaxial visualization.

Expulsive Choroidal Hemorrhage

Expulsive choroidal hemorrhage is one of the most dreaded complications of cataract surgery. Taylor[13] reported an incidence of 0.2% in 1974. Histopathologic studies have demonstrated that rupture of the posterior ciliary arteries is the underlying pathophysiologic event responsible for the development of expulsive choroidal hemorrhage.[14] The leading theory is that the sudden hypotony secondary to surgical decompression of the globe leads to rupture of the blood vessels, most commonly occurring during the delivery of the lens nucleus in an ECCE. Although its cause is most likely multifactorial, reported risk factors include advanced age, uveitis, glaucoma, hypertension, atherosclerotic heart disease, myopia, an acute rise in systemic blood pressure intraoperatively, intrinsic vascular fragility, anticoagulation therapy, and a history of expulsive choroidal hemorrhage in the fellow eye.[10]

The first clinical signs of expulsive choroidal hemorrhage include a suddenly firm eye, with anterior chamber shallowing. The patient may then complain of pain, despite previously adequate anesthesia. The rapidity with which the hemorrhage progresses reflects the briskness of the choroidal bleeding.

If the process is gradual, the surgeon may notice a loss of the red reflex and, through the pupil, may observe a dark mass steadily increasing in size. Indirect ophthalmoscopy may confirm the presence of the hemorrhage in this case.

As the hemorrhage progresses, the intraocular pressure increases, and the intraocular contents start to bulge forward. Initially, the iris, followed by the lens, vitreous, and eventually the retina prolapse anteriorly.

If hemorrhaging is brisk, the intraocular contents may be extruded rapidly, and there may not be sufficient time for suturing. In this case, digital pressure may be the only means available to prevent the complete extrusion of the intraocular contents. A bolus of intravenous mannitol should be given to shrink the intravascular and intravitreal volume. Suturing should be performed as soon as the eye is sufficiently soft to do so, using 7-0 suture material. Smaller-gauge suture material may cut through the tissue or break under positive pressure.

Choroidal blood flow is not autoregulated and is dependent, in part, on intraocular pressure. The rate of choroidal hemorrhage can, therefore, theoretically be diminished by raising intraocular pressure. This result may be accomplished by continuing external pressure on the eye.

Once the eye has been closed by suturing, prolapsed tissue can be reposited into its normal anatomic position. The anterior chamber can be reformed with viscoelastic material or saline.

If the anterior chamber cannot be reformed or if the eye cannot be sutured closed, one should attempt to drain the blood in the suprachoroidal space by radial sclerotomies via the pars plana, 3 to 4 mm posterior to the limbus, in one to four quadrants, depending on the extent of the angle closure.[15] As the suprachoroidal drainage is performed, the anterior chamber is simultaneously reformed with the injection of saline or viscoelastic through a self-sealing limbal stab incision. Once hemostasis has been achieved, the sclerotomy sites should be closed and the case terminated.

Choroidal detachments often extend to the posterior pole, with insertion adjacent to the optic disc. Several authors[16–18] report localized choroidal hemorrhagic detachments, with limited aggregate pooling in the suprachoroidal space. Because the hemorrhage is localized in these cases, there is the chance for sparing of central visual acuity if the choroidal hemorrhage does not involve the fovea. Head positioning may be attempted to prevent gravitational extravasation of the subretinal blood under the fovea. In severer cases, the choroidal detachments adhere centrally to produce a "kissing choroidals" configuration.

The patient should be examined serially by B-scan ultrasound postoperatively for the progression or regression of the choroidal hemorrhage. Numerous studies have shown that the clotted choroidal blood usually diminishes in size over time, as the blood is gradually resorbed by the body.[19] If a large amount of blood persists over time in the subretinal space and in particular subfoveally, a vitrectomy with internal evacuation of the subretinal blood may be considered.

An expulsive choroidal hemorrhage may occasionally occur within the first few days after surgery, with the patient complaining of the sudden onset of severe pain and pressure behind the eye. Maumenee and Schwartz[20] have proposed that this complication is secondary to the gradual enlargement of an intraoperative choroidal detachment, with the eventual rupture of the choroidal blood vessels.

If a patient is thought to be at risk for an expulsive choroidal hemorrhage, several precautionary steps may be undertaken. These include the following: lowering the preoperative intraocular pressure to as close to zero as possible, lowering the patient's systemic blood pressure intraoperatively, adequate lid and globe akinesia, patient positioning to minimize posterior pressure, the use of preplaced sutures, the slow, controlled delivery of the lens nucleus, and the placement of additional sutures at the conclusion of surgery.[10]

In those patients who are at particular risk, one should consider phacoemulsification, given that the incidence of expulsive choroidal hemorrhage is rare with phacoemulsification.[21]

POSTOPERATIVE COMPLICATIONS

Endophthalmitis

Because endophthalmitis is covered in a separate chapter in this book, we discuss only those points regarding endophthalmitis that are pertinent to cataract surgery.

The onset of symptoms of endophthalmitis after cataract surgery is usually sudden, with pain and decreased visual acuity within 1 to 4 days postoperatively. The initial symptoms may be difficult to differentiate from routine postoperative iritis and intraocular inflammation, as both produce conjunctival and episcleral injection, in addition to cells and flare in the anterior chamber.

An evolving endophthalmitis, however, usually declares itself with the rapid progression of intraocular inflammation, with the development of a hypopyon and progressive involvement of the posterior segment. The most common organisms causing acute bacterial endophthalmitis in cataract surgery are *Staphylococcus epidermidis*, *Staphylococcus aureus*, and *Streptococcus viridans*.[10] Gram-negative bacterial organisms are particularly rapid in their presentation, with severe intraocular inflammation present within 24 hours.

Bacterial endophthalmitis may also present as a delayed process, with similar organisms responsible for both the more typical acute and less common delayed presentations. In particular, *Propionibacterium acnes* may cause a delayed-onset, prolonged inflammation after ECCE with posterior chamber lens implantation.[22,23] Histopathologic studies demonstrate that this organism may remain sequestered in the posterior capsular bag,[23] thus making the diagnosis difficult.

The source of bacteria in typical cases of acute bacterial endophthalmitis include the patient's normal flora of the eyelids, cilia, and conjunctiva. Numerous preoperative surgical preparations have been proposed, each of which effectively reduces the incidence of postcataract endophthalmitis.[24]

Potential mechanisms increasing the risk of delayed postoperative endophthalmitis include the "vitreous wick syndrome," full-thickness sutures, loosely placed sutures, overly tight sutures with secondary tissue necrosis, removal of a deep or full-thickness suture, and filtering blebs, whether planned or unplanned. Treatment depends on making a prompt diagnosis. One study reported that a specimen obtained at the time of vitrectomy was significantly more likely to yield a positive culture in cases of clinically apparent endophthalmitis than a specimen obtained by means of a vitreous paracentesis.[25]

Cornea

Wound Leak

Postoperative wound leaks occur less commonly today as a result of improved surgical techniques, instrumentation, and suture materials. However, problems in either the creation or the closure of the wound may increase the possibility of a wound leak.

With small-incision phacoemulsification, wound competence is imparted by the creation of a beveled, self-sealing corneal valve.[26] If, however, repeated instrumentation occurs, the corneoscleral wound may be rendered incompetent, and suturing may be necessary.

In cases of ECCE, it is important to create a precise, uniform groove and beveled entrance into the anterior chamber. Any irregularities in the creation of the wound, including damage to or missing tissue, may predispose to the development of a postoperative wound leak.

Suturing technique, including correct suture depth, spacing, and tightness, are also critical to optimal wound closure. For example, sutures that are not placed radially may result in closure of noncorresponding sections of the wound, with secondary kinking and wound incompetence.

Signs suggestive of a postoperative wound leak include hypotony, a conjunctival bleb or diffuse chemosis, and anterior chamber shallowing. The fundus should be examined to detect the presence of a choroidal detachment.

Management of a postoperative wound leak should start with a trial of pressure patching. Many wound leaks respond to 24 to 48 hours of pressure patching, with the gradual recovery of normal intraocular pressure and anterior chamber depth as wound healing and wound competence ensue.

If pressure patching fails to correct a wound leak, or if there is contact between intraocular structures or the IOL and the corneal endothelium, surgical closure should be undertaken. Viscoelastic material may be injected into the anterior chamber to protect the corneal endothelium, restore the anterior chamber, and prevent peripheral anterior synechiae formation, and to help restore the intraocular pressure to a normal level.

One should consider a prophylactic suture or sutures in patients with known organic brain disease or ambulatory difficulties. These patients are at increased risk of inadvertent trauma to their eye in the postoperative period.

Corneal Edema

Corneal stromal edema is most commonly a transient postoperative phenomenon secondary to compromised endothelial function after intraocular surgery. If, however, corneal edema persists postoperatively, this may reflect irreversible endothelial damage.

Causes of postcataract corneal stromal edema include preexisting endothelial disease, direct surgical trauma to the endothelium, Descemet membrane detachment, vitreous adherence or incarceration, iridocorneal touch, epithelial downgrowth, fibrous downgrowth, uveitis, acute elevations of intraocular pressure, and foreign matter that has inadvertently entered the eye during surgery and has deposited on the corneal endothelium. Many of these entities are discussed elsewhere.

Direct endothelial trauma may occur during phacoemulsification secondary to the ultrasound energy itself. This potential for ultrasound-induced endothelial damage has been shown to be reduced with iris-plane and particularly in situ phacoemulsification, as opposed to anterior chamber phacoemulsification. Kraff and associates[27] and Sugar and colleagues[28] report 29% to 34% endothelial cell loss with anterior chamber phacoemulsification, which decreased to 10% to 15% with posterior chamber phacoemulsification. The magnitude of cell loss also increases with intraocular lens implantation. Katz and coworkers[29] reported that even the slightest contact between the IOL and the corneal endothelium resulted in significant endothelial cell loss. Edelhauser[30] demonstrated that BSS Plus (Alcon Laboratories, Inc., Ft. Worth, TX) more closely matches the composition of aqueous humor than does standard balanced salt solution (BSS) and results in a significantly lower incidence of stromal edema than BSS. This finding is especially important with phacoemulsification, which generally requires much larger volumes of irrigation solution than does ECCE.

Patients with known or suspected corneal endothelial disease should have certain modifications made to their cataract operations. These changes include the avoidance of iris-plane or anterior chamber phacoemulsification, use of the lowest emulsification power sufficient to remove the lens nucleus efficiently, and the generous use of a viscoelastic agent. One should consider the use of a higher-viscosity viscoelastic material.

In those cases in which there is borderline endothelial function and no capsular support, one may choose to consider use of a scleral-fixation IOL instead of an anterior chamber IOL. In an eye with both cataract and corneal edema, cataract extraction combined with penetrating keratoplasty is recommended.

Epithelial Downgrowth

Epithelial downgrowth is a serious but rare complication after cataract surgery, with a reported incidence of less than 0.1% by Weiner and associates[31] in a 30-year clinicopathologic review. Given the vastly improved surgical technique and suture materials that have been incorporated within the last decade or so, the incidence of this grave complication is probably even lower than this reported value.

The underlying pathogenesis of epithelial downgrowth is currently believed to involve a fistulous wound or needle track that allows the migration of conjunctival epithelial cells into these tracks and onto the corneal endothelium. The epithelial cells eventually spread onto the angle structures and iris. Abnormal corneal stromal vascularization and uveal vasculature provide the nutrition and scaffold necessary for the survival and proliferation of these cells.

Presenting symptoms of epithelial downgrowth include decreased visual acuity, pain, photophobia, tearing, and injection. On examination, a retrocorneal membrane is observed, with corneal stromal edema overlying the involved endothelial areas (Fig. 8-5). This membrane is characteristically observed to spread from the superior cornea and iris inferiorly. The intraocular pressure is variably elevated, depending on the degree of angle involvement; paradoxically, hypotony may occur if ciliary body function is compromised. An iritis is usually present, and the Seidel test may yield a positive result.

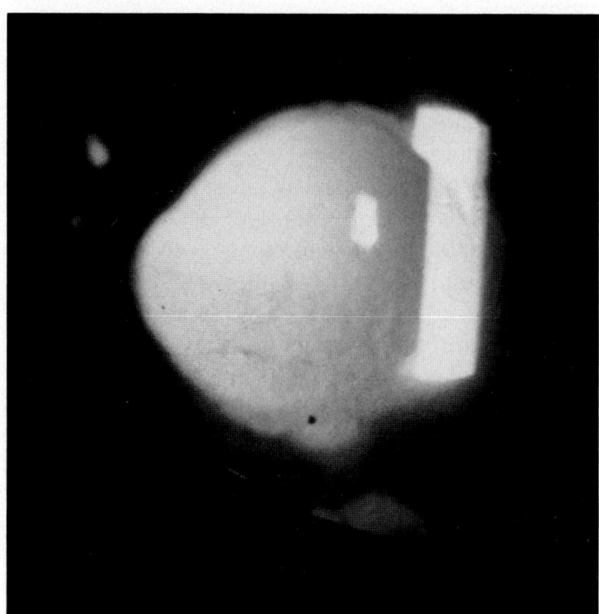

Figure 8-5. Slit-lamp photograph of a patient with epithelial downgrowth. Retroillumination demonstrates the retrocorneal membrane spreading from the superior cornea. (See color plate after page xvi.)

The diagnosis of epithelial downgrowth can be confirmed by laser photocoagulation of the membrane as it overlies the angle or iris.[32] If epithelial cells are present, the argon laser creates a large, white burn with minimal laser power as it destroys the epithelial cells locally; normal angle or iris tissue would be largely unaffected at low-power settings.

Management of epithelial downgrowth is often frustrating because the epithelial membrane inexorably spreads to involve the entire corneal endothelial surface, angle structures, iris, and ciliary body. Surgical management includes the excision of all involved structures, including the fistula, iris, angle structures and ciliary body, with cryotherapy and excision of the cornea; unfortunately, the surgical success in restoring normal corneal, angle, or ciliary body function in these cases has been disappointing.[33]

Another rare complication related to faulty wound closure is epithelial cyst formation, which occurs as a result of the implantation of conjunctival epithelial cells in the anterior chamber. Complications include iridocyclitis and corectopia. It is not clear why in epithelial cysts the passage of conjunctival epithelial cells into the anterior chamber tends to remain relatively stationary, whereas in epithelial downgrowth, the epithelial cells advance aggressively over all intraocular structures. It may be that the cyst formation encapsulates the epithelial cells, preventing their spread. Management involves the aspiration of the cyst, followed by excision; alternatively, the cyst may be obliterated in situ by photocoagulation, cryotherapy, or diathermy.[10]

Fibrous Ingrowth

Fibrous ingrowth is another rare complication related to poor wound closure. The source of the fibroblasts that cause fibrous ingrowth is controversial, with likely sources including subepithelial connective tissue, corneal or limbal stroma, and metaplastic endothelium.[34] The clinical appearance of fibrous ingrowth may be similar to epithelial downgrowth, with a retrocorneal membrane that has advanced over the angle structures, iris, pupil, and ciliary body. One clinical distinction is the presence of an advancing irregular border of fibrous tissue in fibrous ingrowth, as opposed to the generally well-defined border of heaped-up epithelial cells that are seen in epithelial downgrowth.[10]

Secondary complications of fibrous ingrowth include corneal stromal edema, glaucoma, and retinal detachment if the fibrous tissue reaches the posterior segment. Fortunately, eyes with fibrous ingrowth tend to remain quiescent for many years, and specific therapy may be directed at the secondary complications, such as glaucoma, as they arise.

Increased Intraocular Pressure/Glaucoma

Elevated intraocular pressure in the postoperative period is often transient, with restoration of normal intraocular pressure with little or no treatment. Outflow through the trabecular meshwork may be decreased in the early postoperative period by inflammatory cells, blood, fibrin, viscoelastic, and lens and iris debris. In addition, there is usually some component of trabeculitis that occurs after cataract extraction. These forms of secondary glaucoma may be treated with agents that inhibit aqueous production (ie, β-blockers and carbonic anhydrase inhibitors). In addition, topical steroids may be helpful in suppressing the release of inflammatory cells into the aqueous as well as decreasing trabeculitis. Conversely, steroid-induced intraocular pressure elevation may occur, with an increased prevalence in patients with preexisting primary open-angle glaucoma.

More serious are the secondary glaucomas related to angle closure and pupillary block mechanisms. Angle closure after cataract surgery may occur secondary to peripheral anterior synechiae formation, ciliary block, suture compression of the angle, and epithelial downgrowth.

Peripheral anterior synechiae (PAS) formation is the most frequent cause of postcataract glaucoma and is more common in patients with intrinsically shallow anterior chambers. It is most frequently a result of delayed reformation or late shallowing of the anterior chamber, usually associated with a wound leak. PAS formation may also follow episodes of transient angle closure or iris bombé secondary to pupillary block. It is, therefore, important to assess the depth of the anterior chamber as well as the angle postoperatively. If significant narrowing of the angle is observed in the postoperative period, a trial of miotic therapy may be helpful in pulling the peripheral iris more centrally and out of the angle; a potential side effect of miotics, however, is the possibility of inducing pupillary block, which would itself exacerbate the angle narrowing. The concomitant use of epinephrine with the miotic would maximally pull the peripheral iris out of the angle by causing contracture of the iris dilator muscle.

Ciliary block glaucoma is a rare complication after cataract extraction. There is an increased risk in those cases in which the anterior hyaloid face has been broken as well as in patients who are being treated with strong miotics, in whom aqueous becomes trapped posterior to the iris. Diagnosis of ciliary block glaucoma is often a diagnosis of exclusion. Typically, anterior chamber narrowing occurs that is not relieved by laser iridotomy or surgical iridectomy. Although some authors advocate vitreous tap for management of ciliary block glaucoma, the definitive treatment is vitrectomy, with removal of the anterior hyaloid face and the cortical vitreous.[35]

Pupillary block is another important mechanism by which glaucoma may occur postoperatively. In general, any entity that impedes the flow of aqueous from the posterior to the anterior chambers constitutes pupillary block. Pupillary block may itself be caused by two general mechanisms: entities that force the IOL and capsular bag anteriorly (ie, wound leak and choroidal detachment) and entities that physically block the pupillary aperture (ie, inflammatory debris, blood, or fibrin).

The most common cause of pupillary block after cataract extraction is a wound leak, whereby anterior chamber shallowing leads to movement of the capsule and IOL anteriorly. The anterior lens capsule can then adhere to the iris, thus potentially blocking any iridectomy sites, with the IOL optic blocking the pupillary aperture.

Pupillary block may also occur as a result of a choroidal detachment. Choroidal detachment, especially when combined with ciliary body detachment, may push the IOL and capsular bag forward. This result may lead to anterior chamber shallowing, PAS formation, and the potential for pupillary block.

Postoperative inflammation may cause pupillary block in two ways: by means of the presence of a dense fibrinoid coagulum that blocks the pupillary aperture in the early postoperative period or formation of posterior synechiae in cases with prolonged postoperative inflammation. Postoperative hyphema may cause pupillary block in a similar fashion. In either case, frequent postoperative topical steroid application is advocated.

Formed vitreous may block both the pupillary aperture and any iridectomy sites. Therefore, meticulous anterior vitrectomy in the event of vitreous loss is recommended. Visible vitreous strands that occlude or are attached to the pupil may be treated by means of YAG vitreolysis or pars plana vitrectomy.

Residual lens material may also contribute to pupillary block. Both retained lens nuclear and cortical material tend to imbibe fluid if allowed to remain within the capsular bag, thus causing the anterior lens capsule and IOL to bulge anteriorly. Secondary inflammation induced by the retained lens material may exacerbate potential pupillary block. Inflammation promotes the adherence of the anterior lens capsule and IOL to the posterior iris as well as creates the possibility of fibrin-induced pupillary block.[10] An anterior chamber IOL may cause pupillary block; therefore, one or more surgical iridectomies are recommended at the time of anterior chamber IOL insertion.

To prevent pupillary block, a surgical iridectomy is recommended if any intraoperative complication, particularly vitreous loss, occurs.[10] Swan[36] emphasized the importance of transecting both the anterior stromal and posterior pigmented layers of the iris during iridectomy. Swan[37] also advocated basal iridectomy placement, with the rationale that vitreous is usually blocked from contact with the iris periphery by the ciliary body and zonules. Patients with preexisting shallow anterior chambers, known uveitis, and increased posterior pressure are predisposed to pupillary block: one or more surgical iridectomies are advocated in these patients. In addition, patients with diabetes mellitus are more prone to develop postoperative inflammation, which is probably related to diminished vascular integrity, and thus are predisposed to postoperative pupillary block.

Controversy exists regarding a prophylactic surgical iridectomy after an uncomplicated ECCE.[10] Some surgeons advocate such a procedure to minimize the likelihood of IOL or anterior lens capsule–induced pupillary block. Others contend that a surgical iridectomy merely adds the risk of bleeding, increased postoperative inflammation, and secondary IOP elevation, in addition to the potential for glare or diplopia.

Hypotony

The most common causes of postoperative hypotony are wound leak and ciliochoroidal detachment, although these two entities are often found together. Jaffe and coworkers[10] summarized the clinical situations encountered in hypotony as follows: (1) wound leak and a normal anterior chamber depth—no ciliary body detachment; (2) wound leak and shallow anterior chamber depth—probable ciliary body detachment; and (3) no wound leak and shallow anterior chamber depth—probable ciliary body detachment.[10]

Wound leaks have been discussed in a separate section. Ciliary body detachment is thought to be secondary to rapid decompression of the posterior segment during the initial entry into the eye, with consequent hemorrhagic or serous ciliochoroidal detachment. Usually this detachment is only transient, with reattachment occurring when the surgical wound heals sufficiently. If, however, the ciliary body remains detached, organization of the hemorrhage or transudate surrounding the ciliary body may result in permanent hypotony.

Controversy exists regarding the mechanism of hypotony in a ciliochoroidal detachment. Pederson and associates[38] suggested increased uveoscleral outflow as the cause of hypotony associated with ciliochoroidal detachment. Chandler and Maumenee[39] proposed that hyposecretion of the detached ciliary body led to hypotony.

Patients with hypotony are often asymptomatic, and the eye may retain its function indefinitely. In many cases, however, a painful iridocyclitis ensues. Decreased visual acuity may develop, the cause of which is also controversial. Maumenee[40] suggested that secondary macular edema leads to a decline in vision; however, Gass,[41] has challenged this viewpoint. According to the latter, patients with hypotony often develop irregular folding of the choroid and retinal pigment epithelium (RPE), with initial distortion of the photoreceptors and RPE overlying the choroidal folds. These complications are followed by changes in the inner retina.

Medical treatment for hypotony is largely ineffective. Unless decreased visual acuity occurs, observation is sufficient.

If vision is affected, a 24- to 48-hour trial of pressure patching may be initiated. If hypotony persists, then surgical intervention should be considered. Careful gonioscopy should be performed to look for a cyclodialysis cleft, which may be only a few hundred microns in width.

Argon laser treatment of the cyclodialysis is the least invasive procedure. The cleft and surrounding iris and ciliary spur may be treated in multiple sessions to induce closure of the cyclodialysis cleft.[42,43] If this approach is unsuccessful, one may use McCannel suture placement to close the cyclodialysis cleft surgically, with cyclocryotherapy applied after the cleft is closed.[44]

The management of hypotony secondary to a choroidal detachment is discussed later.

Hyphema

Postoperative hyphema usually presents within the first postoperative week. Although the most common source of a postoperative hyphema is blood that was present during surgery and has remained in the eye, there are several causes for new bleeding into the anterior chamber in the postoperative period.

Postoperative bleeding is most frequently a result of defective wound healing. Optimal wound healing is dependent on both a well-created incision and good suture technique. If either of these is deficient, the chances for poor wound healing increase. This complication may lead to an increased likelihood of postoperative bleeding either spontaneously or as a result of minor trauma.

An excessive scleral incision, either in the form of overly long or deep incisions (or in the case of phacoemulsification, a scleral tunnel that is initiated too far posteriorly), increases the risk of transecting a blood vessel.[45,46] If the vessel is of relatively large caliber, initial hemostasis achieved in the operating room may not be sufficient because clot contraction or minor trauma may lead to hyphema in the postoperative period.

The uveitis-glaucoma-hyphema (UGH) syndrome is a relatively uncommon finding now, a result of the near-universal use of posterior chamber intraocular lenses. If an anterior chamber IOL is indicated, however, hyphema as part of the UGH syndrome may manifest itself. This risk is increased in cases in which the anterior chamber intraocular lens is excessively large or has closed-loop haptics.[47]

Swan,[48] and Flaxel and Swan[49] described the "sputtering hyphema syndrome," in which hyphema occurred secondary to corneoscleral wound neovascularization months or even years after cataract surgery. If untreated, neovascular glaucoma may ensue; therefore, careful examination by gonioscopy to localize the source of bleeding should be performed. Abnormal blood vessels should be ablated with the argon[50,51] or transscleral neodymium:yttrium-aluminum-garnet (Nd:YAG) laser.[52]

Most hyphemas are self-limited and absorb spontaneously within the first week after the initial bleeding. Topical and systemic steroids have been shown to have a beneficial effect in diminishing inflammation and the risk of recurrent bleeding.

Surgical intervention, involving anterior chamber washout, is indicated if significant IOP elevation persists or leads to corneal blood staining. Anterior chamber washout is usually performed by means of two paracentesis openings or an automated I–A unit, followed by air injection into the anterior chamber, to help tamponade the bleeding. Evacuation of all visible blood is not recommended because clotted blood is tenacious, and traction on such a strand of clotted blood may dislodge a clot and lead to a new hemorrhage.[53]

Uveitis

Postoperative inflammation is an expected consequence of cataract surgery. In most patients the inflammation is easily managed with topical steroids and dissipates within several weeks, with little or no permanent sequelae. In a few patients, however, inflammation may be more pronounced or more protracted in its course, particularly in those whose complications have occurred during surgery.[54]

Miyake and colleagues[55] described fibrinous iritis as an exuberant postoperative inflammation, with fibrinoid coagula present throughout the anterior chamber. These cause pupil irregularities and a dense fibrinoid membrane anterior or posterior to the intraocular lens. It was postulated that the increased inflammation represented a larger breach of the blood–aqueous barrier than with uncomplicated cataract surgery or a type of hypersensitivity to the surgical manipulation itself. Galin and associates[56] proposed that the lens implant incited a hypersensitivity or foreign-body response in some patients, suggesting that materials or chemicals used in the preparation, polishing, and stabilization of the intraocular lenses were responsible for this reaction.[57] Jaffe and coworkers[10] noted that foreign matter or impurities in the materials used at the time of surgery, including cilia, lint, or talc, may also induce an inflammatory response, which is self-limited in nature.

Residual lens material may also incite a mild postoperative inflammation, as mentioned earlier in this chapter.

IOL Dislocation

Posterior chamber IOLs may become malpositioned in four basic ways: pupil capture, decentration, windshield-wiper syndrome, and sunset syndrome.[58]

Pupil capture occurs when any portion of the IOL optic is present anterior to the iris (Fig. 8-6) and has a reported incidence of 0.6% to 2.6% of cases.[59,60] It is usually a result of sustained pupil dilatation after cataract surgery. Although in many instances it poses merely a cosmetic problem, pupil capture may cause a mild iritis and may limit full pupil dilatation subse-

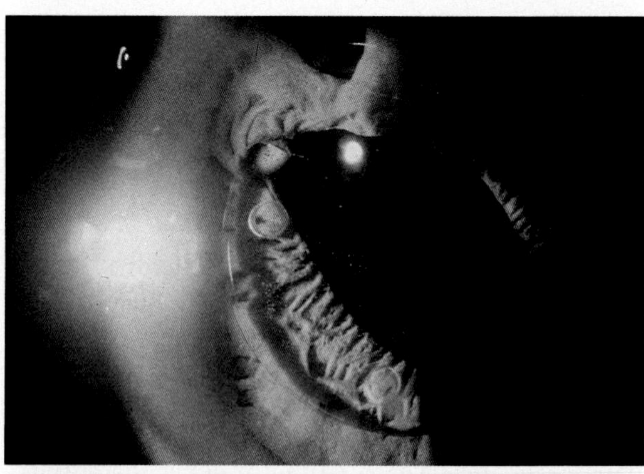

Figure 8-6. Slit-lamp photograph demonstrating a case of pupil capture in which a significant portion of the IOL optic is seen anterior to the iris. (See color plate after page xvi.)

quently. It occurs more commonly with planar posterior chamber lenses; Lindstrom and Herman[61] have demonstrated that anterior angulation of the haptics reduces its incidence. Correction of pupil capture should be initiated soon after surgery, before the development of permanent adhesions between the iris, optic, and posterior capsule.[62] Vigorous pupil dilatation with the patient in the supine position may allow the optic to fall posteriorly into the appropriate position; this should be followed by miotic agents to ensure that pupil capture does not recur. Lindstrom and Herman[61] have recommended the use of applicator-tip pledgets to exert external pressure over the haptics, and Steinert and Puliafito has suggested the use of the YAG laser to push the IOL posteriorly.[61a] Alternatively, if the pupil cannot be sufficiently dilated to clear the anteriorly displaced portion of the optic, a spatula or needle may be used via a corneal stab incision to tap the optic posteriorly. Once permanent adhesions have formed, surgical intervention is not recommended because this approach has been associated with visual loss. Rather, laser iridotomy should be performed as prophylaxis in the event of total pupil capture and consequent pupil block.

Minor degrees of decentration of the IOL optic occur frequently; however, if the position of the IOL remains stable, no intervention is necessary. If the degree of decentration is sufficient to cause an edge of the optic to be visible within the pupil, optical aberrations, most commonly glare, may result. This problem occurs in 0.4% to 3% of cases.[63,64] Decentration is most commonly a result of one haptic (usually the inferior) being fixated within the capsular bag, whereas the other haptic (usually the superior) is fixated within the ciliary sulcus.[65] The best preventive measure is to ensure capsular bag fixation, which is facilitated by performing capsulorhexis.[66] Other causes of decentration include irregular adhesion of the anterior and posterior leaflets of the capsular bag, thickening of the posterior capsule at the edge of the optic, and prolapse of one of the haptics through a break in the zonules. Minor decentration may occur if the optic becomes adherent to the midstromal iris in the postoperative period, an occurrence known as reverse iris tuck (Fig. 8-7); this problem can also be minimized by the use of IOLs with anterior angulated haptics.[60] Decentration can often be successfully managed by the use of miotics to eliminate glare.[67] Alternatively, if decentration is severe, McCannel or scleral-fixation sutures may be considered to reposition and secure the haptics.[44,68]

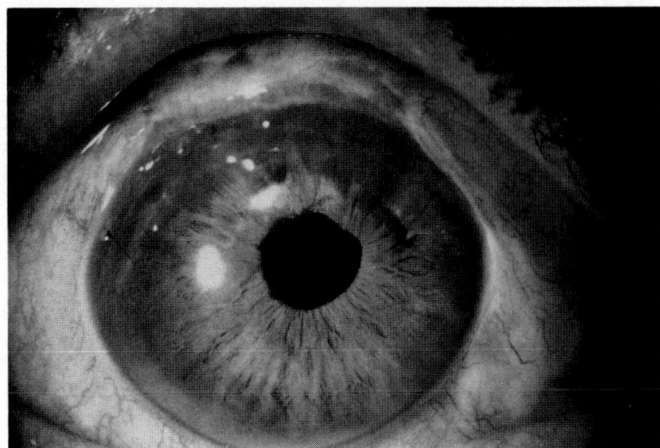

Figure 8-7. Slit-lamp photograph of the right eye demonstrating a case of iris tuck, in which the midstromal iris has become adherent to the intraocular lens (IOL) optic superonasally. This has not resulted in any clinically apparent dislocation of the IOL. This patient had undergone a procedure involving a corneal trephine incision for glaucoma 30 years before cataract extraction. (See color plate after page xvi.)

Windshield-wiper syndrome occurs when the IOL is too small for the eye.[67] In this condition, the superior portion of the IOL moves back and forth horizontally with head movements. This problem occurs most frequently in myopic eyes and in cases in which the haptics are placed in the ciliary sulcus in a vertical orientation. The superior haptic fails to undergo fibrotic adherence to the lens capsule and is consequently free to move. Surgical correction involves the use of a McCannel suture passed through the superior haptic.[44]

Sunset syndrome is the most serious form of IOL dislocation, resulting from inferior zonular dialysis in cases in which the IOL has been placed vertically in the ciliary sulcus[63] (Fig. 8-8). When it is observed shortly after surgery, it is usually due to zonular dialysis occurring at the time of surgery. Later occurrence may occur secondary to globe trauma, including forceful rubbing of the eye. Preventive measures include capsular bag IOL placement and rotation of the haptics to a horizontal configuration. There are various surgical options for the management of sunset syndrome. Several authors advocate iatrogenic pupil capture.[10,53,69] A McCannel suture may be used to fixate the superior haptic to the iris; alternatively, the superior haptic may be sclerally fixated.[70–72] Finally, the IOL may be removed and replaced by an anterior chamber IOL after automated vitrectomy.

Complete dislocation of the IOL into the vitreous cavity may occur, either as a result of complete zonular dialysis or slippage through a break in either the

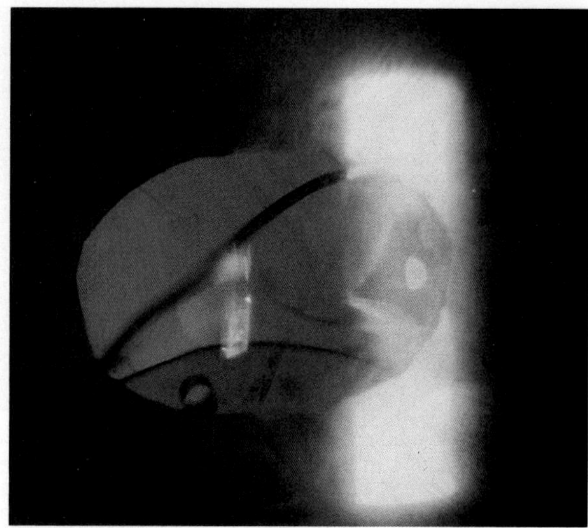

Figure 8-8. Slit-lamp photograph demonstrating a severe case of inferior dislocation of the IOL so that only a small portion of the optic is visible through the pupil (ie, sunset syndrome). (See color plate after page xvi.)

capsular bag or the zonules. Management decisions regarding the IOL are contingent on the mobility of the IOL in the vitreous cavity. If the IOL remains relatively stationary and does not induce inflammatory changes within the vitreous, it may be left in place. If, however, the IOL is observed to move freely with eye movement, or if significant inflammatory changes in the vitreous cavity occur, a vitreoretinal surgeon should be consulted. Management options include pars plana vitrectomy (PPV) with IOL removal, followed by secondary IOL placement in the anterior chamber at the time of surgery or at some future time, or PPV with scleral fixation of the dislocated IOL. In patients in whom corneal endothelial trauma is to be avoided, a scleral- or iris-fixation IOL should be considered.

Anterior chamber IOLs have the least tendency to become malpositioned. Any malposition is usually related to inappropriate lens size. If the IOL is too small, then movement within the anterior chamber may occur, resulting in damage to the angle structures, corneal endothelium, and iris. If the IOL is too large, the UGH syndrome may result. Management in both cases involves IOL exchange.

Choroidal Detachment

Although ciliochoroidal detachments are probably a relatively common occurrence after cataract surgery, they rarely reach clinical significance. They usually occur in the dependent inferior quadrants and may be observed immediately after surgery; most spontaneously resolve within 2 to 3 weeks postoperatively. These patients may be managed by topical steroids and cycloplegic agents.

Less commonly, ciliochoroidal detachment may occur as a consequence of a wound leak, which may occur months or even years after surgery.[10] In these patients, in whom persistent anterior chamber shallowing may occur, a trial of pressure patching should be attempted for up to 48 hours, with surgical repair of the wound leak mandated if adequate anterior chamber depth cannot be achieved with pressure patching. This is to avoid the development of peripheral anterior synechiae and secondary glaucoma.

In the uncommon event of persistent ciliochoroidal detachment without wound leak, a trial of periocular or systemic steroids, as well as cycloplegic agents, may be attempted. If this attempt is unsuccessful, the fluid in the suprachoroidal space may be drained surgically, and the anterior chamber restored by the injection of air, saline, or viscoelastic.

Vitreous Hemorrhage

Vitreous hemorrhage is an uncommon occurrence after cataract surgery. The most common cause of blood in the vitreous cavity after cataract surgery is secondary to the passage of blood from the anterior chamber. The blood may traverse through the zonules if the posterior capsule is intact, or through a break in the posterior capsule or zonular attachments.

Rupture of retinal vessels may occur secondary to a retinal break or posterior vitreous detachment occurring at the time of surgery. This complication may also be a result of zonular traction on the peripheral retinal vessels.[73]

Vitreous hemorrhage usually clears spontaneously over time.[74] If it persists, or if secondary complications, such as hemolytic or ghost cell glaucoma ensue, pars plana vitrectomy is indicated.[75–77]

Retinal Detachment

Approximately 1% to 3% of patients undergoing cataract extraction subsequently develop rhegmatogenous retinal detachment.[78] This compares with an overall incidence of 0.005% to 0.01% in the general population, so that the relative risk among patients undergoing cataract extraction is 100 to 200 times the general risk.

Several theories explain why cataract extraction predisposes the eye to retinal detachment. Cataract extraction is thought to increase the sagittal length of the vitreous cavity, thus allowing the vitreous to project farther anteriorly and, therefore, exert greater traction on the vitreous base and other areas of vitreoretinal adhesion. Foos,[79] and other investigators,[80,81] have reported a significant increase in the prevalence of posterior vitreous detachment after cataract extraction, which may be accompanied by retinal tears or breaks.

Reported risk factors for the development of retinal detachment after cataract surgery include axial myopia, young age, vitreous loss, and retinal detachment in the fellow eye.[82–85]

Surgical treatment of aphakic retinal detachment is beyond the scope of this chapter. Advances in both diagnostic and surgical techniques, however, have improved the reattachment success rate dramatically within the last decade to greater than 90%.

CONCLUSION

The success with which cataract surgery is performed today has been the result of years of improvements in both instrumentation and technique. Ultimately, however, success is dependent on the skills of the surgeon. Appropriate preoperative evaluation of the patient with a cataract as well as attention to the details of the surgical procedure usually results in the avoidance of complications and a successful surgical outcome. However, complications can and do occur, either in the preoperative, intraoperative, or postoperative period. It is hoped that the previous discussion of many of these potential problems assists the cataract surgeon in the prompt identification and treatment of the patient when complications do occur.

References

1. Mackool S. Small pupil enlargement during cataract extraction: a new method. J Cataract Refract Surg 1992;18:523–526.
2. de Juan E Jr, Hickingbotham D. Flexible iris retractor. (Letter) Am J Ophthalmol 1991;111:776–777.

2a. Blumenthal M, Moisseiev J. Anterior chamber maintainer for extracapsular cataract extraction and intracellular lens implantation. J Cataract Refract Surg 1987;13:204.

3. Cionni RJ, Osher RH. Cataract surgery in the face of retrobulbar hemorrhage. Ophthalmology 1991;98: 1153–1155.
4. Zaturansky B, Hyams S. Perforation of the globe during the injection of local anesthesia. Ophthalmic Surg 1987;18:585–588.
5. Little JH, Mallory DB. Cataract surgery. In: Complications in ophthalmic surgery. New York, Churchill Livingstone, 1983:76.
6. Wilson DJ, Jaeger MJ, Green WR. Effects of extracapsular cataract extraction on the lens zonules. Ophthalmology 87;94:467–470.
7. Skuta GL, Parrish RK, Hodapp E. Zonular dialysis during extracapsular cataract extraction in pseudoexfoliation syndrome. Arch Ophthalmol 1987;105: 632–634.
8. Osher RH, Corcoran K. Modification of the IOL power: ciliary sulcus versus capsular bag. Houston, Welsh Cataract Congress, 1986.
9. Cionni RJ, Osher RH. Complications of phacoemulsification surgery. In: Weinstock FJ, ed. Management and care of the cataract patient. Boston, Blackwell Scientific Publications, 1992:198–211.
10. Jaffe NS, Jaffe MS, Jaffe GF. Cataract surgery and its complications, ed 5. St Louis, CV Mosby, 1990.
11. Guzek JP, Holm M, Cotter JB, et al. Risk factors for intraoperative complications in 1000 extracapsular cases. Ophthalmology 1987;94:461–466.
12. McDonald HR, Irvine AR. Light-induced maculopathy from the operating microscope in extracapsular cataract extraction and intraocular lens implantation. Ophthalmology 1983;90:945–951.
13. Taylor DM. Expulsive hemorrhage. Am J Ophthalmol 1974;78:961–965.
14. Manschot WA. The pathology of expulsive hemorrhage. Am J Ophthalmol 1955:40:15–24.
15. Bair HL. Expulsive hemorrhage at cataract operation: report of a case and additional recommendation for its management. Am J Ophthalmology 1966;61:992–994.
16. Davison JA. Acute intraoperative suprachoroidal hemorrhage in extracapsular cataract surgery. J Cataract Refract Surg 1986;12:606–622.
17. Bukelman A, Hoffman P, Oliver M. Limited choroidal hemorrhage associated with extracapsular cataract extraction. Arch Ophthalmol 1987;105:338–441.
18. Hoffman P, Pollack A, Oliver M. Limited choroidal hemorrhage associated with intracapsular cataract extraction. Arch Ophthalmol 1984;102:1761–1765.
19. Michels RG. Complications of retinal detachment. In: Michels RG, ed. Retinal detachment. St Louis, CV Mosby, 1990:1012.

20. Maumenee AE, Schwartz MF. Acute intraoperative choroidal effusion. Am J Ophthalmol 1985;100:147–154.
21. Davison JA. Acute intraoperative suprachoroidal hemorrhage in capsular bag phacoemulsification. J Cataract Refract Surg 1993;19:534–537.
22. Roussel TJ, Culbertson WW, Jaffe NS. Chronic postoperative endophthalmitis associated with *Propionibacterium acnes.* Arch Ophthalmol 1987;105:1199–1201.
23. Jaffe GF, Whitcher JP, Biswell R, et al. *Propionibacterium acnes* endophthalmitis seven months after extracapsular cataract extraction and intraocular lens implantation. Ophthalmic Surg 1986;17:791–793.
24. Allen HF. Prevention of postoperative endophthalmitis. Ophthalmology 1978;85:386–389.
25. Donahue SP, Jewart BH, Kowalski RP, et al. Vitreous tap versus vitrectomy in diagnosing endophthalmitis. Invest Ophthalmol Vis Sci 1992;33(suppl):897.
26. Koch PS. Structural analysis of cataract incision construction. J Cataract Refract Surg 1991;17(Suppl):661–667.
27. Kraff MC, Sanders DR, Lieberman HL. Specular microscopy in cataract and intraocular lens patients. Arch Ophthalmol 1980;98:1782–1784.
28. Sugar J, Mitchelson J, Kraff M. Endothelial trauma and cell loss from intraocular lens insertion. Arch Ophthalmol 1978;96:449–450.
29. Katz J, Kaufman HE, Goldberg EP. Prevention of endothelial damage from intraocular lens insertion. Trans Am Acad Ophthalmol Otolaryngol 1977;83:204–212.
30. Edelhauser H. Intraocular irrigating solution. Alcon Surg Monograph 1987:29.
31. Weiner MJ, Trentacoste J, Pon DM, et al. Epithelial downgrowth: a 30-year clinicopathological review. Br J Ophthalmol 1989;73:6–11.
32. Maumenee AE. Complications of cataract surgery. Highlights Ophthalmol 1968;11:120–132.
33. Brown SI. Results of excision of advanced epithelial downgrowth. Ophthalmology 1979;86:321–328.
34. Swan KC. Fibroblastic ingrowth following cataract extraction. Arch Ophthalmol 1973;89:445–449.
35. Friedman Z, Neumann E. Midcavity vitrectomy for cilio-vitreolenticular block glaucoma. Glaucoma 1982;4:125–126.
36. Swan KC. Relationship of basal iridectomy to shallow chamber following cataract extraction. Arch Ophthalmol 1963;69:191–202.
37. Swan KC. Relationship of basal iridectomy to shallow chamber following cataract extraction. Trans Am Ophthalmol Soc 1962;60:213–235.
38. Pederson JE, Gaasterland DE, MacLellan HM. Uveoscleral aqueous outflow in the rhesus monkey: importance of uveal reabsorption. Invest Ophthalmol Vis Sci 1977;16:1008–1017.
39. Chandler PA, Maumenee AE. A major cause of hypotony. Am J Ophthalmol 1961;52:609–618.
40. Maumenee AE. Glaucoma: hypotony. Highlights Ophthalmol 1966;9:28–53.
41. Gass JDM. The cause of visual loss in hypotony. In: Welsh RC, Welsh J, eds. The new report on cataract surgery. Miami, Miami Educational Press, 1969.
42. Joondeph HC. Management of postoperative and posttraumatic cyclodialysis clefts with argon laser photocoagulation. Ophthalmic Surg 1980;11:186–188.
43. Harbin TS. Treatment of cyclodialysis clefts with argon laser photocoagulation. Ophthalmology 1982;89:1082–1083.
44. McCannel MA. A retrievable suture idea for anterior uveal problems. Ophthalmic Surg 1976;7:98–103.
45. Moses L. Postoperative hyphema in cataract surgery with scleral flap technique. Arch Ophthalmol 1986;104:793.
46. John ME, Noblitt RL, Boleyn KL, et al. Effect of a superficial and a deep scleral pocket incision on the incidence of hyphema. J Cataract Refract Surg 1992;18:495–499.
47. Ellingson FT. Complications with the Choyce Mark VIII anterior chamber implant. J Am Intraocul Implant Soc 1977;3:199–201.
48. Swan KC. Hyphema due to wound vascularization after cataract extraction. Arch Ophthalmol 1973;89:87–90.
49. Flaxel JT, Swan KC. Limbal wound healing after cataract extraction. Arch Ophthalmol 1969;81:653–659.
50. Sharpe ED, Simmons RJ. Argon laser therapy of occult recurrent hyphema from anterior segment wound neovascularization. Ophthalmic Surg 1986;17:283–285.
51. Petreli EA, Wizinia RA. Argon laser photocoagulation of inner wound vascularization after cataract extraction. Am J Ophthalmol 1977;84:59–61.
52. Kramer TR, Brown RH, Lynch MG, et al. Transscleral Nd:YAG photocoagulation for cataract incision vascularization associated with recurrent hyphema. Am J Ophthalmol 1989;107:681–682.
53. Clayman HM, Jaffe NS, Galin MA. Intraocular lens implantation: techniques and complications. St Louis, CV Mosby, 1983.
54. Goodman DF, Stark WJ, Gottsch JD. Complications of cataract extraction with intraocular lens implantation. Ophthalmic Surg 1989;20:132–140.
55. Miyake K, Asakura M, Kobayashi H. Effect on intraocular lens fixation on the blood-aqueous barrier. Am J Ophthalmol 1984;98:451–455.
56. Galin MA, Tuberville AW, Dotson RS. Immunologic aspects of intraocular lenses. Int Ophthalmol Clin 1982;22:227–234.
57. Meltzer DW. Sterile hypopyon following intraocular surgery. Arch Ophthalmol 1980;98:100–104.

58. Obstbaum SA, To K. Posterior chamber intraocular lens dislocations and malpositions. Aust NZ J Ophthalmol 1989;17:265–271.
59. Southwick PC, Olson RJ. Shearing posterior chamber intraocular lenses: five-year postoperative results. Am Intraocul Implant Soc J 1984;10:318–323.
60. Faulkner JD. Advantages and indications for posterior chamber intraocular lens implants. Contact Intraocul Lens Med J 1982;8:50–52.
61. Lindstrom RJ, Herman WK. Pupil capture: prevention and management. Am Intraocular Implant Soc J 1983;9:201–204.

61a. Steinert RF, Puliafito CA. The Nd-Yag Laser in Opthalmology: principles and clinical applications of photodisruption. Philadelphia; WB Saunders, 1985:129–130.

62. Steinert P, Puliafito CA. New applications of the Nd:YAG laser. Am Intraocul Implant Soc J 1984; 10:372–376.
63. Kratz RP. Complications associated with posterior chamber lenses. Ophthalmology 1979;86:659–661.
64. Pallin SL, Walman GB. Posterior chamber intraocular lens implant centration: in or out of "the bag." Am Intraocul Implant Soc J 1982;8:254–257.
65. Hansen SO, Tetz MR, Solomon KD, et al. Decentration of flexible loop posterior chamber intraocular lenses in a series of 222 postmortem eyes. Ophthalmology 1988;95:344–349.
66. Legler UFC, Assia EI, Castaneda VE, et al. Prospective experimental study of factors related to posterior chamber intraocular lens decentration. J Cataract Refract Surg 1992;18:449–455.
67. Smith SG, Lindstrom RL. Malpositioned posterior chamber lenses: etiology, prevention, and management. Am Intraocul Implant Soc J 1985;11:584–591.
68. Smith SG, Lindstrom RL. Report and management of the sunrise syndrome. Am Intraocul Implant Soc J 1984;10:218–220.
69. Shearing S. Posterior chamber lens implantation. Int Ophthalmol Clin 1982;221:135–153.
70. Sternberg P, Michael RG. Treatment of dislocated posterior chamber intraocular lenses. Arch Ophthalmol 1988;104:1391–1393.
71. Price FW, Whitson WE. Visual results of suture-fixated posterior chamber intraocular lenses during penetrating keratoplasty. Ophthalmology 1989;96:1234–1240.
72. Apple DJ, Price FW, Gwin T, et al. Sutured retropupillary posterior chamber intraocular lenses for exchange or secondary implantation: the Twelfth Annual Binkhorst Lecture, 1988. Ophthalmology 1989; 96:1241–1247.
73. Vogt A. Die Operative Therapie und die Pathogenese der Netzhautablosing. Stuttgart, Ferdinand Enke Verlag, 1936.
74. Galli L, Nagy M. Intravitreal hemolysis. Szemeszet 1963;100:76–84.
75. Machemer R. A new concept for vitreous surgery. II. Surgical technique and complications. Am J Ophthalmol 1972;74:1022–1033.
76. Machemer R. A new concept in vitreous surgery. VI. Anesthesia and improvements in surgical techniques. Arch Ophthalmol 1974;92:402–406.
77. Machemer R. A new concept in vitreous surgery: two instrument techniques in pars plana vitrectomy. Arch Ophthalmol 1974;92:407–412.
78. Jaffe NS. Results of intraocular lens implant surgery: the Third Binkhorst Medal Lecture. Am J Ophthalmol 1978;85:13–23.
79. Foos RY. Posterior vitreous detachment. Trans Am Acad Ophthalmol Otolaryngol 1972;76:480–497.
80. Heller MD, Straatsma BR, Foos RY. Detachment of the posterior vitreous in phakic and aphakic eyes. Mod Probl Ophthalmol 1972;10:23–36.
81. McDonnell PJ, Patel A, Green WR. Comparison of intracapsular and extracapsular cataract surgery: histopathologic study of eyes obtained postmortem. Ophthalmology 1985;92:1208–1225.
82. Coonan P, Fung WE, Webster RG, et al. The incidence of retinal detachment following cataract extraction. Ophthalmology 1985;92:1096–1101.
83. Smith PW, Stark WJ, Maumenee AE, et al. Retinal detachments after extracapsular cataract extraction with posterior chamber intraocular lens. Ophthalmology 1987;94:495–504.
84. Javitt JC, Vitale S, Canner JK, et al. National outcomes of cataract extraction. I. Retinal detachment after inpatient surgery. Ophthalmology 1991;98:895–902.
85. Nielsen NE, Naeser K. Epidemiology of retinal detachment following extracapsular cataract extraction: a follow-up study with an analysis of risk factors. J Cataract Refract Surg 1993;19:675–680.

Ophthalmic Surgery Complications: Prevention and Management,
edited by Judie F. Charlton and George W. Weinstein.
J. B. Lippincott Company, Philadelphia © 1995.

9

Marian S. Macsai

Complications of Corneal Surgery

Complications of corneal surgery reflect the broad spectrum of microsurgical and laser techniques used by the corneal surgeon, and new techniques are constantly being developed. This wide range results from the intricacies involved in intraocular and extraocular procedures ranging from penetrating keratoplasty to lamellar keratoplasty or refractive surgery. As with any surgical procedure, a level of comfort and familiarity with the complications that may be encountered enhances the surgical outcome for both surgeon and patient.

PENETRATING KERATOPLASTY

Penetrating keratoplasty is becoming an increasingly popular procedure in the United States. In 1992, more than 42,000 penetrating keratoplasties were performed.[1] Penetrating keratoplasty has unusual potential for intraoperative complications because of the size of the wound. After removal of the host cornea, and before securing the donor corneal button in position, a circular wound remains. This provides excellent opportunity for anterior segment reconstruction and intraocular lens exchange; however, unique complications may occur during these procedures. As a result, it is important to examine the intraoperative complications separately from the early and late postoperative complications.

Intraoperative Complications

Acute Choroidal Detachment

Acute choroidal detachment, whether serous or hemorrhagic in nature, is the most devastating complication of penetrating keratoplasty. Removal of the corneal button creates a hole in the front of the eye approximately 8 mm in diameter. As a result of this large wound, an acute choroidal detachment is more difficult to control during penetrating keratoplasty. The rapid drop of intraoperative pressure after removal of the corneal button may result in a pressure differential that allows for rapid expansion of the suprachoroidal space, by either blood or serous fluid, with subsequent forcing of the intraocular contents through the corneal wound and out of the eye. The overall incidence of this complication ranges from 0.45% to 1.08%.[2,3]

Numerous risk factors for the development of an acute choroidal detachment have been identified. These include increased patient age, increased intraocular pressure, systemic hypertension, previous ocular surgery, previous trauma, intraoperative Valsalva maneuvers, and myopia.[4,5] Presenting signs may include a sudden increase in posterior pressure with anterior displacement of the lens iris diaphragm, loss of the red reflex, or spontaneous prolapse of the iris lens or vitreous. The sequelae of an unrecognized acute choroidal detachment may include extrusion of the entire intraocular contents, including the retina.

Rapid recognition of the signs and symptoms are key to controlling the situation. Immediate closure of the wound, either with digital pressure or securing of the donor cornea must occur to increase the intraocular pressure and thereby decrease the pressure differential. Failure to decrease the pressure differential allows for rapid expansion of the suprachoroidal hemorrhage.

Immediate closure of the wound is best achieved with application of the index finger over the corneal wound and subsequent digital tamponade. Immediately after this procedure, numerous posterior sclerotomies should be performed to release the suprachoroidal blood and prevent further expulsion of the intraocular contents. This is best achieved with a supersharp blade. The blade is passed approximately 4 to 5 mm posterior to the limbus, directly through the conjunctiva and sclera, into the suprachoroidal space. Rotating the blade 90 degrees opens the sclerotomy and allows for outflow of the subchoroidal hemorrhage or serous fluid.[6]

Even with prompt treatment, overall prognosis for a suprachoroidal hemorrhage or acute choroidal detachment is poor. Closure of the wound may result in vitreous incarceration in the wound with subsequent vitreous traction and retinal detachment. Even if the acute intraoperative complication has been managed successfully, postoperative retinal complications may occur.

Anterior Segment Bleeding

Bleeding from the structures of the anterior segment may occur intraoperatively. Structures from which bleeding may occur include the cornea, ciliary body, and anterior chamber angle. The cornea, a normally avascular structure, may frequently be vascularized in diseases that require penetrating keratoplasty. Bleeding from the corneal vessels may be controlled with the application of 2.5% or 10% phenylephrine on a cellulose sponge. Partial trephination of the cornea, to approximately 75% depth, with application of phenylephrine may result in constriction of the corneal vessels and coagulation of the blood, allowing the surgeon to proceed with little bleeding after removal of the corneal button. Cautious use of phenylephrine is advised in patients with hypertension. Any blood that does seep into the anterior chamber should be removed to decrease the postoperative complications of glaucoma and intraocular inflammation.

When an intraocular lens is removed in pseudophakic bullous keratopathy, there is frequently fibrosis with resultant cocoon formation around the haptics. Identification of this condition preoperatively may alert the surgeon to this possibility and allow for formulation of an operative plan. It may be necessary to separate the optic from the haptics, and remove each haptic individually by rotating it out of the cocoon as described by Waring.[7] Careful manipulation of the haptics may result in removal without bleeding. Intraoperative manipulation of the iris, which is required in a pupilloplasty or anterior chamber reconstruction, may also result in bleeding from both the iris root and the ciliary body if excessive force is applied to the iris. In the event of bleeding from the angle, iris root, or ciliary body, simple application of cold Healon to the bleeding site may result in coagulation. If the application of cold Healon or pressure over the bleeding area does not cause coagulation, a cellulose sponge soaked in thrombin in a 1:10,000 dilution for 30 seconds may stop further bleeding.[8] If a vessel has been damaged and is visibly bleeding, endodiathermy may be used to stop the flow of blood in the vessels.

Handling of Donor Tissue

Donor tissue should be handled with extreme care, even while it is still in its storage container. Dropping the storage container could result in cracking and contamination of the donor cornea. When removing the donor cornea from the storage medium, the surgeon should grasp the tissue at the margin to avoid damage to the endothelial cells, or use a spatula. All containers in which the donor cornea is placed should be clearly labeled to avoid possible cross-contamination with other irrigating solutions that might be used during the surgery.

Transfer of donor cornea onto the corneal punch should be done carefully to avoid possible damage to the endothelial cells. Before punching the donor cornea, the surgeon should always check the size of the trephine to assure that no confusion has transpired, resulting in a change in the trephine size. Once the donor cornea has been punched to the correct size, it must remain covered with storage medium and in a moist chamber until the surgeon is ready to suture it into position.

Transferring the donor cornea from the moist chamber to the operative field may be done with spatula or forceps; however, care should be taken to avoid damage to both the epithelial and endothelial surfaces of the donor cornea. Intraoperative damage to the corneal endothelium, either mechanical or chemical (irrigating solutions), may result in postoperative corneal edema or primary graft failure.

Injury or Dislocation of the Lens

In the phakic patient, care must be taken to avoid inadvertent damage to the lens. Contact between the lens and surgical instruments may result in cataract formation or rupture of the anterior lens capsule, and subsequent loss of the lens material. Excessive posterior pressure in the eye may result in anterior displacement of the lens iris diaphragm, thereby increasing the likelihood of damage to the lens. Preoperative ocular massage, either digital or through a Honan balloon, should be used to reduce the intraocular pressure. If the intraocular pressure remains high after these maneuvers, intravenous 20% mannitol, 1.5 to 2.5 g/kg, or acetazolamide (Diamox) may be used to lower the intraocular pressure. An inadequate lid block may result in external pressure on the globe; a misplaced lid speculum may increase the posterior pressure and cause anterior displacement of the lens iris diaphragm. Care should be taken during trephination on a soft eye to avoid possible trephination through the cornea and iris, and into the lens.

Securing a Flieringa ring to the globe with Vicryl sutures provides further support for the globe after removal of the cornea, which may decrease the likelihood of anterior displacement of the lens iris diaphragm. This is especially important in the pediatric penetrating keratoplasty during which the sclera is more likely to collapse because of increased elasticity and resultant dislocation of the intraocular lens. The use of eight sutures to secure the Flieringa ring to the globe may decrease the likelihood of anterior displacement of the lens in these cases. Should inadvertent cataract formation occur during penetrating keratoplasty, it is advisable to delay cataract extraction as long as possible to allow for corneal wound healing. Some authors have recommended at least 9 months' delay.[6]

Wound Misalignment

Misalignment of the donor cornea with the host cornea may result in anterior or posterior displacement of the donor cornea with resultant corneal astigmatism and problems with reepithelialization. Detailed attention should be paid to the placement of the corneal sutures to ensure against wound misalignment. Full-thickness corneal sutures decrease the occurrence of wound misalignment; however, the corneal sutures may act as a tract to allow for intraocular penetration of ocular microorganisms, resulting in endophthalmitis. As a result, most corneal surgeons attempt to place their corneal sutures at 80% to 90% depth on both the donor and host corneas. Because of the presence of corneal edema or corneal scarring as in interstitial keratitis, there may be a significant thickness disparity between the host and donor cornea. Should wound misalignment occur with significant anterior override, the use of a bandage soft contact lens (Plano-T) has been recommended to provide some pressure to the anterior displaced tissue and subsequently help in the realignment of the tissue. In addition, the bandage contact lens may allow for more rapid reepithelialization of the displaced tissue.[9]

Early Postoperative Complications

Endophthalmitis

Endophthalmitis is a rare but devastating complication of penetrating keratoplasty. Numerous reports of postoperative endophthalmitis have given an overall incidence of endophthalmitis following penetrating keratoplasty of approximately 0.23%.[10–12] Recent reports of endophthalmitis have been associated with gentamicin-resistant organisms with the streptococcal and endocococcal species of increasing numbers (Wilhelmus K, Adverse Reactions Committee, Eye Bank Association of America, personal communication, June 1993). The increased incidence of endophthalmitis secondary to organisms resistant to gentamicin may be a result of gentamicin being the sole antibiotic added to corneal storage medium. Recently, corneal storage medium has become available, which is supplemented with both gentamicin, 100 mg/L, and streptomycin, 200 mg/L. However, despite antibiotic augmentation, endophthalmitis following penetrating keratoplasty continues to be a devastating complication.[13,14] Recent reports have isolated endophthalmitis caused by coagulase-negative staphylococci as an endophthalmitis with delayed onset, which is chronic and often painless.[15] The cause of endophthalmitis postkeratoplasty is frequently unknown; however, several sources may be identified. The most obvious source would be contamination of the donor tissue or corneal storage medium. Additional sources include the patient's normal flora from the lids and conjunctiva, or the surgeon performing the surgery. The addition of antibiotics to cornea storage medium may decrease the incidence of contamination from the donor tissue or cornea storage medium. The use of topical antibiotics, topical povidone-iodine preoperatively, and subconjunctival antibiotics immediately postoperatively may also reduce the incidence of postoperative endophthalmitis.[16,17]

The clinical signs and symptoms of endophthalmitis postkeratoplasty vary with the virulence of the causative organism. The most virulent organisms present with symptoms earlier than less virulent organisms, such as coagulase-negative staphylococci. Classically, the patient complains of increased pain, redness of the eye, photophobia, and decreased vision. Clinical signs include increased anterior segment inflammation with a hypopyon and possible vitreous reaction, eyelid swelling, corneal edema, and conjunctival chemosis. Any increase in the inflammatory response disproportionate to the expected postoperative inflammation should alert the clinician to the possibility of postoperative endophthalmitis.

In the event of the possibility of endophthalmitis, immediate institution of therapy is indicated. Most cases of endophthalmitis can be diagnosed within the first 48 hours; however, endophthalmitis caused by less virulent organisms, such as *Proprionibacterium acnes* and coagulase-negative staphylococci may have a delayed onset with signs that include chronic inflammation. Frequently, these infections are painless. The differential diagnosis of delayed endophthalmitis must include fungal infections. However, fungal infections tend to occur somewhat earlier than the endophthalmitis secondary to *P acnes.*

When endophthalmitis is a possible diagnosis, aqueous and vitreous samples must be obtained for Gram stain, culture, and sensitivity. The institution of intravitreal antibiotics is by far the most important aspect of treating bacterial endophthalmitis.[18] Current recommendations as reviewed elsewhere in this book include the use of intravenous and topical antibiotics in addition to intravitreal antibiotics. Despite prompt recognition and treatment, the overall prognosis for postoperative endophthalmitis remains poor.

Primary Graft Failure

Primary graft failure occurs when there is persistent corneal edema for at least 2 weeks after penetrating keratoplasty (Fig. 9-1). The incidence of primary graft failure has been reported up to 5%.[19] The causes of primary graft failure can be subdivided into three groups: (1) abnormal donor endothelium, (2) incorrect corneal storage, and (3) surgical trauma. Abnormal donor endothelium has been attributed to numerous causes, including diabetes, chronic glaucoma, previous surgery, and Fuchs endothelial dystrophy. In addition, prolonged time from patient death to corneal preservation may affect the viability of the endothelium. The Eye Bank Association of America has established criteria for selecting donor tissue to prevent the use of poor cornea tissue. These criteria may be found in the Medical Standards Document of the Eye Bank Association of America.

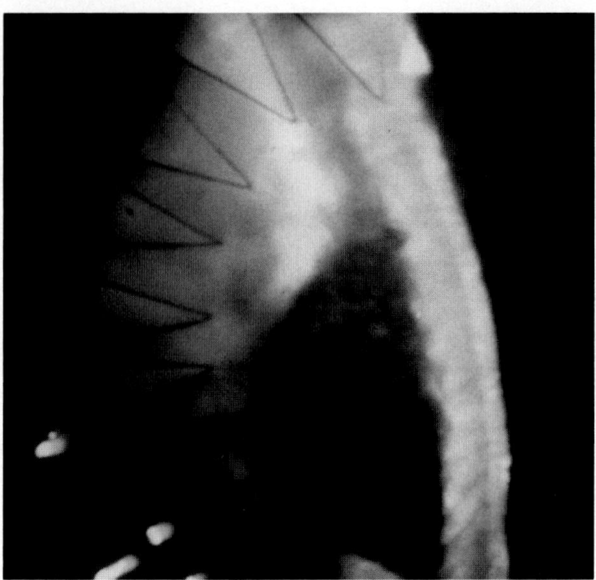

Figure 9-1. Primary graft failure in a patient undergoing penetrating keratoplasty results when corneal edema persists for at least 2 weeks after penetrating keratoplasty. In this patient, the corneal button was cloudy on the table and failed to clear. Repeat penetrating keratoplasty was performed with good visual results.

Incorrect tissue storage may be complicated if there is trauma to the corneal endothelium at the time of procurement. Strict guidelines for corneal storage have been established. The temperature of cornea storage medium should be maintained between 2° to 6°C with a pH of 7 to 7.5. Contamination of the corneal storage medium can also result in damage to the cornea endothelium.

Intraoperatively, surgical trauma may result in primary graft failure. Surgical trauma may result from direct trauma to the endothelium. Before punching the donor material, the corneal block must be adequately cooled because increased temperature of the corneal block may result in endothelial damage. Irrigation fluids used intraoperatively must be the appropriate osmolarity and pH, and increased posterior pressure intraoperatively or postoperatively may result in iris corneal touch or lens corneal touch, which may damage the cornea endothelium. If primary graft failure occurs, regrafting is the only method of restoring the corneal clarity and preventing resultant epithelial edema.

Postoperative Glaucoma

Glaucoma in the immediate postoperative period of penetrating keratoplasty can limit visual recovery by causing significant damage to the corneal graft endothelium and irreversible optic nerve damage.[20–23] The incidence of postoperative glaucoma is variable depending on the patient's preoperative diagnosis and the surgical procedure performed.[24–26] Chien and colleagues[24] have identified an increased incidence of elevated intraocular pressure in patients undergoing vitrectomy at the time of penetrating keratoplasty and patients undergoing combined penetrating keratoplasty, extracapsular cataract extraction, and posterior chamber intraocular lens implantation. In aphakic and pseudophakic patients, an incidence as high as 40% to 50% has been reported.

The cause of glaucoma after penetrating keratoplasty is multifactorial. Preexisting glaucoma, aphakia, and pseudophakia have all been identified as risk factors for the development of postkeratoplasty glaucoma.[27] Postoperative inflammation, pigment dispersion, hemorrhage, pupillary block, and viscoelastic agents have also been identified as factors that contribute to glaucoma in the immediate postoperative period after penetrating keratoplasty. Epithelial downgrowth may result in postkeratoplasty glaucoma; however, the onset is much later.

Numerous causative factors have been identified that may have a mechanical effect on the trabecular meshwork outflow and therefore increase the incidence of glaucoma. A collapse of the trabecular meshwork may result from the incision into Descemet membrane and the removal of the cortical lens.[28] Zimmermann and colleagues[29] identified suture depth as a factor that contributes to trabecular meshwork collapse and resultant decreased aqueous outflow.

As mentioned in the previous discussion of primary graft failure, elevated intraocular pressure has been identified as a causative agent resulting in corneal endothelial damage with resultant corneal edema.[30,31] The degree of intraocular pressure elevation and endothelial cell sensitivity to increased intraocular pressure are both factors that may result in corneal edema. In addition, the elevated intraocular pressure may result in optic nerve damage and, if high enough, retinal vein occlusion.

Treatment of postkeratoplasty glaucoma is dictated by the cause. In the immediate postoperative period, elevated intraocular pressure may be due to inflammation and residual viscoelastic agents. The use of topical corticosteroids may be helpful; however, in patients who develop postkeratoplasty glaucoma after long-term corticosteroid use, the cause-and-effect relation of the topical steroids must always be questioned. In such patients, fluorometholone has the least hypertensive effect of any of the topical steroids, and switching the patient to fluorometholone may result in a significant decrease in the intraocular pressure.

If the pressure does not respond to a change in corticosteroids, medical therapy with aqueous suppressants, such as β-blockers, carbonic anhydrase inhibitors, and apraclonidine, is indicated.[32,33] Miotics may also be used in the late postoperative period when inflammation is no longer contributing to the intraocular pressure. Failure of medical therapy would indicate surgical intervention, such as laser trabeculoplasty, filtration procedures, seton implantation, and cyclodestructive procedures. All of these have been reported to have moderate success rates.

Postoperative Hyphema

Postoperative hyphemas are more common in patients who have had manipulation of intraocular tissues during penetrating keratoplasty. The source of bleeding is frequently the iris root or areas in which iris manipulation has occurred. When an intraocular lens has been removed, the fibrovascular tissue surrounding the haptics may result in postoperative hyphemas. Most hyphemas resorb slowly within the first postoperative week. Elevated intraocular pressure may result from blockage of trabecular meshwork and may be treated with acetazolamide, β-blockers, and apraclonidine. Topical and systemic steroids may also be useful to control intraocular inflammation. Anterior chamber washout is rarely indicated; however, it may be necessary to control elevated intraocular pressure and prevent corneal endothelial cell damage or corneal blood staining. Strict control of the postoperative intraocular pressure is necessary in patients with sickle cell disease or trait. In these patients, anterior chamber washout may be required to prevent optic nerve damage if the intraocular pressure remains higher than 24 mmHg for 24 hours.

Wound Leaks

The best treatment for wound leaks postkeratoplasty is careful examination before completing the surgical procedure. Examination of the wound through the operating microscope at high power with application of pressure to the sclera usually demonstrates areas of wound leaks that may be closed intraoperatively. In one series, 5.4% of eyes undergoing penetrating keratoplasty had a wound dehiscence, and about 50% of these had graft failure.[34] If the intraocular pressure is unrecordable during the 1st postoperative day, a wound leak must be suspected. A Seidel test should be performed to rule out an occult wound leak. Application of undiluted fluorescein to the wound with pressure application to the sclera to increase the intraocular pressure usually demonstrates the area of the wound leak. In patients with scarring or cicatrization of the conjunctiva or fornices, the wound may appear tight in primary gaze. Careful examination of the wound in the extreme field of gaze may demonstrate gaping of the wound with a subsequent leak.

Oversizing the corneal graft may prevent postoperative wound leaks in such patients. Pressure patching, aqueous suppression, and bandage contact lenses may often close small wounds; however, when these measures are unsuccessful, the patient should be taken back to the operating room, and the leak should be repaired with additional 10-0 nylon sutures. Failure to recognize a wound leak may result in persistent apposition of the peripheral iris to the cornea endothelium, resulting in peripheral anterior synechiae and subsequent glaucoma. Persistent areas of wound dehiscence may result in fistulization with resultant epithelial downgrowth, a devastating complication of intraocular surgery.

Excessive Postoperative Inflammation

Most postoperative inflammation results from surgical trauma or intraocular bleeding. Normally, postoperative inflammation can be controlled with topical corticosteroids and a cycloplegic agent. When excessive postoperative inflammation is expected because of preoperative predisposing conditions, such as an inflamed eye or excessive stromal vascularization, administration of oral prednisone, 1 to 1.5 mg/kg, may be started 1 to 2 days preoperatively to decrease the severity and incidence of postoperative inflammation. Intracameral tissue plasminogen activator has been described for the control of excessive postoperative inflammation.[35] Excessive postoperative inflammation may be the earliest indication of postoperative endophthalmitis, and in these patients careful daily observation to separate out the causative agents of the inflammation is necessary when corticosteroid agents have been introduced.

Persistent Epithelial Defects

Persistent epithelial defects following penetrating keratoplasty are a potentially serious complication that may ultimately result in graft failure. Numerous patients with predisposing factors for corneal epithelial defects following penetrating keratoplasty have been identified. These include patients with a history of dry eyes, blepharitis, severe meibomitis, decreased corneal sensation, lagophthalmos, and eyelid abnormalities. In these high-risk patients, the predisposing factors must be treated before performing penetrating keratoplasty. Treatment may include punctal occlusion, intensive lid hygiene with oral tetracycline agents, or surgical repositioning of the eyelids. After adequate treatment of these predisposing factors, penetrating keratoplasty should be performed using only donor tissue that has excellent epithelium. Intraoperative techniques to prevent epithelial cell damage should be used, including careful tissue handling and the avoidance of excessive irrigation. Litoff and Krachmer[6] have recommended the use of donor storage medium as a surface lubricant intraoperatively. Viscoelastic agents may also serve to keep the epithelium hydrated during the intraocular procedure.

Postoperative epithelial defects may be treated with pressure patching or bandage contact lenses. In both cases, extreme care must be taken to avoid the increased risk of corneal infection. Tarsorrhaphy or punctal occlusion in patients with dry eyes may also be necessary to promote healing of the epithelial defect. Herpes simplex viral infections have been identified as a cause of persistent epithelial defect.[36–38] In addition, toxicity of topical medications and preservative agents have been identified as causes of persistent epithelial defects.[39] In some cases, changing to unpreserved medications or less toxic medications may result in healing of the epithelial defect (Fig. 9-2).

Wound Misalignment

Wound misalignment resulting from donor tissue override or underride may result in wound leaks, persistent epithelial defect, or increased postkeratoplasty astigmatism. The management of wound misalignment may be necessary to aid in reepithelial-

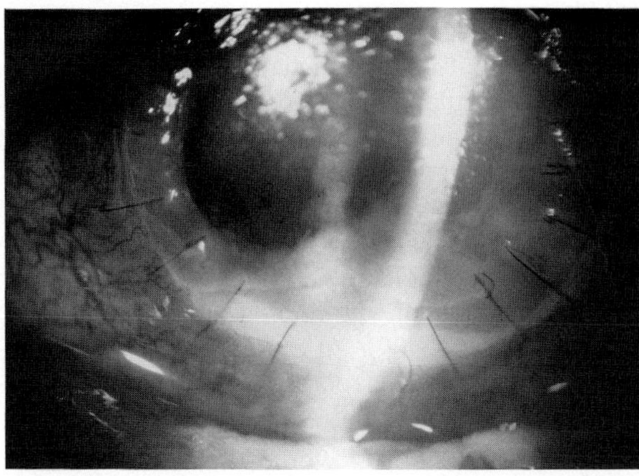

Figure 9-2. A persistent epithelial defect is seen in a patient with inferior override. The corneal epithelium is irregular. The margin of the nonhealing epithelial defect may be seen. The edge of the donor is necrotic with marked corneal infiltrate and loosening of the sutures. Cultures of the wound revealed infectious bacterial keratitis, which responded to treatment with topical fortified antibiotic drops.

ization of the donor graft tissue and prevent postkeratoplasty irregular astigmatism. Realignment of the wound may be performed by taking the patient back to the operating room and replacing or adding interrupted 10-0 nylon sutures. In some cases, application of a bandage soft contact lens may have similar results (Fig. 9-3).[9]

Price and associates[40] have reported an incidence of graft failure as high as 27%, resulting from problems with the external surface of the graft. As previously mentioned, careful attention to suture placement intraoperatively may prevent this early postoperative complication.

Late Postoperative Complications

Graft Rejection

Corneal graft rejection is by far the most common cause of graft failure after penetrating keratoplasty. Alldredge and Krachmer[41] have reported an overall incidence of endothelial graft rejection of 21%. Stromal vascularization or previous allograft rejection have been identified as predisposing factors to corneal graft rejection.[42–44] Overall, corneal graft failure secondary to immunologic graft rejection has been reported as 2% to 5% (Fig. 9-4). The complex immune response that results in corneal graft rejection is only partially understood. Human leukocyte antigens and T lymphocytes may be the primary stimuli in corneal graft rejection. Together with the human leukocyte antigen, T lymphocytes initiate a cascade of

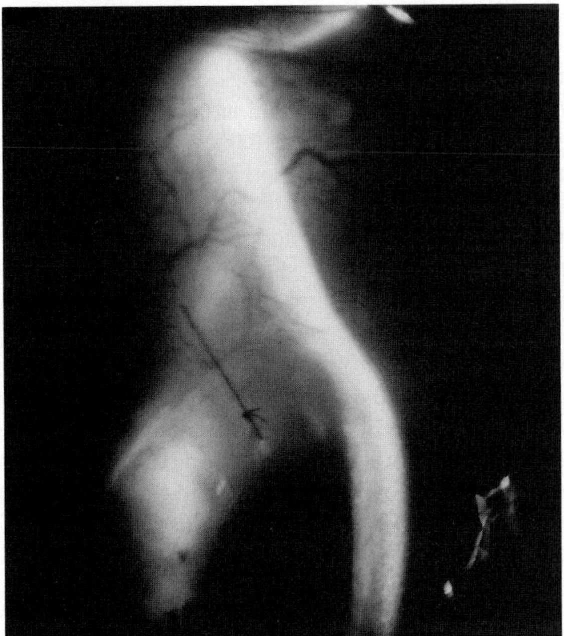

Figure 9-3. Anterior override may be seen with the anterior displacement of the slit beam. In this patient, the override resulted in a persistent epithelial defect, which was successfully treated with a bandage contact lens.

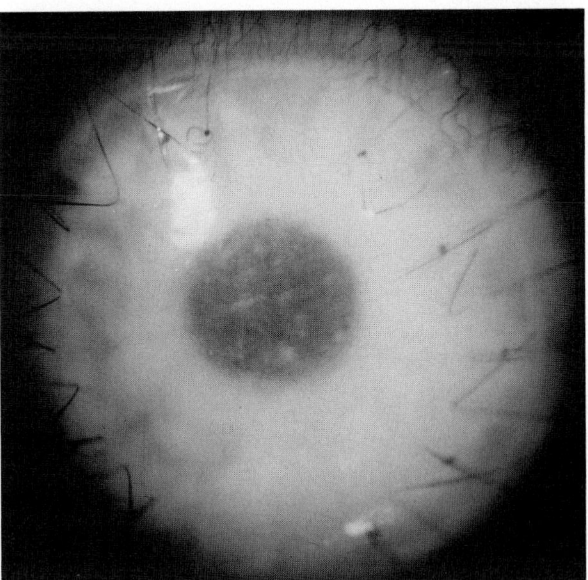

Figure 9-4. Endothelial corneal allograft rejection in a patient who presented with a broken running suture. Note the broken running suture at the 12-o'clock position. Frequently, a broken suture may act as a nidus for infection or rejection. It is not uncommon for patients who ignored the foreign body sensation associated with a broken suture to present with a concomitant graft rejection. Numerous keratic precipitates may be seen in the central aspect of the corneal graft.

cellular interactions that result in the activation and proliferation of cytotoxic T cells, B cells, killer T cells, macrophages, and complement. Belin and colleagues[45] have proposed a model for corneal graft rejection. The Langerhans cells located in the recipient cornea are thought to recognize the foreign antigen in the donor cornea. These Langerhans cells or macrophages then migrate to the regional lymphoid tissue where they present the antigen to helper T cells and release interleukin-1. The activated T cells migrate to the donor cornea and, after recognition, release lymphokines, including interleukin-2. The lymphokines activate cytotoxic T and B cells, which then actively attack the cornea and lead to graft rejection.

Clinically, graft rejection may be associated with pain, redness, and decrease of vision. Some patients may be asymptomatic when undergoing mild graft rejection. Corneal graft rejection has been subdivided into three types—endothelial, subepithelial, and epithelial. Endothelial graft rejection, the most serious type, often leads to graft failure. Clinical signs of endothelial graft rejection may include keratic precipitates, mild iritis, and stromal edema. Classic linear alignment of keratic precipitates has been described as a Khoudadoust line (Fig. 9-5). Endothelial graft rejections have been further subdivided into mild and severe by the collaborative corneal transplantation studies.[46] Subepithelial graft rejection is characterized by multiple subepithelial infiltrates similar to those seen in epidemic keratoconjunctivitis. The subepithelial infiltrates seen in graft rejection are limited to the corneal graft and occur in the absence of any conjunctival hyperemia or inflammation. Epithelial rejection frequently occurs without observation by the clinician. An epithelial rejection line, which may be elevated and stained with fluorescein or rose bengal, may be seen moving from the periphery toward the center of the graft. This represents replacement of the donor epithelium by the recipient epithelium. Early diagnosis and treatment may frequently result in reversal of corneal graft rejections. Education to help patients recognize the signs and symptoms of graft rejection, including pain or discomfort, redness, or loss of vision, is a crucial element in the prevention of corneal graft failure. Patients should be instructed to contact the surgeon if the signs persist for 24 hours. Treatment of endothelial graft rejection involves systemic as well as frequent topical corticosteroids. In a mild corneal allograft rejection, patients are frequently treated with prednisolone acetate every hour while awake and dexamethasone ointment at bedtime, with optional use of a cycloplegic agent. For patients with a severe allograft rejection, immediate institution of corticosteroid therapy is necessary. The Collaborative Corneal Transplant Study (CCTS) protocol recommends 125 mg of methylprednisolone sodium succinate intravenously followed by oral prednisone, 1 mg/kg/d for 5 days. Hourly topical steroids and dexamethasone ointment are also used in severe rejections. A single intravenous dose of 500 mg of methylprednisolone has been shown in one study to have a higher success rate than oral prednisone treatment.[47] An epithelial or subepithelial rejection may be treated with topical steroids every 2 hours followed by a slow tapering. Combined epithelial and subepithelial graft rejection often represent a smoldering endothelial rejection. The success rate of reversing corneal allograft reactions depends on numerous factors. The key factor is patient education; however, the duration of rejection, number of previous episodes of rejection, status of the endothelium, and the amount of the graft that is edematous may all play a role.

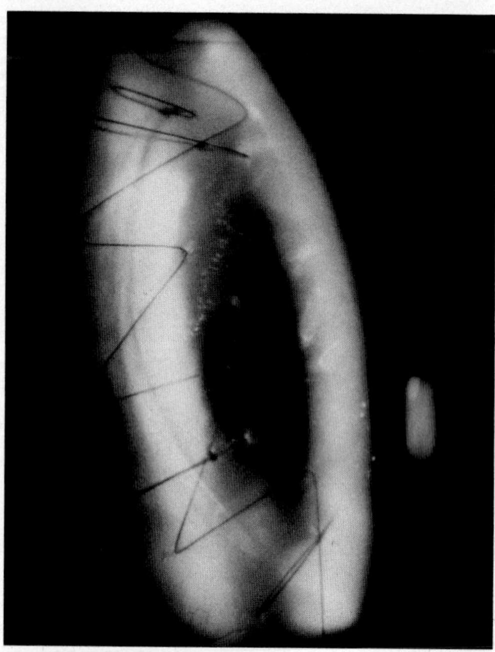

Figure 9-5. A Khoudadoust line may be seen as the keratic precipitates demonstrate a linear alignment near the sutures. Descemet fold and corneal edema may be seen in the slit beam.

Corneal Infections and Suture Abscesses

Microbial keratitis following penetrating keratoplasty may result in corneal graft opacification, corneal graft failure, and endophthalmitis. Fortunately, the incidence of microbial keratitis after penetrating keratoplasty is fairly low, ranging from 1.8% to 5%.[48,49] Numerous risk factors have been identified for the development of postoperative graft infection, including keratoconjunctivitis sicca, blepharitis, meibomianitis, herpes simplex viral infection, contact lens use, ocular cicatricial pemphigoid, lagophthalmos, and eyelid malpositioning. In addition, the use of topical corticosteroids may also predispose a patient to infection by impairing the local host defense mechanisms.

A loose suture may also be a nidus for infection and should be removed immediately (Fig. 9-6).[50] A suture abscess is an infiltrate surrounding a suture with an overlying epithelial defect, and may or may not be accompanied by a hypopyon. This is a potentially serious complication that may result in rapid spread of the infection to involve the entire corneal graft with possible wound dehiscence and endophthalmitis. Therefore, the abscess should be cultured with prompt institution of appropriate antibiotic therapy. Broad-spectrum coverage should be instituted initially with topical tobramycin, 9 mg/mL, and topical fortified cefazolin, 33 mg/mL, until culture results have been obtained. Placement of the removed suture on a blood agar plate may frequently help identify the causative organism.

Regardless of location, all corneal ulcers noted in corneal graft patients should be treated as bacterial unless the patient has a history of herpes simplex keratitis before undergoing penetrating keratoplasty. Herpes simplex keratitis frequently is an indication for penetrating keratoplasty, and recurrence after surgery is common. Recurrence rates after the first year of surgery vary from 10% to 17% and gradually increase during the next several years.[51]

If the recurrence of herpes simplex keratitis is epithelial in nature, diagnosis may be based on the clinical presentation of a dendritic lesion (Fig. 9-7). However, in many cases, recurrent herpetic keratouveitis is difficult to distinguish from corneal graft rejection. In these patients, concomitant treatment for both corneal graft rejection and herpes keratouveitis is indicated. Some authors have advocated the use of oral acyclovir in the perioperative period in patients with herpes simplex keratitis undergoing penetrating keratoplasty.[52] Failure of penetrating keratoplasty from allograft rejection is significantly higher in patients with a history of herpes simplex keratitis when there is significant stromal vascularization. In addition, herpes simplex keratitis has an increased risk of postkeratoplasty epithelial defects, and bacterial or fungal infections.

Recurrent herpetic disease is usually treated with topical antiviral agents for epithelial disease and oral acyclovir for stromal or uveal disease. The concomitant use of topical and systemic steroids is frequently used, but antiviral coverage is necessary under these circumstances. In patients with herpes simplex keratitis who have undergone penetrating keratoplasty,

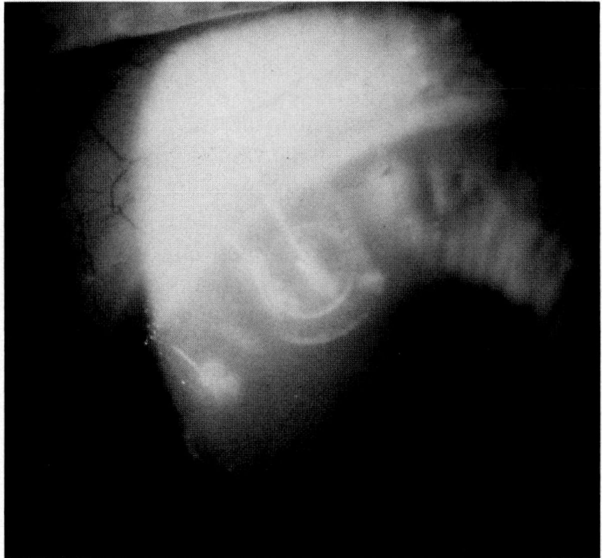

Figure 9-6. A broken interrupted suture is seen acting as a nidus for a suture abscess. Two surrounding ring infiltrates around the abscess may also be seen. Successful treatment involves rapid institution of intensive topical fortified antibiotics.

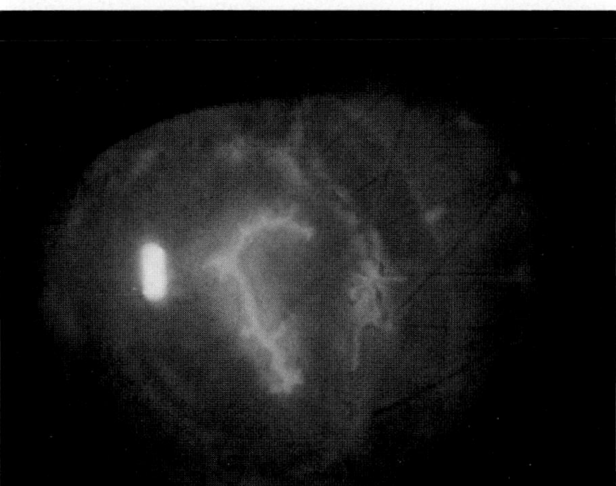

Figure 9-7. Fluorescein staining demonstrates classic dendritic lesion resulting from recurrent herpes simplex viral keratitis in a corneal graft. Treatment includes rapid institution of intensive topical antiviral agents. When the dendrite involves the visual axis, débridement is frequently recommended. (See color plate after page xvi.)

the presentation of an allograft rejection is usually treated with topical and systemic corticosteroids. However, again, these patients must receive antiviral agents to prevent further recurrence of the underlying disease.

Patients who undergo penetrating keratoplasty for infectious keratitis, whether bacterial, fungal, or *Acanthamoeba* in nature, frequently have recurrence of the primary disease in the corneal graft.[53] In this case, aggressive treatment is warranted to prevent decompensation of the transplant and the need for further surgery. Many of these patients have progressive sclerokeratitis, which is an indication for both topical and systemic therapy. The long-term complications of such a severe infectious process include corneal scarring, wound dehiscence, and possible endophthalmitis.

Infectious crystalline keratopathy has been reported in corneal transplants. The characteristic appearance includes a crystalline intrastromal deposit that often resembles a snowflake pattern. This is seen most commonly near the graft–host interface.[54,55] This is a chronic corneal infection with intrastromal bacteria and minimal inflammatory reaction. Numerous organisms have been identified, the most common being α-hemolytic streptococci. Other bacterial species, including *Haemophilus aphrophilus, Staphylococcus aureus, Staphylococcus epidermidis, Pseudomonas* sp, and enterococcus, have been implicated.[56] Therapy includes aggressive topical fortified antibiotics. However, the outcome for many patients is poor because of the intrastromal nature of the bacteria and inadequate penetration of the antibiotics. Regrafting may be necessary if the patients fail to respond to topical medication.

Astigmatism

High postkeratoplasty astigmatism is a difficult and significant problem that can compromise visual rehabilitation despite a clear corneal graft. Causes of high postkeratoplasty astigmatism include the trephine incision, donor–recipient wound misalignment, and variation in suture placement and tension.[57,58] Among the numerous suture techniques advocated to decrease postoperative astigmatism have been single running suture placement with early postoperative suture adjustment, selective suture removal of interrupted sutures, and combined running suture techniques.[59,60]

High postkeratoplasty astigmatism that occurs before suture removal can be treated in one of two ways. If interrupted sutures are present in the steep meridian, the sutures can be removed. The decision as to which sutures require removal is based on keratometry, refraction, retinoscopy, and computer-assisted photokeratoscopy.[61,62] If a continuous running suture remains, the suture in the flat meridian can be tightened and the suture in the steep meridian loosened.[63]

High postkeratoplasty astigmatism that persists after removal of all sutures may frequently be managed with spectacle correction or contact lens wear depending on the severity of the astigmatism. In patients with less than 4 diopters of astigmatism and minimal anisometropia, spectacle correction is frequently tolerated. Contact lenses may correct up to 6 D of postkeratoplasty astigmatism in the average patient. Rigid gas-permeable lenses with or without a soft lens skirt are most successful in these patients. Surgical management of high postkeratoplasty astigmatism may be performed by relaxing incisions with or without compression sutures and wedge resections.[64–66] Relaxing incisions are made in several ways. Some authors recommend placement directly in the corneal wound, whereas others place the relaxing incisions in the corneal graft tissue. A diamond or steel blade has been advocated. The incisions are made approximately 60 degrees in length at both ends of the steep meridian. The incisions are made to a depth of 75% or greater.

Computer-assisted photokeratoscopy can be useful in identifying nonorthogonal astigmatism. In this case, incisions would be made in the appropriate meridians as identified on the photokeratoscopy.

On rare occasions, these methods of reducing postkeratoplasty astigmatism are unsuccessful, and repeated surgery must be performed. Inadvertent perforation may result in endophthalmitis, a flat anterior chamber, or a suprachoroidal hemorrhage. Postoperative bacterial corneal ulcers and infectious crystalline keratopathy have also been reported.[54] All of these risks, including the possible need for repeat penetrating keratoplasty, should be included in the informed consent obtained from the patient.

Epithelial Downgrowth

Epithelial downgrowth is another rare but devastating complication of penetrating keratoplasty. The differential diagnosis includes corneal graft rejection, iridocyclitis, or glaucoma. The origin of epithelial downgrowth involves a fistulous tract, which allows epithelium to proliferate into the anterior chamber. Careful wound closure is a key element in the prevention of epithelial downgrowth.

Epithelial downgrowth may be asymptomatic in nature, or the patient may complain of pain, redness, or photophobia. Early in the course, iridocyclitis may present as clumps of epithelium seen floating in the aqueous. The absence of keratic precipitates should alert the physician to this possibility. Other clinical features include a grayish elevated irregular line on Descemet membrane, glaucoma, corectopia, and an iris membrane.

Frequently, epithelial downgrowth is confused with an endothelial graft rejection. Epithelial downgrowth should be suspected in any patient who does not respond to treatment with topical and systemic corticosteroids in a presumed endothelial graft rejection. Careful documentation with slit-lamp photographs may demonstrate advancement of a posterior corneal line in the face of adequate treatment for endothelial graft rejection.[67,68]

If epithelial downgrowth is suspected, an aqueous aspirate may be examined for cytopathology. Any abnormal areas where an iris membrane is suspected may be confirmed by laser photocoagulation. Large burns may be placed on the iris with the argon laser. If the iris surface turns white, this is considered a positive test for the presence of epithelium on the iris stroma. This method can be used to determine the extent of the epithelial membrane and assist in preoperative planning. The goal of treatment is to remove all of the epithelium from the anterior eye, which may require radical surgery. Some surgeons have advocated various techniques, such as excision of the iris, scraping, and cryotherapy.[69]

Cystoid Macular Edema

Cystoid macular edema is most common after penetrating keratoplasty when performed with intraocular lens exchange. It frequently is present preoperatively; however, the cloudy cornea limits the surgeon's ability to document macular edema. Preoperative discussions with the patient undergoing penetrating keratoplasty should include this possibility and the resultant limited prognosis for visual rehabilitation. It frequently results in poor visual outcome because of damage to the macula.

The incidence of cystoid macular edema after penetrating keratoplasty ranges from 4% to 65%.[70,71] The origin is multifactorial. Cystoid macular edema has been associated with vitreous corneal touch, vitreous incarceration in the wound, vitreous adherence to the iris, chronic intraocular inflammation, and photic damage from the surgical microscope.

The diagnosis is made by clinical examination of the macula with a 90-D lens or contact lens and is confirmed by fluorescein angiography. A classic appearance of a stellate pattern that corresponds to the cystoid spaces on a fluorescein angiogram is diagnostic.

Treatment of cystoid macular edema includes sub-Tenon injection of corticosteroids, topical corticosteroids, topical prostaglandin inhibitors, and systemic carbonic anhydrase inhibitors. Surgical treatment includes complete pars plana vitrectomy. Although numerous different treatments have been recommended for cystoid macular edema, there is no conclusive evidence that any of these agents is effective. Careful intraoperative performance of a vitrectomy can frequently decrease the incidence of postkeratoplasty cystoid macular edema. The bimanual technique, including the use of a light pipe with an automated vitrector, allows better visualization of otherwise clear vitreous strands and more complete removal of the vitreous intraoperatively.

Anisometropia

Significant anisometropia after penetrating keratoplasty may result in a disappointing outcome for both the patient and surgeon. Causes of this anisometropia include miscalculation of intraocular lens power and a steep corneal graft following keratoplasty. In some patients, significant anisometropia may be managed with the use of a monocular contact lens. If there is not significant astigmatism, a soft contact lens may be used. A rigid contact lens may resolve postkeratoplasty astigmatism and anisometropia. Radial keratotomy may be performed after keratoplasty to reduce significant myopia with moderate success.[72]

Recurrent Disease

Numerous indications for penetrating keratoplasty may resurface postoperatively as a recurrent disease. Herpes keratitis after keratoplasty has been reported to occur in from 15% to 47% of cases.[73–75] It does not appear that performing penetrating keratoplasty during active disease puts the patient at risk for recurrence of herpes keratitis in the graft; however, these cases may be complicated by wound healing problems or graft rejection. Therefore, when possible, it is advisable to wait until the herpes keratitis has been quiescent for an extended period (6 months) before performing penetrating keratoplasty. Treatment of graft rejections with intensive topical steroids and prophylactic topical antivirals has improved the results in herpetic keratoplasties and decreased the risk of recurrence of the disease; however, one or more rejection episodes do occur in about half of patients undergoing penetrating keratoplasty for herpes keratitis. In patients with highly vascularized recipient beds, interrupted sutures may decrease the risk of bacterial infection by allowing for removal of loose sutures. Herpes zoster keratitis, which can also recur after keratoplasty, may result in allograft rejection. Patients with herpes zoster frequently have a neurotrophic cornea that may develop problems with persistent epithelial defects. Prophylactic placement of lateral tarsorrhaphies may decrease the incidence of postoperative epithelial defects in these patients. Numerous corneal dystrophies are also known to recur after keratoplasty, including lattice, granular, and Reis-Bückler dystrophy (Fig. 9-8), and hereditary stromal dystrophy. Recurrences occur most commonly in grafts for lattice dystrophy, with 25% to 50% of grafts demonstrating recurrence within 25 years (Fig. 9-9).[76–79] Numerous inflammatory processes, whether bacterial or autoimmune in nature, have also been reported to recur within the graft.

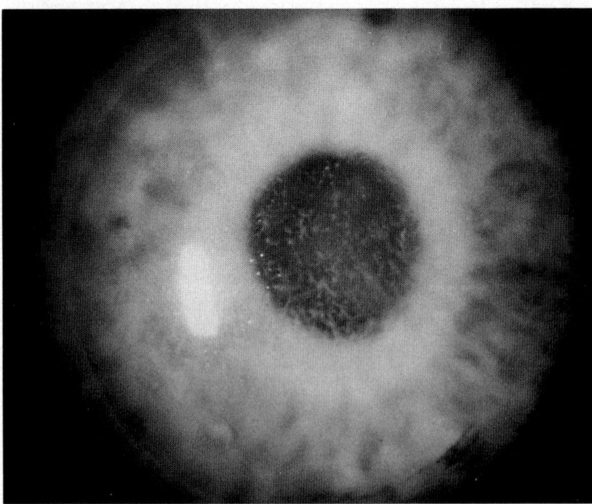

Figure 9-8. Recurrence of Reis-Bücklers corneal dystrophy in a penetrating keratoplasty 8 years after the initial surgery. A honeycomb-like subepithelial pattern may be seen covering the entire surface of the corneal graft. (See color plate after page xvi.)

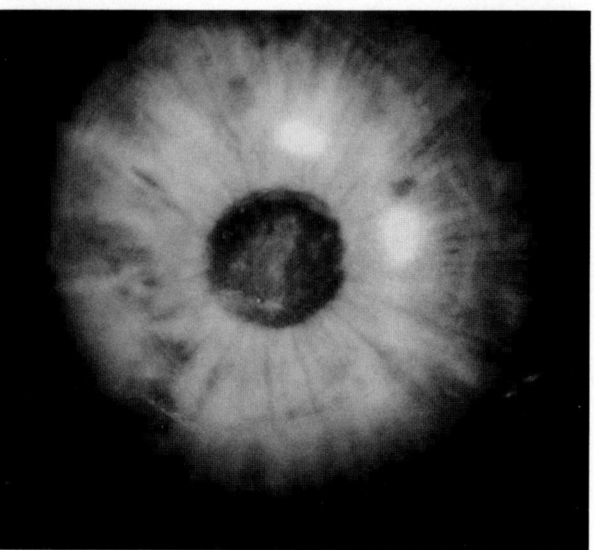

Figure 9-9. Recurrent lattice corneal dystrophy in a penetrating keratoplasty 6 years after the original surgery. The recurrent lattice dystrophy results in an irregular epithelial surface, which is prone to recurrent corneal erosions, as seen here. Methods of treatment modalities have included lamellar keratectomy, excimer laser phototherapeutic keratectomy, and penetrating keratoplasty. (See color plate after page xvi.)

LAMELLAR KERATOPLASTY

The overall number of lamellar grafts has decreased because of the increased availability of donor material and improved surgical instrumentation. Four types of lamellar grafts remain—tectonic lamellar grafts, optical lamellar grafts, therapeutic lamellar grafts, and cosmetic lamellar grafts. The rate of complication decreases with the surgeon's increased experience with the challenging surgical techniques required in lamellar keratoplasty.

Intraoperative Complications

Malpositioning of the Donor Button

Malpositioning of the donor button is obviously a surgeon-related error that may be alleviated with careful preoperative mapping of the corneal disease at the slit lamp (Fig. 9-10). Some surgeons have suggested marking the patient's cornea preoperatively with a fine incision into the corneal epithelium at the slit lamp before performing surgery.

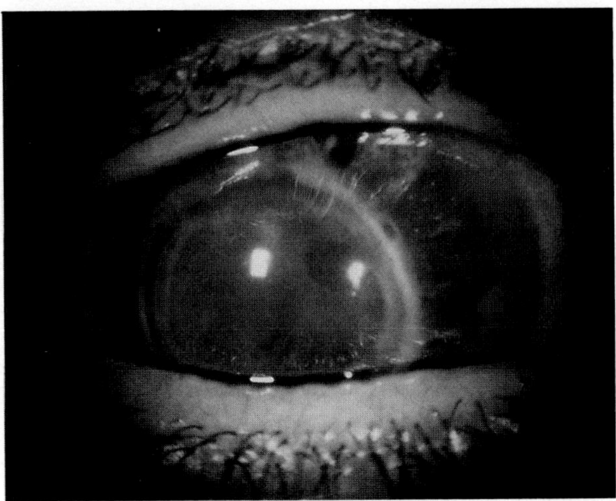

Figure 9-10. A malpositioned lamellar keratoplasty performed for keratoconus. Note that the patient is looking through the edge of the button, causing visually significant distortion.

Inadvertent Perforation

Inadvertent microperforation can and does occur in lamellar keratoplasty. It becomes less likely as the surgeon becomes more experienced with the dissection technique. Injection of air into the stroma may help delineate the corneal stroma from the underlying clear Descemet membrane and allow for dissection of the stroma off of the Descemet membrane without perforation. Should a small perforation occur, the procedure should be completed. The anterior chamber may be formed with air, Healon, or another viscoelastic material to reposition the host tissue against the lamellar graft. A large perforation may allow aqueous to percolate between the two layers and prevent proper wound healing. This may result in a flat anterior chamber. In such cases, a penetrating keratoplasty should be done.

Poor Donor–Host Interface

Uneven dissection may produce a rough recipient bed that results in an optically and structurally poor donor–host interface. This may occur more commonly in patients with a vascularized recipient bed and intrastromal scarring. Incorporation of foreign particles into the recipient bed is a common problem in lamellar keratoplasty. Hamilton and Wood[80] have recommended anchoring the graft with three to four sutures and then irrigating the interface with several milliliters of balanced salt solution using concomitant suction to remove any debris.[80] Lipid deposition is more often seen in vascularized corneas and may contribute to decreased visual acuity. Hemorrhage may also result at the interface in vascularized corneas.

Postoperative Complications

Persistent Epithelial Defects

Persistent epithelial defects lead to increased risk of complication and resultant graft failure. Meticulous attention to the ocular surface before the decision to proceed with lamellar keratoplasty and proper coaptation of the lids may prevent these complications. Aggressive treatment with tarsorrhaphies, bandage contact lenses, and lid hygiene may aid in resolution of these epithelial defects.

Opacification of the Interface

Irregular astigmatism and epithelial ingrowth may result from imperfect alignment of the donor edges at the wound.[81–83] These complications are more commonly encountered when a lamellar graft has been done on a cornea that is still actively inflamed. In some cases, these complications may be treated with the use of a rigid contact lens; however, penetrating keratoplasty may be indicated. Infection of the lamellar bed is greatly increased in patients with persistent epithelial defects and can be reduced by good surgical techniques and careful postoperative follow-up. Graft rejection can occur in lamellar keratoplasty. If the reaction is not properly treated, it may lead to a failed graft.[84]

REFRACTIVE SURGERY

Radial Keratotomy

Radial keratotomy is a growing procedure in the United States to alleviate refractive errors in otherwise normal corneas. This remains an elective procedure in patients who might otherwise be optically corrected with spectacles or contact lenses. Radial keratotomy involves peripheral corneal incisions and thus spares the central visual axis. Procedures that involve surgical intervention in the central visual axis, such as excimer laser keratectomy, lamellar keratoplasty, or epikeratophakia, carry a different set of potential complications than radial keratotomy.

Intraoperative Complications

CORNEAL PERFORATION. Corneal perforation is the most common complication during radial keratotomy. Corneal perforation has been defined as a microperforation or macroperforation. A microperforation that occurs more commonly along the inferior or temporal incision where the cornea is thinnest results in the loss of 1 to 2 drops of aqueous humor.[85,86] Macroperforations result in rapid loss of aqueous humor, flattening of the anterior chamber, and frequently require closure with interrupted 10-0 nylon sutures. The termination of the surgical procedure is required. The prospective evaluation of radial keratotomy (PERK) study reported a rate of microperforations of 2.3%.[87] Macroperforations have been reported to occur with a frequency of 0% to 13%.[88–90] Prolonged corneal dehydration has been cited as a factor that may increase the incidence of corneal perforation.[91]

Perforation may be avoided by setting the depth of the diamond knife to 100% of the thinnest paracentral corneal pachymetry reading; however, the gauge by which the diamond blade is set must also be accurate. The recent development of the micronscope allows calibration of the diamond blade to within 0.001 mm. Numerous postoperative complications may result from corneal perforations during radial keratotomy. Scar formation at all levels of the cornea with damage to the corneal endothelium and peripheral anterior synechiae have all been reported. If the incision is continued in the presence of a shallow anterior chamber, laceration of the iris and anterior lens capsule may occur.[92]

ENDOTHELIAL CELL DAMAGE. A mild decrease in the corneal endothelial cell count has been reported in otherwise uncomplicated radial keratotomy.[93,94] The endothelial cell density has been shown to decrease up to 10%; however, corneal perforation increases the degree of endothelial cell damage.[95,96] Rowsey and associates[96] have demonstrated progressive decrease in the endothelial cell density by specular microscopy and changes in endothelial cell morphology in patients 1 year after radial keratotomy. Clinically, microcystic corneal edema may be seen in the early postoperative period in the cornea immediately adjacent to the incisions. Specular microscopy may demonstrate swelling of the endothelium in these areas. In most patients, clinical evidence of these endothelial cell changes resolves within the first 3 months of the postoperative period.

OPTICAL ZONE DECENTRATION. Failure to identify the central visual axis of the cornea adequately may result in decentration of the incisions. A resultant increase in glare and irregular astigmatism may occur. Numerous techniques have been described to mark the center of the visual axis.[97,98] With the advent of computed corneal topographic analysis, preoperative determinations of both the corneal vertex and pupil may be made on patients undergoing radial keratotomy. These measurements may help the surgeon determine whether the patient has a positive- or negative-angle κ. Placement of the corneal topographic map in the operating room may assist the surgeon in centering the optical zone marker. Caution should be taken to invert the corneal topographic map to correspond to the surgeon's view.

BLEEDING. Intraoperative bleeding into the corneal incisions occurs most commonly when incisions cross the limbus or peripheral corneal pannus. This bleeding into the wound does not enhance the effect of the operation and may stimulate vascularized limbal scar tissue growth into the wound.[99] Placement of incisions within the vascular pannus, which may be present in soft contact lens wearers, decreases the risk of intraoperative bleeding and does not appear to affect the refractive result of the procedure significantly.

EXTENSION OF INCISION. Extension of incisions into the limbus may result in bleeding; however, extension of the incision into the optical clear zone or across the visual axis may result in scar formation and permanent decrease in the visual potential of the patient. Marking of the optical zone with an optical zone marker, which has been stained with gentian violet, may more clearly delineate the optical zone to the surgeon. Placement of incisions from the periphery toward the center may increase the risk of extension of incisions into the optical axis, especially in cases in which the globe is not fixated. The recent development of a duo-track diamond knife allows the surgeon to initiate the cuts from the edge of the optical zone and to move peripherally with a front cutting edge and to backtrack along the incision with a back cutting edge of the diamond knife, which is sharp only at the most distal end. The dullness of the proximal end of the diamond blade prevents extension of the incision into the optical zone during the second pass of the knife.

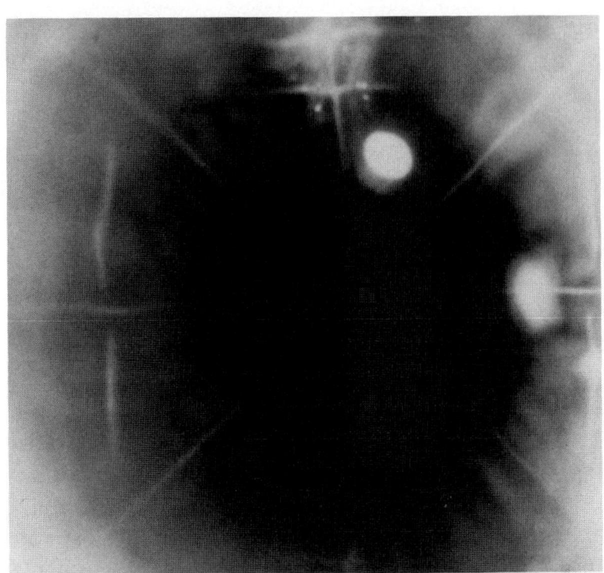

Figure 9-11. An eight-incisional radial keratotomy has been performed with T cuts to reduce corneal astigmatism. Crossing of the incisions may be seen at the 12-o'clock position. Note the significant scarring in this area. In addition, subepithelial opacity is extensive in the area of the crossed incision.

CROSSING INCISIONS. Intersection of incisions during radial keratotomy may produce severe wound gapes and significant amounts of scarring (Fig. 9-11).[100,101] The wound gape that results from intersecting of radial incisions, or radial and transverse incisions eventually fills with epithelium and produce stromal scarring. An extensive subepithelial opacity may extend from this wound. Irregular astigmatism and glare frequently result from such crossing of incisions. The gape created by crossing of incisions may take months to heal and result in significant visual fluctuation and long-term irregular astigmatism.

Postoperative Complications

PAIN. Most patients experience pain or foreign-body sensation after incisional keratotomy. The pain may last for 24 to 72 hours, and patients frequently require analgesics. The topical application of nonsteroidal antiinflammatory drugs may decrease the incidence of postoperative pain as may patching the eye for the first 24 hours. Many patients require pain medication and a sleeping pill during the first 24 hours of the postoperative period.

GLARE. An increase in glare and starburst aberrations when viewing headlights at night has been reported to occur in many patients.[102,103] Most patients note a starburst phenomenon around lights at night, but few have reported a decrease in visual function as a result of this. Mild to moderate glare persists beyond the usual 3 to 6 months in some patients. Rarely, patients report that glare is disabling and disruptive to daily activities, causing them to curtail night driving, use sunglasses, or change their occupations.[104,105] For most patients, glare is minimal and resolves within the first 3 to 6 months of the postoperative period.[106,107]

UNDERCORRECTION AND OVERCORRECTION. Unplanned undercorrection and overcorrection remain the most frequent complications of radial keratotomy. Recent studies using four incisions to correct low to moderate myopia reported a lower incidence of overcorrections than studies using eight incisions.[108–112] Rashid and Waring[105] explained the accommodative problems experienced by the myope who suddenly becomes a hyperope. In addition, patients who are made hyperopic before age 40 experience symptomatic presbyopia at an earlier age as a result of radial keratotomy. Once presbyopic, they require correction for both distance and near vision. Contact lenses may be fit in most patients after radial keratotomy. However, this is generally a more complicated fit. Knowledge of the presurgical keratometry readings may be useful in eliciting a starting point for fitting lenses after radial keratotomy; however, the paracentral steepening of the cornea may tend to decenter the lens. Soft contact lenses may often induce vascularization of peripheral keratotomy scars, especially if they extend to the limbus. Topographic analyses of corneas after radial keratotomy have demonstrated multiple areas of sphericity in the pupil, resulting in a multifocal cornea. In some patients this is beneficial because it allows for both near and distance correction. However, in other patients, multiple confusing visual images have a negative effect.[113–117] Success rates in fitting contact lenses after radial keratotomy have been reported to be only 56% to 58%.[118,119]

Surgical management of overcorrection after radial keratotomy has been described. This technique involves opening of radial incisions followed by placement of continuous purse string sutures, 10-0 nylon sutures, or Mersilene sutures.[120–122] As with corneal wedge resections or relaxing incisions with compression sutures, significant overcorrection needs to be achieved intraoperatively because much of the effect decays with time and suture removal.

Undercorrection is much less problematic than overcorrection. Patients who are used to being myopic have little problem adjusting to mild undercorrections. Recent studies have endorsed a more conservative approach to surgical correction of myopia with a staged procedure allowing for enhancement operations.[123] Using this technique, Werblin[123] reported a 99% uncorrected visual acuity of 20/40 or better in 205 consecutive eyes. Most surgeons intentionally aim for a slightly myopic correction because of the well-documented continued postoperative effect of the procedure. Excimer laser photorefractive keratectomy (PRK) has been reported as a second procedure in eyes that are undercorrected following radial keratotomy.[124] This technique may represent a new future application of purposefully combining radial keratotomy with PRK in the management of myopia.

FLUCTUATIONS IN VISION. Fluctuation of vision has been reported to occur in some patients as long as 5 years after surgery. However, few patients require a separate optical correction during the day. Three and a half years after undergoing radial keratotomy, 31% of eyes in the PERK study showed a change of 0.50 D or more during the course of the day.[125] Most patients underwent a gradual steepening of their corneas during the course of the day, ranging from 0.50 to 1.25 D. Patients with undercorrected defects saw best in the morning, whereas those with overcorrected defects experienced an improvement in visual acuity during the day.[126] Computed video keratography has confirmed these diurnal changes in patients up to 7 years after radial keratotomy.[127] The cause of this diurnal fluctuation is unknown but is thought to be related to long-term wound healing of the keratotomy incisions. In the immediate postoperative period, the sutured wounds are filled with an epithelial plug. The cornea may require more than 5 years to replace the epithelial plug completely with remodeled corneal stroma.[128–130] The constant pressure of the eyelids during sleep, and mild epithelial and stromal edema, are believed to induce a nocturnal flattening of the cornea that may lead to further diurnal fluctuation.[131]

EPITHELIAL CHANGES. Epithelial inclusion cysts, frequently seen within radial keratotomy incisions, do not appear to alter the visual results. Maplike changes consistent with anterior epithelial basement membrane dystrophy may be seen after radial keratotomy.[132] These changes are infrequently associated with clinical symptoms or recurrent epithelial erosions. In most eyes, these changes tend to disappear within the first 3 postoperative months. The epithelial plug is slowly replaced by corneal stroma, and the scars become less dense during the years after surgery. The corneal stroma adjacent to the incisions remodels and becomes more transparent. A single case of epithelial ingrowth after radial keratotomy has been reported.[133] Avoiding the injection of an irrigating stream through the site of corneal perforation may limit the introduction of epithelial cells into the anterior chamber and therefore reduce the likelihood of epithelial ingrowth.[134]

INFECTIONS. Three reports of *S epidermidis* endophthalmitis after radial keratotomy have been made.[135–137] All patients presented with small hypopyon 8 to 10 days postoperatively, and all patients had an excellent visual outcome. Nine otherwise unpublished cases of gram-negative endophthalmitis are reported by Cross and Head.[138] In all cases, corneal perforation with introduction of microorganisms into the eye appears to be the etiology of the endophthalmitis.

The procedure is frequently performed in an office setting; however, strict adherence to sterile surgical technique is required. Bacterial or fungal keratitis may occur in the immediate postoperative period or several years after incisional keratotomy. Causative organisms include *Pseudomonas, Staphylococcus, S epidermidis,* and *Streptococcus pneumoniae.*[139–141] One patient who underwent incisional keratotomy on both eyes within a 24-hour period developed bilateral corneal ulcers. Two cases of *Mycobacterium chelonei* keratitis were reported in one surgeon's office, where outpatient radial keratotomy was performed using cold, sterilized instruments.[142] The risk of infection can be minimized by strict adherence to sterile surgical technique and use of prophylactic topical antibiotics until reepithelialization of the incisions has occurred. Treatment of any blepharitis or condition of the ocular adnexa that might predispose a patient to postoperative infections is required before surgery. Immediate treatment of bacterial keratitis after radial keratotomy may limit the spread of the infection (Fig. 9-12). After corneal scrapings have been taken for culture and Gram staining, therapy should begin with intensive fortified topical antibiotics. Patients unable to administer their own drops may require hospitalization. Daily follow-up of these patients is mandatory to observe the effect of the therapy.

Radial keratotomy in patients with herpes simplex keratitis has been associated with reports of reactivation.[143,144] As a result, some authors think that patients with a history of herpes simplex keratitis should not undergo incisional keratotomy. Late development

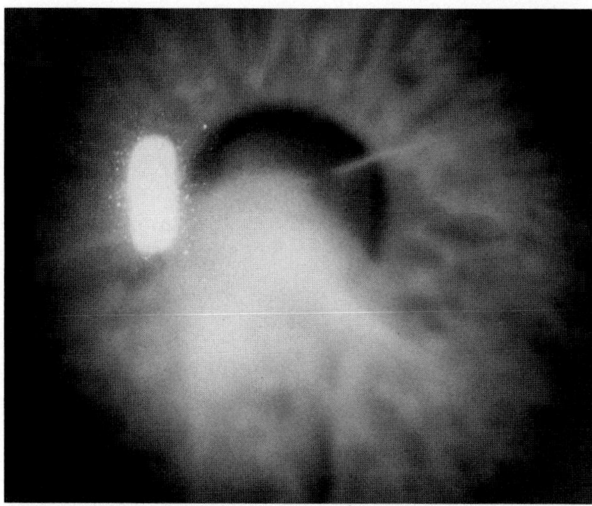

Figure 9-12. Bacterial keratitis after radial keratotomy may result in significant scarring of the visual axis. In this patient, a *Pseudomonas aeruginosa* corneal ulcer resulted in significant corneal scarring despite rapid institution of fortified topical antibiotics.

of bacterial and fungal ulcerative keratitis is an unusual complication of incision keratotomy.[145,146] In all patients, the corneal infiltrates were contiguous with the keratotomy scars, suggesting delayed expulsion of the epithelial plug as a possible cause of a predisposing epithelial defect. Intensive topical fortified antibiotic therapy is necessary regardless of the time of presentation.

CORNEAL RUPTURE. The incisions performed in incisional keratotomy permanently weaken the cornea, making it vulnerable to traumatic rupture of the keratotomy scars (Fig. 9-13).[147–150] The scars from the keratotomy incisions do not appear to have the same tensile strength as the original cornea. There are several reports of traumatic rupture of keratotomy scars after blunt trauma in both human and animal models. The force required to rupture a globe after radial keratotomy is about half that required to rupture control eyes within the first 90 days of healing.[151] After blunt trauma, animal eyes that have undergone radial keratotomy rupture more frequently through the keratotomy incisions, whereas normal eyes rupture most frequently at the equator.[152] Penetrating keratoplasty often produces opening of the scars during trephination, and retinal or vitreal surgery without elevated intraocular pressure may be associated with the opening of keratotomy wounds.[153]

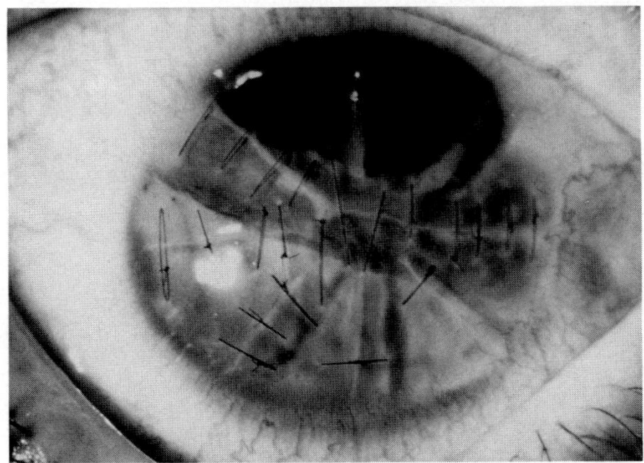

Figure 9-13. Blunt trauma to an eye 2 years after radial keratotomy resulted in disruption of seven of the eight radial keratotomy incisions, and loss of the lens and iris. Primary repair may be seen here.

INDUCED ASTIGMATISM. After radial keratotomy, all corneas demonstrate some degree of irregular astigmatism by keratoscopy. Minimal irregular astigmatism appears to have little effect on vision during daylight conditions; however, during dim illumination, when the pupil dilates, patients have reported increased glare, distortion, and a starburst phenomenon.

After 5 years, the PERK study revealed that 15% of eyes had an increase in astigmatism of 1.00 D or more postoperatively.[154] Functionally significant irregular astigmatism occurs when incisions extend into the visual axis, when radial and transverse incisions intersect, or when eyes have undergone numerous repeat surgeries. Repeated operations may increase the corneal astigmatism, both regular and irregular. In some cases, repeated operations may have no effect or may actually increase the amount of myopia. Visually significant induced astigmatism may be masked by a rigid gas-permeable contact lens or incisional astigmatic keratotomy.

Photorefractive Keratectomy

The 193-nm excimer laser can accurately ablate corneal tissue. The excimer laser destroys Bowman layer in the ablated area, which includes the central visual axis. Phase III clinical trials have been completed on 1400 patients by two companies, Summit Technology, Inc. (Waltham, MA) and Visx Inc. (Fort Worth, TX) The results of these investigational trials await the approval of the Food and Drug Administration. These trials included patients with up to 6 D of myopia and less than 1 D of astigmatism.

Intraoperative Complications

LOSS OF FIXATION. In PRK, fixation of the eye and centration of the laser beam are accomplished by either manual or visual techniques. The visual techniques rely on the patient to fixate on a fixation light, leaving the potential for significant decentration of the ablation. The operation of the laser is through a foot switch controlled by the surgeon, who may visualize the eye through a coaxial operating microscope. This arrangement allows the surgeon to interrupt the procedure at any time, should the patient lose fixation, by merely releasing the foot switch. In the first 700 patients who underwent phase III clinical trials through Summit Technology, Inc, the loss of fixation rate was 2.3% (16 patients). In all patients, refixation was achieved and the procedure completed without complications (Steinert RR, New England Eye Center, personal communication, July 1993).

OPTICAL ZONE DECENTRATION. The optical zone is marked manually by the surgeon during PRK over the constricted pupil. Computerized video keratography may be used to assist in the centering of the excimer laser for PRK.[155] One must consider that the power at the center of the ablation is not a single point value but rather an average measure of the corneal power at the surrounding points.[156] Therefore, the correct centering of PRK is important if a correct refractive result is to be achieved. When no stabilization system is used, small involuntary movements by the patient or surgeon, difficulty fixating on the light by the patient, and pupillary irregularity may all contribute to centering errors. In high myopia, a longer uninterrupted exposure to the laser is required and may cause more frequent loss of fixation and decentration.[157] Calculations show the importance of correct centration for optimal retinal image quality. If a 4-mm optical zone is decentered by 1 mm relative to a 4-mm entrance pupil, 31% of the light rays emanating from a distant object miss the ablated area. These light rays are refracted to a different extent, creating ghost images, glare, or loss of contrast sensitivity.[158–160]

INADEQUATE EPITHELIUM REMOVAL. After the optical zone is marked, complete removal of the epithelium is required. This should occur in a timely manner to prevent dehydration and subsequent change in the corneal thickness from the time of completion of epithelial débridement to activation of the laser. Studies have established that corneal epithelium, Bowman layer, and stroma ablate at different rates.[161] Complete and regular removal of epithelium is essential in PRK, because excimer laser energy applied directly to an uneven corneal surface simply results in a thinner cornea with the same irregular surface.

Postoperative Complications

PAIN. Pain is a problem after PRK. Patients treated in phase III clinical trials experience considerable pain. Recent use of topical nonsteroidal antiinflammatory drops in the postoperative period and a bandage contact lens has shown a decrease in the severity and occurrence of postoperative pain.[162]

CORNEAL HAZE. In virtually every PRK-treated cornea, a faint diffuse subepithelial stromal haze appeared a few months after surgery, gradually diminishing within the first postoperative year (Fig. 9-14*A*). In most patients, the haze does not interfere with vision. Clinically relevant scars occurred in about 2% of cases, usually patients requiring corrections greater than 6 D, and scarring led to reduction of best corrected visual acuity by two or more Snellen lines (see Fig. 9-14*B*).[163–165] In the 585 eyes that had 1-year follow-up in the phase III Summit Technology, Inc, clinical trial, 27.2% of patients had trace haze, 6.5% had mild haze, and 4.1% had moderate haze at the 1-year follow-up. Seiler and colleagues[166] reported success with repeat excimer laser treatment after PRK in patients with visually significant haze. Caubet[167] identified some factors that increase the risk of haze, including higher myopia, smaller ablation diameters, and male gender. These results suggest there exists a significant haze risk group in which the absence or discontinuation of corticosteroids leads to significant haze.[167] Modulating the healing process by steroids, mitomycin C, and other growth inhibiting factors may be promising.[168]

PERSISTENT EPITHELIAL DEFECTS. All patients undergoing PRK appear to reepithelialize within 1 week. One case of a corneal ulcer in a patient with systemic lupus erythematosus has been reported.[169] Seiler[169] has suggested collagen vascular and other autoimmune diseases as contraindications for PRK. Recently, two cases have been reported of patients with traumatic corneal abrasions after excimer laser therapy.[170] No serious sequelae, such as stromal scar-

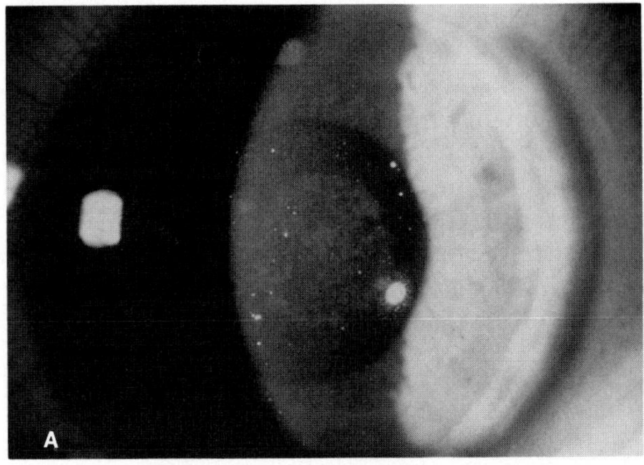
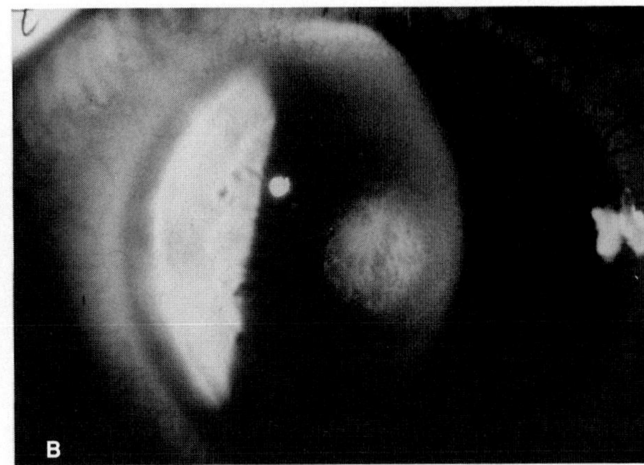

Figure 9-14. (**A**) A patient 6 months after photorefractive keratectomy demonstrating mild central diffuse subepithelial stromal haze. The patient achieved uncorrected 20/20 vision. (**B**) Clinically significant subepithelial stromal haze in a patient who has undergone photorefractive keratectomy for a correction greater than 6 diopters.

ring, recurrent erosions or change in the patient's refractive errors, were reported. Recent studies have suggested that blowing nitrogen gas over the cornea during PRK results in a rougher surface immediately postoperatively, with undesirable effects on surface healing.[171]

Specular microscopy has been used to investigate corneal epithelial changes after excimer laser PRK. Destruction of Bowman membrane caused by PRK does not affect the morphologic characteristics of the most superficial layer of the corneal epithelium in most eyes. However, two patients were identified with abnormal epithelial cell patterns.[172]

PREDICTABILITY AND PROGRESSION OF EFFECT. It is difficult to compare the results of many significant studies on PRK because of differences in inclusion criteria. It is now well known that the predictability of PRK is lower in patients with greater than 6 D of myopia. In the 585 patients of Summit phase III clinical trials, 77.2% had a predictability of +1.00 D at 1 year, and 93.3% had a predictability of +2.00 D at 1 year. It was also found that 90.7% of the patients had a visual acuity greater than or equal to 20/40 (Steinert RR, New England Eye Center, personal communication, July 1993). Tengroth and colleagues[173] included patients with preoperative refraction ranging from −1.25 to −7.50 D, and at 15 months, 87% were within 1 D of ametropia and had uncorrected visual acuity of at least 20/40. Seiler and Wollensak[164] studied patients with preoperative refraction ranging from −1.40 to −9.25 D. They reported that 92% were within ±1.00 D of the intended final refraction, and 96% had an uncorrected visual acuity of 20/40 or better. The variability in refractive outcome might be explained by the mild individual healing response that persists up to 18 months after laser treatment.[174]

Regression of the effect of excimer laser PRK has been well established. A significant overcorrection is common in the early postoperative period and gradually diminishes in the first 3 to 4 months. Rapid regression in the immediate postoperative phase occurs primarily because of the buildup of epithelial cell layers. Some authors recommend dexamethasone or topical steroid application as effective in reversing regression later in the postoperative course. Further studies into this effect are needed.

Phototherapeutic Keratectomy

Phototherapeutic keratectomy (PTK) is used for excision of pathologic superficial lesions of the cornea. It is known to create refractive changes and is considered to be primarily a curative, nonrefractive procedure. At this writing, the 193-nm excimer laser remains under clinical investigation for the purposes of removing superficial corneal opacities and smoothing the anterior corneal surface (or PTK).[175–179] Because PTK has the potential to remove superficial corneal opacities and surface irregularities, it may replace more invasive procedures, such as lamellar or penetrating keratoplasty.

PTK has been used to treat numerous different pathologic conditions, including lattice dystrophy, granular dystrophy, macular dystrophy, Reis-Bücklers dystrophy, Salzmann nodular degeneration, anterior basement membrane dystrophy, band keratopathy, recurrent corneal erosions, and pterygia (Fig. 9-15). It has also proved effective in treating superficial corneal scars and irregularities secondary to such infections as herpes simplex viral keratitis. As previously mentioned, the ablation rates of epithelium, Bowman layer, and corneal stroma are different, and the ablation rate of various corneal pathologic changes are also different. This technique appears to be useful for ablating pathology of 70 to 100 μm in depth, which involves the central or paracentral cornea. The reduced refractive error appears to be dependent on the depth and location of the ablation.

Intraoperative Complications

INADEQUATE REMOVAL OF EPITHELIUM. As previously noted, the excimer laser, applied to an uneven corneal surface, simply results in a thinner cornea with the same irregular surface. This occurs because the peaks and valleys of the pathology generally ablate at the same rate. To avoid complications resulting from this irregular surface, a blocking agent is used to fill in the low spots and leave the high spots exposed so that the high spots may be selectively ablated, achieving a smooth surface. Numerous blocking agents have been tried; however, methylcellulose in varying concentrations (2%, 1%, and 0.5%) appears to have the highest success.[180] For patients in whom the anterior corneal pathology has not disturbed the surface epithelium leaving a smooth preoperative surface, it may be advisable to leave the epithelium intact. Once the pathology is encountered, the treatment should be halted, and methylcellulose should be employed to provide for more even ablation of the now uneven pathologic surface.[181] Patients whose conditions have not improved after PTK may require alternative treatment, such as lamellar or penetrating keratoplasty.

INADEQUATE REMOVAL OF PATHOLOGY. Thompson and colleagues[182] have stated that the golden rule in PRK is "an under-treatment is better than an over-treatment." In other words, PTK may be used to reduce the pathology only to the point at which the epithelium may heal over to create a smooth air–tear interface. A small remaining anterior stromal scar with a smooth air–tear interface frequently allows for dramatic visual improvement in many different corneal pathologic conditions. Overtreatment to remove all of the corneal scar in its entirety increases the risk of inducing large refractive error changes. Intraoperative inspection by moving the patient to the slit-lamp microscope ensures against overtreatment. A corneal scar that persists after PTK and is visually significant may be further treated with the laser at a later date.

LOSS OF FIXATION. Two distinctly different techniques for PTK have been described. In one technique, after removal of the epithelium and application of a blocking agent, the eye is fixated with a

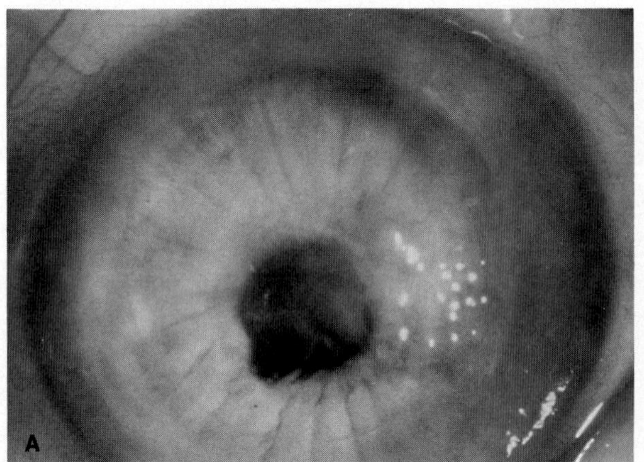

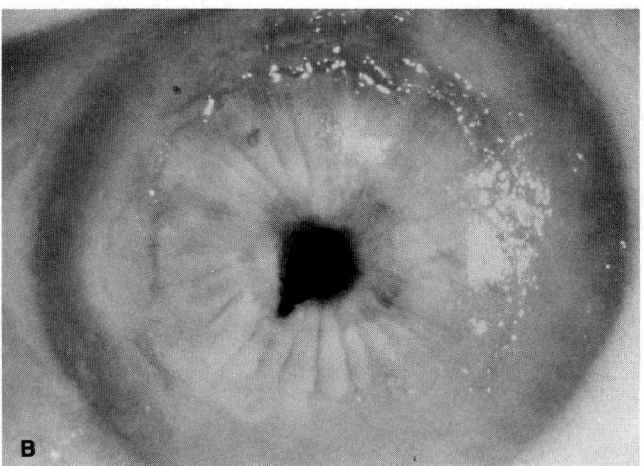

Figure 9-15. (**A**) Recurrent lattice corneal dystrophy 6 years after penetrating keratoplasty. (**B**) The same patient immediately after excimer laser phototherapeutic keratectomy. Note the clearing of the visual axis and the smoothing of the central corneal graft that have transpired. The patient's vision improved from the 20/200 level to 20/25 after phototherapeutic keratectomy. (See color plate after page xvi.)

suction ring and stabilized before and during the laser exposure. In this technique, loss of fixation is not a problem. In the second technique, the surgeon intentionally moves the eye or patient's head during PTK to create a peripheral blend at the edge of the ablation zone. It is thought that movement also helps reduce refractive changes and achieve a smoother transition zone from the area of ablation to the area of no ablation.

Postoperative Complications

PAIN. As with PRK, patients with normal corneal sensation experience significant pain until reepithelialization has occurred after PTK. Simple pressure patching, topical nonsteroidal antiinflammatory agents, and pain medication may all increase patient comfort during the reepithelialization period.

PERSISTENT EPITHELIAL DEFECT. Rates of reepithelialization vary significantly. Stark and colleagues[178] reported 93% reepithelialization within two weeks, whereas Hersh[183] reports one patient who required a bandage soft contact lens and 3 weeks for complete reepithelialization. Both Forster and associates[184] and Fagerholm and colleagues[185] report complete reepithelialization in all patients. The resultant smooth corneal surface after PTK appears to decrease the incidence of persistent epithelial defects significantly.

REFRACTIVE CHANGES. Refractive changes are a known complication of PTK, and the surgeon must be aware of these in preoperative planning. Central ablations create a hyperopic shift, leaving the patient less myopic, whereas paracentral ablations may cause a steeper myopic shift and induce astigmatism. The frequency of hyperopic shift is increased with the treatment of deeper corneal opacities. Therefore, the postoperative hyperopic refraction correlates with the number of stromal pulses expended during excimer treatment. Minimal treatment has been used successfully in the treatment of recurrent corneal erosions. Treatment has been performed with as little as 15 pulses, which treats only Bowman layer and is associated with little or no induced astigmatism. Approximately 0.25 μm of tissue are ablated per pulse. Therefore, a treatment of 15 pulses is thought to partially remove Bowman membrane. Interestingly, this group of patients treated for recurrent erosions, who had the mildest excimer treatment, seemed to have the most difficulty with postoperative pain. This may be a function of decreased innervation in patients with pathologic changes in their cornea, and therefore less postoperative pain. A technique of plain disk ablation has been described that is theoretically designed to remove the same thickness of cornea throughout the ablation area. Some authors argue this may actually result in a more cup-shaped ablation area because of the curvature of the cornea. It also may result in a hyperopic shift. In patients with both corneal and lens opacities, the induced hyperopic shift or refractive error may be compensated for with adjustments of intraocular lens power during cataract extraction after PTK. The postoperative complication of hyperopic shift may mandate contact lens fitting for visual rehabilitation. Both the surgeon and the patient must consider the potential for a significant hyperopic shift and discuss the possibility of requiring a contact lens for visual rehabilitation in the postoperative period. Unwillingness of a patient to accept the possibility of a contact lens postoperatively should exclude this patient from consideration for this procedure.

CORNEAL INFECTIONS. There appear to be no reports of bacterial corneal infection recurring after PTK. Herpes simplex has been cited to recur in several different studies. Animal studies have shown that this virus can be reactivated with the excimer laser.[186] Campos and associates[179] pretreated one patient who had a postherpetic scar with oral acyclovir, 200 mg four times a day, and continued this regimen for 10 days postoperatively.[179] This patient had no disease recurrence during the 15-month follow-up period. Further studies on the efficacy of this treatment in preventing recurrence of herpes simplex keratitis are necessary.

CORNEAL HAZE. Postoperative haze has been reported to be minimal compared with the preoperative level. Several patients have been reported to develop postoperative corneal opacities that appear to be related to the preoperative diagnosis. This is more common in patients who are treated for band keratopathy. Campos and associates[179] report one patient treated for corneal surface disease associated with atopy, who 3 months postoperatively developed a Salzmann-type degeneration with nodular opacities despite the use of corticosteroids and lubricants. Recurrence of herpes simplex has been reported after excimer laser keratectomy.[187] Corneal disorders where the pathologic tissue is resistant to excimer ablation have also been reported.[188] PTK remains an investigational procedure; however, it appears able to improve visual acuity in selected patients with corneal opacities and may be especially helpful in those with corneal dystrophies. The procedure may provide an alternative to penetrating or lamellar keratoplasty. The excimer laser may provide an alternative to conventional surgical techniques in the treatment of superficial corneal opacities and irregularities; however, the long-term effects of excimer laser PTK must be observed, and the suitability of this procedure for various conditions must be carefully evaluated by both the patient and the surgeon.

References

1. EBAA News Release. Washington, DC, March 1993.
2. Khandaker AA, Price FW, Whitson WE. Suprachoroidal hemorrhage in penetrating keratoplasty. Ophthalmology 1991;98:155.
3. Ingraham HJ, Donnenfeld ED, Perry HD. Massive suprachoroidal hemorrhage in penetrating keratoplasty. Am J Ophthalmol 1989;108:670.
4. Speaker MG, Guerriero PN, Met JA, et al. A case-control study of risk factors for intraoperative suprachoroidal expulsive hemorrhage. Ophthalmology 1991;98:202.
5. Purcell JJ, Krachmer JH, Doughman DJ, Bourne WM. Expulsive hemorrhage in penetrating keratoplasty. Ophthalmology 1982;89:41.
6. Litoff D, Krachmer JH. Complications of corneal surgery. Int Ophthalmol Clin 1992;4:797.
7. Waring GO. Management of pseudophakic corneal edema with reconstruction of the anterior segment. Arch Ophthalmol 1987;105;709.
8. Mannis MJ, Sweet E, Landers MB, Lewis RA. Uses of thrombin in ocular surgery: effect on the corneal endothelium. Arch Ophthalmol 1988;106:251.
9. Mannis MJ, Zadnik K. Hydrophilic contact lenses for wound stabilization in keratoplasty. CLAO J 1988;14:191.
10. Kattan HM, Flynn HW, Pflugfelder SC, et al. Nosocomial endophthalmitis. Surv Ophthalmol 1991;98:227.
11. Guss RB, Koenig S, Delapena W, et al. Endophthalmitis after penetrating keratoplasty. Am J Ophthalmol 1983;95:651.
12. Leveille AS, McMullan RD, Cavanaugh HD. Endophthalmitis following penetrating keratoplasty. Ophthalmology 1983;90:38.
13. Insler MS, Cavanaugh HD, Wilson LA. Gentamicin-resistant pseudomonas endophthalmitis after penetrating keratoplasty. Br J Ophthalmol 1985;69:189.
14. Baer JC, Nirankari VS, Glaros DS. Streptococcal endophthalmitis from contaminated donor corneas after keratoplasty: clinical and laboratory investigations. Arch Ophthalmol 1988;106:517.
15. Omerod LD, Ho DD, Becker LE, et al. Endophthalmitis caused by coagulase negative staphylococci. Ophthalmology 1993;100:715.
16. Speaker MG, Menikoff JA. Prophylaxis of endophthalmitis with topical povidone-iodine. Ophthalmology 1991;98:1769.
17. Mindrup EA, Dubbel PA, Doughman DJ. Betadine decontamination of donor globes. Cornea 1993;12:324.
18. Baum J, Peyman GA, Barza M. Intravitreal administration of antibiotic in the treatment of bacterial endophthalmitis: III. Consensus. Surv Ophthalmol 1982;26:204.
19. Harbour RC, Stearn GA. Variables in McCarey-Kaufman corneal storage medium. Ophthalmology 1983;90:136.
20. Irvine AR, Kaufman HE. Intraocular pressure following penetrating keratoplasty. Am J Ophthalmol 1969;68:835.
21. Arentsen JJ, Laibson PR. Surgical management of pseudophakic corneal edema: complications and visual results following penetrating keratoplasty. Ophthalmic Surg 1982;13:371.
22. Foulks GN. Glaucoma associated with penetrating keratoplasty. Ophthalmology 1987;94;871.
23. Simmons RB, Stearn RA, Teekhasaenee C, Kenyon KR. Elevated intraocular pressure following penetrating keratoplasty. Trans Am Ophthalmologic Soc 1989;87:79.
24. Chien AM, Courtland MS, Cohen EJ, et al. Glaucoma in the immediate postoperative period after penetrating keratoplasty. Am J Ophthalmol 1993;115:711.
25. Schanzlin DJ, Robin JB, Gomez DS, et al. Results of penetrating keratoplasty for aphakic and pseudophakic bullous keratopathy. Am J Ophthalmol 1984;98:302.
26. Waring GO, Stulting RD, Street D. Penetrating keratoplasty for pseudophakic corneal edema with exchange of intraocular lenses. Arch Ophthalmol 1987;105:58.
27. Polack FM. Glaucoma and keratoplasty. Cornea 1988;7:67.
28. Olson RJ, Kaufman HE. A mathematical description of causative factors in prevention of elevated intraocular pressure after keratoplasty. Invest Ophthalmol Vis Sci 1977;16:1085.
29. Zimmermann TJ, Krupin T, Grodzki W, et al. The effect of suture depth on outflow facility in penetrating keratoplasty. Arch Ophthalmol 1978;96:505.
30. Svedbergh B. The effects of artificial intraocular pressure elevation on the endothelium of the vervet monkey. Acta Ophthalmol 1975;53:839.
31. Charlin R, Polack FM. The effect of elevated intraocular pressure on the endothelium of corneal grafts. Cornea 1982;1:241.
32. Lass JH, Pavan-Langston D. Timolol therapy in secondary angle closure glaucoma after penetrating keratoplasty. Ophthalmology 1979;86:51.

33. Gardner S. Apraclonidine for intraocular pressure control. Ocular Ther Manag 1990;11.
34. Binder PS, Abel R, Polack FM, Kaufman HE. Keratoplasty wound separations. Am J Ophthalmol 1975;80:109.
35. Snider RW, Sherman MD, Allison RW. Intracameral tissue plasminogen activator for treatment of excessive fibrin response after penetrating keratoplasty. Am J Ophthalmol 1990;109:483.
36. Beyer CR, Byrd TJ, Hill JM, Kaufman HE. Herpes simplex virus and persistent epithelial defects after penetrating keratoplasty. Am J Ophthalmol 1990; 109:95.
37. Mannis MJ, Plotnik RD, Schwab IR, Newton RD. Herpes simplex dendritic keratitis after keratoplasty. Am J Ophthalmol 1991;11:480.
38. Salisbury JD, Berkowitz RA, Gebhardt BM, Kaufman HE. Herpes virus infection of cornea allografts. Ophthalmic Surg 1984;15:406.
39. Stern GA, Schemmerg B, Rarber RD, Gorovoy MS. Effects of topical antibiotic solutions in corneal epithelial wound healing. Arch Ophthalmol 1983;101:644.
40. Price FW, Whitson WE, Collins KS, Marks RG. Five year corneal graft survival. Arch Ophthalmol 1993; 111:799.
41. Alldredge AOC, Krachmer JH. Clinical types of corneal transplant rejection. Arch Ophthalmol 1981; 99:599.
42. Volker-Dieben HJM, D'Amaro J, Kok-Van Alphen CC. Hierarchy of prognostic factors for corneal allograft survival. Aust NZ J Ophthalmol 87;15:11.
43. Volker-Dieben HJM, Kok-Van Alphen CC, Lansbergen Q, Persinjn GG. Different influences in corneal graft survival in 539 transplants. Acta Ophthalmol 1982;60:198.
44. Aaronson JJ. Corneal transplant allograft rejection: possible predisposing factors. Trans Am Ophthalmol Soc 1983;81:361.
45. Belin MW, Bouchard CS, Phillips TM. Update on topical cyclosporin A. Cornea 1990;30:184.
46. Collaborative Corneal Transplantation Studies Research Group. Design and methods of collaborative corneal transplantation studies. Cornea 1993;12:93.
47. Hill JC, Maske R, Watson P. Corticosteroids in corneal graft rejection. Ophthalmology 1991;98:329.
48. Lamensdorf M, Wilson LA, Waring GO, Cavanaugh D. Microbial keratitis after penetrating keratoplasty. Ophthalmology 1982;89:124.
49. Tuberville AW, Wood TO. Corneal ulcers in corneal transplants. Current Eye Research 1981;1:479.
50. Varley GA, Meisler DM. Complications of penetrating keratoplasty: graft infections. Refract Corneal Surg 1991;7:62.
51. Polack FM, Kaufman HE. Penetrating keratoplasty in herpes keratitis. Am J Ophthalmol 1972;73:908.
52. Kaufman HE, Rayfield MS. Viral conjunctivitis and keratitis. In: Kaufman HE, Barron BA, McDonald MD, Waltham SR, eds. The cornea. New York, Churchill Livingstone, 1988:299.
53. Ficker LA, Kirkness C, Wright P. Prognosis for keratoplasty in Acanthamoeba keratitis. Ophthalmology 1993;100:105.
54. Meisler DM, Langston RHS, Naab TJ, et al. Infectious crystalline keratopathy. Am J Ophthalmol 1984; 97:337.
55. Kincaid MC, Fouraker BD, Schanzlin DJ. Infectious crystalline keratopathy after relaxing incisions. Am J Ophthalmol 1991;111:374.
56. Lam S, Meisler D, Krachmer JH. Enterococcal infectious keratitis. Cornea 1993;12:273.
57. Rij GV, Waring GO. Configuration of corneal trephine opening using five different trephines in human donor eyes. Arch Ophthalmol 1988;106:1228.
58. Olson RJ. Corneal transplantation techniques. Kaufman HE, Barron BA, McDonald MD, Waltham SR, eds: The cornea. New York, Churchill Livingstone, 1988:743.
59. Filatov V, Steiner TRF, Talamo JH. Postkeratoplasty astigmatism with single running suture or interrupted sutures. Am J Ophthalmol 1993;115:715.
60. Van Meter WS, Gussler JR, Soloman KD, Wood TO. Post-keratoplasty astigmatism control. Ophthalmology 1991;98:177.
61. Strelow S, Cohen EJ, Leavitt KG, Laibson PR. Corneal topography for selective suture removal after penetrating keratoplasty. Am J Ophthalmol 1991; 112:657.
62. Frangieh GT, Kwitko S, McDonnell PJ. Prospective corneal topographic analysis in surgery for post keratoplasty astigmatism. Arch Ophthalmol 1991; 109:506.
63. McNeill JI, Wessels IF. Adjustment of single continuous suture to control astigmatism after penetrating keratoplasty. Refract Corneal Surg 1989;5:216.
64. Krachmer JH, Fensel RE. Surgical correction of high postkeratoplasty astigmatism. Arch Ophthalmol 1980;98:1400.
65. Mandel MR, Shapiro MB, Krachmer JH. Relaxing incisions with augmentation sutures for correction of postkeratoplasty astigmatism. Am J Ophthalmol 1987;103:441.
66. Geggel HS. Limbal wedge resection at the time of intraocular surgery for reducing postkeratoplasty astigmatism. Ophthalmic Surg 1990;21:102.
67. Maumanee AE. Treatment of epithelial downgrowth and intraocular fistula following cataract extraction. Trans Am Ophthalmol Soc 1964;62:153.
68. Anseth A, Dohlman CH, Elbert DM. Epithelial downgrowth fistula repair and keratoplasty. Refract Corneal Surg 1991:7:23.
69. Feder RS, Krachmer JH. The diagnosis of epithelial

downgrowth after keratoplasty. Am J Ophthalmol 1985;99:697.
70. Kramer SG. Cystoid macular edema after aphakic penetrating keratoplasty. Ophthalmology 1981; 98:682.
71. Busin M, Brauweiler P, Thorsten B, Spitznas N. Complications of sulcus supported intraocular lenses with iris sutures, implanted during penetrating keratoplasty after intracapsular cataract extraction. Ophthalmology 1990;97:401.
72. Shapiro MB, Harrison DA. Radial keratotomy for intolerable myopia after penetrating keratoplasty. Am J Ophthalmol 1993;115:327.
73. Ficker LA, Kirkness CM, Rice NSC, et al. The changing management and improved prognosis for corneal grafting in herpes simplex keratitis. Ophthalmology 1989;96:1587.
74. Fine M, Cignetti FE. Penetrating keratoplasty in herpes simplex keratitis: Recurrence in grafts. Arch Ophthalmol 1977;95:63.
75. Pfister RR, Richards JSF, Dohlman CH. Recurrence of herpetic keratitis in corneal grafts. Am J Ophthalmol 1972;73:192.
76. Olson RJ, Kaufman HE. Recurrence of Reis-Bückler's corneal dystrophy in a graft. Am J Ophthalmol 1978;85:349.
77. Rodrigez MM, McGavic JS. Recurrent corneal granular dystrophy: a clinical pathologic study. Trans Am Ophthalmic Soc 1975;73:300.
78. Meisler DM, Fine M. Recurrence of the clinical signs of lattice corneal dystrophy (type I) in corneal transplants. Am J Ophthalmol 1984;97:210.
79. Robin A, Green WR, Lapsa TP, et al. Recurrence of macular corneal dystrophy after a lamellar keratoplasty. Am J Ophthalmol 1977;84:457.
80. Hamilton W, Wood TO. Inlay lamellar keratoplasty. In: Kaufman HE, Barron BA, McDonald MB, Waltman SR, eds. The cornea. New York, Churchill Livingstone, 1988.
81. Gasset AR. Lamellar keratoplasty in the treatment of keratoconus: conectomy. Ophthalmic Surg 1979; 10:26.
82. Malbran E, Stefani C. Lamellar keratoplasty in corneal ectasia. Ophthalmologica 1972;164:50.
83. Barraquer JI. Lamellar keratoplasty (special techniques). Ann Ophthalmol 1972;4:437.
84. Maumanee AE. Clinical patterns of corneal graft failures. In: Porter R, Knight J, eds. Corneal graft failures, vol 15. Ciba Foundation Symposium. New York, Elsevier/Associated Scientific, 1973:5.
85. Rowsey JJ, Balyeat HD. Preliminary results in complications of radial keratotomy. Am J Ophthalmol 1982;93:437.
86. Rowsey JJ, Balyeat HD. Radial keratotomy: preliminary report of complications. Ophthalmic Surg 1982;13:27.
87. Waring GO, Lin MJ, Gelender H, et al. Results of a prospective evaluation of radial keratotomy (PERK study) one year after surgery. Ophthalmology 1985;92:177.
88. Marmorr H. Radial keratotomy complications. Ann Ophthalmol 1987;19:409.
89. Sawelson H, Marks RG. Two year results of radial keratotomy. Arch Ophthalmol 1985;103:505.
90. Schwab IR, ed. Refractive keratoplasty. New York, Churchill Livingstone, 1987:227.
91. Villaseno RA, Salz J, Steel D, Krasnow MA. Changes in corneal thickness during radial keratotomy. Ophthalmic Surg 1981;12:341.
92. Grady FJ. Experience with radial keratotomy. Ophthalmic Surg 1983;13:395.
93. Hoffer KJ, Darrin JJ, Pettit TH, et al. Three years experience with radial keratotomy: the UCLA study. Ophthalmology 1983;93:627.
94. MacRae SM, Matsuda M, Rich LF. The effects of radial keratotomy on the corneal endothelium. Am J Ophthalmol 1985;100:538.
95. Chiba K, Oak SS, Tsubota K, et al. Morphometric analysis of corneal endothelium following radial keratotomy. J Cataract Refract Surg 1987;13:263.
96. Rowsey JJ, Balyeat HD, Monlux R, et al. Endothelial cell loss after radial keratotomy. Ophthalmology 1987;94:97.
97. Uozat OH, Guyton DL. Centering corneal surgical procedures. Am J Ophthalmol 1987;103:264.
98. Uozat OH, Guyton DL, Waring GO. Centering corneal surgical procedures. In: Waring GO, ed. Refractive keratotomy for myopia and astigmatism. St. Louis, CV Mosby, 1992;491.
99. Ellis W. Radial keratotomy and astigmatism surgery. Irvine, CA, Keith C. Terry & Associates, 1986:117.
100. Lindstrom RL, Lindquist TD. Surgical correction of postoperative astigmatism. Cornea 1988;7:138.
101. Rashid ER, Waring GO. Complications of refractive keratotomy. Waring GO, Ed. Refractive keratotomy for myopia and astigmatism. St. Louis, Mosby, 1992:863.
102. American Academy of Ophthalmology. Radial keratotomy for myopia. Ophthalmology 1993;100:1103.
103. Waring GO, Lynn MJ, Fielding B, et al. Results of a prospective evaluation of radial keratotomy (PERK) study four years after surgery for myopia. JAMA 1990;263:1083.
104. O'Day DM, Feman SS, Elliott JH. Visual impairment following radial keratotomy: a cluster of cases. Ophthalmology 1986;93:319.
105. Rashid ER, Waring GO. Complications of radial and traverse keratotomy. Surv Ophthalmol 1989;34:73.

106. Veraart HG, Vandenberg TJ, Ijspeert JK, Cardozo OL. Stray light in radial keratotomy in the influence of pupil size and stray light angle. Am J Ophthalmol 1992;114:424.
107. Gieser J, Sugar A. Radial keratotomy in corneal scarring. Arch Ophthalmol 1992;110:1527.
108. Salz JJ, Villasenor RA, Elander R, Swinger C, Reader AL. Four incision radial keratotomy for low to moderate myopia. Ophthalmology 1986;93:727.
109. Arrowsmith PN, Marks RG. Four year update on predictability of radial keratotomy. J Cataract Refract Surg 1988;4:37.
110. Salz JJ, Salz MS. Results of four and eight incision radial keratotomy for 6-12 Ds of myopia. J Cataract Refract Surg 1988;4:46.
111. Spigelman AV, Williams PA, Nichols BD, Lindstrom RL. Four incision radial keratotomy. J Cataract Refract Surg 1988;14:125.
112. Spiegelman AV, Williams PA, Lindstrom RL. Further studies of four incision radial keratotomy. Refract Corneal Surg 1989;5:292.
113. Bogan SJ, Waring GO, Ibrahim O, Drew SC, Curtis L. Classification of normal corneal topography based on computer-assisted video keratography. Arch Ophthalmol 1990;108:945.
114. Bogan SJ, Maloney RK, Drews CD, Waring GO. Computer assisted video keratography of corneal topography after radial keratotomy. Arch Ophthalmol 1991;108:834.
115. Maguire LJ, Singer DE, Klyce SD. Graphic presentation of computer analyzed keratoscope photographs. Arch Ophthalmol 1987;105:223.
116. McDonnell PJ, Garbus J. Corneal topographic changes after radial keratotomy. Ophthalmology 1989;96:45.
117. Maguire LJ, Bourne WM. A multi-focal lens effect as a complication of radial keratotomy. Refract Corneal Surg 1989;5:394.
118. Hofmann RF, Starling JC, Masler W. Contact fitting after radial keratotomy. J Cataract Refract Surg 1986;2:155.
119. Shivitz IA, Russell BM, Arrowsmith PN. Contact lenses in the treatment of patients with over corrected radial keratotomy. Ophthalmology 1987; 94:899.
120. Starling J, Hofmann R. A new surgical technique for the correction of hyperopia after radial keratotomy: an experimental model. Refract Corneal Surg 1986;2:9.
121. Lindquist TD, Rubenstein JB, Lindstrom RL. Correction of hyperopia following radial keratotomy: quantification in human cadaver eyes. Ophthalmic Surg 1987;18:432.
122. Lindquist PD, Williams PA, Lindstrom RL. Surgical treatment of over correction following radial keratotomy: evaluation of clinical effectiveness. Ophthalmic Surg 1991;22:12.
123. Werblin TP, Stafford GN. The Casebeer system for predictable keratorefractive surgery: one year evaluation of 205 consecutive eyes. Ophthalmology 1993;100:1095.
124. Seiler T, Jean B. Photorefractive keratectomy as a second attempt to correct myopia after radial keratotomy. Refract Corneal Surg 1992;8:211.
125. Schanzlin DJ, Santos VR, Waring GO, et al. Diurnal change in refraction, corneal curvature, visual acuity, and intraocular pressure after radial keratotomy in the PERK study. Ophthalmology 1986;93:167.
126. Waring GO, Lynn MJ, Culbertson W, et al. Three year results of the prospective evaluation of radial keratotomy (PERK) study. Ophthalmology 1987;94:1339.
127. Kwitko S, Gritz DC, Garbus JJ, Gauderman J, McDonnell PJ. Diurnal variation of corneal topography after radial keratotomy. Arch Ophthalmol 1992;110:351.
128. Binder PS, Nayak SK, Deg JK, et al. An ultrastructural and histochemical study of long term wound healing after radial keratotomy. Am J Ophthalmol 1987;103:432.
129. Yamaguchi T, Tamaki K, Kaufman HE, et al. Histologic study of a pair of human corneas after anterior radial keratotomy. Am J Ophthalmol 1985;100:281.
130. Steinberg EB, Waring GO, Wilson LA. Slit lamp microscopic study of corneal wound healing after radial keratotomy in the PERK study. Am J Ophthalmol 1985;100:218.
131. Lindquist TD. Complications of corneal refractive surgery. Int Ophthalmol Clin 1992;32:97.
132. Nelson JD, Williams P, Lindstrom RL, Doughman DJ. Map finger dot changes in the corneal epithelial basement membrane following radial keratotomy. Ophthalmology 1985;92:199.
133. Binder PS. Presumed epithelial ingrowth following radial keratotomy. CLAO Journal 1986;12:247.
134. MacRae SM, Matsuda M, Rich LF. The effects of radial keratotomy on the corneal endothelium. Am J Ophthalmol 1985;100:538.
135. O'Day DM, Feman SS, Elliott JH. Visual impairment following radial keratotomy: a cluster of cases. Ophthalmology 1986;93:319.
136. Gelender H, Flynn HW, Mandelbaum SH. Bacterial endophthalmitis resulting from radial keratotomy. Am J Ophthalmol 1982;93:323.
137. Manka RL, Gast TJ. Endophthalmitis following Ruiz procedure. Arch Ophthalmol 1990;108:21.
138. Cross WD, Head WJ. Complications of radial keratotomy: an overview. In: Sanders D, Hofmann RF, Salz J, eds. Refractive corneal surgery. Thorofare, NJ, Slack 1986:347.

139. Beldavs RA, Al-Ghamdi S, Wilson LA, Waring GO. Bilateral microbial keratitis after radial keratotomy. Arch Ophthalmol 1993;111:440.
140. Marmor RH. Radial keratotomy complications. Ann Ophthalmology 1987;19:409.
141. Lewicky A, Salz. Special report radial keratotomy survey. J Cataract Refract Surg 1986;2:32.
142. Robin JB, Beatty RF, Dunn S, et al. *Mycobacterium chelonei* keratitis after radial keratotomy. Am J Ophthalmol 1986;102:72.
143. Santos CI. Herpes keratitis after radial keratotomy. Am J Ophthalmol 1982;93:370.
144. Santos CI. Herpetic corneal ulcer following radial keratotomy. Ann Ophthalmol 1983;15:82.
145. Mandelbaum S, Waring GO, Forster RK, et al. Late development of ulcerative keratitis in radial keratotomy scars. Arch Ophthalmol 1986;104:1156.
146. Shivitz IA, Arrowsmith PN. Delayed keratitis after radial keratotomy. Arch Ophthalmol 1986;104:1153.
147. Ingraham HJ, Guber D, Green WR. Radial keratotomy: clinical pathologic case report. Arch Ophthalmol 1985;103:683.
148. Luttrell JK, Jester JV, Smith RE. The effect of radial keratotomy on ocular integrity in an animal model. Arch Ophthalmol 1982;100:319.
149. McKnight SJ, Fitz J, Giangiacomo J. Corneal rupture following radial keratotomy in cats subjected to BB-gun injury. Ophthalmic Surg 1988;19:156.
150. Simmons KB, Linsalata RP. Ruptured globe following blunt trauma after radial keratotomy: a case report. Ophthalmology 1987;94:184.
151. Larson BC, Kremer FB, Eller AW, Bernardino VB. Quantitated trauma following radial keratotomy in rabbits. Ophthalmology 1983;90:660.
152. Rylander HG, Welch AJ, Fleming B. The effect of radial keratotomy on the rupture strength of pig eyes. Ophthalmic Surg 1983;14:744.
153. Beatty RF, Robin JB, Schanzlin DJ. Penetrating keratoplasty after radial keratotomy. J Cataract Refract Surg 1986;2:207.
154. Waring GO, Lynn MJ, Nizam, et al. Results of the prospective evaluation of radial keratotomy (PERK) study five years after surgery. Ophthalmology 1991;98:1164.
155. Spadea L, Sabetti L, Balestrazzi E. Effect of centering excimer laser (PRK) on refractive results: a corneal topography study. Refract Corneal Surg 1993;9:S22.
156. Balestrazzi E, DeMolfetta V, Spadea L. Excimer laser photorefractive keratectomy: histological immunohistochemical and ultrastructural study on human corneas. Ital J Ophthalmol 1992;6:95.
157. Wilson SE, Klyce SD, McDonald MB, et al. Changes in corneal topography after excimer laser photorefractive keratectomy for myopia. Ophthalmology 1991;98:1338.
158. Maloney R. Corneal topography and optical zone location in photorefractive keratectomy. Refract Corneal Surg 1990;6:363.
159. Van Mellaert CE, Missotten L. On the safety of 193 nanometer excimer laser refractive corneal surgery. Refract Corneal Surg 1992;8:235.
160. Lohmann CP, Fitzke F, Obrart D, et al. Corneal light scattering and visual performance in myopic individuals with spectacles, contact lenses, or excimer laser photorefractive keratectomy. Am J Ophthalmol 1993;115:444.
161. Seiler T, Bende T, Wollensac J. Ablation rate of human corneal epithelium in Bowman's layer with the excimer laser (193 nM). Refract Corneal Surg 1990;6:99.
162. Lavery FL. Photorefractive keratectomy in 472 eyes. Refract Corneal Surg 1993;9:S98.
163. Seiler T. Recent development in refractive corneal surgery. Curr Opinion Ophthalmol 1992;3:482.
164. Seiler T, Wollensak J. Myopic photorefractive keratectomy with the excimer laser. Ophthalmology 1991;98:1156.
165. Gartry D, Ker R, Muir M, Marshall J. Photorefractive keratectomy with an argon fluoride excimer: a clinical study. Refract Corneal Surg 1991;7:420.
166. Seiler T, Derse N, Pham T. Repeated excimer laser treatment after photorefractive keratectomy. Arch Ophthalmol 1992;110:1230.
167. Caubet E. Cause of subepithelial corneal haze over 18 months after photorefractive keratectomy for myopia. Refract Corneal Surg 1993;9:S65.
168. Talamo J, Gollamudi S, Green R, et al. Modulation of corneal wound healing after excimer laser keratomileusis using topical mitomycin C and steroids. Arch Ophthalmol 1991;109:1141.
169. Seiler T, Wollensak J. Myopic photorefractive keratectomy with excimer laser. Ophthalmology 1991;98:1156.
170. Vrabec MP, McDonald MB, Chase DS, et al. Traumatic corneal abrasions after excimer laser keratectomy. Am J Ophthalmol 1993;101.
171. Campos M, Cuevas K, Garbus J, et al. Corneal wound healing after excimer laser ablation: effect of nitrogen gas blower. Ophthalmology 1992;99:893.
172. Amano S, Shimizu K, Subota K. Corneal epithelial changes after excimer laser photorefractive keratectomy. Am J Ophthalmol 1993;115:441.
173. Tengroth B, Epstein D, Fagerholm P, et al. Excimer laser photorefractive keratectomy for myopia: clinical results in sighted eyes. Ophthalmology 1993;100:739.
174. Hanna K, Pouliquen Y, Salvodelli M, et al. Corneal wound healing in monkeys 18 months after excimer laser keratectomy. Refract Corneal Surg 1990; 6:340.
175. Gaster RN, Binder PS, Koalwell K, et al. Corneal surface ablation by 193 nanometer excimer laser and

wound healing in rabbits. Invest Ophthalmol Vis Sci 1989;30:90.

176. Steinert RF, Puliafito CA. Excimer laser phototherapeutic keratectomy for a corneal nodule. Refract Corneal Surg 1990;6:352.
177. Sher NA, Bowers RA, Zabel RW, et al. Clinical use of the 193 excimer laser in the treatment of corneal scars. Arch Ophthalmol 1991;109:491.
178. Stark WJ, Chamon W, Kamp MT. Clinical follow-up of 193-nm ArF excimer laser photokeratectomy. Ophthalmology 1992;99:805.
179. Campos M, Nielsen S, Szerenyi K, et al. Clinical follow-up of phototherapeutic keratectomy for the treatment of corneal opacities. Am J Ophthalmol 1993;115:433.
180. Talamo JH, Steinert RF, Puliafido CA. Clinical strategies for excimer laser therapeutic keratectomy. Refract Corneal Surg 1992;8:319.
181. Kornmehl EW, Steinert RF, Puliafito CA. A comparative study of masking fluids for excimer laser phototherapeutic keratectomy. Arch Ophthalmol 1991; 109:860.
182. Thompson V, Dorrie DS, Cavanaugh TB. Philosophy and technique for excimer laser phototherapeutic keratectomy. Refract Corneal Surg 1993;9:581.
183. Hersh PS, Spinak A, Grrana R, Mayers M. Phototherapeutic keratectomy: strategies and results in 12 eyes. Refract Corneal Surg 1993;9:S90.
184. Forster W, Grue S, Atzler U, et al. Phototherapeutic keratectomy in corneal diseases. Refract Corneal Surg 1993;9:S85.
185. Fagerholm P, Fitzsimmons TD, Orndahl M, et al. Phototherapeutic keratectomy: long term results in 166 eyes. Refract Corneal Surg 1993;9:S76.
186. Pepose JS, Laycock KA, Miller JK, et al. Reactivation of latent herpes simplex virus by excimer laser photokeratectomy. Am J Ophthalmol 1992;114:45.
187. Vrabec MP, Durrie DS, Chase DS. Recurrence of herpes simplex after excimer laser keratectomy. Am J Ophthalmol 1992;114:96.
188. McDonnel JM, Garbus JJ, McDonnell PJ. Successful excimer laser phototherapeutic keratectomy. Arch Ophthalmol 1992;110:977.

Ophthalmic Surgery Complications: Prevention and Management,
edited by Judie F. Charlton and George W. Weinstein.
J. B. Lippincott Company, Philadelphia © 1995.

10

Marc F. Lieberman

Complications of Glaucoma Surgery

COMPLICATIONS OF FILTERING PROCEDURES

General Perspectives

Functional Goals

The clinician's dilemma in managing glaucoma is that the many available interventions—medical, laser, and surgical—are all related to modifying the intraocular pressure. The difficulty lies in the imperfect relationship between the control of intraocular pressure and the long-term health of the optic nerve, whose functional preservation must be the final arbiter of successful intervention. A review of the literature on glaucoma surgery reveals that different parameters are applied by different authors to assess the efficacy of their reported procedures and that success is relative. The astute clinician must maintain, however, the larger picture that glaucoma is a long-term disease of many years' duration whose ultimate manifestation depends on the preservation of as much vision and visual field as possible. "Success" and "complication" must be considered from this perspective.

In the literature, the association of surgically reduced intraocular pressure and long-term success in the treatment of glaucoma is mixed. For example, in a 20-year retrospective study of their patients who underwent trabeculectomy,[1] Watson, who was one of the earliest popularizers of this procedure, and his colleagues made several fascinating observations: (1) that the anatomic absence of a bleb was not necessarily related to the failure to reduce intraocular pressure; (2) that the type and frequency of preoperative medications had no effect on the outcome of the operation; (3) that visual fields could be stabilized even if pressures were not reduced below 16 mm Hg; and (4) that long-term reduction in visual acuity and visual field nevertheless occurred in over half of the patients. This loss of visual function was not related to the original height of the intraocular pressure, to the amount of reduction of intraocular pressure, to the form of glaucoma requiring surgery, or to any specific long-term complication. In fact, Watson and his colleagues concluded that "the reduction of intraocular pressure alters the rate of this progress but nothing more." This study certainly suggests that primary open-angle glaucoma is a disease of relentless deterioration and that surgical reduction of pressure can only alter the slope or rate at which this deterioration manifests.

Similar conclusions were presented by other investigators. In one study in which patients were observed for 7 to 10 years, although intraocular pressure was reduced in more than two thirds of patients by trabeculectomy, half of the patients lost visual field at a mean rate of 2.3% per year.[2] In another study, no relationship was reported between intraocular pressure control and progressive field loss in eyes with low-tension glaucoma.[3] Werner and coworkers[4,5] reported a rate of 42% field deterioration despite values for intraocular pressure in the mid-teens, and these eyes were almost indistinguishable from eyes with similar tensions but stable visual fields. The one suspicious factor in the group who showed field deterioration, however, was a tendency for occasional spikes of intraocular pressure. In a study of patients observed for 5 years after filtering procedures a lower, but substantial, rate of 18% progression was reported.[6] Here, too, those patients with progressive field deterioration had a tendency toward slightly higher intraocular pressure than those whose intraocular pressure was stable. A similar retrospective study of 300 trabeculectomies in Amsterdam identified a progression rate for visual field defects in 7% of eyes despite good control of intraocular pressure.[7] A different evaluation of the relationship between intraocular pressure and visual field progression (not restricted to surgical patients) identified overlapping distributions among many variables in patients who had either stable or progressing visual fields, and intraocular pressure was not of use in separating these two groups.[8]

On the other hand, there is substantial documentation in the literature that surgical reduction of intraocular pressure is not without merit. In eyes that had advanced glaucomatous damage with deterioration in the high normal range, and were brought down to pressures of 12 mm Hg or less, the glaucomatous process was shown to be halted.[9] Shirakashi and coworkers[10] also reported a significant trend toward visual field loss unless the intraocular pressure was below 13 mm Hg. Similarly, Odberg[11] found stable visual fields if pressures were under 15 mm Hg for 7 years. Findings in eyes with pigmentary dispersion glaucoma were similar.[12] All these reports echo Grant and Burton's admonition to aim for the lowest range of normal pressures as possible for long-term stability.[13]

Improvement of visual field *may* be seen with pressure reduction. In the study by Akafo,[2] a full 17% of eyes gained visual field at a mean rate of 7% of the preoperative field per year after trabeculectomy. Spaeth[14] has reported patients whose visual field was shown by computerized perimetry to improve after reduction of intraocular pressure, and there was a direct correlation between the amount of reduction and the amount of improvement as measured by static perimetric criteria. A similar improvement in visual field function was reported in patients whose intraocular pressure was reduced by 50% down to the mid-teens at a 12-month follow-up.[15]

Perhaps another measure of the protective effect of surgically reduced intraocular pressure is the fate of eyes with far advanced visual field involvement close to macular fixation. An influential study based on patients with "split fixation" by Goldmann kinetic perimetry suggested that this visual field configuration was an ominous sign for "central snuff out."[16] This retrospective study indicated that there was a high correlation of visual loss with intraocular pressure slightly greater than normal. More recent studies have identified the rarity of "central snuff out" after glaucoma surgery that lowers intraocular pressure. Langerhorst and coworkers[17] reported that the majority of 50 cases with advanced damage were seen to show an increase in the mean radius of the central island after surgery, without any example of central visual loss. Nearly identical results were reported from a cohort of 44 patients with advanced central field loss: there was not a single instance of a patient with split fixation who lost acuity after surgical reduction of pressure.[18]

Other lines of evidence also suggest the value of filtering procedures in stabilizing the visual field in many, if not most, patients. The association noted by Werner and colleagues[4,5] that decreased visual field was more common in eyes with occasional elevations of intraocular pressure was substantiated with home tonometry in a study of a large number of patients, some of whose visual fields were deteriorating. Those patients with the most frequent elevations of intraocular pressure had a greater rate of field loss than patients whose intraocular pressures were more stable.[19] Full-thickness filtering procedures[20] and trabeculectomy[21] can significantly reduce the diurnal variations of intraocular pressure long after surgery.

With respect to visual field stability then, it appears that the literature amply documents that the long-term fate of the majority of eyes with chronic open-angle and angle-closure glaucoma will be stabilized with a lower pressure, though as many as two in five patients may experience further progression. Nevertheless, the resultant dampening of diurnal variation of intraocular pressure, and the reduction of intraocular pressures to the low normal range, may be among the most desirable goals of trabeculectomy.[22]

There are, of course, other positive results from trabeculectomy that have been documented. Katz and associates[23] identified 20% of their patients after glaucoma surgery who showed reversal of their optic nerve cupping by photographic analysis, with nearly one third showing computerized visual field improvement. The strongest correlation was in patients whose intraocular pressure dropped more than 30%. Similar studies with optic nerve image analysis systems have reported improved optic nerve measurements after reduction of pressure: decreased mean cup–disc ratio and mean neural retinal rim area.[24,25] Since protecting the optic nerve from progressive damage is the ultimate goal of any glaucoma intervention, these studies are encouraging.

In assessing the long-term effect on visual acuity following filtering procedures, one must sort out the predictable percentage of patients whose cataract formation will be accelerated (and become visually significant), from a less understood phenomenon of reduced visual acuity, ascribed to progressive glaucomatous damage. The rate of cataract formation following filtering procedures is on the order of one fourth to one third of patients.[26,27] Among the factors that have been implicated in cataract formation are (1) the amount of presurgical lens damage; (2) the appearance and perseverance of shallow or flat anterior chamber following surgery; and (3) the age of the patient. It seems that cataracts are more commonly progressive in eyes that have undergone full-thickness procedures than in eyes that have undergone trabeculectomy.[27]

Even when cataract formation has been taken into account, however, there is evidence that suggests that reduced acuity is related directly to the rate of visual field loss but not to the initial intraocular pressure, the percentage reduction in intraocular pressure, the type of glaucoma or postoperative bleb, or the presence of hypotony.[1] One study with computerized perimetry has substantiated this slight tendency for decreased acuity following a filtering procedure, in which the measured foveal value was seen to be lower after trabeculectomy surgery, despite the apparent increase of the overall visual field.[17]

In conclusion, any discussion on the complications of glaucoma surgery must be cognizant of the "supreme complication": the loss of visual function *despite* otherwise successful surgical intervention. Both the surgeon and patient should share in this knowledge that a certain decrease in visual field and visual acuity may result despite successful pressure reduction. This risk, however, is in the context of a probably *greater* chance of visual field and acuity loss if the pressure remains elevated. In fact, the most recent long-term studies[13] continue to substantiate that the safest pressure is a pressure in the low-normal range. Studies that have gone on from between 7 to 15 years[10,11] have all identified a significant tendency for visual field stabilization in those patients achieving intraocular pressures in this range. Reduced pressure and the reduced tendency toward diurnal variation are likely to be the most substantial achievements of any successful glaucoma surgery, with subsequent equilibrium for optic nerve function.

Filtering Surgical Options: An Overview

The filtering operations for glaucoma can be conveniently divided into those with a scleral flap and those without a scleral flap.[28] Full-thickness procedures refer to a group of techniques that include the posterior lip sclerectomy, thermosclerostomy, and trephination. The partial-thickness procedure usually refers to trabeculectomy. Traditionally, both approaches share a majority of intraoperative steps in common, with the primary distinction being whether a fistula is introduced at the limbus directly under the conjunctiva or underneath a prepared scleral flap. The variations of technique have been extensively elaborated in other sources.[29–32]

The advantages and disadvantages of each of these procedures have evoked an ongoing and productive long-running exchange of views in the literature. In brief, trabeculectomies are the most commonly performed procedure, and they are widely regarded as having a lower rate of complications, especially a reduced rate of shallow chamber and hypotony. On the other hand, there are reports that the full-thickness procedure gives a more robust and long-lived intraocular pressure-lowering effect. Reports with a moderate to long-term follow-up (2.7–5 years) indicated that the results between the two procedures were similar.[33,34] A similar study showed that after a 5-year follow-up nearly twice as many eyes with thermosclerostomies required no medications. With the adjunct use of topical therapy, the rate of intraocular pressure reduction was similar between the two operations, though with a tendency for lower pressures with the full-thickness procedure.[35]

This tendency for lower pressures with the full-thickness procedure has been commented on in several other studies. A 1-year study from the Mayo Clinic reported a mean postoperative pressure of 17 mm Hg after trabeculectomy versus 15 mm Hg after trephination.[36] Other reports have emphasized the viability of the full-thickness procedure: Lamping and coworkers[27] reported a stable reduction of intraocular pressure with disc and field stability over 6 years in 88% of patients after full-thickness procedure versus 76% of patients after trabeculectomy. The advantages of a full-thickness procedure have also been argued by Hutchinson and Robert.[37] When the additional risk factor of African-American race was taken into account, studies comparing the two techniques showed a slightly greater complication rate with a full-thickness procedure (especially cataract) but with consistently lower pressures after the posterior lid sclerectomies.[38,39]

The absolute distinction, however, between full- and partial-thickness procedures is blurring with the innovation of surgical techniques. For example, releasable sutures have been advocated both as a means of controlling the anterior chamber depth after trabeculectomy[40] and as a means to augment filtration in the presence of impaired filtration due to excessive apposition of the scleral flap.[41,42] These techniques have been advocated as providing the surgeon with slightly greater control than when argon laser suture lysis of the scleral flap is performed.

Laser suture lysis after trabeculectomy was initially described using a commonly available four-mirrored gonioscopy lens,[43] and later with a specially designed occlusion device.[44] Suture lysis has been advocated as a means of "salvaging" many trabeculectomies whose filtration is underactive. In the absence of antimetabolite therapy, suture lysis must be performed within a window of 7 to 10 days postoperatively before excessive fibrosis between the scleral flap and the wound edges prevents its effectiveness.[45,46] This "window for suture lysis" is greater if antimetabolites are used, either at the time of surgery or postoperatively, with successful flap opening as long as 2 to 4 weeks in an eye that has received antimetabolites.[47]

The downside of either releasable sutures or laser suture lysis is that the tamponade effect of the scleral flap is sacrificed, sometimes with an "all or nothing" response: either the filtration is impeded before flap release or is suddenly excessive. The consequences of a large bleb, shallow chamber, or choroidal effusion are reminiscent indeed of the problems of full-thickness filtration surgery.

Similarly, the complications common after full-thickness procedures are encountered after a contemporary version of this operation using a holmium laser to make a subconjunctival sclerostomy.[48,49] Although often the hole that is made is only a few hundred microns in diameter, considerably smaller than that which is rendered either surgically or thermally with a traditional full-thickness procedure, it often results in a significant early egress of aqueous and a shallowing of the chamber. On the other hand, such laser techniques have their own profile of procedure-specific complications, notably the predilection for the iris or Descemet flap to plug the small ostium[48,50] and the difficulty of performing an iridectomy at the time of the sclerostomy. Similar problems arise with a novel technique of internal trephination using an automated instrument to create full-thickness filtration. Its use has been reported both with and without the use of antimetabolites to augment the surgical effect, with promising results. Here, too, the issue of iris incarceration in the ostium requires specific surgical attention.[51,52]

Perhaps the greatest blurring now in the distinction between partial- and full-thickness procedures is the widespread use of antimetabolites in glaucoma surgery, specifically 5-fluorouracil (5-FU) and mitomycin-C. These antimetabolites have profoundly augmented the surgeon's ability to inhibit the normal healing process following trabeculectomy. They have thus created a new generation of thin-walled and extensive blebs, similar to those faced by the generation of surgeons trained with full-thickness procedures.[53,54] These techniques and complications are discussed more fully below.

There continues to be an amazing variety of innovations in filtering techniques that expand the definitions of full- and partial-thickness approaches. Procedures have been devised that unroof the Schlemm canal, allowing filtration without full-thickness penetration into the anterior chamber.[55,56] Promising results of an intriguing "selective trabeculectomy" to unroof the Schlemm canal have also been reported.[57] A particularly clever technique that allows for either full-thickness or guarded limbal fistulas, without touching the conjunctiva and operating solely through the cornea, has also been devised.[58] Each of these techniques may be able to avoid certain kinds of difficulties but will, inevitably, share complications with other forms of filtration procedures.

Risk Characteristics for Glaucoma Surgery

Many risk factors have been identified that have the potential to alter the results of filtering surgical intervention. One of the most intriguing is whether the glaucomatous eye has been exposed to a long period of topical antiglaucoma medication. In a series of provocative studies from the United Kingdom,[59–63] patients presenting with primary open-angle glaucoma were assigned either an early surgical intervention, or a conventional topical medication and laser treatment protocol preceding surgical intervention. A higher success rate was observed in eyes that underwent trabeculectomy without any prior exposure to topical antiglaucoma agents. Such drugs were believed to incite an inflammatory effect on the conjunctiva and Tenon tissue with a possible adverse effect on the surgical outcome.[64] More recent research has suggested that reduced numbers of conjunctival goblet cells may correlate with poor bleb function.[65] However, this seemingly adverse effect of topical medications was not appreciated by Watson and his colleagues in their 20-year retrospective study.[1]

Other negative risk factors are reported to increase the possibility of surgical failure. The young age of a patient is believed to be prejudicial to success.[66,67] Glaucoma in patients of African-American ancestry is thought to be a slightly negative risk factor in some reports[68] but unimportant in others.[38,67]

Among the most consistent factors prejudicial to filtration are prior ophthalmic procedures. In particular, a previous surgical procedure for glaucoma or cataract presages a higher risk of failure of filtration surgery, because of previous conjunctival disturbance.[7,67,69,70] Yet not all of the unfavorable results in eyes that are aphakic or pseudophakic are necessarily due to conjunctival scarring. There may be some "healing predilection" of the previously operated eye that makes it more prone to a hyperinflammatory response, and hence filtration failure. This phenomenon, for example, might explain the poor trabeculectomy results following keratoplasty,[71,72] in which there is a very high failure rate despite an open angle and relatively intact conjunctiva.

Specific Disease Entities

UVEITIC GLAUCOMAS. Besides the generalized risk factors mentioned above, there are specific conditions (such as corticosteroid-induced glaucoma)[73] and disease entities that cause secondary glaucoma and require specific planning and anticipation. For example, eyes that have sustained documented herpes zoster uveitis may have good results after surgical intervention for glaucoma and cataract but still have a tendency for prolonged postoperative inflammation.[74] Similarly, eyes of patients with juvenile arthritis may be prone to bilateral, nongranulomatous chronic anterior uveitis. The visual prognosis for these particular uveitic eyes is reported to be good to fair in 75% of cases, with the remaining 25% developing a visual impairment from either complicated cataract or secondary inflammatory glaucoma, the latter of which is difficult to manage.[75]

A larger cohort study of Fuchs heterochromic uveitis has observed that the risk of developing glaucoma is approximately 0.5% per year, substantially falling off after 15 years of follow-up.[76] Chronic open-angle glaucoma is the most common manifestation, though glaucomas with synechial angle closure, rubeosis, lens-induced angle closure, and recurrent hyphema have also been documented. There is a high likelihood that cataract surgery will precipitate the onset of glaucoma and that such glaucoma poorly responds to filtering procedures in the absence of antimetabolites: a failure rate of greater than 55% has been reported.

PSEUDOEXFOLIATION AND PIGMENTARY GLAUCOMAS. The prognosis for glaucoma in pseudoexfoliation was evaluated in a very large series of 519 patients in Australia.[77] More than half of these patients had glaucoma, which presented unilaterally three times more often than bilaterally. The detection of pseudoexfoliation material in the nonglaucomatous eye nevertheless was a serious risk factor: nearly 75% of the fellow eyes developed elevated tensions, and 25% progressed to frank glaucomatous damage. More than 10% of patients with pseudoexfoliation in one or both eyes presented with an acute, usually open-angle, glaucoma. As is well documented in the general literature on glaucoma, the course of glaucoma in patients with pseudoexfoliation can be condensed and aggressive. There may be rapid manifestation of optic disc and visual field loss and rapid tachyphylaxis to medication or laser intervention that often requires surgery and the use of antimetabolites.

A large retrospective study of patients with pigmentary dispersion and pigmentary glaucoma was undertaken to identify risk factors for the development and severity of glaucomatous disease.[78] Patients with the most difficult glaucoma requiring aggressive therapy and surgery tended to be male, younger, and African-American and presented with higher degrees of myopia and more frequent Krukenberg spindles. Such patients should be kept under particularly tight surveillance.

NEOVASCULAR GLAUCOMA. Perhaps the most difficult secondary glaucoma that requires surgical intervention is neovascular angle-closure glaucoma that is secondary either to a retinal vascular occlusion or to diabetic retinopathy. This particular form of glaucoma is notoriously difficult to control with standard procedures because of (1) the risk of hyphema and bleeding; (2) the predilection for closure of the stoma internally from a rubeotic membrane; and (3) the closure of the trabeculectomy bleb at the episcleral surface due to neovascularization, inflammation, or both. Although panretinal ablation by either laser or cryopexy is often helpful at either reducing the rubeosis or causing it to involute, glaucoma control is not always effected.[79]

The surgical strategies for neovascular glaucoma are dealt with in greater detail later in the chapter under the sections on the use of antimetabolites and glaucoma setons. One risk factor of interest, however, is that in patients presenting with an acute onset of neovascular glaucoma, visual acuity was seen to deteriorate at a very high rate 2 years or more after surgery—this factor was completely unrelated to good intraocular pressure control obtained surgically or medically.[80] This grim prognosis should be shared with the patients and kept in mind in evaluating the literature on surgical results for neovascular glaucoma.

IRIDOCORNEAL ENDOTHELIAL SYNDROME. Another difficult group of secondary glaucomas to manage are due to the iridocorneal endothelial syndrome. In a large series of 83 patients with glaucoma related to this syndrome, over half required filtering surgery.[81] Some 24 of 42 of these eyes required a second filtration surgery, and 8 required a third procedure. Similar poor success rates were seen with all three variations of the syndrome: Chandler syndrome, central iris atrophy, and Cogan-Reese syndrome. Accordingly, persistent surgical intervention is recommended, despite a high rate of initial failure.

Intraoperative Complications

Conjunctival Incontinence and Perforation

Although full-thickness filtering procedures are almost invariably performed with the limbus-based conjunctival flap, with trabeculectomy the surgeon has the option of choosing either a limbus-based flap or a fornix-based flap. Although there has been some controversy in the literature as to the equality or superiority of one approach over the other, several generalizations can be drawn. The long-term results of intraocular pressure control show that both the fornix-based flap and limbus-based flap procedures are comparable.[82–85]

The fornix-based conjunctival flap is certainly easier for the surgeon, in terms both of mechanically preparing the flap and in providing visualization of the perilimbal episcleral surface for the elaboration of a scleral flap. After its closure, it can be secured to the limbus with a variety of techniques, such as forming a corneal groove and placing a running Tenon nylon suture[86] or running a mattress suture using a 9-0 nylon vascular needle.[87] Although there is a slight tendency for greater microscopic aqueous leakage ("positive Seidel test") with the fornix flap, this minimal dehiscence is usually self-limited.[88]

The major drawback of the fornix-based flap trabeculectomy approach is when it is combined with antimetabolites either applied at the time of surgery (eg, mitomycin-C) or injected postoperatively (eg, 5-FU). A watertight wound is absolutely necessary when these very powerful antifibrotic agents are used, and most experienced surgeons recommend a limbus-based flap for this very reason. In the absence of antimetabolites, it is wise for the surgeon, at the conclusion of the operation, to inflate the anterior chamber through a paracentesis track to assess the quality of filtration into the bleb and to verify that it is, in fact, watertight at the limbus.

Limbus-flap procedures require much more manipulation of the conjunctiva and Tenon tissue, with the attendant risks of hemorrhage near the filter site or formation of conjunctival buttonholes either at the wound edge (from incomplete closure) or elsewhere (from punctures or tears). Such buttonholes can be minimized with several maneuvers.[89] The first is to maximize the visualization during all moments of the dissection; this is especially crucial when the blunt dissection is being performed to separate the conjunctiva from the episcleral surface. The most typical context for buttonholes is in an eye that has had previous surgery, with conjunctival adhesions that do not easily dissect, or in an eye undergoing limbus-based flap dissection with extremely diaphanous conjunctiva, as can sometimes be seen in very elderly eyes. It is sometimes helpful to balloon up the conjunctiva from the episcleral surface with an injection through a 30-gauge needle of either balanced salt solution or a lidocaine solution containing 1:100,000 epinephrine.

Once a buttonhole has inadvertently been made, the surgeon must assess if it is small enough or eccentric enough from the intended site of filtration to cause abandonment of the procedure at that particular location, or if it can simply be repaired. It is possible, though extremely difficult, to undermine the episcleral surface to which the conjunctiva may be adherent and to proceed anteriorly toward the limbus with an episcleral dissection; usually excessive bleeding is encountered.[89] It should also be cautioned that conjunctival buttonholes can easily be induced when the tissue is weakened by the application of excessive cautery to bleeding areas on the episcleral surface or subconjunctival space.

The repair of the buttonhole may be left to the conclusion of the procedure so that any stress on the wound is minimized during the remainder of the procedure.[29] The specific technique that the surgeon chooses will often depend on the location of the buttonhole. Small circular or linear tears in the area of the actual limbus-based dissection of conjunctiva can sometimes be closed at the time the larger conjunctival wound is being sutured. Dehiscences that are between the limbus and the limbus-based conjunctival wound can be closed either with a mattress suture technique or a pursestring technique. What is perhaps the most useful point is to use the smallest possible tapered needle that can be found, usually called a "vascular" needle; 10-0 nylon suture with such a needle is particularly useful. It is imperative to assess the integrity of the bleb for the absence of leakage from any possible buttonhole sites at the conclusion of the operation, using the highest possible magnification and careful drying of the area with cellulose sponges. As with every step of the procedures dealing with the conjunctiva, nontoothed forceps are imperative to position conjunctiva for both dissection and repair of any dehiscences without causing microperforation.

Disinsertion of the Scleral Flap

Interestingly, the actual size of the scleral flap and corneal block (ostium) is not as crucial for the final results of filtration as one might hypothesize. One prospective study compared trabeculectomies that had large scleral flaps (4×4×4 mm) and a large corneal ostium (3×3 mm) versus smaller scleral flaps (2×2×2 mm) and a small ostium (1×1 mm). After over a 1-year follow-up, there was no significant difference in either the intraocular pressure or the complication rates between the two groups.[90] Nevertheless, one prominent surgical authority has suggested that it is worthwhile to consider making a scleral flap that is less than one-fourth thickness of the sclera, with less than 0.5 mm between the ostium and the edge of the sclera trap door.[91] It is also clear that the use of argon laser suture lysis allows scleral flaps that are initially tightly adherent to the bed, since this occlusive effect can be obviated with the laser cutting of the suture and pressing on the eye.[46]

Whatever the surgeon's choice for fashioning the scleral flap, the most feared complication is the inappropriate dissection or disinsertion of the flap from its limbal insertion. This complication may result from the inappropriate use of a pointed forceps that perforates or tears the scleral flap away from its insertion or the dissection of a scleral flap at such a thin level anteriorly that no constant depth is maintained during the dissection and a portion of the flap amputates. Although an attempt can be made to close the scleral flap with a 10-0 nylon suture,[29] this is not always successful. Another strategy is to dissect a swatch of Tenon tissue that is approximately 4×4 mm from an adjacent site of the limbal-based conjunctival dissection area and to pull it tightly like a trampoline over the torn scleral flap at the conclusion of the trabeculectomy procedure. This can be secured to the corneal edges of the wound with the 10-0 nylon suture at each of the corners and at the posterior edges, forming a tight rectangular patch over the partially amputated scleral flap.[91]

With the conclusion of the conjunctival suturing, the anterior chamber should be assessed for its ability to maintain depth and the bleb should be assessed for the watertight integrity of its surface. If the chamber seems to be shallowing excessively because of the scleral flap dissection, maneuvers that are appropriate for shallow chamber following full-thickness filtering procedures can be contemplated. These could include either a Simmons tamponade shell[92,93] or an occluding symblepharon ring.[94]

Intraoperative Hemorrhage

Hemorrhage that is derived from the dissection of the conjunctiva from the episcleral surface during trabeculectomy is usually limited and controlled with cautery. Conditions that of course would predispose to such an event would be neovascular glaucoma, systemic anticoagulation therapy (eg, with aspirin or warfarin), or eyes exposed to an intense miotic over the long term. Bleeding can be partially reduced by the use of preoperative sympathomimetic drops (eg, neosynephrine or clonidine derivatives), or by intraoperative subconjunctival injection of low-dose (eg, 1 : 100,000) epinephrine.

When the bleeding is at the surface of the episclera, this can often be controlled with a bipolar cautery "pencil," with a flat, elliptical surface of approximately 3 mm length, which can be used with balanced salt solution to paint the surface clear of leaky vessels. If small hemorrhage is encountered at the time of the dissection of the scleral flap or the excision of the corneal block (eg, if the hemorrhage seems to be coming from the underlying ciliary body), this can best be controlled with the pinpoint precision of the coaxial monopolar diathermy probe that uses radiofrequency energy (Simmons-Savage cautery).[95] The lowest possible cautery setting is always advisable, to minimize shrinkage of tissue. This is especially crucial when the Simmons-Savage diathermy probe is used within the eye, to minimize shrinkage of the ostium edges or damage to the lens, zonules, or ciliary body.

Retrospective studies of trabeculectomy suggest that a small amount of hyphema formation is frequently seen postoperatively, often due to bleeding after iridectomy. Its incidence has been reported from 8%[27] to as high as 54%.[1] Such hemorrhage is usually incidental and rarely leads to synechial formation. There is one reported case, however, of extensive staining of the cornea with blood despite low intraocular pressure.[22]

The devastating complication of either intraoperative suprachoroidal or expulsive hemorrhage is fortunately rare. It has an estimated rate of occurrence of between 0.2% and 0.9% in all intraocular operations.[96,97] It is always important for the surgeon to have some strategy in mind in the event of the appearance of such a hemorrhage during surgery. The ominous presenting sign is the sudden shallowing of the anterior chamber with a prolapse of the iris (or unfortunately, vitreous and lens) into the trabeculectomy ostium. The pressure is suddenly seen to go high, and often the loss of the red reflex can be appreciated through the operating microscope. Immediate closure of the wound with multiple, tight sutures is imperative. Consideration should also be given to an emergency sclerostomy over the pars plana in the adjacent or inferior quadrant,[29] as well as intravenous osmotic therapy, such as with mannitol.

A related but rarely recognized complication is acute intraoperative choroidal effusion, which is reported to sometimes precede expulsive hemorrhage.[98] Immediate closure of the wound is advised; it is common that the intraocular pressure may rise at this juncture. It is possible to administer intravenous osmotic agents to reduce the tensions, with expected reduction of pressure within 30 minutes as the effusion is localized. A sclerostomy to drain fluids is not indicated if the wound can be closed before there is prolapse of intraocular tissues.

Intraoperative Lens Damage

Although it has been well documented that glaucoma surgery itself can be cataractogenic in a large number of patients,[99] this complication is usually identified in the long-term follow-up.[26] Of concern here is that during the trabeculectomy there are three critical stages of the surgery when it is possible to mechanically violate the lens capsule and precipitate early cataract formation.

The first such inadvertent opportunity would be during the creation of the corneal block tissue, by incision by either knife, scissors, or punch. The most dangerous moment is the actual entry into the anterior chamber with a sharp blade, during which time there is aqueous egress and shallowing of the chamber often before the knife blade has completed its transverse incision beneath the scleral flap. It is important not to use a "seesaw" or carving motion but to complete the penetration of the Descemet membrane across the full length of the incision as quickly as possible with a single smooth motion as the knife is being pulled out of the eye. This is particularly important in eyes with angle-closure glaucoma, in which the iris and lens may be more anterior than expected.

A second moment of vulnerability for the lens is if the paracentesis has been made in a shallow eye, either because it was inadvertently placed after the entry into the anterior chamber for the corneal block incision or because there was leakage from, for example, a corneal traction stay suture. It is advisable to place a paracentesis site with a sharp blade at the very beginning of the procedure while the anterior chamber is at its deepest. If the chamber is shallow already, a careful incision, parallel to and always above the iris, can be made obliquely (eg, from 11 to 7 o'clock), which would allow insertion of a cannula to re-form the chamber with a viscoelastic agent.

The third critical moment for lens damage is during the iridectomy, when a forceps is often inserted in the eye to procure the iris and bring it through the ostium for cutting. It is important that maximum visualization and the gentlest of touch be used to grasp the iris with a fine-toothed forceps and to avoid touching or penetrating the lens capsule behind the iris itself.[100] Although the use of viscoelastic agents in glaucoma surgery has been explored in an attempt to reduce the incidence of shallow anterior chambers postoperatively, there is no evidence that it decreases the incidence of lens opacification.[101]

Vitreous Loss

Vitreous loss during filtering surgery is rare in phakic eyes that have no history of trauma, prior iridectomy, or other predilection toward lens dislocation. An excessively posterior entry into the eye at the time of the fashioning of the corneal block can actually unroof the ciliary body and allow the presentation of vitreous at the site of a weak zonular ring. Preoperative conditions such as ocular syphilis, Marfan syndrome, pseudoexfoliation, homocystinuria, and high myopia should all be kept in mind as possible contexts in which this complication can arise.

Vitreous loss is more frequent in eyes that are aphakic or in eyes that are pseudophakic in the presence of zonular weakening (eg, pseudoexfoliation). Such factors that increase the risk of vitreous loss are not limited to glaucoma surgery alone and are especially well known to the cataract surgeon. These include a history of vitreous loss in the fellow eye, proptosis, chronic obstructive pulmonary disease, emphysema, increased venous pressure, short and thick neck, and obesity. A particularly high-risk eye is an eye of a child with congenital or juvenile glaucoma undergoing trabeculectomy: a rate of 12% vitreous loss has been reported.[102]

When faced with the appearance of vitreous through a wound that is either inappropriately posterior or at the site of a disturbed zonular face, it is best to close the wound promptly at this point before there is excessive disturbance of the presenting vitreous. Sometimes a minimal intervention with cellulose sponges and scissors vitrectomy is all that is necessary before the scleral flap can be closed and an alternate trabeculectomy site be fashioned. In the event that excessive vitreous presents, it is probably best to proceed with a full anterior vitrectomy, using contemporary surgical technique. The presentation of vitreous may be caused by the sudden expansion of a suprachoroidal effusion or hemorrhage, or even an unsuspected retrobulbar hemorrhage.

Intraoperative Antimetabolite Application

The most important innovation in glaucoma filtering surgery in the past decade is undoubtedly the introduction of antimetabolites, which impair normal wound healing and hence facilitate the formation of highly functional filtering blebs. Commencing with the pioneering studies on the use of 5-FU subconjunctival injections after glaucoma filtering surgery,[103,104] a rigorous prospective study was later reported[105] that led to the widespread appreciation of this technique to maximize bleb function.

A one-time intraoperative antimetabolite strategy using mitomycin-C was later described by Chen.[53] Early reports were later confirmed as showing that just a few minutes of exposure to a cellulose sponge saturated with mitomycin-C and placed between the conjunctiva and episclera resulted in greatly enhanced bleb function.[106] Mitomycin-C, in fact, proved equal if not superior to 5-FU in controlled studies as well.[54,107]

Observations of the use of mitomycin-C during filtering surgery have generated many contradictory recommendations for its most effective usage. Although various studies have used concentrations between 0.2 and 0.5 mg/mL, with exposure times from 1 to 5 minutes, there is as yet no widely accepted dose–response curve to guide the clinician. Moreover, different studies have used different kinds of cellulose sponges in their applications: some have used complete uncut sponges that are saturated with the mitomycin-C solution and applied either beneath the conjunctiva on the episcleral surface[54], or between the bed of the scleral flap and its scleral roof. Other studies have used fragments of a cellulose sponge, bisected horizontally parallel to the flat axis of the sponge and then perpendicularly near the tip, to create a triangular wedge approximately 3 mm in length and 1.5 mm in thickness before being saturated.[108,109] It is probable that there are variations in the saturation capacities and release abilities of various brands of cellulose sponges that make the comparison of different surgeons' techniques complicated.

As a result of these variations in technique, there remains a significant number of questions as to the parameters that are most effective and safe. Initially it was believed that the application of mitomycin-C on the episcleral surface and the conjunctiva should be applied before entering the eye to minimize the possibility of mitomycin-C leaching into the anterior chamber, where its toxicity would be most unwelcome. However, other surgeons have successfully used the mitomycin-C at the completion of phacoemulsification procedures, with wounds that appear watertight at the microscope, without observable consequences from any possible mitomycin-C entry into the eye. One report comparing the effects of mitomycin-C and 5-FU on anterior chamber inflammation found no difference between them.[110] By extrapolation, mitomycin-C has been safely used at the conclusion of a trabeculectomy, when the scleral flap has been tightened with sutures and the surgeon is certain that no inadvertent conjunctival buttonholes have been formed. Similarly, it can be used at the conclusion of a combined phacoemulsification and trabeculectomy. As with the uncertainty regarding dosage and sponge size, the superiority of using mitomycin-C before or after filtering incision into the eye remains to be clarified.

Although mitomycin-C is chemically known to inhibit mitosis and interrupt DNA synthesis,[111] surgeons report on remarkable changes in the conjunctival appearance after just a few minutes of exposure to mitomycin-C. The conjunctiva quickly blanches, as though there is immediate vascular infarction. The conjunctiva can also become suddenly quite thin and tenuous, requiring both the utmost delicacy in its manipulation by nontoothed forceps and minimum stress on the conjunctiva during the closure of its limbal-based wound.

Two other surgical tips using mitomycin-C are worth mentioning. It is also believed judicious to keep the actual edges of the limbus-based conjunctiva flap off of the mitomycin-C–saturated sponge, so that there will be no inhibition of wound healing precisely at the junction of the wound edge to be sutured. Similarly, it is advisable to refrain from tenonectomy until after the placement of the sponge, using the Tenon tissue as a tongue overlying the sponge and protecting the cut edge of the limbus-based conjunctival flap.

In a clever attempt to extrapolate the mitomycin-C experience to the use of 5-FU, Smith and associates[112] used a cellulose sponge saturated with 5-FU (0.5 mg/mL) that was applied for 5 minutes between the episclera and conjunctiva of a limbus-based flap trabeculectomy. Because the 5-FU did not appear to be as potent as mitomycin-C, it was still necessary in a certain number of cases to apply subconjunctival 5-FU injections postoperatively; however, the number of injections was greatly reduced. This technique remains to be clarified, but it is particularly attractive because the total amount of 5-FU that the eye is exposed to can be regulated depending on the vigor of the bleb, in contrast to the "all or nothing" effect that is obtained with mitomycin-C. A variation of this approach used a subconjunctival collagen sponge saturated with either 5-FU or bleomycin, with good long-term results in a small series of patients.[113]

Early Postoperative Complications

The postoperative appearance of the eye in the first days after a filtering procedure depends on many factors, not all of which can be controlled. Although it is customary to conclude a filtration procedure after ascertaining that the chamber is formed and a bleb is present, it is not uncommon that this is not the same appearance 24 hours later. The depth of the chamber and the extent of the bleb will depend on many factors, including whether a full-thickness or guarded procedure (trabeculectomy) was performed, the tightness of the scleral flap, the use of antimetabolites at the time of the surgery, the use of intracameral viscoelastics, and so on. Nevertheless, as many as one third of trabeculectomies will show a pressure near the hypotonous range (under 8 mm Hg) for as long as 2 weeks,[114] a figure that is representative of the experience of most glaucoma surgeons. Reassuringly, however, the low pressure in the first postoperative weeks does not necessarily foretell problems. In fact, in one study that looked at the medium-term follow-up of the eyes sustaining hypotony in the early postoperative period from trabeculectomy, there was no difference in the final intraocular pressure control in eyes between groups that did or did not have early hypotony.[22]

What is particularly useful for the postoperative management of trabeculectomy is the clinical classification of shallow chambers, popularized by Spaeth.[115,116] In the grade 1 chamber, the anterior chamber is peripherally flat, with touch between the peripheral iris and cornea, but with preservation of the anterior chamber adjacent to the pupillary space (Fig. 10-1). The grade 2 shallow chamber describes greater apposition between the mid-iris and the cor-

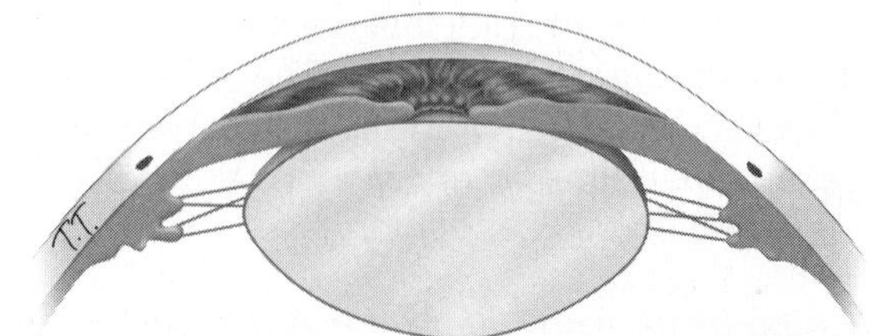

Figure 10-1. *Grade 1 shallow chamber.* Although there is touching of the peripheral iris and cornea, the central anterior chamber surrounding the pupillary area remains formed.

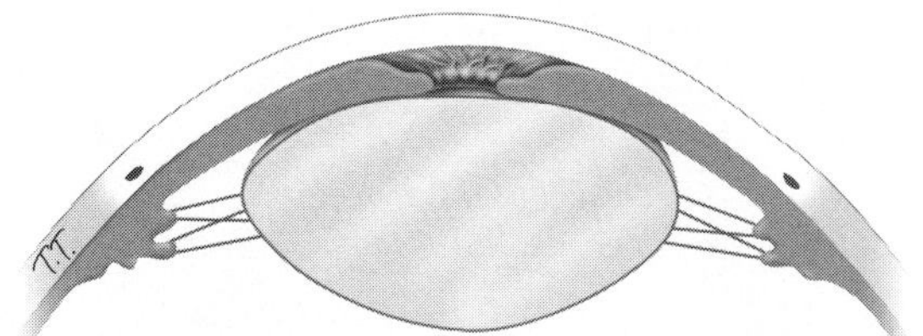

Figure 10-2. *Grade 2 shallow chamber.* The anterior chamber is quite compromised, with iris-to-corneal apposition peripherally and centrally, although the area anterior to the pupil and lens remains formed. To clinically monitor this small chamber over time, its depth can be graded with that of a fraction of the overlying cornea (eg, "central chamber one-half corneal thickness").

nea, but with the retention of some space between the anterior surface of the lens (or vitreous) and the cornea in the pupillary region (Fig. 10-2). (It may be useful for the surgeon to describe the actual depth of the small, central "anterior chamber" in reference to how many "corneal thicknesses," based on the slit-lamp assessment, exist between the cornea and the pupil itself.) The grade 3 anterior chamber is truly flat, with complete contact of the iris and the pupillary space with the posterior surface of the cornea (Fig. 10-3).

Perhaps the most important discrimination after describing the chamber depth is to determine if the intraocular pressure is either higher than expected or excessively low in conjunction with one of these three configurations of shallow chamber. By and large, grades 1 and 2 will almost always spontaneously reverse with time, responding to moderate intervention such as cycloplegia. The grade 3 flat chamber is a "medical urgency," which if not spontaneously resolved within a short period of time (1–2 days) will usually require surgical intervention. The corneal endothelium is the vulnerable structure under such circumstances, with loss of cells greatly increasing if the eye passes from a grade 2 to grade 3.[117,118] Anterior chamber re-formation by intraocular gas has been advocated for grade 3 cases.[119]

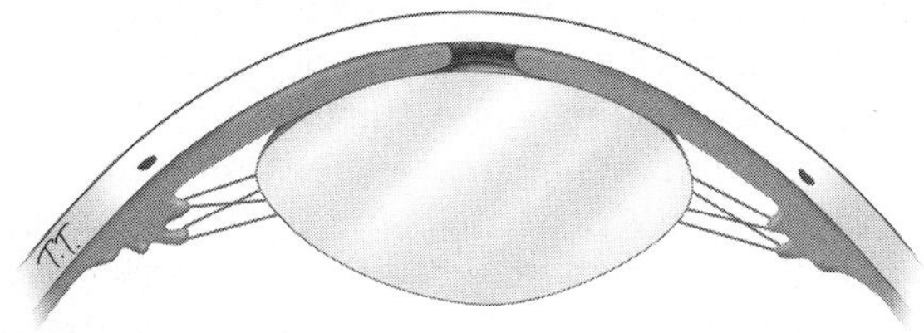

Figure 10-3. *Grade 3 shallow chamber.* The anterior chamber is completely collapsed, with pupillary–corneal touch, and sometimes even lens–corneal touch.

Low Postoperative Intraocular Pressure

WOUND LEAK. Assuming that intraoperative precautions were taken and no conjunctival dehiscence was appreciated at the conclusion of the surgery, wound leaks can nevertheless appear on the first postoperative day. These may be slightly more common with fornix-based conjunctival flaps than limbus-based flaps.[88] A focal leak can be seen in the presence of a formed or shallow anterior chamber and is best appreciated by evaluating the integrity of the wound with the use of fluorescein strips. This Seidel test is usually obvious in the presence of a genuine leak, though sometimes it is necessary to apply light pressure through the eyelid onto the globe to identify an area of inadvertent aqueous drainage.[120]

The standard approach to a leaking point depends in large part on the dimensions of the dehiscence. In the presence of low intraocular pressure it is sometimes possible to medically manage these leaks by further reducing aqueous flow by applying a topical agent (such as a β-blocker), providing long-term cycloplegia (with atropine drops), and reducing the dose of any corticosteroid drops and adding slightly irritating antibiotic drops (eg, gentamicin) (to enhance a modest amount of inflammation, in hopes of promoting wound healing).[115] Especially if antimetabolites have not been used, these small leaks will usually resolve with a simple medical regimen.

Sometimes, however, it is necessary to apply some sort of sustained pressure on the eye, in an attempt to close the wound. This is the rationale for the use of semi-pressure patching of the eye with a leaky bleb, especially in conjunction with the previously mentioned medical regimen. Another option is the use of large soft contact lenses.[121] Lenses are available in sizes from 16 to 24 mm and are usually quite comfortable for the patient. These can be used with or without a semi-pressure patch. Their compressive effect, however, is not always impressive.

Along the same lines there is an extensive literature about the merits of using a shell tamponade technique, originally described by Simmons and Omah[122] and more recently elaborated in extensive detail by Spurny and associates.[93] Although used originally in conjunction with full-thickness filtration techniques to temporarily reduce aqueous flow and prevent shallow chambers in the early postoperative period, it has subsequently been described for postoperative bleb leaks.[123,124] Modifications have been devised to reduce the rotation of the large plastic shell[125] and to minimize the damage to the cornea, which can sometimes result in abrasions or abscesses.[126] The use of the large soft contact lens beneath the shell has proven effective in minimizing corneal trauma.[92] Because there is a considerable amount of technical expertise and time investment for the successful use of the shell tamponade, a less intensive but similar intervention has been proposed using a modified symblepharon ring (Fig. 10-4), which allows compression from the limbus to the fornices but permits the cornea to be unimpeded for measurement of intraocular pressure and visualization.[94]

Leaking blebs can also be approached in other novel fashions. Large-spot argon laser applications to the bleb site have been described as a means of reducing pinpoint leaks or limiting the extent of the blebs (Fig. 10-5).[127] The thermal absorption of the argon light may be enhanced by the use of fluorescein applied to the bleb surface.

Another interesting approach to correct leaking blebs derives from experience in treating irregular corneal lacerations or perforations: the application of cyanoacrylate tissue adhesive glue.[128] This can be done well with an operating microscope in a minor surgery setting, using sterile technique. After carefully drying the leaking area with a cellulose sponge, a drop of medical-grade sterile glue can be applied to

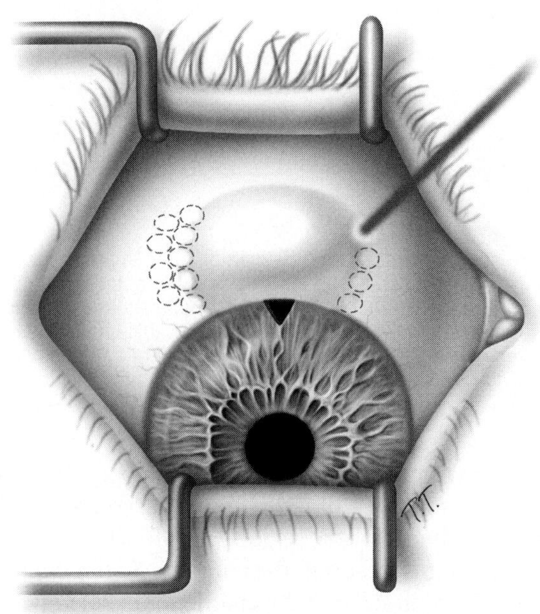

Figure 10-5. *Argon laser bleb treatment.* Under topical anesthesia, foci of bleb leakage (or the margins of large blebs, as illustrated here) can be lightly coagulated with an argon laser, using a large spot size and minimal energy. Topical dyes, such as fluorescein or rose bengal, may enhance the thermal absorption.

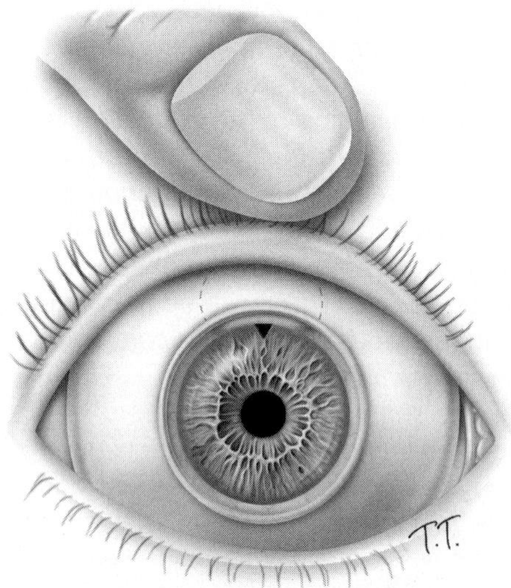

Figure 10-4. *Bleb compression.* As an alternative to the Simmons shell technique, involving tamponade of a bleb with excessive filtration, a modified symblepharon ring can be applied, which leaves the cornea free for intraocular pressure measurements and for the patient's vision. The ring is available in either colored or clear plastic. The surgeon also has the option of using a large soft contact lens beneath the ring for corneal comfort.

the leaking area. One technique uses a "sandwich" arrangement, in which a small dab of sterile ointment is applied at the end of a wooden stick applicator, upon which a 2- to 3-mm disc of sterile plastic (eg, hand-cut from a sterile plastic drape) is balanced (Fig. 10-6). A drop of glue is applied on this plastic disc. Immediately after drying the leaking conjunctival area with a cellulose sponge (Fig. 10-7), the stick with the ointment, disc, and glue is inverted so that the glue is applied to the conjunctival surface. The stick is used to compress the disc over the glue to make a flat area, and after 1 minute's duration the stick can be easily slid off the underlying plastic disc by virtue of the ointment.

An alternative way to deliver cyanoacrylate glue to a leaky bleb is with a microapplicator, with the patient sitting at a slit lamp. The glue is instantly applied after drying the site with a cellulose sponge (Fig. 10–7). To prevent premature "blinking off" of the glue and plastic from the bleb area after either technique of gluing, a large soft contact lens can be applied (Fig. 10-8), obviating the need for a pressure patch. Sometimes this gluing technique needs to be repeated, but it is a well-established and reasonable approach.

Sometimes the simplest technique for repairing leaks is simply to resuture the area with 10-0 nylon

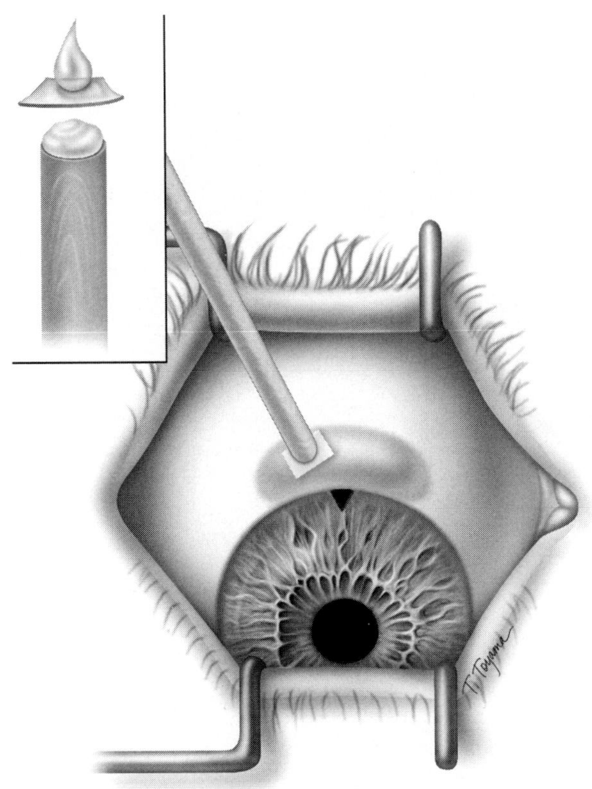

Figure 10-6. *Bleb gluing.* After applying a topical anesthetic to the eye and positioning the patient supine under an operating microscope (or loupes), the surgeon prepares a 2- to 3-mm disk of sterile plastic, cut from the drape material. This piece of sterile plastic is then applied to the end of a wooden applicator and secured by the use of any ophthalmic ointment between the wood and the plastic. Having initially dried the area carefully with a cellulose sponge, the surgeon applies a drop of cyanoacrylate glue to the upper surface of the plastic disk and then applies the entire "sandwich" to the leaky bleb. After pressure is applied for 1 minute, the glue and plastic should adhere to the area of epithelial leak, and because of the ointment, the wooden applicator can easily be slid off the underlying plastic disk. A soft contact lens can then be applied to prevent the plastic itself from being dislodged by blinking.

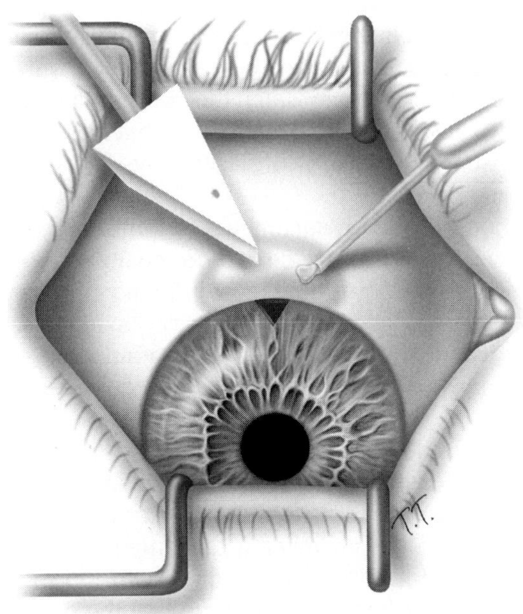

Figure 10-7. *Bleb gluing.* After using a topical anesthetic on the eye and inserting a lid retractor to keep the lids apart while the patient is at the slit lamp, the surgeon meticulously dries the focus of the leaking bleb with a cellulose sponge. Then, a very small drop of cyanoacrylate glue is precisely applied to the dried bleb site, using a pressure-activated micropipette. After 2 minutes, the glue is allowed to dry on the eye.

suture, using a tapered needle to minimize any disruption of the bleb area.[129] In the presence of a chronic or late-onset leak, it is occasionally necessary to excise the entire area of the bleb itself and to mobilize adjacent conjunctiva, bringing it forward to the limbus where it can be sutured in a watertight fashion.[130,131]

CHOROIDAL EFFUSION. Choroidal effusions are fairly ubiquitous after filtering procedures, especially if the pressures are below 10 mm Hg. It has, in fact, been observed that the incidence of choroidal effusions is inversely related to the intraocular pressure level.[115] Such effusions can be observed at frequent

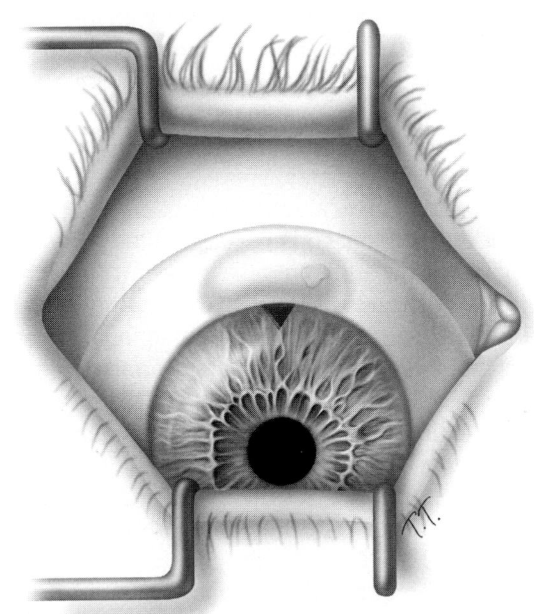

Figure 10-8. *Protecting the glue patch.* Therapeutic soft contact lenses, ranging 16 to 24 mm in diameter, are available to encompass the cornea and perilimbal areas. As illustrated here, such a large lens can amply cover the bleb and the dried site of glue, so that the lid does not blink the glue patch loose before healing has occurred.

observational intervals, appearing as either a low, annular detachment sometimes appreciated only because of the ease with which the ora serrata is visualized, or as large choroidal effusions that may threaten the visual axis when two detachments "kiss" in the mid-vitreal cavity.

The choroidal detachment becomes of greatest clinical concern when the anterior chamber progressively shallows over time, even possibly progressing to a grade 3 "flat chamber." However, in the absence of a wound leak or excessive inflammation, many surgeons prefer to avoid any kind of choroidal drainage procedure. Indications for intervention are usually reserved either for the presence of "kissing choroidals," in which the retinal surfaces are in contact astride large bullous choroidal detachments, or for a flattening of the chamber with compromise of the corneal endothelium. Shy of these two indications, however, it is frequently the case that the choroidal effusions will, with time, resolve, with the vigorous use of atropine cycloplegia and corticosteroids (to reduce inflammation). One particular circumstance that may require early surgical intervention is an eye with chronic angle-closure glaucoma and an extremely shallow chamber after trabeculectomy: in one series, few eyes responded to medical intervention and prompt re-formation was recommended.[119]

Attention should be taken, however, to distinguish choroidal detachments from an overlying serous retinal detachment, which has been seen after a filtering procedure.[132] Similarly, small retinal tears in conjunction with choroidal effusion have led to rhegmatogenous retinal detachments.[133]

In the event that anterior chamber re-formation and choroidal drainage is necessary, the techniques elaborated a decade ago[134] have been only slightly changed in recent years.[135] In brief, one or more sclerostomies are made over the pars plana, the anterior chamber is intraoperatively re-formed with balanced salt solution, and attempts are made to drain the suprachoroidal effusion while maintaining the chamber at as normal a depth as possible. Another elegant approach involves microtrephination through the sclera, anterior to the inferior rectus muscle (Figs. 10-9 and 10-10).[136]

When a choroidal effusion is present, it is difficult to distinguish the role of ciliary hyposecretion in keeping the intraocular pressure low and contributing to a shallowing of the anterior chamber. Most often this is suspected in the presence of intensive inflammation, appreciated in the anterior chamber at the slit lamp. It has been reported that if the pressure re-

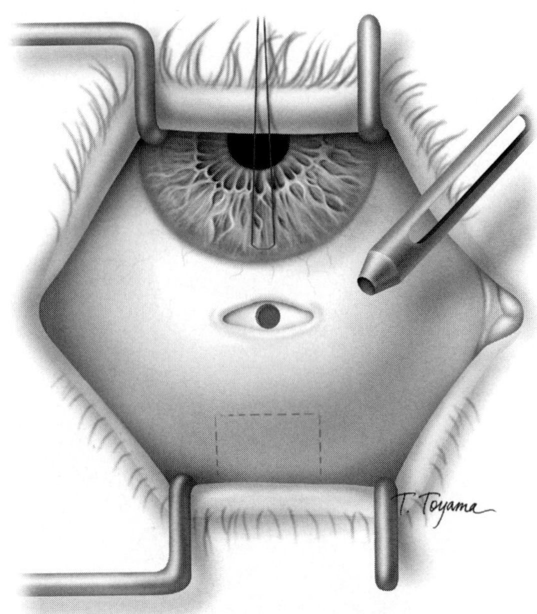

Figure 10-9. *Dellaporta technique for choroidal drainage.*[136] After a conjunctival incision is made 4 mm from the limbus at the 6 o'clock position over the pars plana (and anterior to the inferior rectus muscle), a 1-mm trephine is used to remove a divot of sclera, with great care taken to avoid penetrating the underlying uveal tissue. The divot of sclera can optionally be removed after the drainage of fluid or be lightly sutured into place.

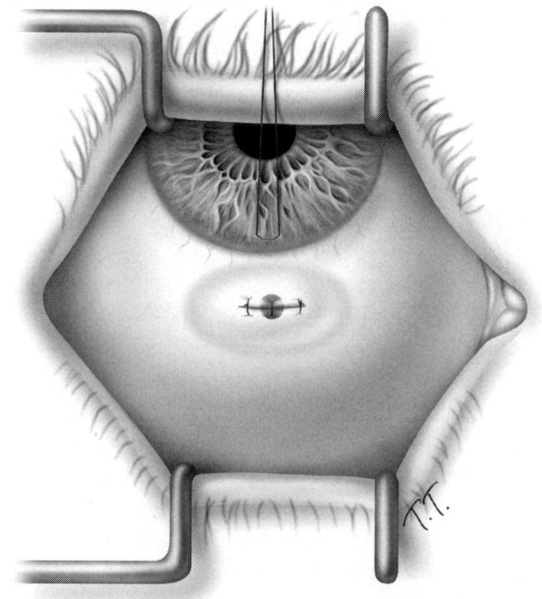

Figure 10-10. *Dellaporta technique (Continued).* After a watertight closure of the conjunctiva wound (eg, using 9-0 Vicryl suture), a dependent bleb forms from the persistent egress of fluid through the 1-mm trephine hole. Uveal prolapse is rarely seen, and the drainage of fluid, activated by the extraocular movements, can sometimes persist for several days, thus reducing the tendency for recurrent accumulation of suprachoroidal effusion.

mains unexpectedly low for more than 4 days without any other obvious explanation, such as large choroidal effusion or Seidel-positive leakage, the hyposecretory mechanism is probably responsible.[115] This may resolve with the intensive use of corticosteroid drops to minimize inflammation. It is also worthwhile to consider the observations of Vela and Campbell[137] in situations in which β-blocker drops continue to be used in the fellow eye. Presumably on the basis of ciliary hypersensitivity, profound reduction in aqueous production with effusion can be seen in the post-trabeculectomy eye by a crossover effect. It is worth considering halting the β-blocker therapy in the fellow eye if hyposecretion and choroidal effusion are not resolving in an appropriate period of time.

HYPERFILTRATION. Especially with the use of antimetabolite applications at the time of surgery, it is possible to see a low intraocular pressure and shallowing anterior chamber on the basis of an excessively large filtering area. Sometimes this takes the appearance of a 360-degree perilimbal "donut ring bleb." Another contributing factor besides antimetabolites might be excessive subconjunctival elevation from the surgeon's irrigation at the conclusion of surgery, which dissects the conjunctiva around the limbus and creates a larger potential filtering space than that which would be obtained by simple filtration pressures alone.

Some of the techniques mentioned earlier for the management of wound leak can be applied to hyperfiltration blebs. A medical regimen would include the reduction of aqueous flow by the use of topical β-blocker or carbonic anhydrase inhibitor or the curtailment of corticosteroid therapy and addition of an "irritative" antibiotic to enhance the adhesion of the conjunctiva to the episcleral surface. A mechanical means to force the conjunctiva back, such as a large soft contact lens, symblepharon ring, or glaucoma tamponade shell, can also be applied. Most often, this complication is short-lived and responds to one of the previously mentioned interventions in the first several weeks after surgery. Excessive blebs that persist beyond this period may be approached with other means, such as freezing, cautery, or chemical irritation (see below).

Elevated Postoperative Intraocular Pressure

ELEVATED PRESSURE WITH A DEEP ANTERIOR CHAMBER. In the immediate postoperative 24 to 36 hours there may be transient obstruction to aqueous flow despite an uncomplicated surgical procedure. In a very important report by Liebmann and associates,[138] it was observed that when intraocular pressures were measured postoperatively 4 to 6 hours after trabeculectomy, nearly one of five eyes showed a pressure elevation of 40 mm Hg or greater. This elevation was considerably higher than what is usually seen in the first postoperative day and had no correlation with the patient's age, glaucoma diagnosis, preoperative intraocular pressure, or the number of sutures used to tie the flap. It is possible that fibrin or a microscopic amount of hemorrhage causes a temporary seal to form around the trabeculectomy flap at or below the episcleral surface, impeding flow and subjecting the eye to an elevated pressure. Although it is theoretically possible that an eye with split fixation and advanced nerve loss could sustain a significant loss of central vision with such a pressure elevation, it has rarely been appreciated in clinical practice.[18] Tissue plasminogen activation has even been used in circumstances with extended clot blockade.[139]

Focal obstruction of the flap may explain the clinical observation that though the pressure may be unexpectedly high on the first postoperative day, a large bleb can be raised and the tension reduced instantaneously by the application of direct massage on the eye. This can be done by either pushing a cotton-tipped applicator or goniolens inward on the cornea and pressing posteriorly toward the optic nerve or by rolling an applicator along the limbal aspect of the filtering site (the "Traverso maneuver").[115]

Viscoelastics retained in the eye can also account for elevated pressures in the period immediately after trabeculectomy.[138,140] In the past several years there have been many reports advocating the use of viscoelastics, such as sodium hyaluronate, at the time of glaucoma surgery. Observers have mentioned that viscoelastic use is associated with fewer choroidal detachments, less postoperative shallowing of the anterior chamber, and a reduced amount of bleeding.[101,141–145]

ELEVATED PRESSURE WITH A SHALLOW ANTERIOR CHAMBER

Pupillary Block. The shallowing of the anterior chamber from pupillary block has been reported under many circumstances, though they are not terribly common. There may be impaired flow between the posterior and anterior segments on the basis of excessively strong miotic usage and sphincter constriction.[115] Pupillary block can also be seen on the basis of an excessively large cataract or dislocated lens, which would be evident by phacodonesis; or there may be a transient blockade of the pupil from either blood, fibrin, vitreous, inflammatory debris, or even viscoelastic agent. It is also possible in the immediate weeks after surgery that adhesions can appear between the hyaloid face and the iris or between a lens implant and the iris.[146]

As with the usual presentation of pupillary block, glaucoma, it is expected that there would be greater shallowing of the periphery of the anterior chamber than centrally. Because trabeculectomies are almost invariably performed with surgical iridectomy, it is important to assess whether the iridectomy is in fact patent, either by transillumination or direct visualization or by gonioscopy. The availability and ease of performing laser iridotomy, either with argon or neodymium:yttrium-aluminum-garnet (Nd:YAG) laser energy, should allow the elimination of this mechanism from consideration in the presence of a shallow chamber and elevated pressure.

Suprachoroidal Hemorrhage. There is a spectrum of clinical severity with the appearance of hemorrhage in the suprachoroidal space, from the much-feared occurrence of an intraoperative expulsive hemorrhage, to the delayed onset of a limited suprachoroidal hemorrhage, usually within the first 2 weeks of surgery.[147] The acute form can lead to particularly devastating consequences in the presence of a large ocular wound, such as at the time of cataract extraction. A more limited form can be seen with the appreciation of an acute intraoperative choroidal effusion.[98] This is often heralded by the rapid shallowing of the anterior chamber and the elevation of the intraocular pressure to as high as 80 mm Hg, with resolution within 15 to 30 minutes of light pressure. Sclerostomies are not necessary for the resolution of this complication, if it in fact is appreciated.

The incidence of intraoperative suprachoroidal hemorrhage is in the range of 0.2% in glaucomatous eyes.[96] Subjectively it is accompanied by a great deal of pain, which usually brings the patient to the surgeon's attention. The chamber may be shallowed, and the pressure may be temporarily high, but it is usually on the low side because of an associated choroidal effusion.

The literature is replete with risk factors for suprachoroidal hemorrhage: the most commonly mentioned are old age, aphakia, postoperative hypotony, myopia, increased venous pressure, and general anesthesia.[97,147–149] Two elegant analyses have, however, claimed to isolate the most important risk factors. In a study reported by the Fluorouracil Filtering Surgery Study Group,[150] 10 of 162 eyes receiving 5-FU were studied in a prospective fashion, and there was a remarkably strong association between the appearance of suprachoroidal hemorrhage and the level of preoperative intraocular pressure. Among the patients with pressures under 30 mm Hg, no incident of suprachoroidal hemorrhage appeared; in eyes with pressures between 30 and 39 mm Hg, the percentage was 6% appearance of suprachoroidal hemorrhage; with pressures of 40 to 49 mm Hg the appearance was 11%; and in three patients with pressures over 50 mm Hg, the appearance was nearly 20%. A different analysis using a case control methodology similarly identified the risk factor of increased elevated intraocular pressure and specifically called attention to the greater risk for suprachoroidal hemorrhage in the presence of an axial length greater than 25.8 mm Hg.[151]

The optimal management of suprachoroidal hemorrhage is controversial. There is no question that an acute intraoperative suprachoroidal hemorrhage requires immediate attention, with secure closure of the incision and decompression sclerostomies. However, it has been reported that the majority of eyes will respond to conservative management without the need for surgical intervention.[96] The outcome may depend, however, on the extent of the hemorrhage. In instances in which massive hemorrhages were appreciated, the best visual acuity was obtained when surgical drainage was undertaken within 14 days.[152]

Another technique that has been advocated is the simultaneous air insufflation of the eye during the time of sclerostomy, to maintain the intraocular pressure at a fairly steady rate; good visual acuity was reported in a significant number of patients.[153] If surgical intervention is to be considered, it is appropriate to wait several days for spontaneous clot lysis, which makes the evacuation of the suprachoroidal blood considerably easier.

Malignant Glaucoma. The term *malignant glaucoma* refers to a spectrum of atypical angle-closure glaucomas that share several essential features.[154] Other terms have been proposed for this condition, many of which purportedly point to the underlying pathophysiology. These terms include *aqueous misdirection glaucoma, hyaloid block glaucoma,* and *posterior aqueous entrapment.* Historically, it was commonly appreciated as a complication of a filtering procedure in eyes with preexisting angle-closure glaucoma or shallow anterior chambers. More recently, a bewildering and diverse number of "trigger events" have been described, occurring even in the absence of opening the eye and including ciliary spasm, laser iridotomy, argon suture lysis, and even uveitis.

There are several essential features of this condition about which there is good agreement in the literature, and there are other features that are more controversial. Clinically, malignant glaucoma is suspected in the presence of a grade 2 or grade 3 shallow chamber, with the prominent simultaneous shallowing of the peripheral *and* central anterior chamber (Fig. 10-11). The pressure is usually higher than expected: in the early postoperative period it may simply be between 15 and 20 mm Hg despite the appearance of what would seem to be an otherwise adequate bleb; in other instances, the pressure can be much higher.

To make the diagnosis of malignant glaucoma, it is essential to eliminate the possibility of pupillary block; hence, a patent iridotomy must be established before this diagnosis can be considered. Sometimes the diagnosis is made only in retrospect, after evaluating the eye's response to several interventions. For example, cycloplegic agents can be curative of malignant glaucoma and miotic agents can be exacerbative. If surgical intervention is necessary, disrupting the hyaloid face or collapsing the vitreous is usually curative but long-term dependence on cycloplegic agents may be necessary.

Other aspects that are sometimes seen with malignant glaucoma include the rarity of spontaneous resolution and hence its "malignant" designation. It is usually bilateral in predisposition, and it is often worsened by conventional glaucoma surgery, such as iridectomy or filtration operation. In the clinical presentation of this condition there is some overlap with other conditions, notably angle-closure glaucoma with ciliary choroidal detachment.[155] Other conditions that may overlap with the appearance of malignant glaucoma include eyes that have undergone cataract extraction, with or without lens implantation, with sequestration of aqueous behind the iris plane: these have been referred to as "iridovitreal block"[146] and "retrocapsular aqueous misdirection" (see Fig. 10-11).[156]

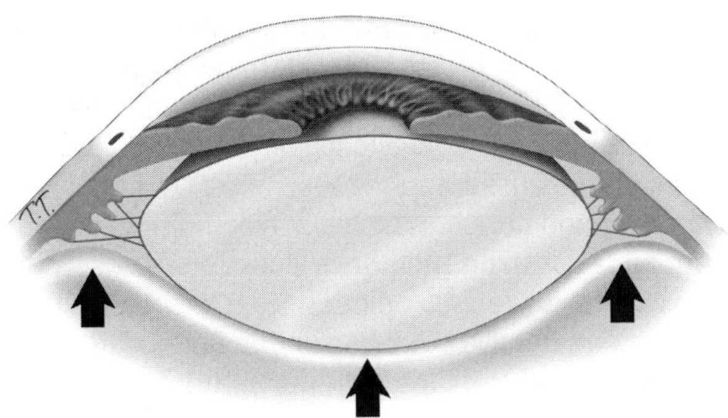

Figure 10-11. *Phakic malignant glaucoma.* With the sequestration of aqueous within the vitreous body, there is compression of the anterior chamber both axially and peripherally, causing central shallowing of the chamber with forward movement of the lens and peripheral angle closure.

Because of the difficulty in identifying a common theme among the various proposed triggers for malignant glaucoma, there nevertheless is some consensus as to the pathophysiologic sequence.[157,158] After some initiating event— shallowing of the chamber from suture lysis,[159] trabeculectomy for chronic open-angle glaucoma in eyes with preexisting central retinal vein occlusion,[160] laser iridotomy,[161–164]—there apparently is some cause for misdirection of the aqueous to circulate into or behind the vitreous body. This leads to an alteration of the vitreous volume and its compaction, with a cycle of increasing vitreous swelling and reduced anterior conductivity of aqueous. The enlarging vitreous body is unable to exchange aqueous across the hyaloid face at the junction of three structures: the zonules, vitreous face, and ciliary processes. This progressive vitreal engorgement results in shallowing both axially and peripherally in the anterior chamber, with increasing apposition of the peripheral iris into the angle, setting up a further cycle of angle-closure glaucoma. The possible overlap of these syndromes with the collection of fluid in the suprachoroidal space has been observed by some authors[154,165] but denied by others.[166]

There is greater unanimity in the management protocol for this condition than in the explanations of pathophysiology. First, it is important to eliminate the possibility of pupillary block glaucoma by verifying or creating a patent iridotomy. Miotic medication should be discontinued, and vigorous cycloplegia should be instituted along with the use of topical corticosteroids. Other reducers of aqueous production, such as topical β-blockers, carbonic anhydrase inhibitors, or osmotic agents, can be applied to reduce the pressure. It has been advised to wait approximately 5 days with this intensive medical regimen to see if there is resolution, with as many as half the cases resolving during this interval.[166] In the event that surgical intervention is necessary, either a needle aspiration[167] or pars plana vitrectomy[168] will usually be curative.

This treatment algorithm is most appropriate for phakic eyes with malignant glaucoma.[154] After cataract extraction, eyes may have either no capsule (Fig. 10-12) or retained posterior capsule, with or without an intraocular lens; this permits a direct incision of the hyaloid face using Nd:YAG laser.[169,170] Epstein and colleagues[169] observed that rupture of the hyaloid face effected resolution of the glaucoma, convincingly demonstrating that aqueous trapped behind the hyaloid can be responsible for the sequence of events in malignant glaucoma. A similar resolution by disrupting the hyaloid can be rarely undertaken in phakic eyes with the fortuitous appearance of a large iridectomy, which allows visualization of the peripheral hyaloid for Nd:YAG laser application.[171] In the presence of a posterior capsule or lens implant, sometimes it is necessary to sequentially eliminate pupillary block, retrocapsular block, and hyaloid block by respectively lasering through iris, the posterior capsule, and hyaloid face (Fig. 10-13).[154]

Vigorous surveillance is still necessary in these eyes, since recurrent cases of malignant glaucoma have been reported, especially after vitreous aspiration or vitrectomy, which in the phakic eye may not be sufficiently anterior to interrupt the obstruction of the hyaloid face. In rare events it is necessary to sacrifice the lens to access the hyaloid itself. Chronic atropine drops may be needed, and great attention should be paid to the fellow eye, which is at a high risk for recapitulating the events of the first eye's malignant glaucoma attack.

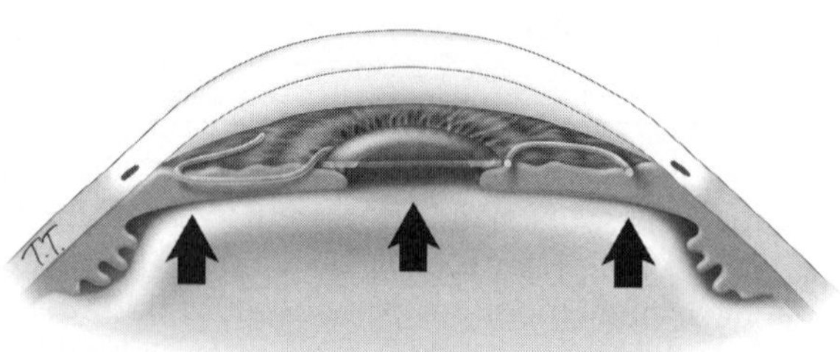

Figure 10-12. *Acapsular malignant glaucoma.* In the absence of a posterior capsule—such as aphakia or, as seen here, an anterior-chamber intraocular lens—the abnormal vitreous forces compress the anterior chamber axially and peripherally, but the abnormal hyaloid surface is accessible to laser or incisional surgery.

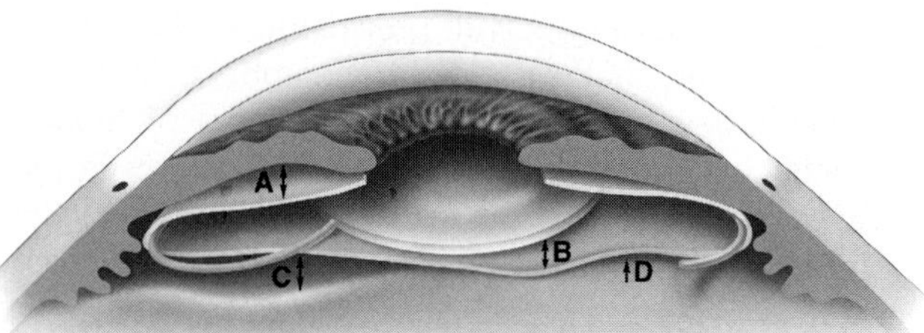

Figure 10-13. *Capsular malignant glaucoma.* In the presence of a posterior capsule with a posterior-chamber intraocular lens there are multiple sites in which aqueous can be sequestered, and these sites must be sequentially eliminated: (**A**) aqueous pockets between the iris and anterior capsule; (**B**) pockets within the capsular bag and lens implant; (**C**) pockets between the posterior capsule and hyaloid face; and (**D**) aqueous trapped within the vitreous cavity behind an intact hyaloid face.

Aspects of Antimetabolite Use in Filtering Surgery

CORTICOSTEROIDS. From the days when topical corticosteroids were first available they have been used as a chemical adjunct to inhibit the scarification of blebs, which is most often due to fibrosis at the level of the episcleral and conjunctival interface.[172] The clinical impression that topical corticosteroids were beneficial for bleb survival was convincingly established in a randomized study from the Wills Eye Hospital.[173] These results stimulated interest in whether preoperative subconjunctival treatment with corticosteroids before trabeculectomy would be beneficial. However, studies using subconjunctival triamcinolone were equivocal in their findings, and this line of pursuit has not been actively pursued.[174]

5-FLUOROURACIL. Probably the most widespread antimetabolite used to retard wound healing and maximize bleb longevity is 5-FU. From the mid-1980s, when it was brought to the attention of clinicians by means of elegantly designed, randomized studies,[104,105,175] a vast literature has been reported on the benefits and side effects of this modality. The initial studies used a large dose of 5-FU: 5-mg doses were injected subconjunctivally twice daily after surgery for 7 days and then once daily for 7 days. Injections were made 180 degrees from the bleb in the inferior conjunctiva, allowing bathing of both the ocular surface and the bleb with the antimetabolite. The total dosage of 5-FU was approximately 105 mg per eye.

The eyes in these early studies had many severe risk factors for failure, most notably either neovascular glaucoma or aphakia. Their success rates reflected the underlying diagnosis. For example, the 3-year success rate for patients with aphakic open-angle glaucoma was 63% versus 75% in phakic eyes with a previously failed trabeculectomy.[175] In part because of the vigorous surveillance, a large number of complications were reported: corneal epithelial defects in over half the patients; conjunctival wound leaks in over one third of the patients; suprachoroidal hemorrhage in over 5% of patients; rhegmatogenous retinal detachment in some 2% of patients; and sporadic instances of late bleb leaks, malignant glaucoma, and tractional retinal detachment.[175]

Other studies have subsequently confirmed the impressive advantage of 5-FU injections over not using antimetabolite in maximizing bleb survival and intraocular pressure control, especially in eyes that are at risk of failure either because of previous surgery or an underlying complicated glaucoma. Results hovering around a 90% success rate were reported by many authors.[176–183]

Two studies in particular deserve special attention. In an elegant 5-year prospective study of 5-FU performed in Japan, eyes were segregated into primary open-angle glaucoma, secondary glaucoma, and refractory glaucoma; results were evaluated by means of the life-table method of Kaplan-Meier.[184] Over 360 eyes were studied, and the total amount of 5-FU that was given subconjunctivally ranged between 36.5 and 49.5 mg. At the 5-year follow-up point, the probability of maintaining intraocular pressure below 21 mm Hg, with or without medication, was significantly higher in eyes that received 5-FU when compared with the control group that did not get 5-FU. In the primary open-angle glaucoma eyes receiving 5-FU, success was achieved in over 92% versus 58% in eyes without 5-FU; over 87% of eyes with secondary glaucoma were successfully treated with 5-FU versus 54% without; in eyes with refractory glaucoma receiving 5-FU, treatment was successful in over 57% versus 28% in eyes that were not treated. When the analysis was performed to identify pressures below 16 mm Hg with or without medication, again the clear superiority was seen for 5-FU in all three groups. Interestingly enough, other than the well-documented surface corneal epithelial defects with 5-FU, no other significant complications, either early or late, were reported in this study.

A different study investigated how effective 5-FU was compared with full-thickness filtering procedure without antimetabolite at obtaining the lowest possible intraocular pressure in eyes either with low-tension glaucoma or far advanced glaucomatous defects near fixation in need of very low postoperative tension.[185] Seventeen patients requiring bilateral surgery were randomized, one receiving a full-thickness procedure with a modified shell tamponade technique on one eye,[92] and the other eye receiving trabeculectomy with 5-FU injections. After a follow-up of more than 9 months, lower pressures were reported in the 5-FU group (average, 7 mm Hg vs. 11 mm Hg in the shell group); but there was a definite trend toward slightly lower visual acuity in the 5-FU–treated eyes. Choroidal detachments were seen with both groups.

There has been a definite movement toward using lower doses of 5-FU postoperatively, and there have been suggestions for new ways of delivering the drug. Smith and coworkers[112] reported the use of 5-FU applied to a cellulose sponge, which was then placed between the conjunctiva and trabeculectomy surface for 5 minutes during surgery, with five to six subsequent subconjunctival injections. This resulted in a very high success rate of pressure control with minimal complications. The authors concluded that 5-FU–saturated sponges at surgery may reduce the total number of subconjunctival injections that are later needed.

Attempts to use lower dosage injections have also been reported, with the surgeon deciding to inject or not depending on the appearance of the bleb. An early report reflecting this approach withheld 5-FU at signs of either excessive corneal symptoms or bleb leaks and reported reasonably good pressure results using doses anywhere between 17 and 60 mg.[186] Other reports have used lower total doses of 5-FU in the 40-mg range,[187] and some have been able to reduce this even lower by using the injections only at the signs of bleb failure and not on a routine prophylactic basis.[188] Indications for injection included a decreasing number of microcysts appreciated at the slit lamp, flattening of the bleb, localization of the bleb, increased vascularization, or elevation of intraocular pressure. An unsuccessful result with 5-FU surgery does not preclude repeat trabeculectomy with 5-FU injections: this has been established both in studies that have looked at reoperations[181] as well as in Pederson needling of the blebs with subsequent 5-FU injections.[189]

The most predictable side effects from subconjunctival 5-FU injections are the effects on the corneal epithelium. Epithelial defects have been well known since the earliest studies,[104,105] and usually these defects heal over a matter of weeks. The final intraocular pressure control bears no relationship to the corneal problems.[190] Patients can experience greater comfort, and possibly experience better bleb healing, with the use of a soft bandage contact lens applied to the eye during the period of 5-FU injections.[191]

Other corneal conditions that bear mentioning are the appearance of filamentary keratitis[186] and striate melanokeratosis[192] following administration of 5-FU. Perhaps of greatest concern, however, are eyes that have concurrent corneal disease undergoing trabeculectomy with antimetabolite. Those with preexisting corneal abnormalities, such as keratoconjunctivitis sicca, exposure keratopathy, or bullous keratopathy, experienced severe complications after administration of 5-FU, including a bacterial corneal ulceration, sterile corneal ulceration, and keratinized corneal plaque.[193] These eyes require special care and attention.

Reports based on a small number of patients with specific kinds of glaucoma have outlined some of the peculiar advantages and caveats with regard to 5-FU filtering. For example, in a series of 21 eyes with preexisting uveitis, 5-FU gave excellent results, with a better response in phakic eyes than aphakic eyes.[194] In another series of eyes with uveitis that had established good intraocular pressure control after 5-FU filtration, recurrent uveitic bouts did not cause loss of the pressure control.[195] In another case involving herpes simplex keratitis, the 5-FU injections seemed to exercise some antiviral activity.[196]

Trabeculectomies with 5-FU have proven their worth in a variety of settings: children with congenital glaucoma who had failed previous goniotomies or trabeculotomies and received subconjunctival injections[197]; patients younger than age 40 with open-angle glaucoma[198]; patients with previous retinal detachment surgery and scarred conjunctiva[182]; and patients undergoing extracapsular cataract extraction, lens implantation, and trabeculectomy augmented with 5-FU, showing superior pressure control to eyes that did not receive the antimetabolite.[199]

In contrast, the literature suggests two circumstances in which the 5-FU augmentation to filtration surgery was disappointing. The first study evaluated eyes with iridocorneal endothelial syndrome secondary glaucoma, in which only 4 of 9 eyes responded to the antimetabolite-augmented filtration surgery and the others progressed to require Molteno glaucoma drainage implantation.[200] The second study was in a large series of patients undergoing 5-FU trabeculectomy in Japan, where a life-table analysis over 30 months' follow-up revealed that there was little difference between the control trabeculectomies and the 5-FU trabeculectomies in terms of pressure control in patients older than the age of 70.[201] This study seems to confirm the clinical impression that elderly patients with very thin conjunctiva and a minimal amount of Tenon tissue may do quite well with trabeculectomy alone, without the need for any antimetabolite.

One complication that was initially reported after 5-FU augmentation but is not specific to this drug reflects the effect of extremely low pressures in certain eyes. Although reported many decades ago during the advent of full-thickness filtering procedures,[202] *hypotonous maculopathy* is being appreciated in large numbers today. It is characterized by persistent hypotony (usually defined as under 5 mm Hg) for many weeks after surgery, with decreased visual acuity.[203] Fundoscopic examination reveals no specific macular edema but rather choroidal wrinkling behind the macula, leading to the appearance of choroidal folds, which are particularly well seen on red-free photography. A series with case controls was reported by Stamper and associates[204] that identified two risk factors associated with hypotonous maculopathy and loss of vision: high myopia and youth (patients younger than 50 years of age). Although it has been established that there is a slight decrease in the axial length of the eye after trabeculectomy without the use of an antimetabolite (on the order of 0.27 mm),[205] the eyes with hypotonous visual loss often required vigorous intervention to reduce the seeming effect of a collapsed posterior pole. When pressures were brought above the level of 6 mm Hg consistently, a return of visual function was seen in many eyes, though sometimes taking 8 to 24 months until restoration to within one or two lines of the preoperative acuity, albeit with some persistent metamorphopsia. This situation has been reported not only with 5-FU[198] but also in several instances of eyes treated with mitomycin-C.[206–208]

MITOMYCIN-C. Although originally described by Chen in 1983[209] as an antimetabolite that could be applied as a single dose at the time of surgery, it was not until several years later that trials reporting successful results appeared from other centers. A prospective randomized study between mitomycin-C and

5-FU was reported by Kitazawa and coworkers,[54] comparing a single application of mitomycin-C, 0.2 mg, at the time of surgery versus a 5-FU regimen including 10 injections over 2 weeks' time. There was a significantly greater pressure reduction in eyes with mitomycin-C (88%) compared with the 5-FU group (47%), achieving pressures of 20 without antiglaucoma medication, with follow-up slightly less than a year. The corneal complications were, as expected, less with the mitomycin-C group (the mitomycin-C was applied only intraoperatively). Similar results were reported from Michigan:[107] a slightly lower intraocular pressure with mitomycin-C, slightly fewer postoperative medications required, and a greatly reduced instance of corneal epithelial defects. A study evaluating whether mitomycin-C or 5-FU caused great anterior chamber reaction found no appreciable difference between them.[110] Similar encouraging results with mitomycin-C were reported in eyes with complicated glaucoma, such as aphakia, rubeosis, or uveitis.[53,106]

The actual dose–response curve for mitomycin-C and the ophthalmic means of application are still unresolved. Early studies used a concentration of 0.5 mg/mL, applied to either an entire cellulose sponge or a wedge of sponge and placed between the conjunctiva and the surface of the episclera before making the incision for trabeculectomy. Other concentration doses have included from 0.1 to 0.5 mg, with many surgeons choosing a "middle of the road" dosage level of 0.3 mg for 2 to 3 minutes. A variant technique applies the antimetabolite-saturated cellulose sponge not beneath the conjunctiva but between the fashioned scleral flap and its bed, avoiding the subconjunctival surface. The flap is closed with a large number of sutures, and the pressure can be incrementally titrated by sequential suture lysis by laser.[210] Mitomycin-C has also been used in conjunction with phacoemulsification at the conclusion of the lens implantation and the fashioning of the trabeculectomy flap by applying the sponge between the conjunctiva and the scleral flap (see below).

Although the biochemical effects of mitomycin-C have been well established,[111,211] it is appreciated by clinicians to be extraordinarily potent and often exercising a toxic effect on the overlying conjunctiva literally within minutes of its application: blanching of the tissue and microvascular infarction suggest a direct effect on the conjunctival matrix. This inhibition of conjunctival responsiveness has been noted to be so profound that even in anecdotal instances of endophthalmitis or zoster inflammation—which would normally be expected to overwhelm a standard filtration bleb—the mitomycin-C blebs remained intact and functioning despite these episodes.[212]

Another feature of delayed ocular healing after mitomycin-C is that argon laser suture lysis can be performed several weeks postoperatively[47,210] instead of within the first 10 to 14 days when an antimetabolite is not used. The prolongation of impaired healing of the bleb has its negative aspects as well. Small bleb leaks have been reported even months after successful surgery.[109,213,214]

Perhaps of greatest concern, however, is the increased observation of hypotonous maculopathy in mitomycin-C–treated eyes.[207,208,211] Although the incidence of the hypotony will depend in part on the surgical technique (eg, how many sutures that are used to close the scleral flap, the size of the scleral flap), the persistence of low pressure for many weeks after surgery has led to identical findings as reported with 5-FU[204]: choroidal folds behind the macula, decreased visual acuity for many months, and clinical resolution not always apparent. Anecdotal evidence suggests that if the pressure can be brought over 6 mm Hg on a long-term basis, there may be long-term resumption of visual acuity in many patients.

The techniques for bleb reduction and reversing hypotony after either mitomycin-C or 5-FU injection are similar to those that have been described in the past for excessive blebs after full-thickness filtering procedures. These would include cryotherapy to the bleb itself,[215] electrocauterization of the bleb,[216] chemical cauterization of the bleb with trichloroacetic acid,[217] and, more recently, argon laser.[218] Regrettably, no one of these techniques is consistently reliable, and often they are used sequentially. These strategies can also be combined with devices to compress the bleb, such as soft contact lenses, Simmons shell tamponade, or a symblepharon ring. In cases of intractable hypotony, surgical revision can be undertaken, with either resuturing of the original scleral flap or even the introduction of donor-sclera grafts over the area of the flap to provide maximal compression. It is possible, of course, that the mere fact of reoperation, with its attendant induction of fibrosis and microscopic bleeding, may exercise some stimulation for bleb scarring. On the other hand, bleb revision surgery after antimetabolite use often reveals profoundly attenuated or "melted" flap tissue, requiring the suturing of additional structural resistance to outflow.

Complications of Bleb Formation

INTERNAL BLOCKAGE OF STOMA AND EXTERNAL BLEB FAILURE. Although obstruction of the trabeculectomy stoma from structure or material in the anterior chamber is an uncommon cause of bleb failure, it nevertheless must be ruled out by gonioscopic evaluation in the event of inadequate pressure control or bleb reduction.[131,172,219]

Debris in the anterior chamber can easily be appreciated visually or by gonioscopy, and strategies to either evacuate the anterior chamber or simply to wait for the dispersion of the material can be chosen accordingly. Hemorrhage, fibrin clot, or lens capsular fragments have all been implicated.[139,220] Perhaps a more frequently seen complication is the appearance of iris blocking the filtration site, either because of an imperforate iridectomy or because of adhesions from peripheral shallowing that have led to iris incarceration into the ostium. This is a particularly common experience with instrumentation that makes small filtration stomas (eg, the automated intracameral trephine[52] or holmium sclerostomy[48]).

In the event that some internal obstructing tissue or material is identified, various interventions have been described. A decade ago, such would include the use of a goniotomy knife or spatula needle inserted into the anterior chamber toward the area of occluded stoma, with mechanical removal of the blockage.[221,222] More recent interventions have used laser energy, either argon[223–225] or Nd:YAG.[226–231] Another technology mentioned in the literature is the use of focused ultrasound, which has been used to revive failed filtering blebs from either internal or external obstruction.[232,233]

It is not always possible to distinguish internal from external scarring, and according to some of the previously mentioned reports, various ultrasonic or laser methods applied at the site of the failed bleb had variable results. If external bleb scarring alone is suspected, a relatively simple surgical alternative[234] uses a disposable 25-gauge needle that is inserted beneath a ballooned conjunctiva (with lidocaine) to lyse the failing or scarred filtering site in the hope of increasing the surface area capable of filtration (Fig. 10-14). This can then be combined with the use of 5-FU injections (Fig. 10-15), often with good results. This technique has been employed successfully even many years after a previously functioning bleb has scarred down.[189] Some clinicians have observed that

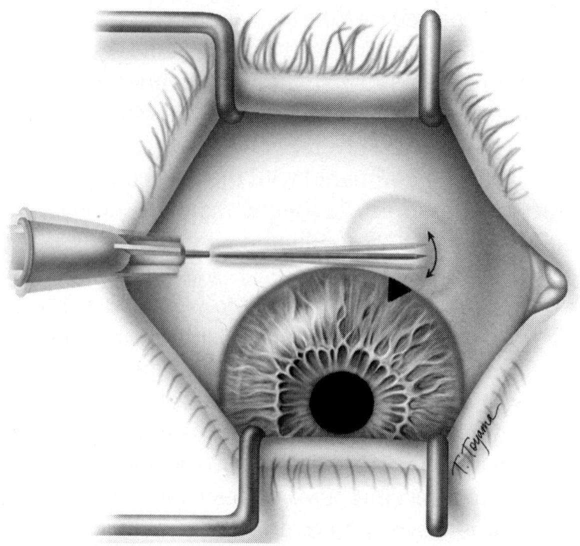

Figure 10-14. *Pederson needling.* A 25-gauge needle is used. The needle is inserted approximately 8 to 10 mm from the failing bleb, and the subconjunctival tissue is ballooned with 1% lidocaine. After entry into the bleb itself, the episcleral fibrosis is lacerated with a sweeping motion, using the sharp edge of the subconjunctival needle. Magnification by an operating microscope or loupe is advised to avoid unintentional perforation of the bleb.

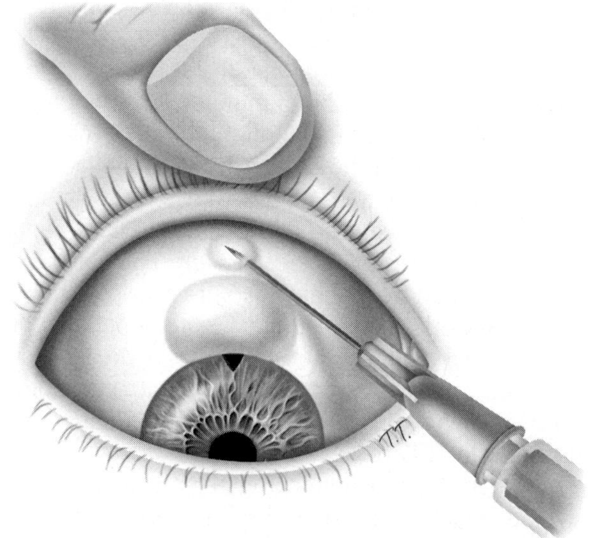

Figure 10-15. *5-FU injection.* After the successful lysing of the bleb scar, evidenced by an obvious reduction of intraocular pressure, an injection of 5-fluorouracil can be given. With a tuberculin syringe containing 0.2 mL of 5 mg/mL solution of 5-fluorouracil and a 30-gauge needle, a small bleb is raised with 0.15 mL injected above the true filtering site.

the needling technique works in a way that is as effective as surgical revision[234] and is appropriate for flat blebs as well as encapsulated blebs.[235]

ENCAPSULATED BLEBS. Many clinicians have commented on the appearance of encapsulated blebs, also referred to as Tenon cysts. These blebs often appear in eyes that have relatively elevated pressures in the first 3 weeks after surgery and have an incidence in the neighborhood of 10% to 15% after trabeculectomies.[234,236–238] Interestingly, the rate of encapsulated bleb formation remains about the same in eyes that do or do not receive 5-FU injections.[238,239]

Multiple studies have tried to identify the risk factors for encapsulation of the bleb. There seems to be evidence that either the appearance of prior Tenon cysts from filtering surgery in the same or fellow eye or the use of sympathomimetic glaucoma medications (particularly nonselective β-blockers) may predispose toward encapsulation. Other factors implicated are prior laser trabeculoplasty, male gender, previous conjunctival surgery, and uveitis.[236,237,240] It has been observed that these are more frequent with the use of limbus-based flaps and are quite rarely seen after the use of fornix-conjunctival flaps for trabeculectomy.[241]

Conservative management of encapsulated blebs frequently seems to result in good pressure control in the long run. Such management consists of antiglaucoma medications, including the use of β-blockers, carbonic anhydrase inhibitors, or miotics; in addition, steroid drops may be helpful to reduce vascular inflammation around the bleb itself.[241,242] The needling technique, mentioned earlier, has also been advocated,[243] as has surgical revision.[131] The decision of whether to intervene with a needling procedure or to persist with simple conservative management depends in large part on the height of the intraocular pressure elevation and the fragility of the optic nerve.

EXCESSIVELY LARGE BLEBS AND CORNEAL SEQUELAE. Especially with the use of the antimetabolites and topical massage to maximize bleb function, it is not uncommon that patients will establish good pressure control, but at the expense of a normalized ocular surface. Large blebs are frequently symptomatic to patients, associated with foreign body sensation and unwanted lacrimation. Often patients can obtain relief by the frequent use of artificial ocular lubricants, either in drop or ointment form. In other instances, attempts to reduce the bleb's height or extent can be attempted, using either freezing techniques (Fig. 10-16), electrocautery (Fig. 10-17),[216] or trichloroacetic acid chemical cautery (Fig. 10-18).[217] But as in attempts to impair exuberant bleb function to reverse hypotonous maculopathy, these techniques are unpredictable in their efficacy. Mechanical alteration of the bleb, such as with the shell tamponade or even surgical revision of the bleb, is sometimes necessary (Figs. 10-19 through 10-24).

One particularly unpleasant consequence of an excessively large bleb is the appearance of a corneal dellen, usually located in the interpalpebral portion of the exposed cornea, adjacent to the bleb at the limbus.[244] This is believed to be due to disrupted tear film integrity and sometimes will respond to conservative measures such as ocular lubrication and patching. The previously mentioned interventions (freezing, cautery, chemical, or needling) to reduce the height of the bleb can also be attempted. Eyes with dellen must be carefully watched for the development

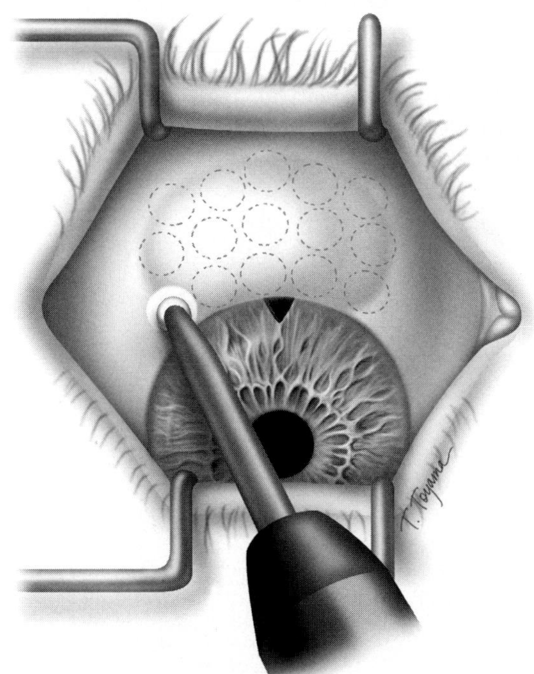

Figure 10-16. *Cryotherapy for bleb reduction.* Under topical anesthesia, a glaucoma probe can be applied on top of and surrounding the exuberant bleb, with a freeze allowed to enlarge approximately 2 mm on each side of the probe, for approximately 5 seconds. Care should be taken for the ice ball to thaw fully before the probe is removed, so as not to disrupt the underlying bleb tissue.

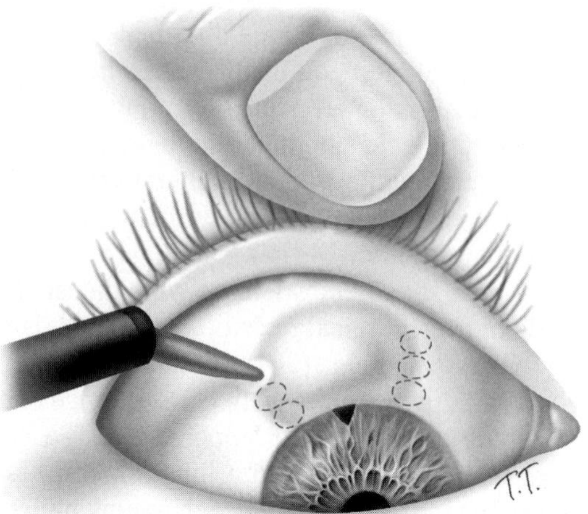

Figure 10-17. *Cautery bleb reduction.* Under topical anesthesia, a standard hyfrecator electrocautery applies mild burns in rows surrounding the exuberant bleb. Applications should be made to barely blanche the conjunctiva, applying light pressure on the device to compress the conjunctiva and its underlying fluid down to the episcleral surface. The cautery is usually not applied to the bleb surface itself.

of either sterile or infectious corneal infiltration, and antibiotic drops may be necessary. Soft contact lenses can also be applied to help in the healing period of the dellen, with the expectation that the lens will provide some compression of the bleb as well as symptomatic relief to the eye.

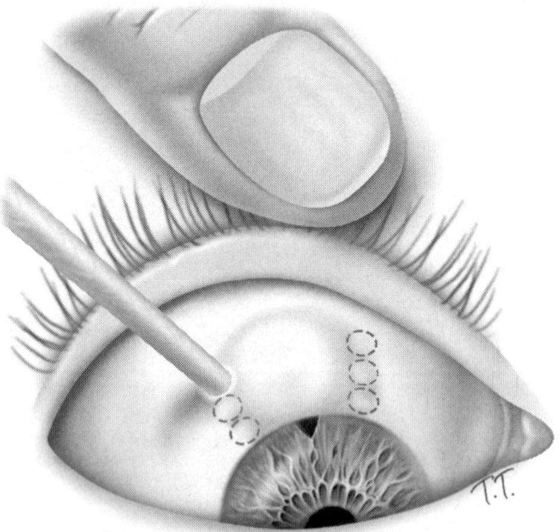

Figure 10-18. *Chemical bleb reduction.* A wooden applicator is dipped into a supersaturated solution of trichloroacetic acid and carefully applied in several rows surrounding the exuberant bleb, with care taken to avoid leakage of the chemical onto the corneal surface. The bleb surface itself is usually avoided. Light chemical blanching and whitening is seen after a few seconds of application. This technique may be uncomfortable for the patient, and topical atropine and patching are often useful.

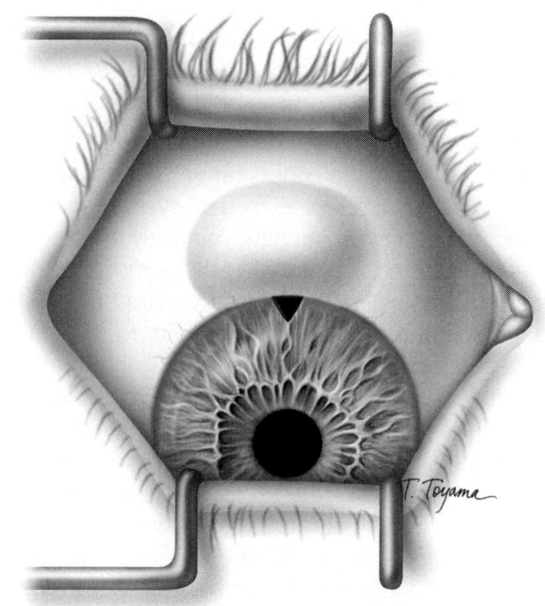

Figure 10-19. *Surgical bleb reduction.* With retrobulbar administration of anesthesia in the operating room, the excessive bleb can be viewed at the operating microscope.

BLEB LEAKS AND BLEB INFECTIONS. It appears that the experience with very thin, avascular blebs that result from antimetabolite trabeculectomies is recapitulating in part the experience of the previous generation of ophthalmic surgeons who observed full-thickness blebs over a long period of time. Microscopic and focal leaks of filtering blebs months to years after the use of 5-FU or mitomycin-C are more and more frequently being observed in glaucoma centers. Sometimes these leaks are seen to be "mi-

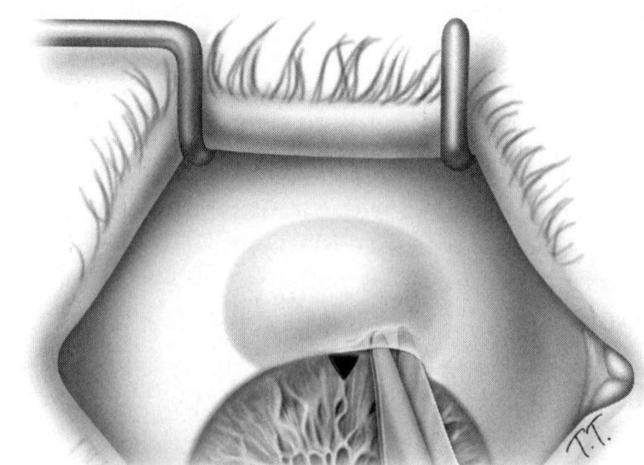

Figure 10-20. *Surgical bleb reduction (Continued).* A fornix-based conjunctival flap is prepared at the base of the excessive bleb.

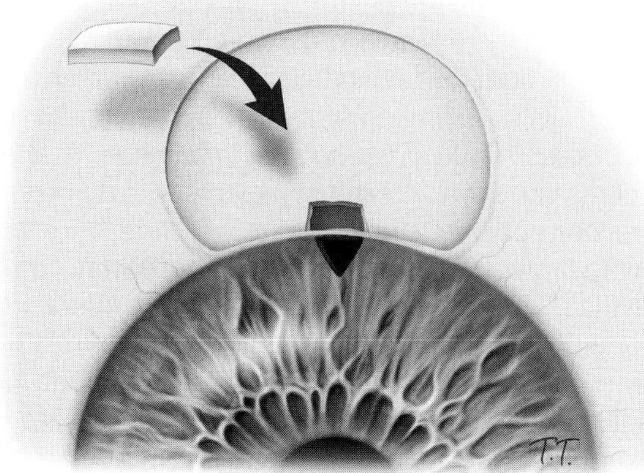

Figure 10-21. *Surgical bleb reduction (Continued).* After removal of the offending bleb structure itself, the episclera is exposed, and the stoma of the original trabeculectomy is evaluated. Sometimes, with the use of antimetabolites such as mitomycin, the scleral flap may have "melted away" (as illustrated here), necessitating the use of a donor scleral-patch graft that is hand-cut and sutured as a secondary trabeculectomy flap.

grating," in the sense that they appear at one locus, seemingly seal down in response to therapy, and then reappear elsewhere on the bleb, several millimeters away. Episoles of breakdown may be separated by weeks or months.

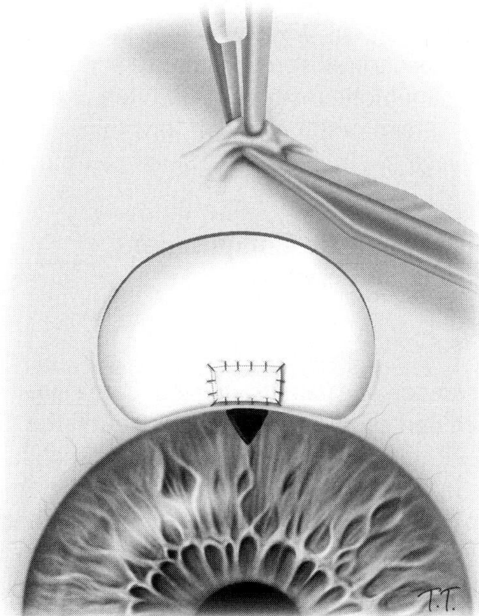

Figure 10-22. *Surgical bleb reduction (Continued).* Once the scleral graft is secured above the trabeculectomy ostium, a relaxing incision can be made peripherally, so as to mobilize the conjunctiva to be drawn down toward the limbus itself.

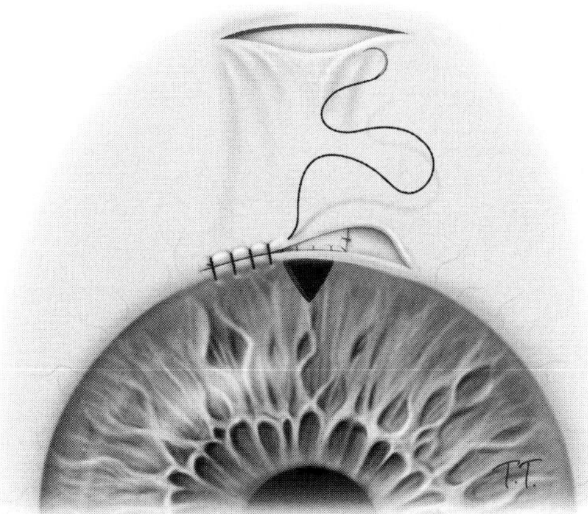

Figure 10-23. *Surgical bleb reduction (Continued).* With the relaxation of the conjunctiva, a watertight fornix flap can be closed (eg, using a 9-0 Vicryl suture), either by attachment to the apron of remaining conjunctiva, as illustrated here, or transcorneally.

How aggressively these bleb leaks are managed depends in large part on whether the intraocular pressure is adversely affected and whether the anterior chamber is shallowed. Conservative measures may be of help, such as reducing the aqueous flow by the use of β-blockers or the withholding of steroid drops. Antibiotic drops that are known to be slightly irritating to the eye, such as gentamicin, can sometimes be used in the expectation that the antibiotic will promote epithelialization at the leaking site. Another technique that has been reported is the injection of

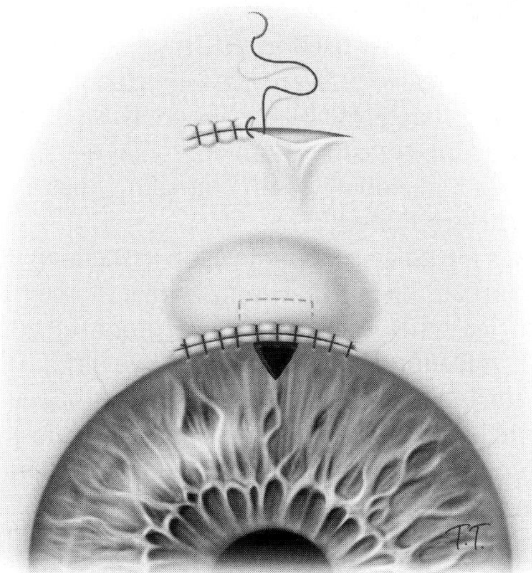

Figure 10-24. *Surgical bleb reduction (Continued).* A Vicryl suture closure of the relaxing incision can be performed, to ensure that the entire wound remains watertight. A bleb can be seen at the site of the revised bleb.

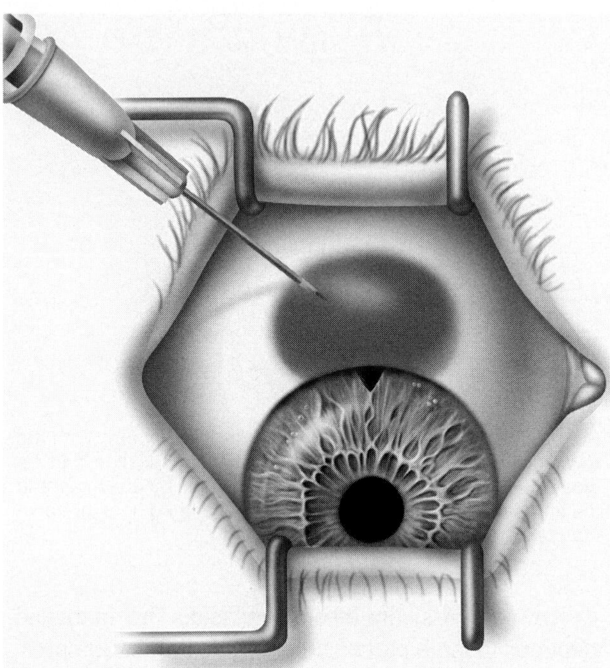

Figure 10-25. *Autologous blood injection.* After a sterile extraction of approximately 1 mL of the patient's blood, a small 27-gauge needle is applied to the same syringe, and under topical anesthetic the autologous blood is injected into the bleb itself. Because of the high likelihood of blood entering the anterior chamber, this technique is sometimes varied to preform the anterior chamber with sodium hyaluronate (Healon), which may produce a "tamponade" effect that minimizes the extent of the iatrogenic hyphema.

autologous blood into the bleb itself (Fig. 10-25). The argon laser has been used as one modality to repair focal wound leaks;[127] cyanoacrylate glue has also been used.[128] Rarely, the bleb leaks are so significant, or the reduction of vision (from choroidal effusion or hypotonous maculopathy) so compelling, that a surgical repair is required.[130,131]

Perhaps the greatest apprehension associated with thin, avascular blebs, however, is that if they are prone to leak they may equally be prone to admit bacterial infection into the bleb or eye itself (Fig. 10-25). The most extensive literature on postoperative endophthalmitis relates to cataract surgery and provides a context. Endophthalmitis here has a 0.05% to 0.3% rate, with the former figure probably more reflective of contemporary surgical technique.[245] The increased risk factor of a thin-walled bleb possibly exposed to microtrauma (from either contact lens or direct injury) may account for the rate of endophthalmitis after filtering surgery to be somewhat higher: somewhere between 0.1% and 2%.[245]

The most common offending organisms are nosocomial,[246] with a large number of reported cases *Streptococcus*[247] and *Haemophilus influenzae.*[248] The risk seems to be even greater in patients with diabetes or a recent upper respiratory tract infection,[246] or in eyes with large axial length, thin blebs, or recent conjunctivitis.[249] The rate of the appearance of infection is frequently many years (on average 7 and up to 18) out from surgery.[249] This fact makes it important to periodically remind the patient with the filtering bleb to have a low threshold of apprehension, so that attention is immediately sought for symptoms of blurred vision, redness, or pain.

It is controversial whether to put patients at risk for infection (eg, those wearing contact lenses or monocular patients with thin blebs) on prophylactic antibiotic therapy. Some unusual bacterial sources for endophthalmitis have been identified (eg, *Moraxella*[250] or *Pseudomonas*[251]), and it is not certain whether the use of routine prophylactic antibiotics would promote or inhibit an infectious tendency of the bleb itself.

The evaluation and treatment of endophthalmitis are covered more thoroughly elsewhere in this volume. It should be noted, however, that sometimes the infection can be identified at an early stage, with the collection of white blood cells confined to within the bleb itself ("blebitis") and with only minimal anterior chamber reaction. Vigorous attempts at culturing and initiating antibiotic treatment can often not only prevent the spread of the infection to within the eye but also salvage the bleb and its glaucoma function.[212]

Miscellaneous Late Complications of Filtering Surgery

Cataracts

The incidence of cataracts after glaucoma surgery depends in part on the choice of procedure: the rate of cataract formation has been reported as high as 34% in eyes undergoing full-thickness procedure, in comparison to 21% of patients undergoing trabeculectomy.[27] The other crucial factor that profoundly influences the reported incidence is the existence of cataract before the filtering surgery. For example, although 51% of one series of patients developed cataracts after trabeculectomy, a full third of these had preoperative cataracts that simply worsened, possibly in an accelerated fashion.[252] The options for dealing with cataract in combination with filtering surgery or in dealing with cataract after an established successful filtering surgery raise many interesting issues, which are more fully discussed later in this chapter.

Chronic Choroidal Detachments

The development of late-onset chronic or recurrent choroidal detachments is a well-documented phenomenon that can occur many years after a filtering procedure.[253,254] One subclassification identified patients with (1) recurrent ciliary choroidal detachments, (2) chronic detachments present for more than 6 months, and (3) detachments associated with obvious inflammation.[253] Intervention often requires intense antiinflammatory therapy, discontinuation of aqueous suppressant therapy, and choroidal drainage. Those patients who underwent cataract extraction often had spontaneous resolution of the choroidal detachment. Of particular interest is the report by Vela and Campbell[137] on eyes sustaining late choroidal detachment and whose fellow eye was still on the topical β-blocker therapy. With the cessation of the β-blocker on the fellow eye, the choroidal detachment resolved and then returned on resumption of the β-blocker. This suggested a supersensitivity to the drug in the operated eye, and it is a worthwhile phenomenon to consider when faced with these circumstances.

Malignant Glaucoma

As mentioned earlier in this chapter, malignant glaucoma can occur many months to years after successful glaucoma surgery, especially when precipitated by the inadvertent use of miotics. The recognition and management of this condition have been discussed earlier.

Hyphema

Another complication that may be seen at some time remote from surgery is the appearance of a late hyphema, allegedly due to fragile vessels that have grown into the wound edge and have, for unknown reasons, broken.[255] These broken vessels can sometimes be treated with laser, but often will disappear on their own.

COMPLICATIONS OF GLAUCOMA DRAINAGE IMPLANT SURGERY

There are a variety of terms used to describe devices that passively shunt aqueous from the anterior chamber to a sequestered subconjunctival space, maintained by some nonbiodegradable plastic, for the establishment of a filtering bleb remote from the interpalpebral fissure. Historically these have been referred to as setons and shunts; occasionally true one-way flow valves have been placed in these devices; the term *glaucoma drainage implant* has widespread use. Historically, imaginative inventions have been attempted to maintain the patency of a surgical fistula, with many forms of materials, both artificial and biologic, having been used.

It was, however, through the pioneering efforts of Molteno that attention was drawn away from preoccupation with keeping the fistula open at the limbus and toward the cultivation of bleb function. The principles that he established have remained the foundation for all subsequent glaucoma drainage implants: (1) the use of nonreactive, synthetic material, which inhibits fibroblast adherence; (2) the establishment of a potential space between the episcleral surface and the conjunctiva, into which the aqueous can pool for incremental absorption; and (3) location of the bleb away from the interpalpebral fissure, to minimize long-term inflammation, reduce palpebral exposure, and maximize bleb survival.[256]

The many designs of these drainage implants share a remarkable number of features, specifically with respect to their results, complications, and limitations. The history of these devices has been reviewed elsewhere.[256–258] Most of the literature revolves around the uses of these implants in eyes with refractory glaucomas that have usually failed previous filtering procedures. By and large, these devices are used as an alternative to trabeculectomy with antimetabolites, though comparable results have been reported when comparing the two procedures.[259]

The largest amount of literature has dealt with devices designed by Molteno, which now appear in four configurations: (1) a single circular silicone plate with a surface area of 135 mm^2; (2) a double-plate composed of two single disks (for a total surface area of 270 mm^2) connected with a silicone tube between them (allowing their placement in adjacent quadrants), with a single tube (right or left) leading into the anterior chamber; and (3) a dual-chamber single plate with an elevation on the disk surface to help impede excessive aqueous outflow in the immediate postoperative period; and (4) a dual-chamber double-plate model.[256,260] These devices are usually placed on the eye by means of a fornix-based flap, with the plates secured to the episcleral surface approximately 9 mm or more away from the limbus and the tube inserted into the anterior chamber approximately 3 mm; there are optional techniques to cover the tube either with donor sclera or under a host flap of sclera, as fashioned with a trabeculectomy.[261]

Because there is no flow valve mechanism in the silicone tubing leaving from the anterior chamber, to the Molteno plate, a multitude of techniques have been devised to occlude the tube either internally or externally, using absorbable or nonabsorbable sutures, either in the anterior chamber or not.[262–271] The interest in devising some means of occluding the silicone tube revolves around an ambivalent desire: to avoid hypotony in the early postoperative phase but to allow the establishment of full filtration once the hypotonous phase has been passed. Another approach to this challenge has been to divide the surgery into two stages: the first stage involves securing of the Molteno plate to the episcleral surface and not inserting the silicone tube into the anterior segment; by waiting several weeks, the Tenon cyst forms around the plate, providing resistance to filtration. With the second stage procedure the tube is inserted into the anterior segment, and hypotony is limited by the now-established cyst around the plate.[272]

Although the square millimeter area that is theoretically available for filtration seems to be large, histopathologic studies have established that a thick collagenous bleb wall forms, allowing only the incremental absorption of aqueous across to the subconjunctival space for removal from the eye.[273] Accordingly, Molteno devised his two-plate devices to literally double the size of absorptive area for better pressure control. The utility of one versus two plates has generated an interesting literature.[274–278] Perhaps the most useful study was a prospective evaluation of one versus two Molteno plates that concluded that there was slightly better pressure control with a double plate, though at the cost of a slightly higher incidence of complications, specifically hypotony.[278]

An equally clever glaucoma drainage device was elaborated by Schocket, based on the potential space for filtration that he observed around circumferential scleral silicone bands placed for retinal buckles.[279,280] As with the Molteno devices, a series of various designs were investigated, using either 360- or 180-degree encircling bands, with passive silicone tubing connecting the anterior chamber to the encircling band that was inverted to make a cavity facing the episcleral surface. Among the attractive features of this device was the simplicity of design and the availability of materials, obviating the need for specially ordered glaucoma implants.

Like the Molteno implants, these Schocket devices, referred to by the acronym ACTSEB (for anterior chamber tube shunt to encircling band), were extensively used with eyes that had failed prior trabeculectomy procedures or had refractory glaucomas with limited prognosis (neovascular or aphakic glaucoma). Results have been reported by many investigators,[281–284] with mixed results. Adequate intraocular pressure control is usually obtained in the majority of patients but often at the expense of a high complication rate or a large number of surgical revisions. Studies that have specifically compared the Molteno to the Schocket devices have found them fairly comparable, though there has been a trend for lower intraocular pressures and perhaps better vision retention with the Molteno implant.[285,286] In another study that compared the ACTSEB device to a Molteno implant and to a valved Joseph glaucoma implant (similar to the ACTSEB design), the Schocket-type tube system had a significantly higher risk of failure when compared with the two other one-piece systems.[287]

Other devices have also been described in the literature, each with its own specific design innovation. Krupin and colleagues,[288] for example, modified a shorter, valved version of a glaucoma implant and incorporated it into an encircling band device, and then later into a soft silicone plastic plate; they have reported results that are comparable to those of other devices. At Moorfields Hospital, a successful device designed by Joseph was similarly based on an encircling band with a valved silicone tube.[289] An intriguing device has been described by White[290] that allows a pumping mechanism to bring aqueous from the anterior segment out to the episcleral surface. Although White's first clinical report was favorable, independent investigators found a very high failure rate with the White pump shunt[291] and an unimpressive track record in eyes with neovascular glaucoma.[292]

Although there may be some slight advantage of one glaucoma implant design over another, many of the results depend on the skill of the surgeon and the status of the glaucoma that is being managed. What is particularly interesting is that there are a ubiquitous number of complications that are shared by nearly all the devices.

Intraoperative Complications

With nearly every type of device that is chosen, the handling of the conjunctiva is almost always an issue that requires great delicacy and attention. The fornix flap is the preferred insertion for most devices; in eyes that have had previous surgery and extensive scarring, it is useful to elevate the conjunctiva with an injection of normal saline or lidocaine with epinephrine to identify and release areas of adhesion. Especially after the securing of the plastic implants to the posterior episcleral surface, it is necessary to pull the conjunctiva over the device, often putting the tissue on stretch and generating the risk of conjunctival buttonholing. Extensive relaxing incisions may obviate this problem.

Identifying the rectus muscles is also important for the placement of most glaucoma implants, and care must be taken to avoid laceration near the muscle insertions, with subsequent hemorrhage. With the placement of devices in the superior quadrants (the most common location), attention should be paid to the superior oblique tendon and its relationship to the superior rectus muscle, to help minimize the possibility of bulk impairment of the extraocular muscular actions. Often the plates or bands have to be secured to the episcleral surface in an awkward position for the surgeon, usually using nonabsorbable sutures of large size with large needles (eg, 5-0 Mersilene). Because of the difficulty working "in a hole," care must be taken to avoid perforation of the sclera and entry into the eye.

The next area of special attention during implant surgery is the securing of the donor scleral flap or donor fascia lata (or the preparation of the trabeculectomy-like flap) that will overlie the tube. If the donor scleral flap has been stored in alcohol or glycerin, it is important that the storage medium has been leached out by soaking for 30 minutes or more in 1 L of normal saline, to which an antibiotic can be added for prophylactic purposes. If a trabeculectomy-like flap is fashioned, it should not be excessively thick so that the tube lies on a thin scleral bed too close to the suprachoroidal space (into which it could erode). Again, securing of the flap with needles requires delicacy so as not to puncture the sclera.

The insertion of the tube into the anterior segment perhaps requires the greatest amount of skill: it is useful to re-form the anterior chamber with a viscoelastic substance to approximate the normal chamber's depth, since it often becomes quite shallow with the extensive manipulations of the globe during the time of the placement of the implant. Although there are various preferences depending on the size of the silicone tube to be inserted, with a Molteno or Baerveldt implant a 23-gauge needle track inserted 2 to 3 mm from the limbus and aimed parallel to the iris surface often allows a very secure fit of the tube into the anterior segment. After insertion, sometimes the tube needs to be pulled out and trimmed; the goal is to prevent its rubbing against the cornea, since it should ideally be equidistant from the endothelial surface and the anterior surface of the iris. On gonioscopy, it is usually seen just anterior to the Schwalbe line. A complication that can occur during this time is that the tube is cut too short: with subsequent elevation of the pressure in the eye and the re-formation of the ocular shape, the tube can retract out from the anterior segment entirely.

There are many strategies to temporarily occlude the plastic tube to forestall hypotony in the early postoperative period. If the tube is to be externally ligated with a suture that needs to be lysed, it should be placed in an area that is easily visible either for incisional or laser access (eg, sutured behind the trabeculectomy flap or through the intracameral tube so it does not dislocate after laser lysis). Similarly, if a tube is to be internally occluded with a suture that will be later pulled from its location in the inferior fornix (eg, a 3-0 Prolene),[266] it is important to secure the trimmed suture to the episclera in the lower fornix to minimize its chance of erosion through the conjunctiva. A novel approach to forestall hypotony used intraocular gas and suture-occlusion of the tube.[293]

Lastly, the conjunctiva should be brought forward and secured in a watertight fashion at the limbus in the common circumstance that a bleb will form from leakage of aqueous around the tube's entry through sclera. Tight conjunctival closure will prevent a wound leak that could lead to an excessive and prolonged period of hypotony. With glaucoma implants as with all intraoperative procedures in glaucomatous eyes, especially those with aphakia or neovascular disease there are the usual common intraoperative risks of hyphema, retinal phototoxicity,[294] choroidal effusion, iris damage, and suprachoroidal hemorrhage.

Early Postoperative Complications

The most common postoperative appearance of the eye with glaucoma implants is with a shallow chamber and relative ocular hypotony. This is seen even in the presence of valved devices, which are specifically designed to minimize this hypotony.[256,289,295] Although it is helpful to try and identify the source of the hypotony, this is not always possible. Leakage around the tube can be surmised if a large bleb is seen between the limbus and the plate itself, but this may be difficult to distinguish from postoperative chemosis. Similarly, it is difficult to discern whether a bleb is forming over the sequestered plastic plate area; B-scan ultrasonography may be of use.[275]

As a consequence of the frequent shallowing of the anterior chamber and low intraocular pressure there may be touch of the tube to the cornea or occlusion of the tube by iris. Equally worrisome is touch of the tube to the actual lens surface. Re-formation of the anterior chamber with viscoelastic, or even reoperation to limit tube flow by ligation or occlusion, may be necessary.

As with other intraocular procedures for glaucoma, the surgeon must always be aware of the possibility of postoperative pupillary block, excessive inflammation, hyphema (especially with neovascular glaucoma), suprachoroidal hemorrhage, wound leaks, early endophthalmitis, graft failure, or malignant glaucoma. Depending on the type of procedure that has been undertaken, other complications may be evident: for example, when Molteno implants are combined with vitrectomy for neovascular glaucoma, a large number of complications have been reported.[296]

Late Postoperative Complications

Perhaps the most ubiquitous late complication seen with glaucoma implants is the failure of the device to function as intended, with return of elevated pressures. This needs to be distinguished from two phenomena: (1) a predictable "ocular hypertensive phase" that can occur between 4 and 16 weeks after surgery and that is allegedly due to collagen remodeling of the bleb[272,275] (a similar phenomenon has been described with trabeculectomy blebs[22]); and (2) late steroid response of elevated intraocular pressure.[256]

Failure of the Schocket procedure most commonly involves the blockage of the tube either in the anterior segment or at its insertion into the encircling band.[281] However, if a bleb is present (indicating no blockage) and intraocular pressure remains uncontrolled, it is often necessary to resume glaucoma medications or perform supplemental implant, filtering, or ciliary body surgery. In our experience, bleb revision (ie, removing the thick-walled cysts encapsulating the plates) even with antimetabolites rarely succeeds.

Late complications such as retinal detachment,[297] sterile endophthalmitis,[298] tube erosion,[299] infectious endophthalmitis,[300,301] or cellulitis[302] have all been documented with all devices.[303] Late intraocular complications such as pupillary block glaucoma, malignant glaucoma, chronic choroidal detachments, vitreous hemorrhage, hyphema, phthisis bulbi, and retraction of the tube from the anterior segment have also been described.[256] As with all cases of difficult glaucomas, there may be a postoperative loss of vision whose specific etiology remains obscure,[304] or visual failure due to the underlying ocular disease.[305,306]

One particular area of concern is the potential for impaired ocular motility following the healing of the glaucoma implants, especially if implanted inferiorly; these have been reported both with Molteno implants[307] and a soft-silicone modification of the Molteno implant called the Baerveldt implant.[308–312] Deficits are most frequently seen with the vertical motility, resulting in hypertropia or hypotropia; lateral motility disturbances have also been reported. It is surmised that there is either a bulk effect of a large filtering bleb that impairs motility of the eye or a Fadden-like adhesion between the posterior aspect of the muscle and the globe, induced by the fibrosis around the large filtering bleb. Diplopia should be explained to patients as a potential complication. Unfortunately, it is usually noncomitant and restrictive and may be amenable only to surgical implant removal at the expense of the glaucoma control.

Another important area of the literature dealing with glaucoma implants has been the relationship between the glaucoma control and its effect on penetrating keratoplasties.[72] There seems to be a high rate of nonimmunologic graft failure in the presence of a Molteno or Schocket implant, and this seems to exist if the implant is placed either before the grafting procedure or afterward.[313–316] Sometimes the graft failure can be salvaged with intensive corticosteroid therapy; in other instances, repeat grafting is required.[317] From a glaucoma point of view, however, the pressure reduction in grafted eyes is usually achieved by the implants, but the exact toll and mechanism for the fragility of corneal grafts remains uncertain.

Despite the well-documented list of complications following glaucoma implants,[256,257,295] this operative technique is a valuable asset in the armamentarium for glaucomas that are difficult to control. It has been established to be of use in patients with epithelial ingrowth[318] and in cases of either congenital glaucoma or juvenile glaucoma.[319–321] Although glaucoma shunts have been compared with noncontact transscleral Nd:YAG cyclophotocoagulation in one study,[322] the ultimate role for glaucoma drainage implants either with respect to trabeculectomies with antimetabolites[259] or ciliary body destruction by laser remains to be clarified.

COMPLICATIONS OF SURGERY FOR CONGENITAL AND JUVENILE GLAUCOMAS

The classification of glaucomas that appear in infancy, childhood, and adolescence comprises a large spectrum of conditions, including congenital defects, infectious etiologies, traumas, and mixed mechanisms of disease. A particularly useful approach to glaucomas in early childhood was devised by Hoskins and simply describes combinations of involvement of iris, trabeculum, and cornea: syndromes of iridodysgenesis, trabeculodysgenesis, and corneodysgenesis, with various mixtures of these three features.[323] What is of particular concern here is that there are specific forms of glaucoma surgery that are usually confined to the treatment of elevated pressures in youthful eyes: goniotomy, trabeculotomy ab externo, and trabeculodialysis. These are discussed with respect to the specific complications that may be seen with their use.

Goniotomy

Goniotomy is a time-honored surgical intervention, the first that was responsible for reversing the devastation of congenital glaucoma. It seems to be an increasingly uncommon operation, which makes it all the more crucial that the surgeon be familiar with all operative details and possible complications. In brief, the procedure requires the use of a specialized goniolens and specialized incisional knife-needles: either the Barkan goniotomy knife, Swan knife (tapered), or Swan needle-knife (nontapered).[324] With the help of an assistant, and with the surgeon aligning either a microscope or loupes for appropriate magnification, the anterior chamber is entered and the trabecular tissue is incised for 4 to 8 clock hours just below the insertion of the Schwalbe line. The procedure can be greatly enhanced for the occasional goniotomist by the use of an intraoperative viscoelastic agent, which both maintains the anterior depth and allows an unhurried intervention.[141]

The complications of goniotomy depend in part on the skill of the surgeon. Visualization must be maintained at all times so that the penetrating knife enters neither too posteriorly with the risk of iris or lens damage nor too anteriorly with the risk of corneal injury. Hyphema is almost invariably encountered during the procedure, though the risk of a total "8-ball" hyphema is quite low (approximately 0.5%).[325] If the visualization of the incision is imperfect, a resulting disinsertion of the iris (iridodialysis) or even of the ciliary body (cyclodialysis) can be incurred. It is very common that as the patient is gonioscopically followed, peripheral anterior synechiae are seen to appear, especially in the incised area. Complications of postoperative uveitis, cataract formation, shallow chamber (in the event that the corneal wound is not appropriately closed), and even retinal detachment (in high myopes) have also been reported.

The utility of goniotomy remains somewhat unclear: an older generation of glaucomatologists, whose experience with the procedure was vast, recommend its use in instances of infantile glaucoma (primary congenital open-angle glaucoma or isolated trabeculodysgenesis). Shaffer and Hoskins[323] report success with over a 15-year follow-up, achieving excellent pressure control in most eyes if the goniotomy was performed between months 1 and 24. Nevertheless, after 15 years, nearly one of seven eyes showed complications, including corneal decompensation and retinal detachment. Draeger and coworkers[326] reported a follow-up of 3 to 22 years, with nearly three of four eyes retaining good pressure control. It was their experience that the key determinant of a successful goniotomy was the age at onset of the condition: the worst prognosis was seen in patients whose glaucoma appeared before the age of 2 months. Some surgeons have recommended the use of two simultaneous goniotomies in the same eye, one to augment the other, but results have been comparable to the use of a solitary intervention.[327]

It is common that more than one goniotomy is subsequently needed for intraocular pressure control. And as with all glaucomas in children, the potential for devastating amblyopia must be anticipated and vigorously managed.

Trabeculotomy Ab Externo

This procedure has become progressively more popular in the management of congenital glaucoma, largely because it is a variation of the familiar surgical approach of trabeculectomy. The procedure consists of either a limbus or fornix-based conjunctival flap, the elaboration of a one-half thickness scleral triangular flap, and the identification of the canal of Schlemm; this is then threaded with specialized trabeculotomes, which when rotated internally cause a rupture of the tissue posterior to the Schwalbe line.[328] The other significant advantage of this procedure is that it can be performed in the presence of a cloudy cornea, which otherwise would completely preclude the angle visualization necessary for goniotomy.

There is considerable challenge in maintaining the proper tissue depth during the dissection of the scleral flap, and it is always imperative that a meticulous identification of the canal of Schlemm be undertaken. This often can be verified by the use of a 5-0 or 6-0 nylon suture, which is introduced into what is presumed to be the canal; sometimes this can be identified immediately below the site of microscopic droplets of percolating aqueous that are seen emerging on the episcleral surface. If the suture can be easily threaded, the surgeon can be fairly certain that this is not a false passage and the trabeculotome can accordingly be inserted. Again the use of a viscoelastic agent in the anterior chamber is very useful here, since after the rotation of the first trabeculotome into the anterior chamber there is a tendency for the chamber to collapse, making the introduction of the second trabeculotome more difficult.

Common complications resulting from the introduction of the trabeculotome into a false passage with rotation interiorly include a resultant iridodialysis, cyclodialysis, and rupture of the Descemet membrane. The detachment of the Descemet membrane is sometimes seen as a very localized scroll, but in other instances a tear can result in focal corneal edema.[329] Hyphemas are almost invariably encountered with a trabeculotomy, with a rate as high as 68%.[330]

In the case of a buphthalmic eye, with stretched sclera and abnormal landmarks, it is possible to inadvertently introduce the trabeculotome well behind the iris insertion, with possible involvement of the lens, causing either immediate cataract or even vitreous loss. If the rotation of the trabeculotome is inappropriately posterior, rupture of vessels in the choroidal area can be encountered, resulting in suprachoroidal hemorrhage. Postoperative infections and trophic corneal ulcers have also been reported.[328]

There has been some discussion in the literature as to the comparative value of trabeculotomy versus goniotomy. Anderson[331] reported that both were efficacious. Other authors have reported a superiority of trabeculotomy in reducing the intraocular pressure and the number of surgical interventions that are required.[332,333] The trabeculotomy ab externo has also been compared with the use of trabeculectomy in childhood glaucomas, the trabeculotomy having a slightly greater intraocular pressure reduction with fewer complications in one series[334] and good long-term results.[335]

Postoperative complications of trabeculotomy, like most glaucoma operative procedures, include in the short-term a flat chamber from leakage, inadvertent bleb formation, or a black "total" hyphema and subsequent peripheral anterior synechiae.

The risk of endophthalmitis following pediatric anterior segment surgery has been elegantly addressed by Wheeler and colleagues,[336] who did an elaborate survey of pediatric ophthalmic surgeons to establish an incidence of approximately seven infections per 10,000 cases—an incidence of infection that is comparable to that following adult extracapsular cataract surgery. The complications reported were devastating: greater than four of five infections appeared by the third postoperative day; nearly two of three were culture positive; and nearly two of three infected eyes went on to lose vision. It was also thought that there were increased risks of nasolacrimal duct obstruction and upper respiratory tract infection predisposing to the endophthalmitis. This information should be considered when weighing the risks and benefits of binocular surgery in a single surgical sitting.

Miscellaneous Procedures

Although goniotomy and trabeculotomy are the mainstays for managing most congenital and childhood glaucomas, the need to repeat each of these procedures often arises on more than one occasion. Standard trabeculectomy filtering procedures have also been reported in this age group but with only modest results. In one series of 38 eyes, 54 procedures were done, including both thermal sclerostomies and trabeculectomies; control of intraocular pressure was obtained in 52% of cases.[337] In one very small series, 5-FU injections were given postoperatively after trabeculectomy, with good results in all 4 eyes.[197] Because of the obvious difficulty in obtaining a child's cooperation for subconjunctival 5-FU injections, it remains to be seen whether the use of mitomycin-C at the time of trabeculectomy in children will prove to be a viable alternative. Molteno glaucoma implants have also been used successfully in several series in the pediatric age group,[319–321] although use of these implants is often reserved until other procedures have failed.

Of particular interest are reports on the use of various forms of Nd:YAG laser energy, either to incise the trabecular tissue (as is done with the goniotomy knife) or to puncture through to the canal of Schlemm (to allow greater outflow). Most of the laser devices that have been reported have been experimental, but preliminary series are intriguing. Nd:YAG trabeculopuncture was reported to be useful in 75% of eyes in bringing pressures down below 19 mm Hg in a small series of eight cases.[338] A goniotomy-like use of the Nd:YAG laser to separate the dysgenic iris was reported in two series,[339,340] with results comparable to surgical goniotomy. The utility and availability of these laser modalities remain to be established.

Specific childhood glaucoma syndromes have bearing on particular kinds of procedures and complications. Aniridia can present as an infantile form of glaucoma, though more commonly it appears later in childhood. Prophylactic goniotomies have been reported, with encouraging results.[324,341] In a large series of eyes reported by Wiggins and Tomey,[342] 17 aniridic eyes required 45 operations, with variations of trabeculectomy, cryotherapy, and Molteno surgery all being required, and with the use of glaucoma implants appearing particularly promising. Because of the absence of iris in these instances, there is always a significant risk of cataract formation with any intracameral intervention such as goniotomy or trabeculotomy.

Sturge-Weber syndrome glaucomas can also present as an early infantile form, but more commonly a later childhood form manifests, related to elevated episcleral venous pressure. The various interventions that have been useful have been well summarized by Iwach and coworkers,[343] who observed 36 eyes over a long-term period. The most specific complications related to surgical procedures in these eyes are a tendency for bleeding and a tendency toward intraoperative choroidal effusion. The latter was reported in 25% of the eyes, but it rarely occurred with goniotomies or trabeculotomies. The risk of effusion with repeat trabeculectomy led others to recommend prophylactic sclerostomies.[344] (See discussion at the end of the chapter.)

Trabeculodialysis

Although not a technique strictly confined to infantile and childhood glaucomas, trabeculodialysis is historically associated with the treatment of aphakic glaucomas in patients with juvenile rheumatoid arthritis. Most of these operations occur in the second decade of life. This technique is very similar to that of goniotomy, with the modification that the tissue posterior to the edge of the goniotomy knife is peeled downward, rather than simply incised.

In a report of 25 eyes of patients with secondary glaucoma from chronic anterior uveitis, Williams and colleagues[345] reported intraocular pressure control by trabeculodialysis in 56% of patients, with follow-up from 1 to 10 years. Two thirds of these eyes were aphakic but showed results no different from those of phakic eyes. Although suprachoroidal hemorrhage was seen as one complication, it was recommended that this procedure be considered in this particular subset of uveitic glaucomatous eyes.

COMPLICATIONS OF CILIARY BODY INTERVENTIONS

In a comprehensive review of cyclodestructive procedures, Shields[346] appropriately distinguished three approaches that have been historically used to reduce aqueous production by destroying its tissue of origin: transscleral, transpupillary, and intraocular. Older approaches, such as penetrating and nonpenetrating diathermy, were supplanted by cyclocryotherapy. By necessity these interventions are *transscleral* in their approach, with the inherent disadvantage of being unable to actually visualize the tissue that is being treated (and hence unable to quantitate the damage). There is also the potential for inadvertent damage to adjacent tissue (specifically the lens, sclera, and non–aqueous-producing uveal tract).

In a very rare number of circumstances, when there is a large sector iridectomy or partial aniridia of either traumatic, surgical, or congenital origin, a laser cyclophotocoagulation of the ciliary processes through a *transpupillary* approach has been described. In eyes that are either aphakic or rendered aphakic for the specific purpose, *intraocular cyclophotocoagulation* has also been established, using endolasers either with vitrectomy surgery[347,348] or with specially designed endoscopes.[349] Most contemporary efforts now are concentrating on laser delivery systems that can focus a very discrete beam of energy in the region of the ciliary processes and hence avoid the difficulty of extensive damage to adjacent structures.[350]

Each of these approaches, with their concurrent complications, is discussed below, after first considering an alternative and time-honored approach to altering ciliary body dynamics by mechanically disinserting it from its adjacent sclera surface: the cyclodialysis operation procedure.

Cyclodialysis Surgery

Although currently out of favor, cyclodialysis remains an alternative procedure worthy of study. Because a cyclodialysis spatula is deliberately inserted between the ciliary body and the sclerai and maneuvered forward into the anterior chamber, there is almost invariably an unavoidable amount of bleeding and mechanical disruption of the angle and structures below the iris. Accordingly it has been reserved primarily for patients who are aphakic and who are free of hemorrhagic predilection (ie, excluding patients with neovascular glaucoma or on anticoagulant therapy).

When intracapsular cataract extraction (ICCE) was the normative procedure for cataract, the cyclodialysis procedure was sometimes combined with an ICCE to control concurrent open-angle glaucoma. Conversely, contraindications to cyclodialysis include secondary angle-closure glaucomas, glaucomas with active uveitis, patients who are intolerant of long-term parasympathomimetics (eg, echothiophate), and patients with eyes in which zonular support of the capsule (with or without posterior chamber lens implant) is deemed important.[351]

The literature reports a modest success rate with this procedure: approximately 50% has been quoted by Sugar,[352,353] and oddly enough a higher rate of success (75%) has been reported in eyes in which it was combined with cataract extraction.[354] More recent studies have identified a high rate of failure, and severe visual loss after the procedure: as high as 20% in one series.[70]

The complications following cyclodialysis are ubiquitous. Hemorrhage in the anterior chamber and stripping of the Descemet membrane are seen in as many as 50% of cases.[355] Other complications occurring at the time of the surgery include inadvertent penetration of the ciliary body, disinsertion of the root of the iris (iridodialysis), and rupture of the hyaloid face with vitreous loss.

If performed in phakic eyes, cataract is extremely common, so much in fact that a clear lens is probably a contraindication to this procedure. Because the creation of a cyclodialysis cleft is in fact the successful titration point of the procedure, it must be carefully nurtured with the use of very strong-acting miotic drops (eg, echothiophate). Accordingly, there is a certain amount of inflammation and discomfort associated with the postoperative course. The amount of cleft available to augment the uveal scleral outflow of aqueous is not subject to precise control, and hypotony is frequently seen—with concomitant reduction of vision, corneal striae, shallowing of the anterior chamber, choroidal detachments, and striae of the choroid. Sometimes persistent cyclodialysis clefts require intervention to reduce their effectiveness, with many techniques described (eg, laser, suturing).[355]

Other infrequent complications of this procedure include phthisis, reduction of central acuity, and retinal detachment. With the inadvertent and spontaneous closure of the cyclodialysis clefts, extremely high spikes of intraocular pressure have been described.

Cryotherapy

Cyclocryotherapy is probably the most commonly used technique for limiting ciliary body function. In part because it has been usually reserved for eyes with glaucomatous damage that have resisted other means of intervention or eyes that have a very poor prognosis (eg, neovascular glaucoma), there are many reports in the literature testifying to the profound destructive and often sight-threatening complications following this intervention.

The technique of cyclocryotherapy is fairly straightforward, simply requiring a cryounit with nitrous oxide as the freezing source, a probe that is 2.5 to 4 mm as the delivery system, and retrobulbar anesthesia. Although many application techniques have been described, a particularly reproducible approach is to restrict applications to six equally spaced freezes placed over 180 degrees of the ciliary body.[356] If repeat sessions are needed, additional 90-degree quadrants can be treated. Some authorities recommend that one quadrant always remain untreated throughout the repeat applications, so that there is a dependable source of aqueous production.[357]

The results of cyclocryotherapy depend in large part on the underlying disease being treated, with neovascular glaucoma having the worst prognosis and aphakic open-angle glaucoma the best.[358] The selection of patients and the duration of follow-up often reflect the variable results reported in the literature: from a 91% success rate over 3 years of follow-up without any serious complications[359] to a more sobering report of 114 patients in which 16% lost vision during the follow-up period and 12% went into phthisis.[360] A longer 10-year follow-up study by Benson and Nelson[361] on 68 eyes reported an overall success rate of 29% in terms of reduction of pressure, but with 30% of eyes going on to no light perception and a full 17% going on to phthisis or requiring enucleation. Again, neovascular eyes fared the worst in this long-term study.

The complications of cyclocryosurgery have been well documented and can regularly be expected. Intense ocular discomfort is commonly encountered and often requires the use of long-term cycloplegics (eg, atropine) and systemic analgesia. Iridocyclitis, hyphema, vitreous haze, and corneal edema are all frequently seen. Acute pressure elevation is almost to be expected with standard techniques of application, with the highest pressure spikes occurring momentarily between the freeze and the thaw.[362] Infrequent complications include corneal ulcers, rhegmatogenous retinal detachments, anterior segment necrosis, and staphyloma formation.[357]

With a careful selection of patients, it is obvious that many complications can be avoided. For example, aphakic eyes with primary open-angle glaucoma seem to respond well to the cyclocryotherapy, and multiple treatments with a few freezing applications may be useful.[357] In contrast, eyes with neovascular glaucoma have a dismal prognosis, with a high rate of hyphema and eventual phthisis; both patients and surgeons should be braced for this eventuality.

Therapeutic Ultrasound of the Ciliary Body

Beginning with the pioneering work of Coleman and colleagues[363,364] in developing an ultrasonic transducer assembly that would allow the delivery of highly focused ultrasonic energy into the ciliary body, various studies have attempted to establish the viability of this technology for transscleral ciliary destruction. Three mechanisms have been invoked for the effect of the therapeutic ultrasound: (1) direct destruction of the secretory ciliary epithelium; (2) scleral thinning, which enhances uveal scleral outflow; and (3) separation of the ciliary body from the sclera, again enhancing uveal scleral outflow.[365]

As with many of the transscleral ciliary body destructive techniques, the results often reflect both the underlying disease and the length of follow-up. In aggregating the results from a multicenter trial by life-table analysis, there is an approximately 50% success rate in reducing intraocular pressure at 1 year out and an approximately 62% success rate with multiple treatments.[364] These studies have been substantiated in large part by other investigators, with most results in the 50% to 70% range.[233,366–368]

The actual technique requires an elaborate water bath delivery system for the ultrasonic device to focus on the sclera adjacent to the limbus. The standard protocol consists of six applications performed 2.5 mm from the limbus, over an approximately 180-degree area.

The technical complexity, cost, and alleged complication rate of the ultrasonic ciliary destructive procedure have contributed to this device's limited clinical adoption. Acute symptoms include corneal edema, iritis, choroidal effusions, and even phthisis. Many of these reactions persist at 6 months, with the most common being the persistence of uveitis and corneal edema, with late cataract and scleral thinning also reported.[364] Staphylomata have also been seen,[369] and attention has been called to the tendency toward a very high intraocular pressure spike in 80% of eyes undergoing re-treatment.[367] The long-term phthisis rate is approximately 0.6%, and hypotony has been seen in 2.5% of eyes.[364]

It remains to be seen whether therapeutic ultrasonography will become a more viable technique. Currently it appears limited both by the complexity of its instrumentation and the only moderate advantage it seems to offer over standard cyclocryotherapy.

Laser Cyclotherapy

Beginning with the pioneering work of Beckman and Waeltermann[370] with ruby laser cyclocoagulation, the advent of multiple lasers for transscleral ciliary ablation has awaited the refinement of laser technology. For example, the advantages of Nd:YAG and diode lasers include the fact that their longer wavelengths have better scleral penetration, with less backscatter.[350] Moreover, both the Nd:YAG and diode lasers have applications beyond that of cyclodestruction, and hence their machinery is less expensive and widely available for clinical use. This is a rapidly changing field, however, and it remains to be seen whether the ultimate efficacy of the laser cycloablation will depend on the specifics of one type of laser delivery system or on the limited responses of the ciliary body to nonvisualized laser destruction. A concise history of the laser development for cyclodestruction is authoritatively summarized by Schuman.[350]

An important distinction to make in assessing the literature is between a noncontact laser delivery device (usually the Lasag MR2 Microruptor 2) and a fiberoptic contact probe device (Surgical Laser Technology Nd:YAG). The standard technique for delivery of noncontact laser with the Lasag instrument requires the patient to be placed at a slit lamp, with or without a specially designed contact lens. Because of the discomfort of the procedure, either a retrobulbar or peribulbar anesthetic is routinely used. The laser is adjusted to an "offset" that will maximally bring the laser beam to focus deep within the ciliary body tissue, and not on the surface of the conjunctiva. Eight spots per quadrant are usually applied, and 360 degrees is frequently treated, with a duration of approximately 20 ms.

The ability to mechanically adapt the widely available Lasag Nd:YAG laser (used for iridotomy and postcataract capsulotomy) has been responsible in part for the large literature based on noncontact Nd:YAG ciliodestructive procedures. Once again it is necessary to articulate the caveat that the reported results reflect as much the types of glaucoma being treated and the duration of follow-up as the technology applied.

One interesting finding is that a more prominent intraocular pressure-lowering effect is seen by focusing the laser beam 1.5 mm from the limbus, rather than 3 mm posteriorly (where it might be expected to allow greater contact with the ciliary processes).[371] In a prospective and large study performed in North Carolina,[372] 100 eyes were observed for at least 6 months, with 68% of eyes showing intraocular pressure response with one treatment (with or without medications), with success increasing to 95% of eyes when more than one treatment was applied. However, 45% of eyes were seen to experience visual loss during the follow-up, though half of these instances could be explained on grounds other than the laser treatment itself. Other studies have substantiated this impressive pressure reduction in the range of 50% to 75% from baseline with follow-up of over 2 years.[373–375] But the rather disturbing trend of frequent visual loss was also suggested by a study of 28 eyes in Toronto, nearly one third of whom went on to experience decreased acuity and in 10% of whom phthisis developed.[376]

The noncontact transscleral Nd:YAG laser was reported in two different studies to be useful in the treatment of patients who had undergone keratoplasty. In one series, 13 eyes were treated, with excellent pressure control at over 18 months but with the necessity to repeat the graft in 5 of these eyes.[377] In another series, various energy settings were investigated, and it was found that applications of under 256 J achieved an adequate intraocular pressure reduction in postkeratoplasty eyes.[378] It was also advised to anticipate fibrinous iritis, which was seen on rare occasion to lead to pupillary block in the absence of a patent iridectomy.

The use of a fiberoptic probe to deliver laser energy (contact Nd:YAG laser) has generated a similar profile of success. Here, too, a retrobulbar or peribulbar anesthetic is required, but the patient is put in a supine position. With the lids held apart by a speculum, the probe is applied eight times per quadrant to either three of four quadrants, with the probe positioned 1.5 mm from the limbus. Typical settings are 0.7 second at 7 W, for a total delivery of 4.9 J per application. In a large study of 14 eyes, over 70% achieved pressures of under 25 mm Hg, and half the eyes achieved pressures of under 19 mm Hg.[379] The maximum pressure reduction was usually obtained within 1 month, which was predictive of the value at 6 months. In this series, it was interesting that there was no significant visual loss. Similar results were reported by others.[380–382] However, eyes with neovascular glaucoma, congenital glaucoma, and uveitis were often in need of repeat treatment.

A similar technology has been devised using a diode laser system, with a fiberoptic probe.[383,384] The intraocular pressure results are comparable to those described with the other contact laser cyclodestructive procedures.

Complications seem to be ubiquitous across all the various laser technologies. These include iritis, pain, hyphema, corneal edema, elevated intraocular pressure, vitreous hemorrhage, and shallow anterior chamber. Sterile hypopyon and cataracts have also been reported with long-term follow-up.[385,386] It remains to be seen if any of the various laser technologies will demonstrate a superior margin of efficacy and safety.

Two issues deserve careful investigation and are of great clinical interest. The first is whether there is in fact a discrepancy in the rate of visual loss following noncontact transscleral Nd:YAG cyclophotocoagulation compared with eyes that have been treated with a contact laser cyclophotocoagulation.[372,379] These different results simply may reflect differences in patient selection. The other issue is whether there is an unacceptably high rate of sympathetic ophthalmia after laser cycloablation therapy. Five cases of sympathetic ophthalmia were observed in the Chicago area, and four of these patients were treated with noncontact Nd:YAG laser cryoablation. All had had cataract operations, and none had had trabeculectomy.[387] Although an earlier report of sympathetic ophthalmia[388] was reported from the same group, subsequent histopathologic evaluation suggested that this event may have been due to other surgical procedures preceding the use of the laser treatment.[389] The clarification of this issue is of considerable interest since it needs to be mentioned when discussing informed consent with patients. Fortunately, however, this cluster of cases has not been appreciated in other locations.

Miscellaneous Ciliary Destructive Procedures

There are other interventions that have been described in the literature to control glaucoma by altering ciliary body function. None of these have achieved wide popularity. Transpupillary destruction of ciliary processes, delivered through large iridectomies, was reported to be effective in less than one fourth of patients treated.[390]

A more challenging technique of vitrectomy and endolaser of ciliary processes was reported with the observation that more than 180 degrees of the ciliary body required ablation for approximately 80% of patients to obtain pressure control under 20 mm Hg.[347,348] As expected with any retinal vitreous surgery, complications such as vitreous hemorrhage and failure to control intraocular pressure were encountered. Similar attempts were described by Shields using an endoscopic laser,[349] with a discouraging number of successes in a small series of patients.

A radical approach was described by Demeler[391] in which a section of the ciliary body was surgically excised for secondary angle-closure glaucoma in aphakic eyes, resulting in a reduction of intraocular pressure in 80% of the patients treated. The surgery was fairly complicated, requiring the use of a Flieringa ring, and was accompanied by complications such as vitreous loss and vitreous hemorrhage.

LASER TECHNIQUES IN GLAUCOMA

Laser Iridotomies

Although the surgical iridectomy was the first definitively curative intervention for glaucoma, described over 100 years ago in Europe, the advent of lasers in the 1970s has for all practical purposes supplanted the incisional technique. There are multiple conditions that respond to laser iridotomy, and the ease of laser treatment has led to earlier ophthalmic care and resolution of many of these circumstances.[392] When the laser iridotomy remains patent, it is usually capable of addressing all aspects of pupillary block that would be addressed by surgery, with comparable efficacy.[393] There are several laser devices available for treating a multitude of conditions.

The most obvious types of glaucoma that respond to laser are those with some element of pupillary block. These may be eyes that have shallow anterior chambers but elevated pressures, often without symptoms, and which are treated to prevent chronic angle embarrassment. In one series of such patients, it was discovered that the pressure reduction was achieved only if preexisting peripheral anterior synechiae were observed; in the absence of these synechiae there was no reduction of intraocular pressure, with follow-up from 1½ to 3 years.[394] In eyes that were similarly selected for the narrowness of their angles, deepening of the anterior chamber was achieved with good pressure control and without the development of frank glaucoma; no mention of the predictive significance of peripheral anterior synechiae was made.[395]

If eyes present with acute angle-closure glaucoma, attempts should be made to reduce the intraocular pressure as quickly as possible. However, those patients with a long history of symptoms or a history of intermittent attacks in the past may not respond as well. In one series of 78 such patients, only 15 acute angle-closure glaucomas responded to laser iridotomy without the need for further attention, and the remainder required either medicines or surgery.[396] There is one report that eyes with "acute congestive angle-closure glaucomas" lasting from 3 to 14 days are usually not responsive to the laser procedure and that surgical sector iridectomies are indicated.[397]

In a similar series of 40 patients presenting with acute angle-closure glaucoma, 3 experienced recurrent acute glaucoma despite patent iridotomy, requiring further laser treatment. Among the 40 patients were 23 patients who had previously tested positive during a provocative test with mydriatic drops; after iridotomy these provocative tests reverted to negative.[398] These studies seemed to substantiate the impression that long duration of angle embarrassment from pupillary block can lead to irreversible changes in the outflow tract that subsequently may not reverse with a patent iridotomy.

Another group of patients with glaucoma who respond well to the laser iridotomy are those with either chronic narrow-angle glaucoma or mixed-mechanism glaucoma. In one series of patients with chronic narrow-angle glaucoma that had completely failed to respond to argon iridotomy, the Nd:YAG laser was able to penetrate through iris.[399] In another series of patients with chronic narrow-angle glaucoma that had responded to argon iridotomy, if visual field loss was present at the time of their treatment, one third of the eyes required subsequent trabeculectomies—again indicating chronic structural changes to the angle.

Sometimes these trabecular structural changes do not require full filtration surgery. Shirakashi and colleagues[400] looked at 16 patients after iridotomy whose intraocular pressure was not controlled and who had less than 50% peripheral anterior synechiae closure of the angle. They received argon laser trabeculoplasty, and two thirds of them responded with excellent pressure control and did not require trabeculectomy. This is a particularly important observation, indicating that once the pupillary block mechanism is eliminated then the visible angle that remains available for filtration can respond to nonsurgical treatment with either medications or laser trabeculoplasty.

There are many techniques that have been described for making a patent iridotomy.[49,401] The suitability of an argon or Nd:YAG device over another often depends on the availability of the machines. There are several authors who recommend a sequential use of argon laser, first to minimize bleeding from the iris, followed some time later by an Nd:YAG iridotomy through the same site.[402,403] Some specifically recommend the sequential use of the argon laser followed by Nd:YAG iridotomy for all eyes that are not blue, with blue eyes being treated with Nd:YAG iridotomy alone.[401] Another author has reported little merit in argon laser pretreatment preceding the Nd:YAG iridotomy.[404]

The question of how large to make an iridotomy was addressed in a study reporting four cases that had patent Nd:YAG iridotomies but required further laser treatment to eliminate pupillary block. It was thought that a minimum size of 150 to 200 μm is necessary to prevent recurrent attacks of angle-closure glaucoma.[405]

Complications

The argon and Nd:YAG laser iridotomy techniques share many complications, with one or two exceptions. The most important complication is the tendency toward elevated intraocular pressure in the first several hours after iridectomy. This has been reported by nearly all observers; for example, when eyes with chronic narrow-angle glaucoma were treated, 35% of them were seen to have pressures of greater than 30 mm Hg, or 40% over baseline pressure; 20% of eyes with narrow angles only (without peripheral anterior synechiae) showed a similar rise.[406] An equally crucial observation was that if the pressure did not rise in the first 2 hours after laser treatment, pressure elevation was not detected 24 hours later. This certainly substantiates the importance of early surveillance to detect this particular problem. Other studies have also reported pressure elevations greater than 40%, with some symptoms of transitory corneal edema.[407]

Fortunately this pressure spike can be aborted with the use of several different pharmacologic preparations. Preoperative timolol and acetazolamide administered 1 hour before iridotomy were able to reduce the number of patients experiencing pressure spikes to 5% versus 55% in a control group.[408] More recently, apraclonidine, an α_2-agonist, has greatly reduced both the frequency of pressure spikes and the magnitude of pressure elevations.[409–412]

With the introduction of lasers for perforating the iris, there was initially great concern that the lens would be affected and cataract progression would be unavoidable. These fears, fortunately, have not proven to be true. In one large series of patients observed for several years after iridotomy, no progressive cataract was ascribed to the laser; instead, all changes were believed to be due to preexistent cataracts.[413] After argon laser iridotomies, small, punctate, white superficial lenticular opacities have been noted in as many as 35% of eyes.[414] These do not progress to a larger cataract change and are of no clinical significance; they are due to focal thermal necrosis of the anterior epithelium of the lens capsule.

In contrast, the nonthermal explosive energy of the Nd:YAG laser has given rise to concern regarding lens capsule integrity. Although cataract formation following Nd:YAG iridotomy is extremely rare,[415] there are two references in the literature documenting rupture of the lens capsule with rapid progression to cataract.[416,417] Such an exceptional event can almost certainly be avoided by the very careful focusing of the Nd:YAG energy so as to impinge on only the iris and not to be aimed at a more posterior plane.

Attention has also focused on corneal responses to laser. After argon laser treatment for iridotomy, especially in the presence of a narrow chamber where the thermal energy being absorbed by the iris is considerably closer to the endothelial surface than in a normal depth chamber, thermal absorption by the cornea with focal transient changes is often noted. There is a risk, however, that focal changes can progress to significant corneal edema in the presence of preexisting guttae (as with Fuchs dystrophy) or with a history of acute angle-closure glaucoma, especially with the additional risk of elevated pressure.[418–422] Yet the corneal decompensation can appear anywhere from 1½ to 3 years after laser treatment. Other risk factors that have been implicated include excessive amounts of laser energy at the time of the iridotomy and the preexistence of diabetes. In studies using endothelial microscopy after laser treatment, it is believed that there may be some decreased numbers of cells in the periphery, near the site of the iridotomy, but not in the center of the cornea.[421] One study interestingly reported no greater tendency for corneal endothelial changes after Nd:YAG iridotomy than after an Nd:YAG capsulotomy.[423]

Understandably, there is a small amount of iritis induced by iridotomy; patients can experience blurred vision and inflammatory discomfort for several hours to days. In some instances this can lead to the development of peripheral anterior synechiae; 37% of one series were seen to show progressive synechiae if miotics were continued after the iridotomy.[424] Two cases of sterile hypopyon have been reported after iridotomy, substantiating that inflammation can be quite severe.[425] In a related manner, pigmented pupillary membranes have been seen to form over the pupil itself. This was thought to be related to both the use of miotics and an intense inflammatory response.[426]

Depending on the placement of the iridotomy, patients may experience either monocular diplopia or monocular blur. These symptoms are more likely to occur if the iridotomy is in the interpalpebral fissure and not hidden by the upper lid; sometimes tinted lenses are required. It has been advised that the iridotomies be placed with great care so as to avoid this potential difficulty.[427]

Malignant glaucoma has also been reported after laser iridotomy, yet it is not always clear whether its onset was related actually to the breaking of the pupillary block or to the fact that these patients were on miotic therapy before or after the iridotomy.[161,162,428] As mentioned earlier in this chapter in the section on malignant glaucoma, this particular syndrome is particularly paradoxical, and the nature of the triggering event is not always obvious; spontaneous events without any medicine or intervention have been reported.[429] Nevertheless, malignant glaucoma is classically associated with eyes with angle-closure glaucoma, and this possibility must be kept in mind during the surveillance of patients requiring iridotomy.

As technology progresses, newer forms of laser devices are available. It is presumed that many of the side effects observed with argon and Nd:YAG iridotomies will appear with these new instruments as well. For example, the diode laser has been reported to be successfully used for iridotomies, using a two-stage technique. However, identical complications have been reported, such as elevations of intraocular pressure, focal cataract, and pupillary distortion.[430]

Not only are new devices on the horizon, but there are also potential new indications for the use of iridotomy. A particularly intriguing story that continues to unfold is the possible role of peripheral laser iridotomy in the management of pigment dispersion syndrome eyes at risk for developing pigmentary open-angle glaucoma. A "reverse pupillary block" has been described, in which the peripheral concave appearance of the peripheral iris in eyes with pigment dispersion is reversed after iridotomy: the iris flattens anteriorly, losing its concave bowing.[431] It remains to be seen, however, whether this intervention will reliably lift the iris off of the zonules where it is presumably being rubbed, thereby reducing the pigment dispersion into the trabecular meshwork. It is also unclear whether patients with dispersion syndrome but without glaucoma should be prophylactically treated, or whether an iridotomy should be first used in eyes that begin to show elevated intraocular pressures and early glaucomatous disease.

Argon Laser Trabeculoplasty

Although argon treatment of the trabecular meshwork was first described in 1974,[432] it was another 6 years before it was adopted by the ophthalmologic world after a successful series reported by Wise and Witter.[433] Because of a high success rate immediately after its use, and a very appealing risk–benefit ratio,[434] argon laser trabeculoplasty quickly became incorporated in the management of glaucomas as a technique that was initially prescribed after exhausting medical options but before proceeding to filtration surgery.

The recent literature on argon laser trabeculoplasty and its permutations is vast. There are many series that have follow-ups of 4 to 10 years,[435–443] and there is a remarkable amount of agreement among these different studies as to the essential features of the treatment's effects, complications, and favorable factors.

By and large, most eyes that will fail argon laser trabeculoplasty will fail in the first year, and this rate may be as high as 25%.[435] The failure rate thereafter is approximately 10% per year.[435,444] Certain eyes show a more vigorous response than others: eyes with pseudoexfoliation are often seen to show a remarkable pressure reduction.[438,443,445–450] Other series suggest that the common denominator for a dramatic response might be pigmentation of the angle, with eyes with pigment dispersion also showing favorable responses.[442] Another condition that has shown good responsiveness and is possibly related to a tendency toward greater pigmentation of the trabecular meshwork is mixed-mechanism glaucoma (ie, chronic angle-closure glaucoma following laser iridotomy).[442,448]

There is also some consensus as to which eyes do poorly: eyes with aphakia, juvenile open-angle glaucoma, uveitis, or angle recession.[447,449–451] There is some uncertainty as to the response of eyes with either high pressure or with very low pressure. Some report that it is unlikely that laser trabeculoplasty will reduce pressure by more than 30% or if the pressure is over 28 mm Hg.[452] This could explain the few negative reports of patients with pseudoexfoliation who often present with elevated intraocular pressures.[445,453] Eyes that have "low-tension glaucoma" have been reported by some researchers to have favorable responses with long-term follow-up[442,443,454]; but in another series, laser trabeculoplasty was thought not to be particularly useful when the intraocular pressure before argon laser trabeculoplasty was already in the mid-teens.[77,436]

Concerns that argon laser trabeculoplasty contributed to a higher failure rate of subsequent filtration surgery was refuted by Schoenleber and associates.[455] Conversely, patients with failed trabeculectomies who subsequently went on to laser trabeculoplasty showed a success rate comparable to patients with eyes that had never been operated on at all.[456]

Complications

The most ubiquitous complication following argon laser trabeculoplasty is an early elevated intraocular pressure, a complication reported in the earliest studies.[434] Various strategies have been designed to address this issue. At one point it was recommended that argon laser trabeculoplasty be divided into two sessions, in which 180 degrees of the trabecular meshwork is treated separately, to minimize both the incidence of elevation and the magnitude of spikes.[457,458] Later, pharmacologic interventions were described that reduced the frequency and severity of intraocular pressure elevations.[459] Preoperative pilocarpine,[460] timolol,[461] and acetazolamide[462] have all been reported to be useful. With the availability of apraclonidine, it was appreciated that 360-degree laser treatment with this α_2-agonist had as safe and favorable a post-laser intraocular pressure profile as did laser treatment of 180 degrees of the trabecular meshwork without apraclonidine.[463,464]

Other investigators studied the power settings for the laser treatment that differed from the standard parameters (0.1 second × 600 to 1000 mW) originally described by Wise and Witter.[433] Longer duration treatments of 0.2 second were reported to be as effective as 0.1 second.[465–468] Others have used lower wattage,[469] and still others have treated even as little as one fourth of the trabecular meshwork[470] with favorable results.

With the well-known fall-off of efficacy of the trabeculoplasty, some researchers have looked at repeating the intervention to see if the first laser's effect can be duplicated. This strategy has equivocal results, with most observers reporting at best a response profile comparable to the initial treatment[471,472] and others reporting less long-term success.[473] In contrast to earlier reports suggesting that the course following treatment of one eye was not necessarily predictive of the other,[449] more recent studies suggest that there is good bilateral correlation of responsiveness.[474]

Another common complication that may occur after argon laser trabeculoplasty includes the development of peripheral anterior synechiae. This has been reported to be as high as 46% of treated eyes.[440,458] These synechiae tend to be very small and peaked and rarely progress to become significant impediments of outflow. An associated phenomenon with the development of peripheral anterior synechiae is postoperative iritis. This may in part depend on the surgeon's skill and success at discretely focusing the laser beam into the trabecular meshwork and away from iris and uveal tissue.[475,476] In fact, one histopathologic study showed almost 50% of the applied laser burns either affected the adjacent corneal endothelium or showed an oblique and confluent effect on the trabecular meshwork.[477]

A sophisticated means of looking at inflammation by the laser flare meter suggested that the peak post-therapeutic inflammation was approximately 48 hours after the treatment, and greater in eyes with pigmentation, including pigment dispersion and pseudoexfoliation.[478] There was some correlation with increasing flare and low intraocular pressure, but this was usually reversed with several days' worth of corticosteroids. In rare instances, elevated intraocular pressures have been seen in combination with trabecular precipitates and were believed to be inflammatory.[386]

Visual loss is extremely rare after laser trabeculoplasty, but patients may experience significant blurred vision immediately after the procedure because of the laser flashes and possibly because of the goniogel solution used by the contact lens.[479] A comprehensive review by Levene[480] suggested a 3% rate of visual loss and an almost 2% rate of emergency trabeculectomy. Fortunately, this high incidence of complications has not been confirmed elsewhere. There is one reported case of lost central field because of a prolonged pressure elevation after laser trabeculoplasty.[481] I personally have observed a case of visual loss from anterior ischemic optic neuropathy 24 hours after trabeculoplasty, presumably related to extremely labile systemic hypertension in a patient experiencing great perioperative anxiety.

Minor corneal endothelial and epithelial burns are uncommon after laser trabeculoplasty, unlike laser iridotomy. Corneal damage has not been a feature of this particular modality. A similarly rare occurrence is that of microhemorrhage into the anterior chamber, which can be controlled by low-power photocoagulation.[479]

In conclusion, argon laser trabeculoplasty is usually a benign intervention whose efficacy is comparable to that of adding a medication to a patient's regimen for glaucoma.[449] The most predictable complications of elevated pressure and inflammation can usually be anticipated and pharmacologically addressed. Patient selection is important for best results. The long-term reduction of pressure spikes during diurnal curves[482] and the ability to reduce the intraocular pressure by 3 to 8 mm Hg in half the patients for 5 years make argon laser trabeculoplasty a worthy addition to the glaucomatologist's armamentarium.

Miscellaneous Laser Treatments

Laser Iridoplasty (Gonioplasty)

The use of argon laser to cause thermal contraction and shrinkage of the peripheral iris is useful in eyes with cramped angles, either on the basis of chronic narrow-angle glaucoma, large lenses, or short eyes.[401] It has also been used in eyes with plateau iris and nanophthalmos, and even in the retraction of recently detected peripheral anterior synechiae.[49,483]

The iridoplasty can be applied either obliquely through a prismatic goniolens or perpendicularly to the iris plane by use of a high-density magnifying contact lens, such as the Abraham iridotomy lens. The shrinkage of the iris depends in large part on the intensity of the settings and the tolerance of the patient. Sometimes repeat procedures are required. It can also be efficacious in improving outflow in eyes with angle-closure glaucoma on the basis of ciliary choroidal effusion, where there is no pupillary block component.[155,484] Its use for the treatment of nanophthalmos may reduce the need for surgical intervention.[485]

Laser Sclerostomies

The development of many kinds of lasers that can deliver highly focused energy with minimal thermal effect is responsible for a variety of exciting innovations in creating sclerostomies.[486] These have been applied in three fashions: (1) sclerostomies that are made through an intracameral probe; (2) sclerostomies that are made through a contact lens into the angle; and (3) sclerostomies that are made by directly applying a probe subconjunctivally at the limbus from an external approach. Most lasers capable of being used in this way are not clinically available.

Perhaps the most familiar device is the holmium laser thermal sclerostomy procedure, which uses a subconjunctival approach to create a sclerostomy at the limbus.[48] Because in effect a full-thickness ostium is created with a very small hole, complications include those expected from excessive filtration: shallow anterior chambers, peripheral anterior synechiae, cataract formation, as well as potential occlusion of the small stoma by either the iris or the Descemet flap.[50] For reasons that are not entirely clear, there has even been a report of a cyclodialysis cleft after holmium laser sclerostomy.[487]

Because the availability of these devices is limited, there is not a large body of clinical experience. It is likely, however, that strategies needed for dealing with classic full-thickness filtration complications will be applicable to these innovative ways of fashioning filtration ostia.

COMPLICATIONS OF CATARACT SURGERY AND GLAUCOMA SURGERY

There are many facets and issues regarding the management of cataract and glaucoma in the same eye. First, there is the congruence of risk factors for both diseases: both cataracts and glaucoma are more frequently seen in the elderly population. Second, eyes with a combination of glaucoma and even mild cataract may have reduced vision simply on the basis of decreased pupillary diameter from miotic usage. And similarly, eyes that have undergone filtration procedures often sustain an acceleration of the natural tendency toward cataract formation, requiring that the cataract eventually be addressed surgically. There are many interesting aspects to the management approaches to these issues,[488] and some of these issues of ophthalmic surgical complications are addressed here.

Implications of Pseudophakia and Aphakia on Subsequent Glaucoma Management

Eyes that have already undergone cataract extraction, and are rendered either aphakic or pseudophakic, present many interesting challenges for glaucoma management. It is a surgical truism in ophthalmology that aphakic eyes do much worse than phakic eyes in terms of standard glaucoma surgery, with a much higher rate of complication.[69] There are multiple mechanisms that have been invoked: secondary angle closure as a result of the cataract surgery (eg, following postoperative shallow chamber), pupillary block (eg, caused by anterior chamber lens implant), and postsurgical iritis.[489–491] In children who have had congenital cataract surgery there is a somewhat mysterious but frequent appearance of glaucoma often several years after surgery.[492,493]

The predilection toward developing glaucoma after lens implant surgery can depend in part on the type of intraocular lens that has been used. For example, rigid anterior chamber lens implants have been associated with increased pigment dispersion, peripheral anterior synechiae, iris atrophy, neovascularization of the iris, and lens-corneal touch.[494] One estimate of the incidence of secondary glaucoma after anterior chamber lenses is approximately 8%; this is in contrast to the lower incidence of secondary glaucoma after posterior chamber lens implants of approximately 2%.[495,496]

In the presence of surgery that is technically uncomplicated, there may be subtle aspects of the pseudophakic state that contribute toward progressive embarrassment of angle outflow. For example, the preoperative use of miotic agents, in combination with an anterior vaulted haptic of a posterior chamber lens, can contribute to the formation of peripheral anterior synechiae.[497,498] Sometimes the synechiae can even progress to involve the angle beyond that which overlies the haptic behind the iris surface.

The choice of filtration surgery with an aphakic and pseudophakic eye must take into consideration the quality of the conjunctiva where the intended bleb is to form. Especially in eyes that have undergone relatively large limbal incisions, such as for intracapsular or extracapsular cataract extraction, there may be extensive conjunctival adhesions at the limbus that might require specific attention at the time of filtering procedure. Sometimes the conjunctiva can be elevated with a subconjunctival injection at the time of surgery using hemostatic fluid (eg, 2% lidocaine with 1:100,000 epinephrine). Such evidence of episcleral scarring should influence the surgeon's choice for the actual location of the intended filtering operation, with care to avoid conjunctival buttonholing.

Multiple considerations must be remembered during filtering surgery in aphakic or pseudophakic eyes.

Because of the scarring at the limbus that often occurs with the use of the fornix-based flap from cataract surgery, it is sometimes difficult when using a limbus-based conjunctival flap to be anterior enough during the formation of the scleral flap: the entry into the eye can be more posterior than intended, ending up over the ciliary body. This can predispose to hyphema and, unfortunately, even to the presentation of vitreous, especially at the site of the surgical iridectomy from the cataract operation. Inadvertent posterior entry over the ciliary body, with or without vitreous involvement, can also affect zonular support in that region, which could place a posterior chamber lens implant at risk for dislocation.

In the presence of an anterior chamber lens implant with filtering surgery, great care must be taken to maintain as deep an anterior chamber as possible during filtering surgery, because of the risk of corneal endothelial damage from shallowing or IOL touch. Moreover, there is the significant risk of suprachoroidal hemorrhage in aphakic eyes, which can be encountered either intraoperatively or postoperatively. In such a circumstance, aggressive therapy may sometimes be necessary to maximize the chance of restoring the best possible vision.[499] Lastly, there is the significant issue of how well a bleb will form under conjunctiva that has been operated on twice. It is the dismal outcome of aphakic and pseudophakic filtering surgery that led in large part to the elaboration of antimetabolite regimens for glaucoma management.[500,501]

Cataract-Related Risk Factors for Developing Glaucoma

Certain preexisting eye conditions increase the chance of glaucoma developing after cataract operation, with or without lens implantation. Diabetic patients pose the most common challenge. In the days of intracapsular cataract extraction, neovascular glaucoma was reported to be as high as 9% after intracapsular surgery, which was nearly identical to the rate of neovascular glaucoma appearing with extracapsular surgery in the presence of a capsulotomy (11%).[502] These rates are in contrast to the much reduced risk of a rubeotic glaucoma in the presence of an intact capsule. Similar findings were reported by Aiello,[503] but an important distinction was made as to whether proliferative diabetic retinopathy was present before cataract surgery: if so, there was a 40% rate of neovascular glaucoma and a greater than 20% rate of vitreous hemorrhage related to the cataract extraction.

Often the violation of the capsule is unavoidable at the time of extracapsular (or phacoemulsification) surgery; at other times it is unavoidable because of the need for a capsulotomy to maximize either vision or ophthalmologic visualization of the fundus. Nevertheless, these risk factors must be shared with the patient, and if it is at all possible to address a preproliferative retina with panretinal photocoagulation before cataract extraction, this should be undertaken.

Another feature of the diabetic eye that should be kept in mind is the higher likelihood of developing pupillary block glaucoma at the time of lens implantation.[504] Although peripheral iridectomies are not commonly placed by most lens implant surgeons in routine cases, it is highly advisable that it be a routine part of any cataract extraction, with either anterior or posterior chamber lens implantation, in eyes with diabetes.

Eyes that present with pseudoexfoliation are certainly more prone to develop cataracts and have a much higher association of glaucoma as well; this condition needs to be detected before cataract extraction is undertaken.[505] There are many features of the pseudoexfoliation eye that make cataract surgery particularly challenging: (1) a tendency toward incomplete mydriasis, with a subsequent small pupil that can complicate cataract extraction; (2) a tendency toward zonular dehiscence or even rupture, with lens dislocation during surgery; (3) a cornea that may be more subject to endothelial damage; (4) a tendency toward hyphema during surgery; and (5) a tendency for total zonular loss, such that even an in-the-bag lens implant can fall into the vitreous.[506] Undiagnosed lens subluxation from weak zonules has been noted by many authorities and should accordingly be anticipated by the surgeon.[507]

Even with the anticipation of complications, however, one series reporting the use of flexible anterior chamber lens implants noted that half the patients requiring these were eyes with pseudoexfoliation, which had a 60% rate of anterior vitrectomy because of lenticular instability during extracapsular surgery.[508] In addition, nearly one third of these eyes subsequently had elevated pressures over 30 mm Hg, though by 2 years the vast majority no longer manifested a secondary glaucoma.

Although some sources have reported no particular tendency toward complications in eyes with Fuchs heterochromic uveitis,[509] others have observed several specific features of this condition that bear directly on the management of the eye with cataract.[510] In over 103 patients with this condition, over one fourth had glaucoma, most of which was of the chronic open-angle glaucoma variety.[76] However, many eyes presented with inflammation and peripheral anterior synechiae, rubeosis of the iris and angle, pupillary block, and recurrent hyphemas. When these eyes underwent glaucoma surgery, more than half failed standard filtration operations (in the absence of antimetabolites). Accordingly, the cataract surgeon should be on the lookout for these many manifestations of this disease.

Another aspect of cataract surgery that has direct bearing on the development of glaucoma is the problem of inadvertent capsular rupture during extracapsular surgery or phacoemulsification, with subsequent loss of nuclear or cortical fragments into the vitreous cavity. There is good agreement among retina-vitreous surgeons that several guidelines be followed: (1) that the lost fragment not be pursued during the cataract operation, because of the high risk of retinal tears at the vitreous base[511]; (2) that any postoperative elevation of pressure and inflammation following the loss of a lens fragment should be medically controlled before vitrectomy is undertaken[512]; and (3) that a standard pars plana vitrectomy by a vitrectomist can be undertaken when the eye is stable, with a reasonably good chance of visual recovery.[513]

Elevated Pressure After Nd:YAG Laser Capsulotomy

After extracapsular cataract extraction with or without posterior chamber lens implantation, there is a predictable rate of capsular opacification, which increases with the length of follow-up.[514,515] This can be addressed by either surgical discission or laser, but it is the Nd:YAG capsulotomy that has the high association with elevated pressures. Multiple risk factors have been identified for the tendency for an elevated pressure after a capsulotomy: (1) history of prior glaucoma or elevated intraocular pressure; (2) myopia; (3) prior retinal-vitreous disease; (4) large capsulotomy; (5) vitreous prolapse into the anterior chamber; and (6) absence of posterior chamber lens implant.[516,517]

Although the intraocular pressure elevation can be profoundly blunted by the use of apraclonidine drops,[518] special attention still must be paid to the exceptional patient. For example, two patients with a history of uveitic glaucoma sustained ciliary choroidal effusions after Nd:YAG capsulotomy.[519] In another unusual case, a patient whose intraocular pressure was not elevated 2 hours after laser treatment (when most patients experience a tension rise[520]) reported 24 hours later with a pressure of over 60 mm Hg.[521] Although the mechanisms remain unclear, it seems that there is a higher incidence of secondary glaucoma after capsulotomies than in patients who do not undergo the laser procedure; as many as 3.6% have been reported to develop a glaucomatous condition requiring management.[517]

Glaucomatous Eyes Requiring Cataract Operations

There are multiple factors that go into the consideration of what type of cataract surgery to offer a patient with glaucoma and what sequence of events to follow.[488] Issues include the type of glaucoma that is present, the efficacy of and compliance with the medical regimen, the financial costs or possible side effects of the medical regimen, the surgeon's skill and options, the status of the optic nerve and visual field, and the visual requirements and the quality of life that the patient wishes to obtain.

For example, eyes with primary angle-closure glaucoma often show a significant improvement in their intraocular pressure control after the removal of cataract, implying that there is some phacomorphic component to their underlying disease, even in the presence of an iridotomy.[522–524] Accordingly, if a patient with this kind of glaucoma presents with relatively good intraocular pressure measurements using a minimal medical therapy, it may be sufficient to proceed with cataract extraction and lens implantation alone, reasonably anticipating a greater than 50% chance that the glaucoma will remain controlled if not improved. On the other hand, reference was made earlier to the significant complication rate that can be seen in eyes with pseudoexfoliative open-angle glaucoma undergoing cataract extraction.[508] Accordingly, cataract surgery should be undertaken with the full spectrum of possible outcomes known to both patients and surgeon.

For the vast majority of patients with primary chronic open-angle glaucoma who must decide about cataract surgery, there are basically three choices: (1) undergo cataract extraction alone and pay no surgical attention per se to the glaucomatous condition; (2) undergo glaucoma filtering surgery first and allow full healing before undergoing a second operation for cataract removal; or (3) undergo a single combined cataract and lens implantation operation at the time of the glaucoma filtering procedure.

It is certainly appropriate to strive for the best possible intraocular pressure control before cataract extraction, and this can include the application of argon laser trabeculoplasty, whose beneficial effects are not likely to change after cataract surgery.[525,526] But then the question arises: how much pressure reduction can be expected with extracapsular or phacoemulsification surgery and lens implantation alone? There is remarkable agreement among various authorities that the pressure reduction from contemporary cataract surgical techniques alone is on the order of 1.5 to 2.5 mmHg at best.[527–529] In a patient with minimal disc and field changes, and reasonably well-controlled intraocular pressures on a simple medical regimen, these results may suggest a course of cataract extraction alone.

In the event, however, that there are other compelling factors to either eliminate medications or to obtain better pressure control, there are those who have suggested that glaucoma control be surgically obtained first and that cataract extraction be subsequently undertaken.[530] In one such study, however, Levene[531] reported on a series of eyes with blebs that were well functioning and at the time of cataract extraction had additional filtration procedures applied—but in which a loss of control resulted nevertheless. Reports in the older literature suggest a bleb failure rate of 30% to 40% after cataract surgery.[532,533]

The observation has been made that the correlation is very poor between the intraocular pressure level and the physical appearance of the bleb after combined surgery.[534] The assumption is that the intraocular inflammation attendant to the healing of the cataract extraction and lens implantation is sufficient to tilt the factors against the preservation of a preexisting filtering bleb. Even with a clear corneal approach to removing the cataract,[535] and avoiding the conjunctiva altogether, these blebs must be carefully watched. Anecdotally, some blebs are subsequently treated with 5-FU injections after cataract extraction, but the data for whether this practice enhances bleb survival are not yet available.

The argument for combining trabeculectomy with cataract extraction is compelling on many fronts. In the absence of posterior pole disease, there is every expectation that decent visual acuity will be obtained in the overwhelming majority of patients.[536,537] But perhaps the most persuasive argument is that eyes that have preexisting glaucoma and undergo cataract extraction are extremely likely to sustain significant elevations of intraocular pressure after surgery that a concomitant filtering procedure may help to abort.

There is ample evidence on the relationship of cataract extraction and pressure spikes in glaucomatous eyes. One series reported a two and one-half times greater incidence of elevated pressures in the absence of trabeculectomy than when the combined procedure was performed.[529] Other reports have indicated a pressure spike in nearly two thirds of eyes with preexisting glaucoma, in contrast to 10% of eyes without.[538] In another study that investigated strategies to reduce these spikes, the perioperative use of acetazolamide (Diamox; 500-mg sequels) and intraoperative acetylcholine (Miochol) reduced pressure significantly more when both drugs were used than when either alone was used; and yet 7% of the maximally treated patients still experienced a mild intraocular pressure elevation.[539] Similar results were reported with the use of intraoperative carbachol, reducing intraocular tensions the first 3 days after surgery.[540]

The presence of a trabeculectomy with cataract extraction does not, however, guarantee the prevention of a pressure rise. Although a pressure spike is three times less likely to appear in the absence of a trabeculectomy, Krupin and colleagues[541] reported that many patients with glaucoma continued to experience elevated pressures after combined procedures, with as many as 80% of patients experiencing fluctuating tensions for the first month after surgery. Similarly, it was reported that as many as half the patients sustained intraocular pressures over 20 mm Hg on the first day with a combined procedure.[542]

Naturally the question arises as to whether there are attendant complications to combining cataract extraction with trabeculectomy. Some authors have reported few problems indeed.[543,544] Other studies have suggested that although a trabeculectomy alone may effect a lower pressure than a combined procedure and more medications may be required after cataract extraction with trabeculectomy than filtration alone, nevertheless there is considerable benefit to the combined approach.[531,545–547]

Intraoperative Considerations of the Combined Procedure

There are several superbly detailed references regarding the surgical techniques for extracapsular cataract extraction combined with lens implantation and trabeculectomy.[548–550] In this section we wish to highlight some of those factors that have the greatest bearing on successful outcome and avoiding postoperative complications.

It is certainly important to prepare the patient for the fact that a combined cataract and glaucoma operation may take longer to heal than a simple lens implant operation. Similarly, in the event that the patient is on a carbonic anhydrase inhibitor and filtration surgery is undertaken, it is usual to stop the systemic medication to enhance filtration. But this risks possible loss of intraocular pressure control in the fellow, unoperated eye. Accordingly, the patient may have to consider the decision to undergo filtration surgery in one eye as ultimately a decision to undergo filtration surgery in both eyes.

Before surgery it is often useful to stop miotic therapy a short time before surgery, because the most challenging aspect of combined procedures is working with the small pupil that the glaucomatous eye is likely to have. A preoperative dilation by the surgeon should provide information as to the maximum pupillary dilation that can be expected in the operating room. Sometimes the pupillary diameter will be enhanced by the use of cardiac epinephrine in intraocular irrigating fluids.[551]

There are multiple approaches that have been offered for the intraoperative mechanical enlargement of the pupil. Sector iridectomies can be performed that then can subsequently be resutured at the end of the surgery to restore a round pupil, which has both optical benefits for the patient and may reduce the incidence of posterior chamber lens capture.[552] Multiple small radial sphincterotomies can be performed with scissors intraoperatively, which in combination with mechanical stretching of the sphincter, can result in a large enough pupillary diameter to proceed with surgery. Another surgical strategy is the introduction of four transcorneal iris retractors, either made of metal or of Prolene-suture material, which can produce a square, 8-mm pupil that is ample for the performance of the capsulotomy and management of the nucleus; these retractors can then be removed for the implantation of a lens implant (Figs. 10-26 through 10-38.)

Another cascading complication that can be seen with small pupils is that the capsulotomy is sometimes extremely difficult; and imperfect capsulotomies can sometimes lead to unreliable capsular support for in-the-bag lens implantation. It is equally important to anticipate a shallow chamber, as seen in chronic angle-closure glaucoma. Even with the use of protective viscoelastic agents, corneal damage can still be sustained under such circumstances.

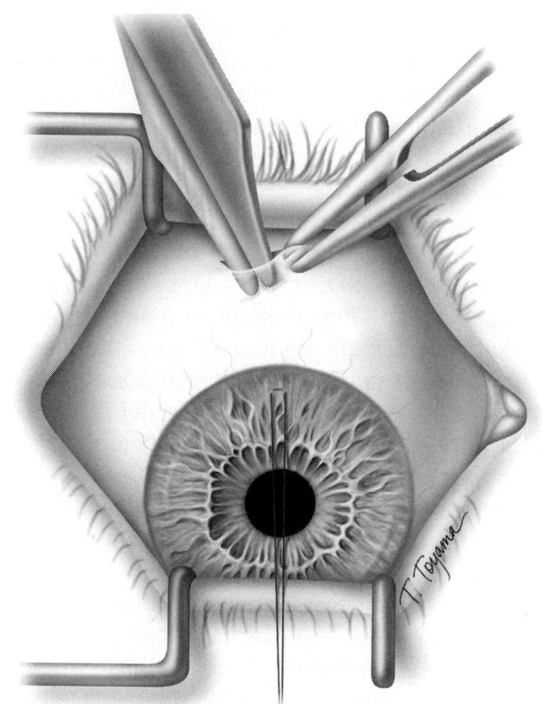

Figure 10-26. *Phacoemulsification with IOL and trabeculectomy with mitomycein-C.* Preparation of limbus-based conjunctival flap approximately 8 mm from the superior limbus, with dissection of conjunctiva and Tenon tissue anteriorly to expose superior 6 mm of the limbal tissue. A 7-0 Vicryl traction suture to the clear cornea is used to spare unnecessary perforation of the superior conjunctiva.

Another consideration is that if viscoelastic agents are used at the time of surgery, they can cause elevated pressure in normal eyes and especially in glaucomatous eyes.[553,554] Accordingly, the strategies of preoperative acetazolamide and intraoperative acetylcholine[539] are worth considering, even in the presence of a trabeculectomy. The use of perioperative medications, either adrenergic or miotic agents, may result in a slightly greater tendency toward hyphemas in the immediate postoperative period.

Lastly, the surgeon will have decided to proceed with either a fornix-based flap or a limbus-based flap for the combined procedure, with each technique having its advantages.[555] The overall results are, in the long run, comparable.

The natural historical development following the introduction of extracapsular cataract extraction and posterior chamber lens implantation was the use of phacoemulsification in a combined trabeculectomy procedure. The logic of this is compelling: the small wound possible with the phacoemulsification device, often 3 to 5 mm, is comparable to the size of a standard trabeculectomy flap; in fact, with the use of fold-

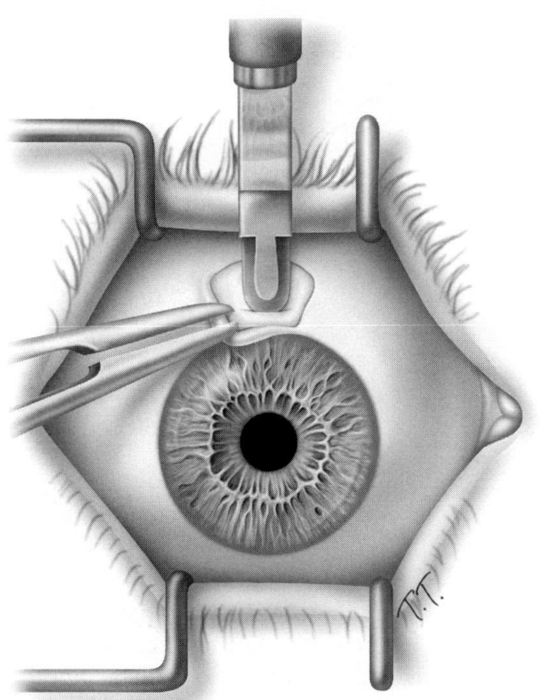

Figure 10-27. *Phaco/filter (Continued).* Preparation of standard phacoemulsification scleral tunnel, which is approximately 2 mm from the limbus surface posteriorly, 3.5 mm in width, and at a depth of one-half the scleral thickness.

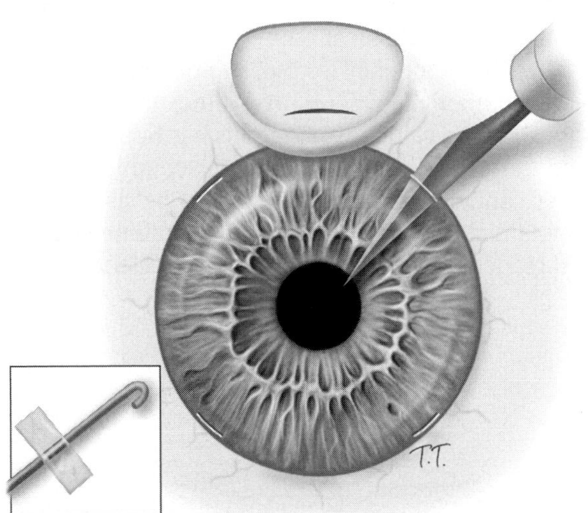

Figure 10-28. *Phaco/filter (Continued).* If the pupil fails to dilate, four Prolene transcorneal iris retractors (seen in the inset) can be used. (The retractor shafts are available as either metal or suture material, with soft silicone, rectangular sleeves.) Creation of four separate paracentesis "stab wounds" with a 15-degree sharp blade, anterior to the limbal vessels and with each insertion 90 degrees apart, allows placement of the retractors.

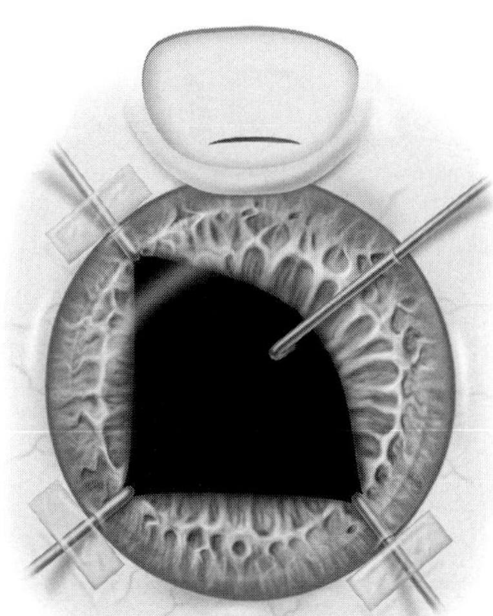

Figure 10-29. *Phaco/filter (Continued).* Introduction of transcorneal iris retractors. Each hook is introduced to grasp the pupillary edge and pull it peripherally to the limbus. The large, square pupil is secured by sliding the clear plastic sleeves forward along the shaft of the retractor up to the limbus itself.

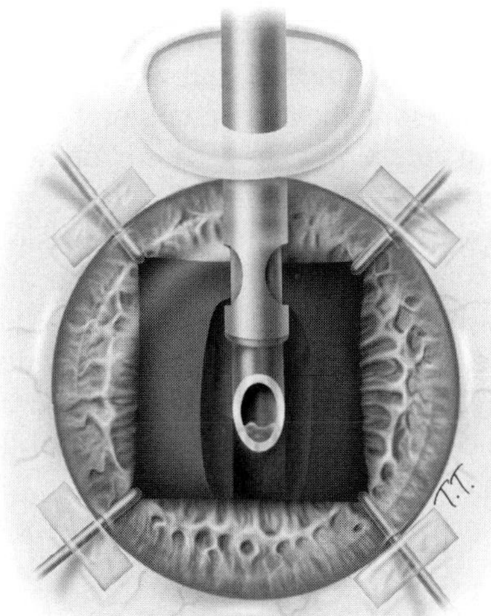

Figure 10-30. *Phaco/filter (Continued).* With the enlargement of the pupil, a standard phacoemulsification can proceed, with capsulorhexis and cataract removal. The superior iris is sometimes "tented" between the two superior iris retractors: care is necessary to avoid trauma to the superior iris when entering the eye and when intracamerally manipulating the phacoemulsification unit.

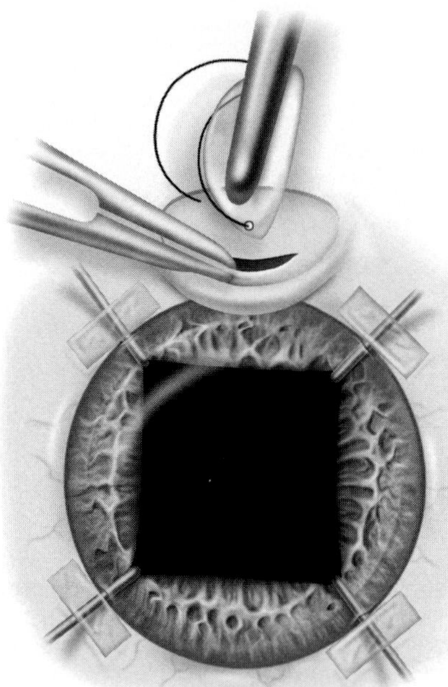

Figure 10-31. *Phaco/filter (Continued).* After completion of the irrigation and aspiration of the lens, the scleral tunnel can be enlarged horizontally in preparation for foldable lens implantation.

able posterior chamber lens implants, the entire cataract extraction and glaucoma procedure can be confined to a 5.5-mm maximal wound.[556–559] Results of the phacoemulsification combined with trabeculectomy are very similar to those reported with filtering surgery and extracapsular cataract extraction, with most patients obtaining excellent vision and decent pressure control,[496,560] even in the absence of anatomically impressive bleb structures.[534,557,561]

In his very thorough review of phacoemulsification technique in eyes with glaucoma, Davison[552] lists the specific features of the different types of glaucoma

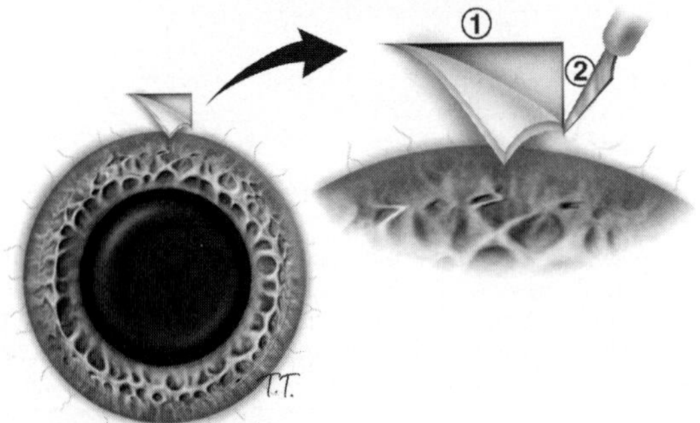

Figure 10-32. *Phaco/filter (Continued).* After placement of the posterior chamber lens implant in the capsular bag, the surgeon converts the phacoscleral tunnel (1) into a nonstandard trabeculectomy flap. This is simply fashioned by making a radial cut (2) from the corner of the scleral tunnel anteriorly to the limbus itself.

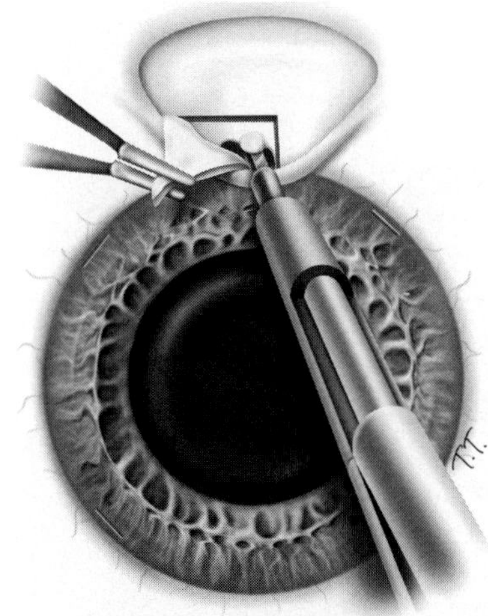

Figure 10-33. *Phaco/filter (Continued).* At the phacoemulsification site at the limbus, a Descemet punch is used to remove the trabeculectomy ostium, which is approximately 2 x 2 mm in size.

that have bearing on this surgical approach. For example, eyes with chronic narrow-angle glaucoma are likely to have shallow anterior chambers, and hence the complication of stripping of the Descemet membrane or iris prolapse must be considered; eyes with pigmentary dispersion glaucoma, being myopic, may have deeper anterior chambers, and hence those ramifications of phacoemulsification surgery at a slightly steeper angle should be considered; eyes with neovascular glaucoma often have nonreactive pupils and a propensity for bleeding; and eyes with angle recession are often likely to have zonular weakening and lens dislocation.

Given the tendency for blebs to become small in a large number of patients over time, the natural response of the glaucoma surgeons has been to investigate the use of antimetabolites in combined procedures, anticipating that they would be as useful in maintaining bleb function with the combined cataract and glaucoma surgery as they are with glaucoma sur-

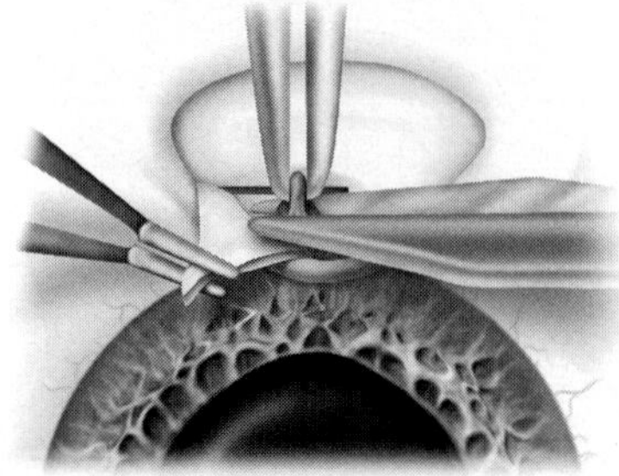

Figure 10-34. *Phaco/filter (Continued).* A basal peripheral iridectomy is performed at the site of the trabeculectomy.

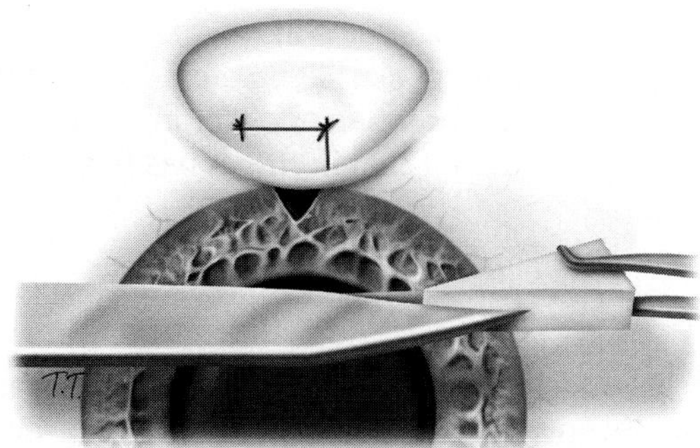

Figure 10-35. *Phaco/filter (Continued).* After suturing the phacoemulsification wound with one 10-0 nylon suture at the corner, and an optional suture along the length of the bed of scleral tunnel, the surgeon prepares for the placement of the antimetabolite: either mitomycin-C or 5-fluorouracil. A one-half thickness of the triangular cellulose sponge is cut parallel to the surface of the sponge (shown here), and this triangular element is again cut so that the triangular sides are approximately 3 to 4 mm in length. The sponge fragment is then saturated with the antimetabolite, using a few drops delivered via syringe and a small needle.

gery alone.[199] Hurvitz[562] performed an interesting evaluation of eyes that had undergone phacoemulsification with trabeculectomy and 5-FU injections, compared both with eyes that had undergone phacoemulsification and trabeculectomy without antimetabolite and with eyes that had undergone extracapsular cataract extraction and trabeculectomy without antimetabolite. Final visual acuities were quite good in all groups, but there was a strong tendency for better bleb survival with the use of 5-FU, with lower intraocular pressures.

Although the foundations for understanding the utility and complications of antimetabolites have

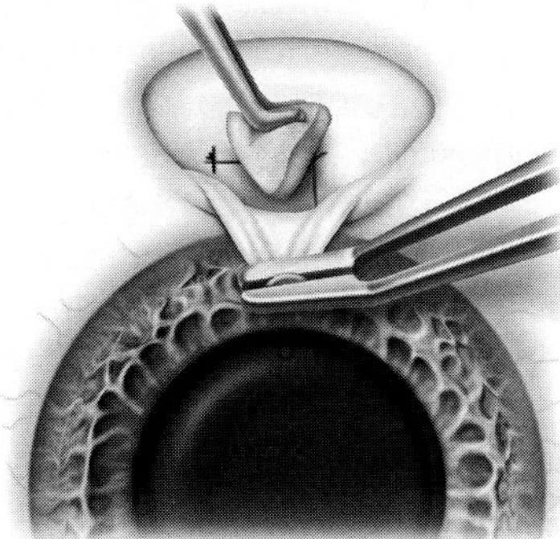

Figure 10-36. *Phaco/filter (Continued).* The saturated cellulose sponge fragment is carefully placed over the trabeculectomy flap, with care taken to lift the Tenon tissue and overlying conjunctiva on top of the saturated sponge but to avoid contact between the conjunctival wound edge and the sponge. The exposure of the antimetabolite to the wound depends on several factors but is approximately 1 to 5 minutes, depending on the concentration and antimetabolite chosen.

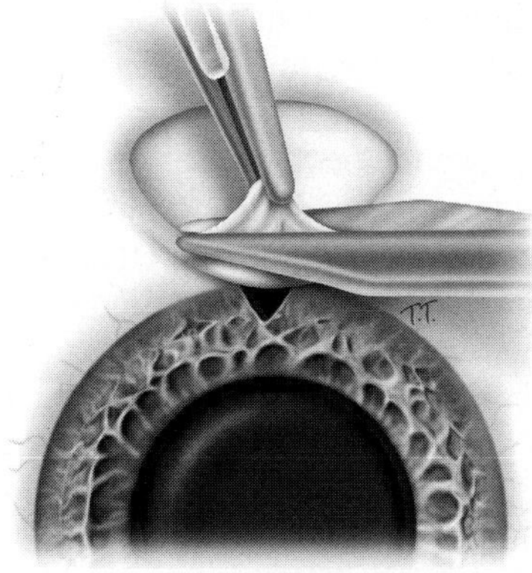

Figure 10-37. *Phaco/filter (Continued).* After removal of the antimetabolite sponge from the area, followed by irrigation with saline solution, the limbus-based conjunctival flap is prepared for closure. Any excess Tenon tissue is excised from the edge of the wound (as shown here), but the excision need not be extensive.

been well established,[108,111] long-term results on the use of these agents with combined cataract and trabeculectomy are still being reported. We prefer to use a limbus-based conjunctival flap, to fashion a 3.2-mm scleral tunnel at the superior limbus, to proceed with a standard phacoemulsification after enlarging the pupil to at least 5 mm, and to insert a foldable posterior chamber lens implant. At this point a single incision is made radially from the edge of the scleral tunnel down toward the limbus and the corner of this flap reflected toward the limbus. This allows the insertion of a Descemet punch to excise an approximately 1.5×2-mm posterior lip from the wound. The corner of the flap is then sutured with a solitary 10-0 nylon suture and a parallel suture in the bed of the scleral tunnel is placed. A fragment of cellulose sponge saturated with 0.5 mm/mL of mitomycin-C is placed over the sclera and beneath the conjunctiva for 1 to 3 minutes, then removed and the site irri-

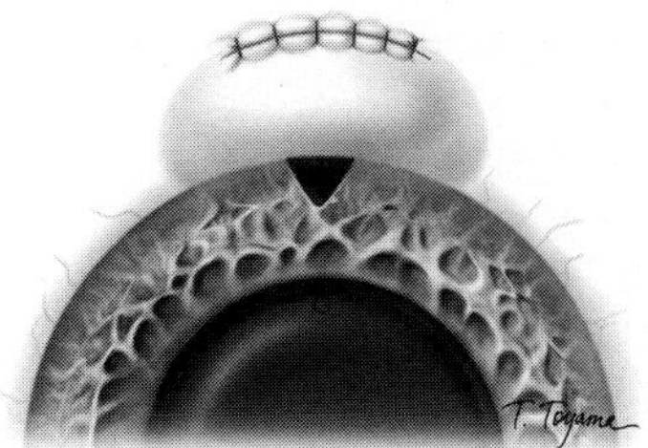

Figure 10-38. *Phaco/filter (Continued).* With a meticulous running suture, preferably using a small-tapered needle (eg, BV–100 on a 9-0 Vicryl suture), the wound is made watertight. This is verified by reforming the anterior chamber, pressing adjacent to the bleb, and checking for bleb integrity.

gated. The limbus-based flap is then closed with a meticulous 9-0 Vicryl suture (see Figs. 10-26 through 10-38).

This has proven to be a very satisfactory approach, although there was some initial trepidation about corneal changes that were were feared using the mitomycin-C after the fashioning of the wound; no such complication has been seen in over 2 years. As with any antimetabolite filtration procedure, great care must be taken to avoid conjunctival buttonholing and excessive antimetabolite leakage into the anterior chamber. In the unfortunate event that there is a ruptured posterior capsule and an anterior chamber lens implant is placed, it may be appropriate to avoid the use of an antimetabolite to minimize the chance of excessive filtration, and shallowing of the chamber, and chronic problems of a large wound incision healing. For these reasons, we elect to use the antimetabolite at the conclusion of the procedure.

Miscellaneous Combinations of Cataract and Glaucoma Surgery

Because of the proliferation of high-technology surgical devices, there are anecdotal reports of many strategies to address combined cataract and glaucoma surgery. For example, there are accounts of phacoemulsification with foldable lens implants that are performed with an adjunctive holmium full-thickness sclerostomy, either applied externally or ab interno.[487,563] Another approach is a combined phacoemulsification with lens implantation in combination with trabeculotomy ab externo.[564] Another technique has combined cataract extraction with cyclodialysis, but with failure in more than half the patients.[353] Yet another strategy is the use of separate incisional sites for both cataract extraction and trabeculectomy.[565] It is unclear whether these innovations will remain surgical oddities or in fact generate sufficiently compelling results to influence their adoption by other surgeons.

COMPLICATIONS OF INFREQUENTLY PERFORMED GLAUCOMA PROCEDURES

With the completion of our review of the many complications from laser and incisional glaucoma interventions, nearly all forms of complications and strategies for their avoidance have been touched on. The following sections simply emphasize aspects of several less common procedures in which specific kinds of complications may be encountered. They tend to differ perhaps only in frequency and intensity rather than in kind, and their management has been elaborated earlier.

Surgical Iridectomy

Surgical iridectomy as an operation performed by itself has been largely superseded with the advent of the argon and Nd:YAG lasers. There are instances, however, when surgical iridectomies are still preferred, if not needed, and the surgeon should be familiar with this particular intervention.

Among the indications for surgical iridectomy are (1) repeated closure of laser iridotomies (usually from inflammatory glaucomas); (2) inability to perform laser iridotomy because of difficulties with patient positioning (eg, age of patient, musculoskeletal disease, or inability of patient to cooperate); and (3) the need for iris biopsy.[566,567]

Without recapitulating the superbly detailed literature on the techniques of performing surgical iridectomy,[566–568] let us simply indicate some of the most common complications that are encountered. Intraoperatively, it is sometimes difficult to induce a prolapse of the iris through the limbal wound—a desirable maneuver that can forestall excessive instrumentation within the anterior chamber. Such factors that contribute to the failure of iris presentation include loss of the posterior pressure gradient (eg, intraocular pressure too low before surgery or excessively long decompression of the eye during surgery), anterior position of the incision, excessively shelved incision, preexisting anterior synechiae, and fibrosed iris.[568] Some of these circumstances can be anticipated with gonioscopy. Another consideration is the size and extent of the iridectomy that is desired; there are multiple directions in which the scissors can be applied to fashion the appropriate iridectomy shape.

The postoperative complications of iridectomy are similar to those seen after a filtration surgery. Hyphema, especially in the presence of neovascularization of the iris, or excessive traction of the ciliary body during the iridectomy can be encountered; systemic factors, such as the patient being on anticoagulants or aspirin, also may be contributory. A flat anterior chamber can be seen if there is inappropriate closure of the wound. As mentioned earlier, malignant glaucoma is more likely to manifest in eyes with chronic narrow-angle glaucoma or acute angle-closure glaucoma, which are precisely the eyes that are most likely to receive surgical iridectomy; surveillance is thus advised. The inflammatory sequelae of any intraoperative procedure, especially with a peripheral iris that may be anatomically in close conjunction to the peripheral angle, makes the complication of peripheral anterior synechiae likely and requires long-term observation.

Inadvertent touch of the lens during the procedure, from instrumentation in the anterior segment poking either through the iridectomy or through the iris, can contribute to increased risk of cataract formation. Incomplete iridectomy can lead to the recurrence of pupillary block glaucoma, necessitating either laser or repeat surgery.

Perhaps the most difficult problem to sort out in advance is how adequate the intraocular pressure control will be after surgical iridectomy. Although anterior chamber deepening and evaluation procedures have been described to assess whether the angle has been sufficiently damaged to require filtration surgery in addition to the iridectomy,[569] the true pressure status is not known until after the operation is completed. Unless there is an inadvertent formation of a filtration bleb, insufficient intraocular pressure control can be, in effect, a complication of not combining the iridectomy with a filtration procedure that is only discovered in retrospect. And finally, as with all intraoperative surgery, there is the finite risk of endophthalmitis.

Goniosynechialysis

Goniosynechialysis is a surgical technique that is used to control intraocular pressure in eyes that either have recently developed peripheral anterior synechiae or have failed to respond to surgical or laser iridectomy. Although advocated over 50 years ago, the technique was abandoned for several decades until revived with the advent of microsurgical instrumentation that prevented the more common complications of hypotony, cataracts, and cyclodialysis cleft formation.[570] The surgical technique is similar to that which can be performed with the argon laser[571] but is considerably more definitive in causing iris retraction from the angle, and in fact can even reverse peripheral anterior synechiae.

Campbell and Vela[572] revitalized the technique in their report describing four patients whose synechial angle closure was less than 1 year in duration. They used a viscoelastic agent to deepen the anterior chamber and inserted an irrigating cyclodialysis spatula to posteriorly retract the synechia and iris under direct visualization. Their positive experience was partially confirmed in a report in which the goniosynechialysis was performed as the solitary procedure in 5 of 15 eyes, with the other 10 requiring some additional procedure.[573] The surgical results were nevertheless impressive: reduction of peripheral anterior synechiae from an average of 340 to 80 degrees of the angle and a mean intraocular pressure drop of 26 mm Hg. A larger series by Tanihara and associates[574] reported 70 cases of primary angle-closure glaucoma whose intraocular pressure was elevated despite either surgical iridectomy or laser iridotomy. There was a distinct response rate depending on the lens status of the eye: 80% of aphakic eyes responded with a reduction of intraocular pressure versus only 42% of phakic eyes. Many of the phakic eyes, however, obtained good pressure control with a second goniosynechialysis combined with cataract extraction.

The most common complications from the procedure are hyphema induced at the time of the surgery, fibrinous iritis, and elevated intraocular pressure postoperatively. Other potential complications include the formation of an inadvertent cyclodialysis cleft, iris perforation, corneal damage, and cataract induction. It is a technique that is promising but needs very specific criteria for intervention: the documented progression of peripheral anterior synechiae within a relatively short time frame, paralleled by elevated intraocular pressures despite patent iridectomy.

Iridencleisis

Although iridencleisis was a popular operation in the 1940s, it has subsequently fallen into disuse because of the association with chronic iritis and possibly a genuinely higher association with sympathetic ophthalmia. Nevertheless, it has been recently described as being a useful adjunct with the classic trabeculectomy technique described by Cairns. In two series of patients (white and black African), intraocular pressure results were well over 90% with minimal complications reported.[575] It has been advocated by others as well[576] and was also found to be the most effective glaucoma procedure in the management of a large number of glaucoma cases occurring within a single family.[577]

Choroidal Drainage Procedures

The presentations of the two major forms of choroidal detachment that occur after glaucoma surgery—effusions and suprachoroidal hemorrhage—were elaborated on earlier in this chapter. These conditions can be ubiquitous after any kind of intraocular surgery, be it for cataract, glaucoma, or retinal surgery. The complications of these events are manifold: flattening of the anterior chamber with development of peripheral anterior synechiae and possible embarrassment of corneal function; failure of filtration bleb; development of cataract; and even retinal adhesions in the presence of "kissing" choroidal detachments.[135]

There are a variety of responses that are appropriate to a choroidal effusion and suprachoroidal hemorrhage. On the one hand, choroidal effusions are extraordinarily common after any lowering of intraocular pressure from filtration surgery.[114] Recurrent detachments are usually associated with ocular inflammation,[253] and these may best be managed by addressing the underlying uveitis. On the other hand, suprachoroidal hemorrhages can be ocular emergencies, requiring intervention within 2 weeks for the maximum preservation of acuity.[499]

Whether there is a need to evacuate suprachoroidal effusion fluid or hemorrhage, the surgical techniques are comparable. It is necessary both to establish a paracentesis to maintain intraocular fluid flow and to establish some access to the suprachoroidal space, using either a radial sclerotomy[135] or a small trephination placed inferiorly, which enhances the flow of suprachoroidal effusion for several hours to days after surgery.[136]

The complications of this technique can be formidable: perforation of the retina with subsequent detachment; initiation of a new hemorrhage; creation of cyclodialysis clefts anteriorly; and failure to decompress the eye, with subsequent postoperative anterior chamber shallowing and possible contribution to cataract formation. Chronic hypotony may be seen after this procedure if there is more than a simple mechanistic basis for the condition, such as chronic inflammation.

SPECIFIC OCULAR CONDITIONS WITH SPECIFIC INTERVENTIONS AND COMPLICATIONS

Nanophthalmos

Nanophthalmos refers to an isolated form of congenital microphthalmus in the absence of systemic abnormalities. It is presumably due from an arrest in embryonic development of the eye, and it has characteristic clinical features: a normal-sized crystalline lens within an eye of profoundly reduced intraocular volume; moderate to extreme hyperopia (greater than 12 diopters); reduced corneal diameters (under 10.5 mm); shallow anterior chambers (1–2 mm centrally); short axial length (14–20 mm); and thickened sclera (usually over 2 mm).[578,579] There is a high association with angle-closure glaucoma, especially in patients older than the age of 40. Because of the profound cramping of the anterior segment, it is crucial that these eyes not be dilated and that they be carefully observed for the development of angle-closure glaucoma.

Although pilocarpine may be used in the management of this condition, laser is often helpful in managing the peripheral iris by means of direct gonioplasty, as well as providing an iridotomy to prevent pupillary block. In the event of an angle-closure glaucoma or cataract that requires removal, the great fear is of the onset of nonrhegmatogenous retinal detachment from uveal effusion.

Surgical recommendations include a prophylactic sclerectomy before proceeding with any intracameral surgery. The sclera is known to be abnormally thick in these eyes, and the glaucoma may in part be due to decreased uveal scleral outflow, which the sclerotomy may help address. Along similar lines, a 4×4-mm one-half thickness scleral flap may also be fashioned, which simply reduces the overall thickness of the sclera, allowing normal transudation of fluid from the choroid in this region.

The anticipatory sclerectomy surgery often leads to the resolution of the choroidal detachment several weeks after surgery. There is a very reasonable chance that no effusion will be present if sclerectomies are done before performing cataract or glaucoma surgery.[485] There are two reports documenting the association of nanophthalmos with pseudoexfoliation as well.[485,580]

Surgical Techniques on Eyes with Enlarged Episcleral Vessels

There are many associations of glaucoma with elevated episcleral venous pressure and enlarged episcleral vessels. The most common are idiopathic, although circumstances that lead to venous obstruction (eg, thyroid ophthalmopathy, retrobulbar tumors, superior vena cava syndrome, cavernous sinus thrombosis), venous communications (orbital varices), and arterial venous communication (eg, carotid-cavernous fistula, dural shunt) are well described.

The most common condition that relates to complications of glaucoma surgery, however, is the Sturge-Weber syndrome, which is a congenital hamartomatous malformation producing hemangiomas in the skin, meninges, and eye.[581,582] Sturge-Weber glaucoma occurs in approximately 30% of eyes on the affected side, and nearly two thirds of these cases will present before the age of 2. The surgical complication rate is related to two factors: (1) the prominent vascularity of all the ocular coats, with subsequent bleeding and associated failure of glaucoma filtration; and (2) the propensity for suprachoroidal effusion; often intraoperatively, with potentially catastrophic effects. Anecdotal reports on the recurrence of choroidal effusion in patients with Sturge-Weber syndrome with a second trabeculectomy bear keeping in mind.[344] Such unfortunate events make reports of Nd:YAG goniotomy[583] or trabeculopuncture[338] well worth considering, although the results are mixed.

Before filtration surgery can be undertaken, it is important, as in nanophthalmic eyes, to perform an anticipatory sclerotomy.[581,584] Complications that have been reported include massive suprachoroidal effusion, flattening of the anterior chamber with or without lens-corneal touch; prolapse of iris into the filtration site from posterior pressure; rotation of ciliary processes in the filtering site because of vitreous pressure; vitreous loss; cataract; serious retinal detachment; hyphema; and expulsive hemorrhage.[581]

Nevertheless, in the event that surgery is required, a report on the long-term follow-up on these patients is surprisingly encouraging.[343] Thirty-six eyes with follow-up between 2 and 10 years were reported on, evaluating both medical and surgical interventions. Nearly one fourth of eyes sustained intraoperative choroidal effusion during trabeculectomy, but no effusion was seen during the performance of goniotomy or trabeculotomy. It was suggested that the sequence of minimal interventions, such as goniotomy and trabeculotomy, be attempted first before proceeding with trabeculectomy. It is unclear whether filtration with antimetabolite or glaucoma implants will be able to sustain sufficient filtration in the presence of elevated episcleral venous pressure and improve the chances for surgical success in the long term.

References

1. Watson PG, Jakeman C, Ozturk M, et al. The complications of trabeculectomy (a 20-year follow-up). Eye 1990;4(pt 3):425–438.
2. Akafo SK, Goulstine DB, Rosenthal AR. Long-term post trabeculectomy intraocular pressures. Acta Ophthalmol 1992;70:312–316.
3. Noureddin BN, Poinoosawmy D, Fietzke FW, et al. Regression analysis of visual field progression in low tension glaucoma. Br J Ophthalmol 1991;75:493–495.
4. Werner EB, Drance SB. Progression of glaucomatous field defects despite successful filtration. Can J Ophthalmol 1977;12:275–280.
5. Werner EB, Drance SM, Schulzer M. Trabeculectomy and the progression of glaucomatous field loss. Arch Ophthalmol 1977;95:1374–1377.
6. Kidd MN, O'Connor M. Progression of field loss after trabeculectomy: a five-year follow-up. Br J Ophthalmol 1985;69:827–831.
7. Veldman E, Greve EL. Glaucoma filtering surgery, a retrospective study of 300 operations. Doc Ophthalmol 1987;67:151–170.
8. Chauhan BC, Drance SM. The relationship between intraocular pressure and visual field progression in glaucoma. Graefes Arch Clin Exp Ophthalmol 1992;230:521–526.
9. Abedin S, Simmons R, Grant W. Progressive low-tension glaucoma: treatment to stop glaucomatous cupping and field loss when these progress despite normal intraocular pressure. Ophthalmology 1982;89: 1–6.
10. Shirakashi M, Iwata K, Sawaguchi S, et al. Intraocular pressure-dependent progression of visual field loss in advanced primary open-angle glaucoma: a 15-year follow-up. Ophthalmologica 1993;207:1–5.
11. Odberg T. Visual field prognosis in advanced glaucoma. Acta Ophtalmologica 1987;65:27–29.
12. Mao L, Stewart W, Shields M. Correlation between intraocular pressure control and progressive glaucomatous damage in primary open-angle glaucoma. Am J Ophthalmol 1991;111:51–55.
13. Grant WM, Burton JF. Why do some people go blind after glaucoma? Ophthalmology 1982;89:991–998.
14. Spaeth GL. The effect of change in intraocular pressure on the natural history of glaucoma: lowering the intraocular pressure in glaucoma can result in improvement of the visual fields. Trans Ophthalmol Soc UK 1985;104:256–263.
15. Yildrim E, Bilge A, Leker S. Improvement of the visual field following trabeculecomy for open angle glaucoma. Eye 1990;4:103–106.
16. Kolker A. Visual prognosis in advanced glaucoma: a

comparison of medical and surgical therapy for retention of vision in 101 eyes with advanced glaucoma. Trans Am Ophthalmol Soc 1977;75:539.

17. Langerhorst CT, de Clercq B, van den Berg TJ. Visual field behavior after intra-ocular surgery in glaucoma patients with advanced defects. Doc Ophthalmol 1990;75:281–289.
18. Martinez JA, Brown RH, Lynch MG, et al. Risk of postoperative visual loss in advanced glaucoma. Am J Ophthalmol 1993;115:332–337.
19. Zeimer RC, Wilensky JT, Gieser DK, et al. Association between intraocular pressure peaks and progression of visual field loss. (Comments) Ophthalmology 1991;98:64–69.
20. Saiz A, Maquet JA, Pinon R. Reduced variation of the diurnal curve after the subscleral Scheie procedure for primary open-angle glaucoma. Ann Ophthalmol 1993;25:16–19.
21. Saiz A, et al. Pressure-curve variations after trabeculectomy for chronic primary open-angle glaucoma. Ophthalmic Surg 1990;21:799–801.
22. Miller E, Caprioli J. The basis for surgical treatment of open-angle glaucoma. In: Caprioli J, ed. Contemporary issues in glaucoma. Philadelphia, WB Saunders, 1991:839–851.
23. Katz J, Spaeth G, Cantor L. Reversible optic disc cupping and visual field improvement in adult patients with glaucoma. Am J Ophthalmol 1989;107:485–492.
24. Shin D, M B, Hong Y. Reversal of glaucomatous cupping optic disc cupping in adult patients. Arch Ophthalmol 1989;107:1599–1603.
25. Funk J. Increase of neuroretinal rim area after surgical intraocular pressure reduction. Ophthalmic Surg 1990;21:585–588.
26. D'Ermo F, Bonomi L, Doro D. A critical analysis of the long-term results of trabeculectomy. Am J Ophthalmol 1979;88:829–835.
27. Lamping KA, et al. Long-term evaluation of initial filtration surgery. Ophthalmology 1986;93:91–101.
28. Belcher CD III. Filtering operations: an overview. In: Thomas JV, Belcher CD, Simmons RJ, eds. Glaucoma surgery. St. Louis, Mosby–Year Book, 1992:17–25.
29. Thomas JV. Filtering operation with scleral flap. In: Thomas JV, Belcher CD, Simmons RJ, eds. Glaucoma surgery. St. Louis, Mosby–Year Book, 1992:27–56.
30. Thomas JV. Filtering operation without scleral flap. In: Thomas JV, Belcher CD, Simmons RJ, eds. Glaucoma surgery. St. Louis, Mosby–Year Book, 1992:57–60.
31. Hitchings RA. Full-thickness versus guarded procedures. In: Sherwood MB, Spaeth GL, eds. Complications of glaucoma surgery. Thorofare, NJ, Slack, 1990:169–176.
32. Savage JA. Glaucoma filtration surgery. In: Higginbotham EJ, Lee DA, eds. Management of difficult glaucomas: a clinician's guide. Boston, Blackwell Scientific, 1994:325–391.
33. Blondeau P, Phelps C. Trabeculectomy and thermal sclerostomy. Arch Ophthalmol 1981;99:810–816.
34. Lewis RA, Phelps CD. Trabeculectomy v thermosclerostomy: a five-year follow-up. Arch Ophthalmol 1984;102:533–536.
35. Spaeth G, Poryzees E. A comparison between peripheral iridectomy with thermal sclerostomy and trabeculectomy: a controlled study. Br J Ophthalmol 1981;65:783–789.
36. Watkins PJ, Brubaker R. Comparison of partial thickness and full thickness filtration procedures in open angle glaucoma. Am J Ophthalmol 1978;86:756–761.
37. Hutchinson BT, Robert BA. Glaucoma filtration surgery. In: Krupin T, Wax MB, eds. New techniques in glaucoma surgery. Philadelphia, WB Saunders, 1988:181–186.
38. Shingleton BJ, Distler JA, Baker BH. Filtration surgery in black patients: early results in a West Indian population. Ophthalmic Surg 1987;18:195–199.
39. Wilson MR. Posterior lip sclerectomy vs trabeculectomy in West Indian blacks. Arch Ophthalmol 1989;107:1604–1608.
40. Johnstone MA, Wellington DP, Ziel CJ. A releasable scleral-flap tamponade suture for guarded filtration surgery. Arch Ophthalmol 1993;111:398–403.
41. Cohen JS, Osher RH. Releasable scleral flap suture. In: Krupin T, Wax MB, eds. New techniques in glaucoma surgery. Philadelphia, WB Saunders, 1988: 187–197.
42. Wilson RP. Releasable sutures in filtration surgery. In: Sherwood MB, Spaeth GL, eds. Complications of glaucoma surgery. Thorofare, NJ, Slack, 1990:199–209.
43. Lieberman M. Suture lysis by laser and goniolens. (Letter) Am J Ophthalmol 1983;95:257.
44. Hoskins H Jr, Migliazzo C. Management of failing filtering blebs with the argon laser. Ophthalmic Surg 1984;15:731–733.
45. Savage JA, et al. Laser suture lysis after trabeculectomy. Ophthalmology 1988;95:1631–1638.
46. Melamed S, et al. Tight scleral flap trabeculectomy with postoperative laser suture lysis. (Comments) Am J Ophthalmol 1990;109:303–309.
47. Pappas K, et al. Late argon suture lysis after mitomycin C trabeculectomy. Ophthalmology 1993;100: 1268–1271.
48. Iwach A, et al. Subconjunctival THC:YAG ("holmium") laser thermal sclerostomy ab externo. Ophthalmology 1993;100:356–365.
49. Lederer CM Jr, Thomas JV. Laser surgery for glau-

coma. In: Thomas JV, Belcher CD, Simmons RJ, eds. Glaucoma surgery. St. Louis, Mosby–Year Book, 1992:157–194.
50. Wong V, et al. Late detachment of Descemet's membrane after subconjunctival THC:YAG laser thermal sclerostomy ab externo. Am J Ophthalmol 1993; 116:514–515.
51. Brown RH, et al. Internal sclerectomy with an automated trephine for advanced glaucoma. Ophthalmology 1988;95:728–734.
52. Brown RH, et al. Internal sclerectomy for glaucoma filtering surgery with an automated trephine. Arch Ophthalmol 1987;105:133–136.
53. Chen CW, et al. Trabeculectomy with simultaneous topical application of mitomycin-C in refractory glaucoma. J Ocul Pharmacol 1990;6:175–182.
54. Kitazawa Y, et al. Trabeculectomy with mitomycin: a comparative study with fluorouracil. Arch Ophthalmol 1991;109:1693–1698.
55. Zimmerman TJ, et al. Effectiveness of nonpenetrating trabeculectomy in aphakic patients with glaucoma. Ophthalmic Surg 1984;15:44–50.
56. Zimmerman TJ, et al. Trabeculectomy vs. nonpenetrating trabeculectomy: a retrospective study of two procedures in phakic patients with glaucoma. Ophthalmic Surg 1984;15:734–740.
57. Skjaerpe F. Selective trabeculectomy: a report of a new surgical method for open angle glaucoma. Acta Ophthalmol 1983;61:714–727.
58. Van Buskirk EM. Trabeculectomy without conjunctival incision. Am J Ophthalmol 1992;113:145–153.
59. Migdal C, Hitchings R. Control of chronic simple glaucoma with primary medical, surgical and laser treatment. Trans Ophthalmol Soc UK 1986;105:653–656.
60. Migdal C. Rational choice of therapy in established open angle glaucoma. Eye 1992;6:346–347.
61. Jay JL, Murray S. Early trabeculectomy versus conventional management in primary open angle glaucoma. Br J Ophthalmol 1988;72:881–889.
62. Jay JL, Allan D. The benefits of early trabeculectomy versus conventional management in primary open angle glaucoma relative to severity of disease. Eye 1989;3:528–535.
63. Jay JL. Rational choice of therapy in primary open angle glaucoma. Eye 1992;6:243–247.
64. Sherwood MB, et al. Long-term morphologic effects of antiglaucoma drugs on the conjunctiva and Tenon's capsule in glaucomatous patients. Ophthalmology 1989;96:327–335.
65. Gwynn D, et al. Conjunctival structure and cell counts and the results of filtering surgery. Am J Ophthalmol 1993;116:464–468.
66. Gressel M, Heuer D, Parrish R II. Trabeculectomy in young patients. Ophthalmology 1984;91:1242–1246.
67. Levene RZ. Glaucoma filtering surgery: factors that determine pressure control. Ophthalmic Surg 1984; 15:475–483.
68. Miller R, Barber J. Trabeculectomy in black patients. Ophthalmic Surg 1981;12:46–50.
69. Bellows AR, Johnstone MA. Surgical management of chronic glaucoma in aphakia. Ophthalmology 1983;90:807–813.
70. Gross RL, et al. Surgical therapy of chronic glaucoma in aphakia and pseudophakia. Ophthalmology 1988;95:1195–1201.
71. Gilvarry AM, et al. The management of post-keratoplasty glaucoma by trabeculectomy. Eye 1989;3:713–718.
72. Lee P, Allingham R, McDonnell P. Penetrating keratoplasty and glaucoma. In: Albert DM, Jakobiec FA, eds. Principles and practice of ophthalmology. Philadelphia, WB Saunders, 1993:1541–1551.
73. Yaldo MK, Lieberman MF. The management of secondary glaucoma in the uveitis patient. Ophthalmol Clin North Am 1993;6:147–157.
74. Marsh RJ, Cooper M. Ocular surgery in ophthalmic zoster. Eye 1989;3:313–317.
75. Kanski JJ. Juvenile arthritis and uveitis. Surv Ophthalmol 1990;34:253–267.
76. Jones NP. Glaucoma in Fuchs' heterochromic uveitis: aetiology, management and outcome. Eye 1991;5:662–667.
77. Brooks AM, Gillies WE. The presentation and prognosis of glaucoma in pseudoexfoliation of the lens capsule. Ophthalmology 1988;95:271–276.
78. Farrar SM, et al. Risk factors for the development and severity of glaucoma in the pigment dispersion syndrome. Am J Ophthalmol 1989;108:223–229.
79. Katz LJ, Spaeth GL. Surgical management of the secondary glaucomas: I. Ophthalmic Surg 1987;18:826–834.
80. Fernandez-Vigo J, et al. Treatment of diabetic neovascular glaucoma by panretinal ablation and trabeculectomy. Acta Ophthalmol 1988;66:612–616.
81. Kidd M, Hetherington J, Magee S. Surgical results in iridocorneal endothelial syndrome. Arch Ophthalmol 1988;106:199–201.
82. Brincker P, Kessing SV. Limbus-based versus fornix-based conjunctival flap in glaucoma filtering surgery. Acta Ophthalmol 1992;70:641–644.
83. Khan AM, Jilani FA. Comparative results of limbal based versus fornix based conjunctival flaps for trabeculectomy. Indian J Ophthalmol 1992;40(2):41–43.
84. Grehn F, Mauthe S, Pfeiffer N. Limbus-based versus fornix-based conjunctival flap in filtering surgery: a randomized prospective study. Int Ophthalmol 1989;13:139–143.
85. Traverso CE, Tomey KF, Antonios S. Limbal- vs

fornix-based conjunctival trabeculectomy flaps. Am J Ophthalmol 1987;104:28–32.
86. Pfeiffer N, Grehn F. Improved suture for fornix-based conjunctival flap in filtering surgery. Int Ophthalmol 1992;16:391–396.
87. Liss RP, Scholes GN, Crandall AS. Glaucoma filtration surgery: new horizontal mattress closure of conjunctival incision. Ophthalmic Surg 1991;22:298–300.
88. Shuster JN, et al. Limbus- v fornix-based conjunctival flap in trabeculectomy: a long-term randomized study. Arch Ophthalmol 1984;102:361–362.
89. Spaeth GL. Management of conjunctival buttonholes. In: Sherwood MB, Spaeth GL, eds. Complications of glaucoma surgery. Thorofare, NJ, Slack, 1990:211–222.
90. Starita RJ, et al. Effect of varying size of scleral flap and corneal block on trabeculectomy. Ophthalmic Surg 1984;15:484–487.
91. Spaeth GL. Difficulties with the scleral flap in trabeculectomy. In: Sherwood MB, Spaeth GL, eds. Complications of glaucoma surgery. Thorofare, NJ, Slack, 1990;223–227.
92. Wilson RP. The use of the Simmons shell tamponade technique and attendant complications. In: Sherwood MB, Spaeth GL, eds. Complications of glaucoma surgery. Thorofare, NJ, Slack, 1990:189–197.
93. Spurny RC, Thomas JV, Simmons RJ. Shell tamponade technique. In: Thomas JV, Belcher CD, Simmons RJ, eds. Glaucoma surgery. St. Louis, Mosby–Year Book, 1992:61–73.
94. Hill RA, et al. Use of a symblepharon ring for treatment of overfiltration and leaking blebs after glaucoma filtration surgery. Ophthalmic Surg 1990;21:707–710.
95. Savage JA, Simmons RJ. Coaxial radio frequency (RF) diathermy in anterior segment surgery. Ophthalmic Surg 1985;16:333–336.
96. Cantor LB, Katz LJ, Spaeth GL. Complications of surgery in glaucoma: suprachoroidal expulsive hemorrhage in glaucoma patients undergoing intraocular surgery. Ophthalmology 1985;92:1266–1270.
97. Davison JA. Acute intraoperative suprachoroidal hemorrhage in extracapsular cataract surgery. J Cataract Refract Surg 1986;12:606–622.
98. Maumenee AE, Schwartz MF. Acute intraoperative choroidal effusion. Am J Ophthalmol 1985;100:147–154.
99. Katz LJ. Cataract formation following filtering surgery. In: Sherwood MB, Spaeth GL, eds. Complications of glaucoma surgery. Thorofare, NJ, Slack, 1990:301–305.
100. Swann K, Lindgren T. Unintentional lens injury in glaucoma surgery. Trans Am Ophthalmol Soc 1980;78:55–69.
101. Raitta C, Vesti E. The effect of sodium hyaluronate on the outcome of trabeculectomy. Ophthalmic Surg 1991;22:145–149.
102. Beauchamps G, Parks M. Filtering surgery in children: Barriers to success. Ophthalmology 1979; 86:170.
103. Gressel MG, Parrish RK II, Folberg R. 5-Fluorouracil and glaucoma filtering surgery: I. An animal model. Ophthalmology 1984;91:378–383.
104. Heuer DK, et al. 5-Fluorouracil and glaucoma filtering surgery: II. A pilot study. Ophthalmology 1984; 91:384–394.
105. Heuer DK, et al. 5-Fluorouracil and glaucoma filtering surgery: III. Intermediate follow-up of a pilot study. Ophthalmology 1986;93:1537–1546.
106. Palmer S. Mitomycin as adjunct chemotherapy with trabeculectomy. Ophthalmology 1991;98:317–321.
107. Skuta G, et al. Introperative mitomycin vs. post-operative 5-fluorouracil in high risk glaucoma filtering surgery. Ophthalmology 1992;99:438–444.
108. Deuker DK, Higginbotham E. Pharmacologic modulation of filtration surgery wound healing. In: Higginbotham EJ, Lee DA, eds. Management of difficult glaucomas: a clinician's guide. Boston, Blackwell Scientific 1994:414–427.
109. Wand M. Minimizing conjunctival wound leaks in filtration surgery with mitomycin-C. Ophthalmic Surg 1993;24:708–709.
110. Kawase K, et al. Anterior chamber reaction after mitomycin and 5-fluorouracil trabeculectomy: a comparative study. Ophthalmic Surg 1993;24:24–27.
111. Rader JR, Parrish RK II. Update on adjunctive antimetabolites in glaucoma surgery. In: Caprioli J, ed. Contemporary issues in glaucoma. Philadelphia, WB Saunders, 1991:861–888.
112. Smith MF, et al. Results of intraoperative 5-fluorouracil supplementation on trabeculectomy for open-angle glaucoma. Am J Ophthalmol 1992;114:737–741.
113. Herschler J. Long-term results of trabeculectomy with collagen sponge implant containing low-dose antimetabolite. Ophthalmology 1992;99:666–670.
114. Migdal C, Hitchings R. Morbidity following prolonged postoperative hypotony after trabeculectomy. Ophthalmic Surg 1988;19:865–867.
115. Spaeth GL. Complications of glaucoma surgery. In: Spaeth GL, ed. Ophthalmic surgery: principles & practice, ed 2. Philadelphia, WB Saunders, 1990: 334–353.
116. Spaeth GL. Flat anterior chamber. In: Sherwood MB, Spaeth GL, eds. Complications of glaucoma surgery. Thorofare, NJ, Slack, 1990:229–236.
117. Smith DL, et al. The effect of glaucoma filtering surgery on corneal endothelial cell density. Ophthalmic Surg 1991;22:251–255.
118. Fiore PM, et al. The effect of anterior chamber depth

on endothelial cell count after filtration surgery. Arch Ophthalmol 1989;107:1609–1611.

119. Fourman S. Management of cornea-lens touch after filtering surgery for glaucoma. (Comments) Ophthalmology 1990;97:424–428.
120. Varma R, Spaeth GL, Nicholl J. Detection of conjunctival leaks following filtration surgery. (Letter) Ophthalmic Surg 1988;19:293–294.
121. Blok MD, et al. Use of the Megasoft Bandage Lens for treatment of complications after trabeculectomy. Am J Ophthalmol 1990;110:264–268.
122. Simmons RJ, Omah S. Shell tamponade technique in glaucoma surgery. In: Symposium on glaucoma: transactions of the New Orleans Academy of Ophthalmology. St. Louis, CV Mosby, 1981:266–267.
123. Melamed S, et al. The use of glaucoma shell tamponade in leaking filtration blebs. Ophthalmology 1986;93:839–842.
124. Ruderman JM, Allen RC. Simmons' tamponade shell for leaking filtration blebs. Arch Ophthalmol 1985; 103:1708–1710.
125. Joiner DW, Liebmann JM, Ritch R. A modification of the use of the glaucoma tamponade shell. Ophthalmic Surg 1989;20:441–442.
126. Rajeev B, Thomas R. Corneal hazards in use of Simmons shell. (Comments) Aust NZ J Ophthalmol 1991;19:145–148.
127. Hennis HL, Stewart WC. Use of the argon laser to close filtering bleb leaks. Graefes Arch Clin Exp Ophthalmol 1992;230:537–541.
128. Zalta AH, Wieder RH. Closure of leaking filtering blebs with cyanoacrylate tissue adhesive. Br J Ophthalmol 1991;75:170–173.
129. Bellows AR. Complications of filtering surgery. In: Albert DM, Jakobiec FA, eds. Principles and practice of ophthalmology. Philadelphia, WB Saunders, 1993: 1646–1655.
130. O'Connor DJ, Tressler CS, Caprioli J. A surgical method to repair leaking filtering blebs. Ophthalmic Surg 1992;23:336–338.
131. Van Buskirk E. Assessment and management of filtering blebs. In: Mills R, Weinreb R, eds. Glaucoma surgical skills: Ophthalmology Monographs 4. San Francisco, American Academy of Ophthalmology, 1991:99–116.
132. Lavin M, Franks W, Hitchings RA. Serous retinal detachment following glaucoma filtering surgery. Arch Ophthalmol 1990;108:1553–1555.
133. Laatikainen L, Syrdalen P. Tearing of retinal pigment epithelium after glaucoma surgery. Graefes Arch Clin Exp Ophthalmol 1987;225:308–310.
134. Bellows A, Chylack L, Hutchinson B. Choroidal detachment: clinical manifestations, therapy, and mechanisms of formation. Ophthalmology 1981; 88:1107–1115.
135. Spurny RC, Thomas JV. Choroidal tap and anterior chamber reformation. In: Thomas JV, Belcher CD, Simmons RJ, eds. Glaucoma surgery. St. Louis, Mosby–Year Book, 1992:205–214.
136. Dellaporta A. Scleral trephination for subchoroidal effusion. Arch Ophthalmol 1983;101:1917–1919.
137. Vela MA, Campbell DG. Hypotony and ciliochoroidal detachment following pharmacologic aqueous suppressant therapy in previously filtered patients. Ophthalmology 1985;92:50–57.
138. Liebmann JM, et al. Early intraocular pressure rise after trabeculectomy. Arch Ophthalmol 1990;108: 1549–1552.
139. Szymanski A. Promotion of glaucoma filter bleb with tissue plasminogen activator after sclerectomy under a clot. Int Ophthalmol 1992;16:387–390.
140. Barak A, et al. The protective effect of early intraoperative injection of viscoelastic material in trabeculectomy. Ophthalmic Surg 1992;23:206–209.
141. Draeger J, Winter R, Wirt H. Viscoelastic glaucoma surgery. Trans Ophthalmol Soc UK 1983;103:270–273.
142. Yamashita H, et al. Trabeculectomy: a prospective study of complications and results of long-term follow-up. Jpn J Ophthalmol 1985;29:250–262.
143. Alpar JJ. Sodium hyaluronate (Healon) in glaucoma filtering procedures. Ophthalmic Surg 1986;17:724–730.
144. Raitta C, Setala K. Trabeculectomy with the use of sodium hyaluronate: a prospective study. Acta Ophthalmol 1986;64:407–413.
145. Wilson RP, Lloyd J. The place of sodium hyaluronate in glaucoma surgery. Ophthalmic Surg 1986;17:30–33.
146. Shrader CE, et al. Pupillary and iridovitreal block in pseudophakic eyes. Ophthalmology 1984;91:831–837.
147. Frenkel RE, Shin DH. Prevention and management of delayed suprachoroidal hemorrhage after filtration surgery. Arch Ophthalmol 1986;104:1459–1463.
148. Canning CR, et al. Delayed suprachoroidal haemorrhage after glaucoma operations. Eye 1989;3:327–331.
149. Givens K, Shields MB. Suprachoroidal hemorrhage after glaucoma filtering surgery. Am J Ophthalmol 1987;103:689–694.
150. Fluorouracil Filtering Surgery Study Group. Risk factors for suprachoroidal hemorrhage after filtering surgery. Am J Ophthalmol 1992;113:501–507.
151. Speaker MG, et al. A case-control study of risk factors for intraoperative suprachoroidal expulsive hemorrhage. Ophthalmology 1991;98:202–209.
152. Gressel MG, Parrish RK II, Heuer DK. Delayed nonexpulsive suprachoroidal hemorrhage. Arch Ophthalmol 1984;102:1757–1760.

153. Abrams GW, et al. Management of postoperative suprachoroidal hemorrhage with continuous-infusion air pump. Arch Ophthalmol 1986;104:1455–1458.
154. Lieberman MF. Diagnosis and management of malignant glaucoma. In: Higginbotham EJ, Lee DA, eds. Management of difficult glaucomas: a clinician's guide. Boston, Blackwell Scientific, 1994:183–194.
155. Fourman S. Angle-closure glaucoma complicating ciliochoroidal detachment. Ophthalmology 1989;96: 646–653.
156. Karim F, et al. Mechanisms of pupillary block: in reply. Arch Ophthalmol 1988;106:167.
157. Epstein DL, et al. Experimental perfusions through the anterior and vitreous chambers with possible relationships to malignant glaucoma. Am J Ophthalmol 1979;88:1078–1086.
158. Quigley HA. Malignant glaucoma and fluid flow rate. Am J Ophthalmol 1980;89:879–880.
159. Di Sclafani M, Liebmann JM, Ritch R. Malignant glaucoma following argon laser release of scleral flap sutures after trabeculectomy. Am J Ophthalmol 1989;108:597–598.
160. Weder W, Lissel U, Stoltzing M. Complications and results after trabeculotomy. Dev Ophthalmol 1987; 13:78–84.
161. Fourman S. "Malignant" glaucoma post laser iridotomy. (Letter) Ophthalmology 1992;99:1751–1752.
162. Brooks AM, Harper CA, Gillies WE. Occurrence of malignant glaucoma after laser iridotomy. (Comments) Br J Ophthalmol 1989;73:617–620.
163. Geyer O, Rothkoff L, Lazar M. Malignant glaucoma after laser iridectomy. (Letter; comment) Br J Ophthalmol 1990;74:576.
164. Robinson A, et al. The onset of malignant glaucoma after prophylactic laser iridotomy. Am J Ophthalmol 1990;110:95–96.
165. Luntz MH, Rosenblatt M. Malignant glaucoma. Surv Ophthalmol 1987;32:73–93.
166. Simmons RJ, Thomas JV, Yaqub MK. Malignant glaucoma. In: Ritch R, Shields MB, Krupin T, eds. The glaucomas. St. Louis, CV Mosby, 1989:1251–1263.
167. Simmons RJ, Thomas JV. Surgical therapy of malignant glaucoma. In: Thomas JV, Belcher CD, Simmons RJ, eds. Glaucoma surgery. St. Louis, Mosby–Year Book, 1992:251–260.
168. Lynch MG, et al. Surgical vitrectomy for pseudophakic malignant glaucoma. Am J Ophthalmol 1986; 102:149–153.
169. Epstein DL, Steinert RF, Puliafito CA. Neodymium-YAG laser therapy to the anterior hyaloid in aphakic malignant (ciliovitreal block) glaucoma. Am J Ophthalmol 1984;98:137–143.
170. Halkias A, Magauran D, Joyce M. Ciliary block (malignant) glaucoma after cataract extraction with lens implant treated with YAG laser capsulotomy and anterior hyaloidotomy. Br J Ophthalmol 1992;76:569–570.
171. Brown RH, et al. Neodymium-YAG vitreous surgery for phakic and pseudophakic malignant glaucoma. Arch Ophthalmol 1986;104:1464–1466.
172. Skuta GL, Parrish RK II. Wound healing in glaucoma filtering surgery. Surv Ophthalmol 1987;32:149–170.
173. Starita RJ, et al. Short- and long-term effects of postoperative corticosteroids on trabeculectomy. Ophthalmology 1985;92:938–946.
174. Ball SF. Corticosteroids, including subconjunctival triamcinolone, in glaucoma filtering surgery. In: Krupin T, Wax MB, eds. New techniques in glaucoma surgery. Philadelphia, WB Saunders, 1988;143–155.
175. Rockwood EJ, et al. Glaucoma filtering surgery with 5-fluorouracil. Ophthalmology 1987;94:1071–1078.
176. Ruderman JM, et al. A randomized study of 5-fluorouracil and filtration surgery. Am J Ophthalmol 1987;104:218–224.
177. Ruderman JM, et al. A prospective, randomized study of 5-fluorouracil and filtration surgery. Trans Am Ophthalmol Soc 1987;85:238–253.
178. Liebmann JM, et al. Initial 5-fluorouracil trabeculectomy in uncomplicated glaucoma. (Comments) Ophthalmology 1991;98:1036–1041.
179. Kitazawa Y, et al. 5-Fluorouracil for trabeculectomy in glaucoma. Graefes Arch Clin Exp Ophthalmol 1987;225:403–405.
180. Taniguchi T, Kitazawa Y, Shimizu U. Long-term results of 5-fluorouracil trabeculectomy for primary open-angle glaucoma. Int Ophthalmol 1989;13:145–149.
181. Ophir A, Ticho U. Filtering surgery with 5-fluorouracil: a second course. Eye 1990;4:819–822.
182. Ophir A, Ticho U. Trabeculectomy with 5-fluorouracil subsequent to circular buckling operation and cataract extraction. Ann Ophthalmol 1992;24:386–390.
183. Ophir A, Ticho U. A randomized study of trabeculectomy and subconjunctival administration of fluorouracil in primary glaucomas. Arch Ophthalmol 1992;110:1072–1075.
184. Araie M, et al. Postoperative subconjunctival 5-fluorouracil injections and success probability of trabeculectomy in Japanese: results of 5-year follow-up. Jpn J Ophthalmol 1992;36:158–168.
185. Wilson RP, Steinmann WC. Use of trabeculectomy with postoperative 5-fluorouracil in patients requiring extremely low intraocular pressure levels to limit further glaucoma progression. Ophthalmology 1991; 98:1047–1052.
186. Weinreb RN. Adjusting the dose of 5-fluorouracil after filtration surgery to minimize side effects. Ophthalmology 1987;94:564–570.
187. Rabowsky JH, Ruderman JM. Low-dose 5-fluorouracil and glaucoma filtration surgery. Ophthalmic Surg 1989;20:347–349.
188. Krug J Jr, Melamed S. Adjunctive use of delayed and

adjustable low-dose 5-fluorouracil in refractory glaucoma. Am J Ophthalmol 1990;109:412–418.

189. Ewing RH, Stamper RL. Needle revision with and without 5-fluorouracil for the treatment of failed filtering blebs. Am J Ophthalmol 1990;110:254–259.
190. Loane ME, Weinreb RN. Reducing corneal toxicity of 5-fluorouracil in the early postoperative period following glaucoma filtering surgery. (Comments) Aust NZ J Ophthalmol 1991;19:197–202.
191. Beckman RL, et al. Bandage contact lens augmentation of 5-fluorouracil treatment in glaucoma filtration surgery. Ophthalmic Surg 1991;22:563–564.
192. Peterson M, et al. Striate melanokeratosis following trabeculectomy with 5-fluorouracil. Arch Ophthalmol 1990;108:216.
193. Knapp A, et al. Serious corneal complications of glaucoma filtering surgery with postoperative 5-fluorouracil. Am J Ophthalmol 1987;103:183–187.
194. Patitsas CJ, et al. Glaucoma filtering surgery with postoperative 5-fluorouracil in patients with intraocular inflammatory disease. Ophthalmology 1992; 99:594–599.
195. Jampel HD, Jabs DA, Quigley HA. Trabeculectomy with 5-fluorouracil for adult inflammatory glaucoma. Am J Ophthalmol 1990;109:168–173.
196. Ophir A, Ticho U. Subconjunctival 5-fluorouracil and herpes simplex keratitis. Ophthalmic Surg 1991;22: 109–110.
197. Zalish M, Leiba H, Oliver M. Subconjunctival injection of 5-fluorouracil following trabeculectomy for congenital and infantile glaucoma. Ophthalmic Surg 1992;23:203–205.
198. Whiteside-Michel J, Liebmann JM, Ritch R. Initial 5-fluorouracil trabeculectomy in young patients. Ophthalmology 1992;99:7–13.
199. Cohen JS. Combined cataract implant and filtering surgery with 5-fluorouracil. Ophthalmic Surg 1990; 21:181–186.
200. Wright MM, et al. 5-Fluorouracil after trabeculectomy and the iridocorneal endothelial syndrome. Ophthalmology 1991;98:314–316.
201. Watanabe J, et al. Trabeculectomy with 5-fluorouracil. Acta Ophthalmol 1991;69:455–461.
202. Dellaporta A. Fundus changes in post-operative hypotony. Am J Ophthalmol 1955;40:781–785.
203. Detry-Morel M, Kittel B. Surface-wrinkling maculopathy as a potential complication of trabeculectomy: a case report. Ophthalmic Surg 1991;22:38.
204. Stamper RL, Mcmenemy MG, Lieberman MF. Hypotonous maculopathy after trabeculectomy with subconjunctival 5-fluorouracil. Am J Ophthalmol 1992; 114:544–553.
205. Nemeth J, Horoczi Z. Changes in the ocular dimensions after trabeculectomy. Int Ophthalmol 1992;16: 355–357.
206. Jampel HD, Pasquale LR, Dibernardero C. Hypotony maculopathy following trabeculectomy with mitomycin-C. (Letter) Arch Ophthalmol 1992;110:1049–1050.
207. Costa V, et al. Hypotony maculopathy following the use of topical mitomycin C in glaucoma filtration surgery. Ophthalmic Surg 1993;24:389–394.
208. Zacharia P, Deppermann S, Schuman J. Ocular hypotony after trabeculecetomy with mitomycin C. Am J Ophthalmol 1993;116:314–326.
209. Chen C. Enhanced intraocular pressure controlling effectiveness of trabeculectomy by local application of mitomycin-C. Trans Asia Pacif Acad Ophthalmol 1983;9:172.
210. Geijssen HC, Greve EL. Mitomycin-C, suture lysis and hypotony. Int Ophthalmol 1992;16:371–374.
211. Jampel H. Effect of brief exposure to mitomycin-C on viability and proliferation of cultured human Tenon's capsule fibroblasts. Ophthalmology 1992;99:1471–1476.
212. Yaldo M, Stamper R. Long-term effects of mitomycin on filtering blebs: lack of fibrovascular proliferative response following severe inflammation. Arch Ophthalmol 1993;111:824–826.
213. Keller C, To K. Bleb leak with hypotony after laser suture lysis and trabeculectomy with mitomycin. (Letter) Arch Ophthalmol 1993;111:427–428.
214. Schwartz AL, Weiss H. Bleb leak with hypotony after laser suture lysis and trabeculectomy with mitomycin-C. Arch Ophthalmol 1992;110:1049.
215. Cleasby G, Fung W, Webster R. Cryosurgical closure of filtering blebs. Arch Ophthalmol 1972;84:319.
216. Kirk H. Cauterization of filtering blebs following cataract extraction. Trans Am Acad Ophthalmol Otolaryngol 1973;77:573.
217. Gehring J, Ciccarelli E. Trichloroacetic acid treatment of filtering blebs following cataract extraction. Am J Ophthalmol 1972;74:662.
218. Fink AJ, Boys-Smith JW, Brear R. Management of large filtering blebs with the argon laser. Am J Ophthalmol 1986;101:695–699.
219. Maumenee A. External filtering operations for glaucoma: Mechanisms of function and failure. Trans Am Ophthalmol Soc 1960;58:319.
220. Katz LJ. Blockage of internal sclerostomy. In: Sherwood MB, Spaeth GL, eds. Complications of glaucoma surgery. Thorofare, NJ, Slack, 1990:277–281.
221. Swan K. Reopening of non-functioning filters: simplified surgical techniques. Trans Am Acad Ophthalmol 1975;79:342–348.
222. Sofinski S, Thomas JV, Simmons RJ. Filtering bleb revision techniques. In: Thomas JV, Belcher CD, Simmons RJ, eds. Glaucoma surgery. St. Louis, Mosby–Year Book, 1992:75–82.
223. Ticho U, Ivry M. Reopening of occluded filtering blebs by argon laser photocoagulation. Am J Ophthalmol 1977;84:413.

224. Van Buskirk E. Reopening filtration fistulas with the argon laser. Am J Ophthalmol 1982;94:1–3.
225. Kurata F, Krupin T, Kolker AE. Reopening filtration fistulas with transconjunctival argon laser photocoagulation. Am J Ophthalmol 1984;98:340–343.
226. Latina MA, Rankin GA. Internal and transconjunctival neodymium:YAG laser revision of late failing filters. Ophthalmology 1991;98:215–221.
227. Cohn HC, Whalen WR, Aron-Rosa D. YAG laser treatment in a series of failed trabeculectomies. Am J Ophthalmol 1989;108:395–403.
228. Rankin GA, Latina MA. Transconjunctival Nd:YAG laser revision of failing trabeculectomy. Ophthalmic Surg 1990;21:365–367.
229. Dailey RA, Samples JR, Van Buskirk EM. Reopening filtration fistulas with the neodymium-YAG laser. Am J Ophthalmol 1986;102:491–495.
230. Prywes AS, Lo Pinto RJ. Temporary visual loss with ciliary body detachment and hypotony after attempted YAG laser repair of failed filtering surgery. Am J Ophthalmol 1986;101:305–307.
231. Praeger DL. The reopening of closed filtering blebs using the neodymium:YAG laser. Ophthalmology 1984;91:373–377.
232. Yablonski M, et al. Use of therapeutic ultrasound to restore failed trabeculectomies. Am J Ophthalmol 1987;103:492–496.
233. Valtot F, Kopel J, Haut J. Treatment of glaucoma with high intensity focused ultrasound. Int Ophthalmol 1989;13:167–170.
234. Pederson JE, Smith SG. Surgical management of encapsulated filtering blebs. Ophthalmology 1985;92: 955–958.
235. Gillies WE, Brooks AM. Restoring the function of the failed bleb. Aust NZ J Ophthalmol 1991;19:49–51.
236. Richter CU, et al. The development of encapsulated filtering blebs. Ophthalmology 1988;95:1163–1168.
237. Sherwood MB, et al. Cysts of Tenon's capsule following filtration surgery: medical management. Arch Ophthalmol 1987;105:1517–1521.
238. Ophir A, Ticho U. Encapsulated filtering bleb and subconjunctival 5-fluorouracil. Ophthalmic Surg 1992;23:339–341.
239. Ophir A. Encapsulated filtering bleb: a selective review—new deductions. Eye 1992;6:348–352.
240. Feldman RM, et al. Risk factors for the development of Tenon's capsule cysts after trabeculectomy. Ophthalmology 1989;96:336–341.
241. Scott DR, Quigley HA. Medical management of a high bleb phase after trabeculectomies. Ophthalmology 1988;95:1169–1173.
242. Shingleton BJ, et al. Management of encapsulated filtration blebs. Ophthalmology 1990;97:63–68.
243. Hodge W, et al. Treatment of encapsulated blebs with 30-gauge needling and injection of low-dose 5-fluorouracil. Can J Ophthalmol 1992;27:233–236.
244. Soong HK, Quigley HA. Dellen associated with filtering blebs. Arch Ophthalmol 1983;101:385–387.
245. Katz LJ. Endophthalmitis. In: Sherwood MB, Spaeth GL, eds. Complications of glaucoma surgery. Thorofare, NJ, Slack, 1990:265–276.
246. Kattan HM, et al. Nosocomial endophthalmitis survey: current incidence of infection after intraocular surgery. (Comments) Ophthalmology 1991;98:227–238.
247. Lee K, Pien F. Endophthalmitis caused by nutrient variant streptococci after filtering bleb surgery. Ann Ophthalmol 1993;25:51–53.
248. Mandelbaum S, et al. Late onset endophthalmitis associated with filtering blebs. Ophthalmology 1985; 92:964–972.
249. Ashkenazi I, et al. Risk factors associated with late infection of filtering blebs and endophthalmitis. Ophthalmic Surg 1991;22:570–574.
250. Lipman RM, Deutsch TA. Late-onset *Moraxella catarrhalis* endophthalmitis after filtering surgery. Can J Ophthalmol 1992;27:249–50.
251. Del Piero E, Pennett M, Leopold I. *Pseudomonas cepacia* endophthalmitis. Ann Ophthalmol 1985;17: 753–756.
252. Razzak A, al Samarrai A, Sunba MS. Incidence of posttrabeculectomy cataract among Arabs in Kuwait. Ophthalmic Res 1991:23:21–23.
253. Berke SJ, et al. Chronic and recurrent choroidal detachment after glaucoma filtering surgery. Ophthalmology 1987;94:154–162.
254. Burney EN, Quigley HA, Robin AL. Hypotony and choroidal detachment as late complications of trabeculectomy. Am J Ophthalmol 1987;103:685–688.
255. Wilensky JT. Late hyphema after filtering surgery for glaucoma. Ophthalmic Surg 1983;14:227–228.
256. Lieberman MF, Ewing RH. Drainage implant surgery for refractory glaucoma. Int Ophthalmol Clin 1990; 30:198–208.
257. Williams AS. Setons in glaucoma surgery. In: Albert DM, Jakobiec FA, eds. Principles and practice of ophthalmology. Philadelphia, WB Saunders, 1993: 1655–1667.
258. Melamed S, Fiore PM. Molteno implant surgery in refractory glaucoma. Surv Ophthalmol 1990;34:441–448.
259. Bluestein E, Stewart W. Trabeculectomy with 5-fluorouracil vs single-plate Molteno implantation. Ophthalmic Surg 1993;24:669–673.
260. Freedman J. Clinical experience with the Molteno dual-chamber single-plate implant. Ophthalmic Surg 1992;23:238–241.
261. Melamed S. Implantation of setons in glaucoma. In: Higginbotham EJ, Lee DA, eds. Management of difficult glaucomas: a clinician's guide. Boston, Blackwell Scientific, 1994:401–413.
262. Price FW, Whitson WE. Polypropylene ligatures as a

means of controlling intraocular pressure with Molteno implants. Ophthalmol Surg 1989;20:781–783.

263. Rose GE, Lavin MJ, Hitchings RA. Silicone tubes in glaucoma surgery: the effect of technical modifications on early postoperative intraocular pressures and complications. Eye 1989;3:553–561.
264. Stewart W, Feldman RM, Gross RL. Collagen plug occlusion of Molteno tube shunts. Ophthalmic Surg 1993;24:47–48.
265. Susanna R Jr. Modifications of the Molteno implant and implant procedure. Ophthalmic Surg 1991; 22:611–613.
266. Sherwood MB, Smith MF. Prevention of early hypotony associated with Molteno implants by a new occluding stent technique. Ophthalmology 1993;100: 85–90.
267. el-Sayyad F, et al. The use of releasable sutures in Molteno glaucoma implant procedures to reduce postoperative hypotony. Ophthalmic Surg 1991;22: 82–84.
268. Egbert PR, Lieberman MF. Internal suture occlusion of the Molteno glaucoma implant for the prevention of postoperative hypotony. Ophthalmic Surg 1989;20: 53–56.
269. Kapetansky FM. Prevention of early over-filtration. Molteno Implant Newsl 1989;1(1):3.
270. Nairne JEAH, et al. Single stage insertion of the Molteno tube for glaucoma and modifications to reduce postoperative hypotony. Br J Ophthalmol 1988;72:846–851.
271. Molteno AC, Polkinghorne PJ, Bowbyes JA. The Vicryl tie technique for inserting a draining implant in the treatment of secondary glaucoma. Aust NZ J Ophthalmol 1986;14(4):343–354.
272. Molteno ACB. Use of Molteno implants to treat secondary glaucoma. In: Cairns JE, ed. Glaucoma. London, Grune & Stratton, 1986:211–238.
273. Minckler DS, et al. Experimental studies of aqueous filtration using the Molteno implant. Trans Am Ophthalmol Soc 1987;55:368–392.
274. Traverso CE, Tomey KF, al-Kaff A. The long-tube single plate Molteno implant for the treatment of recalcitrant glaucoma. Int Ophthalmol 1989;13:159–162.
275. Minckler DS, et al. Clinical experience with the single-plate Molteno implant in complicated glaucomas. Ophthalmology 1988;95:1181–1188.
276. Lloyd MA, et al. Clinical experience with the single-plate Molteno implant in complicated glaucomas: update of a pilot study. Ophthalmology 1992;99:679–687.
277. Mermoud A, et al. Use of the single-plate Molteno implant in refractory glaucoma. Ophthalmologica 1992;205:113–120.
278. Heuer DK, et al. Which is better? One or two? A randomized clinical trial of single-plate versus double-plate Molteno implantation for glaucomas in aphakia and pseudophakia. Ophthalmology 1992;99: 1512–1519.
279. Schocket SS, et al. Anterior chamber tube shunt to an encircling band in the treatment of neovascular glaucoma and other refractory glaucomas: a long-term study. Ophthalmology 1985;92:553–562.
280. Schocket SS. Investigations of the reasons for success and failure in the anterior shunt-to-the-encircling-band procedure in the treatment of refractory glaucoma. Trans Am Ophthalmol Soc 1986;54:743–798.
281. Sherwood MB, Joseph NH, Hitchings RA. Surgery for refractory glaucoma: Results and complications with a modified Schocket technique. Arch Ophthalmol 1987;105:562–569.
282. Mandelkorn RM, Olander KW. Valves and draining implants used in the treatment of neovascular glaucoma. In: Weinstein GW, ed. Open-angle glaucoma. New York, Churchill Livingstone, 1986:251–265.
283. Omi CA, et al. Modified Schocket implant for refractory glaucoma: experience of 55 cases. Ophthalmology 1991;98:211–214.
284. Watanabe J, Sawaguchi S, Iwata K. Long-term results of anterior chamber tube shunt to an encircling band in the treatment of refractory glaucomas. Acta Ophthalmol 1992;70:766–771.
285. Wilson R, et al. Aqueous shunts: Molteno versus Schocket. Ophthalmology 1992;99:672–676.
286. Smith MF, Sherwood MB, McGorray SP. Comparison of the double-plate Molteno drainage implant with the Schocket procedure. Arch Ophthalmol 1992; 110:1246–1250.
287. Lavin MJ, et al. Clinical risk factors for failure in glaucoma tube surgery: a comparison of three tube designs. Arch Ophthalmol 1992;110:480–485.
288. Krupin T, et al. A long Krupin-Denver valve implant attached to a 180 degrees scleral explant for glaucoma surgery. Ophthalmology 1988;95:1174–1180.
289. Hitchings RA, et al. Use of one-piece valved tube and variable surface area explant for glaucoma drainage surgery. Ophthalmology 1987;94:1079–1084.
290. White T. Clinical results of glaucoma surgery using the White glaucoma pump shunt. Ann Ophthalmol 1992;24:365–373.
291. Davidovski F, Stewart RH, Kimbrough RL. Long-term results with the White glaucoma pump-shunt. (Comments) Ophthalmic Surg 1990;21:288–293.
292. Chihara E, et al. Outcome of White pump shunt surgery for neovascular glaucoma in Asians. Ophthalmic Surg 1992;23:666–671.
293. Franks WA, Hitchings RA. Injection of perfluoropropane gas to prevent hypotony in eyes undergoing tube implant surgery. Ophthalmology 1990;97:899–903.
294. Kramer T, et al. Molteno implants and operating mi-

croscope-induced retinal phototoxicity: a clinicopathologic report. Arch Ophthalmol 1991;109:379–383.
295. Melamed S, et al. Postoperative complications after Molteno implant surgery. Am J Ophthalmol 1991; 111:319–322.
296. Lloyd MA, et al. Combined Molteno implantation and pars plana vitrectomy for neovascular glaucomas. Ophthalmology 1991;98:1401–1405.
297. Huna R, et al. Retinal detachment adherent to posterior chamber IOL after Molteno implant surgery. Ophthalmic Surg 1990;21:854–856.
298. Siegel MJ. Molteno rip-cord related suture hypopyon. (Letter; comment) Ophthalmic Surg 1990;21:812.
299. Lieberman MF. Late infectious endophthalmitis from exposed glaucoma setons. (Letter) Arch Ophthalmol 1992;110:1685.
300. Perkins TW. Endophthalmitis after placement of a Molteno implant. Ophthalmic Surg 1990;21:733–734.
301. Krebs DB, et al. Late infectious endophthalmitis from exposed glaucoma setons. (Letter) Arch Ophthalmol 1992;110:174–175.
302. Karr DJ, Weinberger E, Mills RP. An unusual case of cellulitis associated with a Molteno implant in a 1-year-old child. J Pediatr Ophthalmol Strabismus 1990;27:107–110.
303. Sherwood MB. Complications of silicone tube drainage devices. In: Sherwood MB, Spaeth GL, eds. Complications of glaucoma surgery. Thorofare, NJ, Slack, 1990:307–326.
304. Lotufo DG. Postoperative complications and visual loss following Molteno implantation. Ophthalmic Surg 1991;22:650–656.
305. Wellemeyer M, Price FJ. Molteno implants in patients with previous cyclocryotherapy. Ophthalmic Surg 1993;24:395–398.
306. Mermoud A, et al. Molteno tube implantation for neovascular glaucoma: long-term results and factors concerning outcome. Ophthalmology 1993;100:897–902.
307. Kooner K, et al. Eye movement restrictions after Molteno implant surgery. (Letter) Ophthalmic Surg 1993;24:498–499.
308. Christmann LM, Wilson ME. Motility disturbances after Molteno implants. J Pediatr Ophthalmol Strabismus 1992;29:44–48.
309. Wilson-Holt N, et al. Hypertropia following insertion of inferiorly sited double-plate Molteno tubes. Eye 1992;6:515–520.
310. Munoz M, Parrish R. Strabismus following implantation of Baerveldt drainage devices. Arch Ophthalmol 1993;111:1096–1099.
311. Smith S, et al. Early clinical experience with the Baerveldt 350-mm^2 glaucoma implant and associated extraocular muscle imbalance. Ophthalmology 1993; 100:914–918.
312. Ball S, et al. Brown's superior oblique tendon syndrome after Baerveldt glaucoma implant. (Letter) Arch Ophthalmol 1992;110:1368.
313. McDonnell PJ, et al. Molteno implant for control of glaucoma in eyes after penetrating keratoplasty. Ophthalmology 1988;95:364–369.
314. Beebe WE, et al. The use of Molteno implant and anterior chamber tube shunt to encircling band for the treatment of glaucoma in keratoplasty patients. Ophthalmology 1990;97:1414–1422.
315. Kirkness CM, Ling Y, Rice NS. The use of silicone drainage tubing to control post-keratoplasty glaucoma. Eye 1988;2:583–590.
316. Kirkness CM, Moshegov C. Post-keratoplasty glaucoma. Eye 1988;2:S19–S26.
317. Sherwood M, et al. Drainage tube implants in the treatment of glaucoma following penetrating keratoplasty. Ophthalmic Surg 1993;24:185–189.
318. Fish LA, et al. Molteno implantation for secondary glaucomas associated with advanced epithelial ingrowth. Ophthalmology 1990;97:557–561.
319. Billson F, Thomas R, Aylward W. The use of two-stage Molteno implants in developmental glaucoma. J Pediatr Ophthalmol Strabismus 1989;26:3–8.
320. Munoz M, et al. Clinical experience with the Molteno implant in advanced infantile glaucoma. J Pediatr Ophthalmol Strabismus 1991;28:68–72.
321. Hill RA, et al. Molteno implantation for glaucoma in young patients. Ophthalmology 1991;98:1042–1046.
322. Noureddin BN, et al. Advanced uncontrolled glaucoma. Nd:YAG cyclophotocoagulation or tube surgery. Ophthalmology 1992;99:430–436.
323. Shaffer RN, Hoskins HD. Montgomery lecture: Goniotomy in the treatment of isolated trabeculodysgenesis (primary congenital [infantile] developmental glaucoma). Trans Ophthalmol Soc UK 1983;103:581–585.
324. Walton DS. Goniotomy. In: Thomas JV, Belcher CD, Simmons RJ, eds. Glaucoma surgery. St. Louis, Mosby–Year Book, 1992:107–121.
325. Litinsky S, Shaffer R, Hetherington J. Operative complications of goniotomy. Trans Am Acad Ophthalmol Otolaryngol 1977;83:78.
326. Draeger J, Wirt H, Ahrens V. Long-term results following goniotomy in congenital glaucoma. Klin Monatsbl Augenheilkd 1984:185:481–489. (in German)
327. Catalano RA, et al. One versus two simultaneous goniotomies as the initial surgical procedure for primary infantile glaucoma. J Pediatr Ophthalmol Strabismus 1989;26:9–13.
328. Shrader CE, Cibis GW. External trabeculotomy. In: Thomas JV, Belcher CD, Simmons RJ, eds. Glaucoma surgery. St. Louis, Mosby–Year Book, 1992: 123–131.
329. Katz LJ. Congenital glaucoma. In: Sherwood MB,

Spaeth GL, eds. Complications of glaucoma surgery. Thorofare, NJ, Slack, 1990:355–364.

330. Harms H, Dannheim R. Epicritical consideration of 300 cases of trabeculotomy ab externo. Trans Ophthalmol Soc UK 1969;89:491.
331. Anderson DR. Trabeculotomy compared to goniotomy for glaucoma in children. Ophthalmology 1983;90:805–806.
332. Martin BB. External trabeculotomy in the surgical treatment of congenital glaucoma. Aust NZ J Ophthalmol 1989;17:299–301.
333. McPherson S Jr, Berry DP. Goniotomy vs external trabeculotomy for developmental glaucoma. Am J Ophthalmol 1983;95:427–431.
334. Debnath SC, Teichmann KD, Salamah K. Trabeculectomy versus trabeculotomy in congenital glaucoma. Br J Ophthalmol 1989;73:608–611.
335. Kjer B, Kessing S. Trabeculotomy in juvenile primary open-angle glaucoma. Ophthalmic Surg 1993;24: 663–668.
336. Wheeler DT, Stager DR, Weakley D Jr. Endophthalmitis following pediatric intraocular surgery for congenital cataracts and congenital glaucoma. J Pediatr Ophthalmol Strabismus 1992;29:139–141.
337. Cadera W, et al. Filtering surgery in childhood glaucoma. Ophthalmic Surg 1984;15:319–322.
338. Melamed S, Latina MA, Epstein DL. Neodymium:YAG laser trabeculopuncture in juvenile open-angle glaucoma. Ophthalmology 1987;94:163–170.
339. Mishima S, Kitazawa Y, Shirato S. Laser therapy for glaucoma. Aust NZ J Ophthalmol 1985;13:225–235.
340. Senft SH, Tomey KF, Traverso CE. Neodymium-YAG laser goniotomy vs surgical goniotomy: A preliminary study in paired eyes. Arch Ophthalmol 1989;107:1773–1776.
341. Walton DS. Aniridic glaucoma: the results of goniosurgery to prevent and treat this problem. Trans Am Ophthalmol Soc 1986;84:59–70.
342. Wiggins R Jr, Tomey KF. The results of glaucoma surgery in aniridia. Arch Ophthalmol 1992;110:503–505.
343. Iwach AG, et al. Analysis of surgical and medical management of glaucoma in Sturge-Weber syndrome. Ophthalmology 1990;97:904–909.
344. Shihab ZM, Kristan RW. Recurrent intraoperative choroidal effusion in Sturge-Weber syndrome. J Pediatr Ophthalmol Strabismus 1983;20:250–252.
345. Williams RD, Hoskins HD, Shaffer RN. Trabeculodialysis for inflammatory glaucoma: A review of 25 cases. Ophthalmic Surg 1992;23:36–37.
346. Shields MB. Cyclodestructive surgery for glaucoma: past, present, and future. Trans Am Ophthalmol Soc 1985;83:285–303.
347. Patel A, et al. Endolaser treatment of the ciliary body for uncontrolled glaucoma. Ophthalmology 1986; 93:825–830.
348. Zarbin M, et al. Endolaser treatment of the ciliary body for severe glaucoma. Ophthalmology 1988; 95:1639–1648.
349. Shields MB. Intraocular cyclophotocoagulation. In: Krupin T, Wax MB, eds. New techniques in glaucoma surgery. Philadelphia, WB Saunders, 1988:167–173.
350. Schuman JS. Cycloablation. In: Albert DM, Jakobiec FA, eds. Principles and practice of ophthalmology. Philadelphia, WB Saunders, 1993:1667–1677.
351. McAllister J. Complications of cyclodialysis. In: Sherwood MB, Spaeth GL, eds. Complications of glaucoma surgery. Thorofare, NJ, Slack, 1990:333–341.
352. Sugar H. Experiences with some modifications of cyclodialysis for aphakic glaucoma. Ann Ophthalmol 1977;9:1045–1052.
353. Hansen S, Laursen AB. Visualized cyclodialysis—an additional option in glaucoma surgery. Acta Ophthalmol 1986;64:142–145.
354. McAllister J, Spaeth G. Intracapsular cataract extraction with cyclodialysis: a useful procedure. Klin Monatsbl Augenheilkd 1984;184:283–286.
355. Singh OS, Simmons RJ. Cyclodialysis. In: Thomas JV, Belcher CD, Simmons RJ, eds. Glaucoma surgery. St. Louis, Mosby–Year Book, 1992:133–147.
356. Caprioli J. Cyclotherapy. In: Sherwood MB, Spaeth GL, eds. Complications of glaucoma surgery. Thorofare, NJ, Slack, 1990:343–354.
357. Brown SVL, Deppermann SR, Thomas JV. Cyclocryosurgery. In: Thomas JV, Belcher CD, Simmons RJ, eds. Glaucoma surgery. St. Louis: Mosby–Year Book, 1992:149–155.
358. Caprioli J, et al. Cyclocryotherapy in the treatment of advanced glaucoma. Ophthalmology 1985:92:947–954.
359. Devreese M, Belgrado G, Hennekes R. Cyclocryotherapy in primary glaucoma: intraocular pressure reducing effects and complications. Bull Soc Belge Ophtalmol 1991;241:105–111.
360. Brindley G, Shields MB. Value and limitations of cyclocryotherapy. Graefes Arch Clin Exp Ophthalmol 1986;224:545–548.
361. Benson MT, Nelson ME. Cyclocryotherapy: a review of cases over a 10-year period. Br J Ophthalmol 1990;74:103–105.
362. Caprioli J, Sears M. Regulation of intraocular pressure during cyclocryotherapy for advanced glaucoma. Am J Ophthalmol 1986;101:542–545.
363. Coleman D, et al. Therapeutic ultrasound in the treatment of glaucoma: II. Clinical applications. Ophthalmology 1985;1985:347.
364. Harmon GK, Yablonski ME, Coleman DJ. Ultrasonic treatment of glaucoma. In: Krupin T, Wax MB, eds. New techniques in glaucoma surgery. Philadelphia, WB Saunders, 1988:157–162.
365. Haut J, et al. Indications and results of Sonocare (ultrasound) in the treatment of ocular hypertension:

A preliminary study of 395 cases. Ophtalmologie 1990:4:138–141.

366. Maskin SL, et al. Therapeutic ultrasound for refractory glaucoma: a three-center study. Ophthalmic Surg 1989;20:186–192.
367. Silverman RH, et al. Therapeutic ultrasound for the treatment of glaucoma. Am J Ophthalmol 1991; 111:327–337. (Published erratum appears in Am J Ophthalmol 1991;112(1):105.)
368. Sterk CC, Borsje RA, van Delft JL. The effect of high-intensity focused ultrasound on intraocular pressure in therapy-resistant glaucoma 3–4 months and 1 year after treatment. Int Ophthalmol 1992;16:401–404.
369. Wilensky JT. Staphyloma formation as a complication of ultrasound treatment in glaucoma. (Letter) Arch Ophthalmol 1985;103:1113.
370. Beckman H, Waeltermann J. Transscleral ruby laser cyclocoagulation. Am J Ophthalmol 1984;98:788–795.
371. Crymes BM, Gross RL. Laser placement in noncontact Nd:YAG cyclophotocoagulation. Am J Ophthalmol 1990;110:670–673.
372. Hampton C, et al. Evaluation of a protocol for transscleral neodymium:YAG cyclophotocoagulation in one hundred patients. Ophthalmology 1990;97:910–917.
373. Balazsi G. Noncontact thermal mode Nd:YAG laser transscleral cyclocoagulation in the treatment of glaucoma: Intermediate follow-up. Ophthalmology 1991;98:1858–1863.
374. McAllister J, O'Brien C. Neodymium:YAG transscleral cyclocoagulation: a clinical study. Eye 1990;4:651–656.
375. Devenyi RG, et al. Neodymium:YAG transscleral cyclocoagulation in human eyes. Ophthalmology 1987;94:1519–1522.
376. Trope GE, Ma S. Mid-term effects of neodymium:YAG transscleral cyclocoagulation in glaucoma. Ophthalmology 1990;97:73–75.
377. Wheatcroft S, et al. Treatment of glaucoma following penetrating keratoplasty with transscleral YAG cyclophotocoagulation. Int Ophthalmol 1992;16:397–400.
378. Levy NS, Bonney RC. Transscleral YAG cyclocoagulation of the ciliary body for persistently high intraocular pressure following penetrating keratoplasty. Cornea 1989;8:178–181.
379. Schuman JS, et al. Contact transscleral continuous wave neodymium:YAG laser cyclophotocoagulation. Ophthalmology 1990;97:571–580.
380. Royal G, et al. One year follow-up of Nd:YAG contact transscleral laser cyclophotocoagulation (#2878-19 ARVO). Invest Ophthalmol Vis Res 1992;33/34:1268.
381. Brancato R, et al. Contact transscleral cyclophotocoagulation with Nd:YAG laser in uncontrolled glaucoma. Ophthalmic Surg 1989;20:547–551.
382. Kermani O, et al. Contact cw-Nd:YAG laser cyclophotocoagulation for treatment of refractory glaucoma. Ger J Ophthalmol 1992;1:74–78.
383. Gaasterland DE, Pollack IP. Initial experience with a new method of laser transscleral cyclophotocoagulation for ciliary ablation in severe glaucoma. Trans Am Ophthalmol Soc 1992;90:225–243.
384. Hennis HL, Stewart WC. Semiconductor diode laser transscleral cyclophotocoagulation in patients with glaucoma. Am J Ophthalmol 1992;113:81–85.
385. Fiore PM, Melamed S, Krug J Jr. Focal scleral thinning after transscleral Nd:YAG cyclophotocoagulation. Ophthalmic Surg 1989;20:215–216.
386. Fiore PM, Melamed S, Epstein DL. Trabecular precipitates and elevated intraocular pressure following argon laser trabeculoplasty. Ophthalmic Surg 1989; 20:697–701.
387. Lam S, et al. High incidence of sympathetic ophthalmia after contact and noncontact neodymium:YAG cyclotherapy. Ophthalmology 1992;99:1818–1822.
388. Edward D, et al. Sympathetic ophthalmia following Nd:YAG cyclotherapy. Ophthalmic Surg 1989;20:544.
389. Minckler D. Does Nd:YAG cyclotherapy cause sympathetic ophthalmia? Ophthalmic Surg 1989;20:543.
390. Shields S, Stewart WC, Shields MB. Transpupillary argon laser cyclophotocoagulation in the treatment of glaucoma. Ophthalmic Surg 1988;19:171–175.
391. Demeler U. Ciliary surgery for glaucoma. Trans Ophthalmol Soc UK 1986:105:242–245.
392. Rivera AH, Brown RH, Anderson DR. Laser iridotomy vs surgical iridectomy. Have the indications changed? Arch Ophthalmol 1985;103:1350–1354.
393. Go FJ, et al. Argon laser iridotomy and surgical iridectomy in treatment of primary angle-closure glaucoma. Jpn J Ophthalmol 1984;28:36–46.
394. McGalliard JN, Wishart PK. The effect of Nd:YAG iridotomy on intraocular pressure in hypertensive eyes with shallow anterior chambers. Eye 1990;4:823–829.
395. Schwartz GF, et al. Surgical and medical management of patients with narrow anterior chamber angles: comparative results. Ophthalmic Surg 1992; 23:108–112.
396. Saunders DC. Acute closed-angle glaucoma and Nd-YAG laser iridotomy. Br J Ophthalmol 1990;74:523–525.
397. Newhouse RP, Schutz S. Sector iridectomy in the management of prolonged attacks of acute congestive glaucoma. Ann Ophthalmol 1987;19:340–342.
398. Gray RH, Nairne JH, Ayliffe WH. Efficacy of Nd-YAG laser iridotomies in acute angle closure glaucoma. Br J Ophthalmol 1989;73:182–185.
399. Robin AL, Pollack IP. Q-switched neodymium-YAG laser iridotomy in patients in whom the argon laser fails. Arch Ophthalmol 1986;104:531–535.
400. Shirakashi M, Iwata K, Nakayama T. Argon laser tra-

beculoplasty for chronic angle-closure glaucoma uncontrolled by iridotomy. Acta Ophthalmol 1989; 67:265–270.

401. Belcher CD III, Greff LJ. Laser therapy of angle-closure glaucoma. In: Albert DM, Jakobiec FA, eds. Principles and practice of ophthalmology. Philadelphia, WB Saunders, 1993:1597–1609.
402. Ho T, Fan R. Sequential argon-YAG laser iridotomies in dark irides. Br J Ophthalmol 1992;76:329–331.
403. Goins K, Schmeisser E, Smith T. Argon laser pretreatment in Nd:YAG iridotomy. Ophthalmic Surg 1990; 21:497–500.
404. Fleck BW, Wright E, McGlynn C. Argon laser pretreatment 4 to 6 weeks before Nd:YAG laser iridotomy. Ophthalmic Surg 1991;22:644–649.
405. Fleck BW. How large must an iridotomy be? Br J Ophthalmol 1990;74:583–588.
406. Krupin T, et al. Acute intraocular pressure response to argon laser iridotomy. Ophthalmology 1985;92: 922–926.
407. Naveh N, Zborowsky-Gutman L, Blumenthal M. Neodymium-YAG laser iridotomy in angle closure glaucoma: preliminary study. Br J Ophthalmol 1987; 71:257–261.
408. Hsieh JW. Effects of timolol and acetazolamide on intraocular pressure elevation following argon laser iridotomy. Taiwan I Hsueh Hui Tsa Chih 1992;91:29–33.
409. Robin AL. The role of apraclonidine hydrochloride in laser therapy for glaucoma. Trans Am Ophthalmol Soc 1990;87:729–761.
410. Hong C, et al. Effect of apraclonidine hydrochloride on acute intraocular pressure rise after argon laser iridotomy. Korean J Ophthalmol 1991;5:37–41.
411. Fernandez-Bahamonde JL, Alcaraz-Michelli V. The combined use of apraclonidine and pilocarpine during laser iridotomy in a Hispanic population. Ann Ophthalmol 1990;22:446–449.
412. Kitazawa Y, Taniguchi T, Sugiyama K. Use of apraclonidine to reduce acute intraocular pressure rise following Q-switched Nd:YAG laser iridotomy. Ophthalmic Surg 1989;20:49–52.
413. Tomey KF, Traverso CE, Shammas IV. Neodymium-YAG laser iridotomy in the treatment and prevention of angle closure glaucoma: a review of 373 eyes. Arch Ophthalmol 1987;105:476–481.
414. Robin A, Pollack I. A comparison of neodymium:YAG and argon laser iridotomies. Ophthalmology 1984; 91:1011.
415. Haut J, et al. Study of the first hundred phakic eyes treated by peripheral iridotomy using the Nd:YAG laser. Int Ophthalmol 1986;9:227–235.
416. Fernandez-Bahamonde JL. Iatrogenic lens rupture after a neodymium: yttrium aluminum garnet laser iridotomy attempt. Ann Ophthalmol 1991;23:346–348.
417. Berger CM, Lee DA, Christensen RE. Anterior lens capsule perforation and zonular rupture after Nd:YAG laser iridotomy. Am J Ophthalmol 1989; 107:674–675.
418. Wilhelmus KR. Corneal edema following argon laser iridotomy. Ophthalmic Surg 1992;23:533–537.
419. Jeng S, Lee JS, Huang SC. Corneal decompensation after argon laser iridectomy—a delayed complication. Ophthalmic Surg 1991;22:565–569.
420. Zabel RW, Mac Donald IM, Mintsioulis G. Corneal endothelial decompensation after argon laser iridotomy. Can J Ophthalmol 1991;26:367–373.
421. Wishart PK, et al. Corneal endothelial changes following short pulsed laser iridotomy and surgical iridectomy. Trans Ophthalmol Soc UK 1986;105:541–548.
422. Wishart PK, Hitchings RA. Neodymium:YAG and dye laser iridotomy—a comparative study. Trans Ophthalmol Soc UK 1986;105:521–540.
423. Canning CR, et al. Neodymium:YAG laser iridotomies—short-term comparison with capsulotomies and long-term follow-up. Graefes Arch Clin Exp Ophthalmol 1988;226:49–54.
424. Lederer C Jr, Price PK. Posterior synechiae after laser iridectomy. Ann Ophthalmol 1989;21:61–64.
425. Cohen JS, Bibler L, Tucker D. Hypopyon following laser iridotomy. Ophthalmic Surg 1984;15:604–606.
426. Geyer O, et al. Pigmented pupillary pseudomembranes as a complication of argon laser iridotomy. Ophthalmic Surg 1991;22:162–164.
427. Murphy PH, Trope GE. Monocular blurring: a complication of YAG laser iridotomy. (Comments) Ophthalmology 1991;98:1539–1542.
428. Aminlari A, Sassani JW. Simultaneous bilateral malignant glaucoma following laser iridotomy. Graefes Arch Clin Exp Ophthalmol 1993;231:12–14.
429. Fanous S, Brouillette G. Ciliary block glaucoma: malignant glaucoma in the absence of a history of surgery and of miotic therapy. Can J Ophthalmol 1983;18:302–303.
430. Emoto I, Okisaka S, Nakajima A. Diode laser iridotomy in rabbit and human eyes. Am J Ophthalmol 1992;113:321–327.
431. Karickhoff JR. Pigmentary dispersion syndrome and pigmentary glaucoma: a new mechanism concept, a new treatment, and a new technique. Ophthalmic Surg 1992;23:269–277.
432. Worthen D, Wickham M. Argon laser trabeculotomy. Trans Am Acad Ophthalmol Otolaryngol 1974;78: 371.
433. Wise J, Witter S. Argon laser therapy for open-angle glaucoma. Arch Ophthalmol 1979;97:319.
434. Schwartz A, Del Priore L. The evolving role of argon laser trabeculoplasty in glaucoma. In: Caprioli J, ed. Contemporary issues in glaucoma. Philadelphia, WB Saunders, 1991:827–838.
435. Shingleton BJ, et al. Long-term efficacy of argon laser

trabeculoplasty. Ophthalmology 1987;94:1513–1518.
436. Brooks AM, West RH, Gillies WE. Argon laser trabeculoplasty five years on. Aust NZ J Ophthalmol 1988;16:343–351.
437. Moulin F, Le Mer Y, Haut J. Five-year results of the first 159 consecutive phakic chronic open-angle glaucomas treated by argon laser trabeculoplasty. Ophthalmologica 1991;202:3–9.
438. Elsas T, Johnsen H. Long-term efficacy of primary laser trabeculoplasty. Br J Ophthalmol 1991;75:34–37.
439. Reiss GR, Wilensky JT, Higginbotham EJ. Laser trabeculoplasty. Surv Ophthalmol 1991;35:407–428.
440. Richardson LE. Argon laser trabeculoplasty: a review. J Am Optom Assoc 1992;63:252–256.
441. Amon M, et al. Long-term follow-up of argon laser trabeculoplasty in uncontrolled primary open-angle glaucoma: a study with standardized extensive preoperative treatment. Ophthalmologica 1990:200:181–188.
442. Eendebak GR, Boen-Tan TN, Bezemer PD. Long-term follow-up of laser trabeculoplasty. Doc Ophthalmol 1990;75:203–214.
443. Ticho U, Nesher R. Laser trabeculoplasty in glaucoma: ten-year evaluation. (Comments) Arch Ophthalmol 1989;107:844–846.
444. Moulin F, Haut J, Abi Rached J. Late failures of trabeculoplasty. Int Ophthalmol 1987;10:61–66.
445. Gillies WE, Brooks AM. The presentation of acute glaucoma in pseudoexfoliation of the lens capsule. Aust NZ J Ophthalmol 1988;16:101–106.
446. Psilas K, et al. Comparative study of argon laser trabeculoplasty in primary open-angle and pseudoexfoliation glaucoma. Ophthalmologica 1989;198:57–63.
447. Goldberg I. Argon laser trabeculoplasty and the open-angle glaucomas. Aust NZ J Ophthalmol 1985;13:243–248.
448. Robin AL, Pollack IP. Argon laser trabeculoplasty in secondary forms of open-angle glaucoma. Arch Ophthalmol 1983;101:382–384.
449. Lieberman MF, Hoskins HD, Hetherington J. Laser trabeculoplasty and the glaucomas. Ophthalmology 1983;90:790–795.
450. Brooks AM, Gillies WE. Do any factors predict a favourable response to laser trabeculoplasty? Aust J Ophthalmol 1984;12:149–153.
451. Wilensky JT, Weinreb RN. Early and late failures of argon laser trabeculoplasty. Arch Ophthalmol 1983;101:895–897.
452. Coakes R. Laser trabeculoplasty. Br J Ophthalmol 1992;76:624–626.
453. Higginbotham EJ, Richardson TM. Response of exfoliation glaucoma to laser trabeculoplasty. Br J Ophthalmol 1986;70:837–839.
454. Schulzer M. Intraocular pressure reduction in normal-tension glaucoma patients: the Normal Tension Glaucoma Study Group. Ophthalmology 1992;99:1468–1470.
455. Schoenleber DB, Bellows AR, Hutchinson BT. Failed laser trabeculoplasty requiring surgery in open-angle glaucoma. Ophthalmic Surg 1987;18:796–799.
456. Fellman RL, et al. Argon laser trabeculoplasty following failed trabeculectomy. Ophthalmic Surg 1984;15:195–198.
457. Weinreb RN, et al. Influence of the number of laser burns administered on the early results of argon laser trabeculoplasty. Am J Ophthalmol 1983;95:287–292.
458. Glaucoma Laser Trial Research Group. The Glaucoma Laser Trial: I. Acute effects of argon laser trabeculoplasty on intraocular pressure. Arch Ophthalmol 1989;107:1135–1142.
459. Robin A. Argon laser trabeculoplasty medical therapy to prevent the intraocular pressure rise associated with argon laser trabeculoplasty. Ophthalmic Surg 1991;22:31.
460. Elsas T, Johnsen H, Stang O. Pilocarpine to prevent acute pressure increase following primary laser trabeculoplasty. Eye 1991;5:390–394.
461. Odberg T. Primary argon laser trabeculoplasty after pretreatment with timolol: a safe and economic therapy of early glaucoma. Acta Ophthalmol 1990;68:317–319.
462. Brooks AM, et al. Preventing a high rise in intraocular pressure after laser trabeculoplasty. Aust NZ J Ophthalmol 1987;15:113–117.
463. Allf BE, Shields MB. Early intraocular pressure response to laser trabeculoplasty 180 degrees without apraclonidine versus 360 degrees with apraclonidine. Ophthalmic Surg 1991;22:539–542.
464. Elsas T, Johnsen H, Brevik TA. The immediate pressure response to primary laser trabeculoplasty—a comparison of one- and two-stage treatment. Acta Ophthalmol 1989;67:664–668.
465. Hugkulstone CE. Standard and long duration repeat argon laser trabeculoplasty. Acta Ophthalmol 1990;68:575–578.
466. Hugkulstone CE. Argon laser trabeculoplasty with standard and long duration. Acta Ophthalmol 1990;68:579–581.
467. Hugkulstone CE. The effects of different energy levels in argon laser trabeculoplasty. Acta Ophthalmol 1989;67:271–274.
468. Blondeau P, Roberge JF, Asselin Y. Long-term results of low power, long duration laser trabeculoplasty. Am J Ophthalmol 1987;104:339–342.
469. Shirakashi M, et al. Long-term efficacy of low power argon laser trabeculoplasty. Acta Ophthalmol 1990;68:23–28.
470. Takenaka Y, Yamamoto T, Shirato S. One-quadrant argon laser trabeculoplasty and its indication. Jpn J Ophthalmol 1987;31:483–488.

471. Weber PA, Burton GD, Epitropoulos AT. Laser trabeculoplasty retreatment. Ophthalmic Surg 1989; 20:702–706.
472. Grayson DK, et al. Long-term reduction of intraocular pressure after repeat argon laser trabeculoplasty. Am J Ophthalmol 1988;106:312–321.
473. Feldman RM, et al. Long-term efficacy of repeat argon laser trabeculoplasty. Ophthalmology 1991;98: 1061–1065.
474. Bishop KI, et al. Bilateral argon laser trabeculoplasty in primary open-angle glaucoma. Am J Ophthalmol 1989;107:591–595.
475. Eguchi S, et al. Methods of argon laser trabeculoplasty, complications and long-term follow-up of the results. Jpn J Ophthalmol 1985;29:198–211.
476. Hoskins H Jr, et al. Complications of laser trabeculoplasty. Ophthalmology 1983;90:796–799.
477. Starita RJ, et al. Histopathologic verification of position of laser burns in argon laser trabeculoplasty. Ophthalmic Surg 1984;15:854–858.
478. Mermoud A, Pittet N, Herbort CP. Inflammation patterns after laser trabeculoplasty measured with the laser flare meter. Arch Ophthalmol 1992;110:368–370.
479. Richter CU. Laser therapy of open-angle glaucoma. In: Albert DM, Jakobiec FA, eds. Principles and practice of ophthalmology. Philadelphia, WB Saunders, 1993:1588–1597.
480. Levene R. Major early complications of laser trabeculoplasty. Ophthalmic Surg 1983;14:947–953.
481. Thomas J, Simmons R, Belcher C. Argon laser trabeculoplasty in the presurgical glaucoma patient. Ophthalmology 1982;89:187.
482. Greenidge KC, Spaeth GL, Fiol-Silva Z. Effect of argon laser trabeculoplasty on the glaucomatous diurnal curve. Ophthalmology 1983;90:800–804.
483. Matai A, Consul S. Argon laser iridoplasty. Indian J Ophthalmol 1987;35:290–292.
484. Burton TC, Folk JC. Laser iris retraction for angle-closure glaucoma after retinal detachment surgery. Ophthalmology 1988;95:742–748.
485. Jin JC, Anderson DR. Laser and unsutured sclerotomy in nanophthalmos. Am J Ophthalmol 1990; 109:575–580.
486. Latina MA, Charles J-B. Laser filtration surgery. In: Albert DM, Jakobiec FA, eds. Principles and practice of ophthalmology. Philadelphia, WB Saunders, 1993:1609–1618.
487. Terry SA. Cyclodialysis cleft following holmium laser sclerostomy, treated by argon laser photocoagulation. Ophthalmic Surg 1992;23:825–826.
488. Gross RL. Cataracts and glaucoma: approach to management. In: Higginbotham EJ, Lee DA, eds. Management of difficult glaucomas: a clinician's guide. Boston, Blackwell Scientific, 1994:155–160.
489. Tomey KF, Traverso CE. The glaucomas in aphakia and pseudophakia. Surv Ophthalmol 1991;36:79–112.
490. Lamping KA. Management of the aphakic and pseudophakic patient with glaucoma. In: Higginbotham EJ, Lee DA, eds. Management of difficult glaucomas: a clinician's guide. Boston, Blackwell Scientific, 1994:144–154.
491. Krug J. Glaucoma following cataract surgery. In: Albert DM, Jakobiec FA, eds. Principles and practice of ophthalmology. Philadelphia, WB Saunders, 1993: 1511–1520.
492. Chrousos GA, Parks MM, O'Neill JF. Incidence of chronic glaucoma, retinal detachment and secondary membrane surgery in pediatric aphakic patients. Ophthalmology 1984;91:1238–1241.
493. Pressman SH, Crouch E Jr. Pediatric aphakic glaucoma. Ann Ophthalmol 1983;15:568–573.
494. Moses L. Complications of rigid anterior chamber implants. Ophthalmology 1984;91:819–825.
495. Downing J. Ten-year follow up comparing anterior and posterior chamber intraocular lens implants. Ophthalmic Surg 1992;23:308–315.
496. Kooner KS, et al. Intraocular pressure following ECCE, phacoemulsification, and PC-IOL implantation. Ophthalmic Surg 1988;19:643–646.
497. Van Buskirk EM. Late onset, progressive, peripheral anterior synechiae with posterior chamber intraocular lenses. Ophthalmic Surg 1987;18:115–117.
498. Evans R. Peripheral anterior synechia overlying the haptics of posterior chamber lenses: occurrence and natural history. Ophthalmology 1990;97:415–423.
499. Lakhanpal V, et al. A new modified vitreoretinal surgical approach in the management of massive suprachoroidal hemorrhage [see comments]. Ophthalmology 1989;96:793–800.
500. Fluorouracil Filtering Surgery Study Group. Fluorouracil Filtering Surgery Study one-year follow-up. (Comments) Am J Ophthalmol 1989;108:625–635.
501. Fluorouracil Filtering Surgery Study Group. Fluorouracil filtering surgery study one-year follow-up (Letter; comment). Am J Ophthalmol 1990; 109:613–616.
502. Poliner LS, et al. Neovascular glaucoma after intracapsular and extracapsular cataract extraction in diabetic patients. Am J Ophthalmol 1985;100:637–643.
503. Aiello LM, Wand M, Liang G. Neovascular glaucoma and vitreous hemorrhage following cataract surgery in patients with diabetes mellitus. Ophthalmology 1983;90:814–820.
504. Weinreb R, et al. Pseudophakic pupillary block with angle-closure glaucoma in diabetic patients. Am J Ophthalmol 1986;102:325–328.
505. Hietanen J, et al. Exfoliation syndrome in patients scheduled for cataract surgery. Acta Ophthalmol 1992;70:440–446.

506. Pignalosa B, Toni F, Liguori G. Considerations on posterior chamber intraocular lens implantation in patients with pseudoexfoliation syndrome. Doc Ophthalmol 1989;71:49–53.
507. Raitta C, Setala K. Intraocular lens implantation in exfoliation syndrome and capsular glaucoma. Acta Ophthalmol 1986;64:130–133.
508. Bergman M, Laatikainen L. Intraocular pressure level in glaucomatous and nonglaucomatous eyes after complicated cataract surgery and implantation of an AC-IOL. (Comments) Ophthalmic Surg 1992;23:378–382.
509. Jakeman CM, et al. Cataract surgery with intraocular lens implantation in Fuchs' heterochromic cyclitis. Eye 1990;4:543–547.
510. Jones NP. Extracapsular cataract surgery with and without intraocular lens implantation in Fuchs' heterochromic uveitis. Eye 1990;4:145–150.
511. Lambrou FJ, Stewart W. Management of dislocated lens fragments during phacoemulsification. Ophthalmology 1992;99:1260–1262.
512. Fastenberg D, et al. Management of dislocated nuclear fragments after phacoemulsification. Am J Ophthalmol 1991;112:535–539.
513. Gilliland GD, Hutton WL, Fuller DG. Retained intravitreal lens fragments after cataract surgery. Ophthalmology 1992;99:1263–1267.
514. Moisseiev J, Bartov E, Schochat A. Long-term study of the prevalence of capsular opacification following extracapsular cataract extraction. J Cataract Refract Surg 1989;15:531–533.
515. Stamper R, Sugar A, Ripkin D. Complications of intraocular lenses. In: Intraocular lenses: basics and clinical applications. San Francisco, American Academy of Ophthalmology, 1993:93–111.
516. Schubert HD. A history of intraocular pressure rise with reference to the Nd:YAG laser. Surv Ophthalmol 1985;30:168–72.
517. Keates RH, et al. Long-term follow-up of Nd:YAG laser posterior capsulotomy. J Am Intraocul Implant Soc 1984;10:164–168.
518. Robin AL. Medical management of acute postoperative intraocular pressure rises associated with anterior segment ophthalmic laser surgery. Int Ophthalmol Clin 1990;30:102–110.
519. Schaeffer AR, Ryll DL, O'Donnell F Jr. Ciliochoroidal effusions after neodymium:YAG posterior capsulotomy: association with pre-existing glaucoma and uveitis. J Cataract Refract Surg 1989;15:567–569.
520. Flohr MJ, Robin AL, Kelley JS. Early complications following Q-switched neodymium:YAG laser posterior capsulotomy. Ophthalmology 1985;92:360–363.
521. Nesher R, Kolker AE. Failure of apraclonidine to prevent delayed IOP elevation after Nd:YAG laser posterior capsulotomy. Trans Am Ophthalmol Soc 1990;88:229–232.
522. Civerchia LL, Balent A. Intraocular lens implantation in acute angle closure glaucoma associated with cataract. J Am Intraocul Implant Soc 1985;11:171–173.
523. Gunning FP, Greve EL. Uncontrolled primary angle closure glaucoma: results of early intercapsular cataract extraction and posterior chamber lens implantation. Int Ophthalmol 1991;15:237–247.
524. Wishart PK, Atkinson PL. Extracapsular cataract extraction and posterior chamber lens implantation in patients with primary chronic angle-closure glaucoma: effect on intraocular pressure control. Eye 1989;3:706–712.
525. Obstbaum SA, Orlando F. Glaucoma and its relationship to intraocular lens implantation. Aust NZ J Ophthalmol 1989;17:303–308.
526. Brown SV, et al. Effect of cataract surgery on intraocular pressure reduction obtained with laser trabeculoplasty. Am J Ophthalmol 1985;100:373–376.
527. Gunning FP, Greve EL. Intercapsular cataract extraction with implantation of the Galand disc lens: a retrospective analysis in patients with and without glaucoma. Ophthalmic Surg 1991;22:531–538.
528. Handa J, et al. Extracapsular cataract extraction with posterior chamber lens implantation in patients with glaucoma. Arch Ophthalmol 1987;105:765–769.
529. Brooks AM, Gillies WE. The effect of cataract extraction with implant in glaucomatous eyes. Aust NZ J Ophthalmol 1992;20:235–238.
530. Burratto L, Ferrari M. Extracapsular cataract surgery and intraocular lens implantation in glaucomatous eyes that had a filtering bleb operation. J Cataract Refract Surg 1990;16:315–319.
531. Levene R. Triple procedure of extracapsular cataract surgery, posterior chamber lens implantation, and glaucoma filter. J Cataract Refract Surg 1986;12:385–90.
532. Sugar H. Post-operative cataract in successfully filtering glaucomatous eyes. Am J Ophthalmol 1970; 69:740.
533. Kass M. Cataract extraction in an eye with a filtering bleb. Ophthalmology 1982;89:871.
534. Simmons ST, et al. Extracapsular cataract extraction and posterior chamber intraocular lens implantation combined with trabeculectomy in patients with glaucoma. Am J Ophthalmol 1987;104:465–470.
535. Oyakawa R, Maumenee A. Clear-cornea cataract extraction in eyes with functioning filtering blebs. Am J Ophthalmol 1982;93:294–298.
536. Longstaff S, et al. Glaucoma triple procedures: efficacy of intraocular pressure control and visual outcome. Ophthalmic Surg 1990;21:786–793.
537. Percival SP. Glaucoma triple procedure of extracapsular cataract extraction, posterior chamber lens implantation, and trabeculectomy. Br J Ophthalmol 1985;69:99–102.
538. McGuigan LJ, et al. Extracapsular cataract extraction

and posterior chamber lens implantation in eyes with preexisting glaucoma. Arch Ophthalmol 1986;104:1301–1308.

539. West J, et al. Prevention of acute postoperative rises in glaucoma patients undergoing cataract extraction with posterior chamber implants. Br J Ophthalmol 1992;76:534–537.
540. Wood TO. Effect of carbachol on postoperative intraocular pressure. J Cataract Refract Surg 1988;14:654–656.
541. Krupin T, Feitl ME, Bishop KI. Postoperative intraocular pressure rise in open-angle glaucoma patients after cataract or combined cataract-filtration surgery. Ophthalmology 1989;96:579–584.
542. Vu MT, Shields MB. The early postoperative pressure course in glaucoma patients following cataract surgery. Ophthalmic Surg 1988;19:467–470.
543. Kriger SH, Tuberville A, Hamilton RS. A review of extracapsular cataract extraction and intraocular lens implantation combined with trabeculectomy. Ann Ophthalmol 1989;21:266–268.
544. Binkhorst CD. Preexisting primary glaucoma and intraocular lenses. Trans Ophthalmol Soc UK 1985; 104:567–569.
545. Naveh N, et al. The long-term effect on intraocular pressure of a procedure combining trabeculectomy and cataract surgery, as compared with trabeculectomy alone. Ophthalmic Surg 1990;21:339–345.
546. Savage JA, et al. Extracapsular cataract extraction and posterior chamber intraocular lens implantation in glaucomatous eyes. Ophthalmology 1985;92: 1506–1516.
547. Murchison J Jr, Shields MB. An evaluation of three surgical approaches for coexisting cataract and glaucoma. Ophthalmic Surg 1989;20:393–398.
548. Mills R. Combined cataract extraction and trabeculectomy. In: Mills R, Weinreb R, eds. Glaucoma surgical techniques. San Francisco, American Academy of Ophthalmology, 1991:59–71.
549. Thomas JV, Savage JA, Albuquerque M. Surgical management of coexisting glaucoma and cataract. In: Thomas JV, Belcher CD, Simmons RJ, eds. Glaucoma surgery. St. Louis, Mosby–Year Book, 1992: 263–294.
550. Gross R. Cataracts and glaucoma: technique of combined procedures. In: Higginbotham EJ, Lee DA, eds. Management of difficult glaucomas: a clinician's guide. Boston, Blackwell Scientific, 1994:392–400.
551. Freeman J, Gettelfinger T. Maintaining pupillary dilation during lens implant surgery. Am Intraocul Implant Soc J 1981;7:172–173.
552. Davison JA. Phacoemulsification in glaucomatous eyes. In: Thomas JV, Belcher CD, Simmons RJ, eds. Glaucoma surgery. St. Louis, Mosby–Year Book, 1992:295–314.
553. Lane S, et al. Prospective comparison of the effects of Occucoat, Viscoat, and Healon on intraocular pressure and endothelial cell loss. J Cataract Refract Surg 1991;17:21–26.
554. Lane SS, Lindstrom RL. Viscoelastic agents: formulations, clinical applications and complication. In: Ostbaum SA, ed. Cataract and introcular lens surgery. Philadelphia, WB Saunders, 1991:313–330.
555. Murchison J Jr, Shields MB. Limbal-based vs fornix-based conjunctival flaps in combined extracapsular cataract surgery and glaucoma filtering procedure. Am J Ophthalmol 1990;109:709–715.
556. Allan B, Barrett G. Combined small incision phacoemulsification and trabeculectomy. J Cataract Refract Surgery 1993;19:97–102.
557. Lyle A, Jin J. Comparison of a 3- and 6-mm incision in combined phacoemulsification and trabeculectomy. Am J Ophthalmol 1991;111:189–196.
558. Wedrich A, et al. Combined small-incision cataract surgery and trabeculectomy—technique and results. Int Ophthalmol 1992;16:409–414.
559. Whitsett J, Stewart R. A new technique for combined cataract/glaucoma procedures in patients on chronic miotics. Ophthalmic Surg 1993;24:481–485.
560. Pasquale LR, Smith SG. Surgical outcome of phacoemulsification combined with the Pearce trabeculectomy in patients with glaucoma. J Cataract Refract Surg 1992;18:301–305.
561. Galin MA, et al. Trabeculectomy, cataract extraction and intra-ocular lens implantation. Trans Ophthalmol Soc UK 1985;104:570–573.
562. Hurvitz L. 5-FU–supplemented phacoemulsification, posterior chamber intraocular lens implantation, and trabeculectomy. Ophthalmic Surg 1993:24:674–680.
563. Kendrick RM, Kollarits CR. Combined cataract-glaucoma surgery using the THC:YAG (holmium) laser ab interno without gonioscopy. Ophthalmic Surg 1992;23:697–699.
564. Gimbel HV, Meyer D. Small incision trabeculotomy combined with phacoemulsification and intraocular lens implantation. J Cataract Refract Surg 1993; 19:92–96.
565. Gillies WE, Brooks AM. The results of combined cataract extraction and trabeculectomy using separate incisions. Aust NZ J Ophthalmol 1992;20:239–242.
566. Sherwood MB, Tolat N, Sando R. Complications of surgical iridectomy: prevention and management. In: Sherwood MB, Spaeth GL, ed. Complications of glaucoma surgery. Thorofare, NJ: Slack, 1990:327–332.
567. Sharpe ED, Belcher CD III, Thomas JV. Surgical iridectomy. In: Thomas JV, Belcher CD, Simmons RJ, eds. Glaucoma surgery. St. Louis, Mosby–Year Book, 1992:97–105.
568. Spaeth GL. Iridectomy. In: Spaeth GL, ed. Ophthalmic surgery: principles and practice, ed 2. Philadelphia, WB Saunders, 1990:273–286.

569. Smith PD, Belcher CD III, Thomas JV. Anterior chamber deepening with intraoperative gonioscopy. In: Thomas JV, Belcher CD, Simmons RJ, eds. Glaucoma surgery. St. Louis, Mosby–Year Book, 1992: 215–221.
570. Sharpe ED, Thomas JV, Simmons RJ. Goniosynechialysis. In: Thomas JV, Belcher CD, Simmons RJ, eds. Glaucoma surgery. St. Louis, Mosby–Year Book, 1992:245–249.
571. Fu YA, Liaw ZC. Argon laser gonioplasty with trabeculoplasty for chronic angle-closure glaucoma. Ann Ophthalmol 1987;19:419–422.
572. Campbell DG, Vela A. Modern goniosynechialysis for the treatment of synechial angle-closure glaucoma. Ophthalmology 1984;91:1052–1060.
573. Shingleton BJ, et al. Surgical goniosynechialysis for angle-closure glaucoma. Ophthalmology 1990;97: 551–556.
574. Tanihara H, Nishiwaki K, Nagata M. Surgical results and complications of goniosynechialysis. Graefes Arch Clin Exp Ophthalmol 1992;230:309–313.
575. Gess LA, Koeth E, Gralle I. Trabeculectomy with iridencleisis. Br J Ophthalmol 1985;69:881–885.
576. Holland G, Seeth T. Clinical experience with iridencleisis. Klin Monatsbl Augenheilkd 1983;182:281–285. (in German)
577. Wyatt HT, et al. Autosomal dominant iridogoniodysgenesis: glaucoma management. Can J Ophthalmol 1983;18:11–14.
578. Singh OS, Simmons RJ. Glaucoma surgical techniques in nanophthalmos. In: Thomas JV, Belcher CD, Simmons RJ, eds. Glaucoma surgery. St. Louis, Mosby–Year Book, 1992:223–233.
579. Singh O, Sofinski S. Nanophthalmos: guidelines for diagnosis and therapy. In: Albert DM, Jakobiec FA, eds. Principles and practice of ophthalmology. Philadelphia, WB Saunders, 1993:1528–1540.
580. Diehl DL, et al. Nanophthalmos in sisters, one with exfoliation syndrome. Can J Ophthalmol 1989; 24:327–330.
581. Lytle RA, Thomas JV, Simmons RJ. Glaucoma surgical techniques in eyes with enlarged episcleral vessels. In: Thomas JV, Belcher CD, Simmons RJ, eds. Glaucoma surgery. St. Louis, Mosby–Year Book, 1992:235–243.
582. Goldstick B, Weinreb R. Glaucoma associated with elevated episcleral venous pressure. In: Higginbotham EJ, Lee DA, eds. Management of difficult glaucomas: a clinician's guide. Boston, Blackwell Scientific, 1994:282–290.
583. Yumita A, et al. Goniotomy with Q-switched Nd:YAG laser in juvenile developmental glaucoma: a preliminary report. Jpn J Ophthalmol 1984;28:349–355.
584. Sherwood MB. Filtering procedures: the patients. In: Sherwood MB, Spaeth GL, eds. Complications of glaucoma surgery. Thorofare, NJ, Slack, 1990:159–168.

Ophthalmic Surgery Complications: Prevention and Management,
edited by Judie F. Charlton and George W. Weinstein.
J. B. Lippincott Company, Philadelphia © 1995.

11

Jeffrey M. Lehmer
Hilel Lewis

Complications of Vitreoretinal Surgery

Modern vitreous surgery is an important and effective means of intervention in many ocular diseases. As new advances are made, the list of indications for vitrectomy grows longer, and results improve as experience is gained with each new technique.[1,2] Advances in vitreoretinal surgery have led to an improvement in the complete long-term retinal reattachment rate from 63% to 80% between 1978 and 1988.[2,3] The use of perfluorocarbon liquids (PFLs), one of these advances, has made a significant impact on the prognosis of eyes with giant retinal tears (GRTs). Before their use, only 11% of eyes achieved better than 20/200 vision, compared with 60% today.[4]

As the scope of vitreoretinal surgical applications increases, so does the potential for complications. Identifying complications and the risk factors associated with them can help reduce the likelihood of poor anatomic or visual results. For instance, the incidence of de novo iris neovascularization after vitrectomy for diabetic retinopathy dropped from 29% to 11% between 1974 and 1983.[5] The complications associated with vitreoretinal surgery result from both intraoperative factors such as mechanical or toxic damage and postoperative factors such as the late effects of intraoperative damage and inflammation. The type, incidence, and severity of complications depend on several factors, including the indication for surgery, the underlying ocular and systemic disease, the materials and techniques used in surgery, and the degree to which the surgical objectives are met intraoperatively.

This chapter first addresses complications that can be encountered in vitreoretinal surgery for any indication, including discussion on management and prevention. Complications most commonly seen during and after vitreous surgery for specific disease entities are then discussed, and a final section is devoted to special tools such as retinal tacks, glue, and PFLs.

GENERAL INTRAOPERATIVE COMPLICATIONS

Corneal Abnormalities

Most corneal abnormalities are noted postoperatively but result from intraoperative mechanical or toxic insults. The most common intraoperative problem is epithelial edema secondary to the intraocular pressure elevation often necessary to control bleeding during dissection of fibrovascular tissue. Its incidence in all cases is estimated at 14%.[6] Diabetic eyes are especially prone to epithelial edema because they have basement membrane abnormalities that weaken epithelial adhesion to the underlying Bowman membrane.[6] The incidence of intraoperative epithelial edema in nondiabetic eyes is 10% versus 20% in diabetic eyes.[6] Aphakic and pseudophakic eyes commonly develop epithelial edema, even though endothelial cell loss rates in pseudophakic eyes appear significantly lower than those of aphakic eyes.[7] The highest endothelial cell loss occurs in aphakic eyes undergoing fluid–gas exchange as a part of the initial vitrectomy.[8] Topical phenylephrine has been shown to be toxic to endothelium intraoperatively, and to lead to epithelial edema, especially in the presence of an epithelial defect.[8]

Management

If visualization is impaired, the corneal epithelium can be removed with a blade, but care must be taken to avoid trauma to the Bowman membrane; such trauma can lead to prolonged postoperative healing time.[6] Epithelial removal improves visibility but increases the risk of developing posterior stromal edema, manifested as folds in the Descemet membrane. These can be visually significant for the surgeon, especially during air–fluid exchange. The optical effect of the folds can be neutralized by coating the corneal endothelium with a thin layer of sodium hyaluronate before fluid–air exchange.[9]

Cataract Formation

Direct damage to the crystalline lens during vitreous surgery occurs in less than 1% of cases.[8] It most often occurs from direct contact with the shaft of the endoilluminator during excision of the anterior vitreous gel. This is best avoided by using caution when working near the lens, by using retroillumination for anteroperipheral vitreous, and by switching hands to reach vitreous that is 180 degrees away from the cutter's position rather than reaching across the eye.

The crystalline lens in diabetic eyes is susceptible to low-glucose irrigating solutions.[9] Fern-like posterior subcapsular opacities may occur under balanced-salt irrigation. Adding glucose to achieve a concentration of 400 mg/dL can prevent this.

Management

Prolonged contact between the gas and the lens is the most common cause of postoperative cataract formation. Intraoperative air–fluid exchange occasionally leads to the development of posterior subcapsular opacities that are opaque enough to require lensectomy to complete the posterior segment surgery. It is therefore advisable to minimize the time of contact between the air and the lens during the procedure.

Iatrogenic Retinal Breaks and Dialyses

Retinal breaks are a frequent complication of vitreous surgery, occurring in up to 69% of eyes with complicated retinal detachments from proliferative diabetic retinopathy.[10] The incidence varies depending on the condition being treated and the area of the retina concerned. In simple vitrectomy with membrane peeling for macular pucker, posterior retinal breaks have occurred in 1% to 5% of eyes, compared with 0% to 6% for breaks in the peripheral retina.[11–15] Posterior retinal breaks are more frequent (19%) during removal of epiretinal membranes occurring after retinal detachment surgery than those of the idiopathic variety (5%).[14] The reason is unclear but may be related to ultrastructural differences of epiretinal membranes that occur under varying circumstances.[16] During vitrectomy with use of PFLs to remove dislocated crystalline lenses, iatrogenic retinal breaks were seen in 11% of eyes.[17] In vitrectomy for progressive proliferative diabetic retinopathy, 18% of eyes suffered intraoperative breaks.[18] The rate for repair of diabetic traction retinal detachment is the highest and varies from 22% to 69%.[10,19,20] Breaks are generally a result of direct damage from cutting or suction devices or indirect damage from traction on epiretinal tissue or the vitreous base.

Management

Peripheral retinal tears are most common (76%) in the meridians of the pars plana sclerotomies, occurring in 4% to 25% of cases.[10,19] The breaks tend to occur along the posterior margin of the vitreous base, where traction is exerted from the placement and removal of surgical instruments. Breaks at the posterior vitreous base insertion elsewhere in the eye are less common and usually result from suction forces.[9] Treatment generally involves transscleral cryotherapy and postoperative tamponade with an intraocular gas bubble. A low circumferential scleral buckle may be applied for peripheral breaks but is not needed in most cases.[9] The incidence of peripheral breaks may be minimized by the gentle insertion and removal of instruments, paying particular attention to removal of vitreous or other tissue remnants from the instrument tips as they are introduced into the vitreous cavity. Careful examination of the retinal periphery with scleral depression must be done before closure to detect and treat all peripheral breaks.

Prevention

Posterior retinal breaks are usually caused by direct trauma from the vitrectomy probe or scissors during cutting or removal of opaque tissue near an area of retinal detachment or by traction on epiretinal tissue or cortical vitreous during its removal. This can be minimized by using the second instrument as a guard between the mobile, detached retina and the vitreous cutter and by maximizing visualization of vitreoretinal adhesions before cutting them. Posterior tears are treated with photocoagulation and gas tamponade.

Retinal Incarceration

Complications

There are no definitive reports on the incidence of retinal incarceration as a complication of vitreoretinal surgery, but it is uncommon and is usually encountered as a result of penetrating trauma rather than the surgery itself. Incarcerations that result from surgical complications most commonly occur when the retina is highly elevated and mobile. In this setting, the retina can become incarcerated into the sclerotomy wound during the exchange of surgical instruments, especially if the infusion pressure to the eye is not temporarily lowered or interrupted (Fig. 11-1). Vitreous base adjacent to a sclerotomy wound can also become incarcerated, causing secondary retinal incarceration. Loosely fitting scleral wound plugs can become dislodged due to pressure from scleral depression if indirect ophthalmoscopy is done before air–fluid exchange, leading to incarceration of mobile retina.

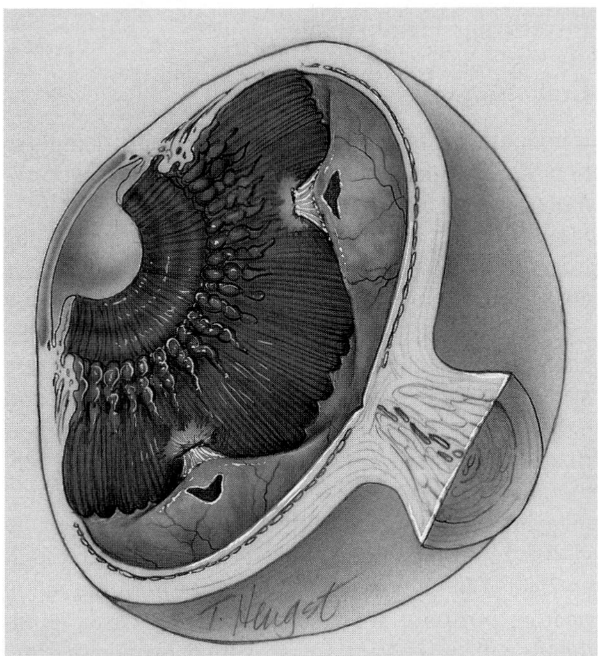

Figure 11-1. Vitreous base gel incarceration into two sclerotomy wounds with resulting iatrogenic retinal flap tears.

Management and Prevention

If vitreous incarcerates into a sclerotomy wound, causing peripheral retinal distortion, or if there is frank retinal incarceration, air–fluid exchange can free the tissues after blunt instruments are used to tease them free gently from an external approach. If the eye is aphakic or pseudophakic, the internal approach can be used; this involves placing a silicone-tipped extrusion cannula through the uninvolved sclerotomy and gently teasing the tissue back into the vitreous cavity with intermediate suction. This maneuver obviates the need to perform an air–fluid exchange in the middle of the operation but requires removal of the lens in a phakic eye. This type of tissue incarceration is best avoided by lowering the infusion pressure to the eye before withdrawing instruments or plugs.[9]

Choroidal Hemorrhage

Complications

Reports of the incidence of significant choroidal hemorrhage vary. Piper and associates reported a 1.9% incidence of operative or immediately postoperative choroidal hemorrhage for vitreous surgery.[21] They identified these possible risk factors: placement of a scleral buckle, increasing age at surgery (especially more than 55 years), elevated preoperative intraocular pressure, and nonphakic status. Their figure is much higher than the risk reported for intraocular surgery in general (0.7%)[22] or for cataract surgery in particular (0.2%).[23] A smaller series studying the risks of silicone oil removal reported a 1% rate of expulsive choroidal hemorrhage.[24] Lakhanpal and associates reported a series of seven cases of massive suprachoroidal hemorrhage; all the patients had undergone vitrectomy, scleral buckling, and laser and cryoretinopexy with fluid–gas exchange for complicated retinal detachments.[25] Risk factors identified were multiple surgical procedures, high myopia, aphakia, and intraocular inflammation. Other contributing factors include placement of a broad posterior scleral buckle with intraoperative hypotony and transscleral cryotherapy.[25]

Management

Significant intraoperative suprachoroidal hemorrhage is best managed conservatively. Intraoperative drainage is not generally recommended, because doing so only decompresses the suprachoroidal space, leading to further hemorrhaging. Leaving the suprachoroidal space unviolated allows the hemorrhage to tamponade itself. The recommended mode of management includes closure of the eye and use of hyperosmolar agents with aqueous suppressants such as acetazolamide to lower intraocular pressure.[25] Drainage sclerotomies combined with pars plana vitrectomy, if indicated, may be performed after 10 to 14 days of medical management, when the risk of rebleeding has decreased.[26]

Prevention

Prevention of massive hemorrhage involves identifying high-risk patients (aphakic myopes with a history of multiple surgeries, including large scleral buckles), using laser instead of cryotherapy, and using long-acting gas instead of a scleral buckle or buckle revision whenever possible.[25]

Macular Phototoxicity

Complications

Microscope light-induced phototoxic maculopathy is well recognized in cataract surgery.[27] The microscope has also been the source of the same damage in vitreoretinal surgery,[28] but the endoilluminator has been the perpetrator of most phototoxic maculopathy reported in the literature.[29–32] This complication, although obviously produced intraoperatively, cannot be identified until several days afterward, when vision fails to improve to expected levels and the characteristic white, edematous outer retinal and retinal pigment epithelium (RPE) lesion is seen clinically, with corresponding window defects on the fluorescein angiogram (Fig. 11-2). This lesion can be detected within 1 week and usually occurs during surgery for macular pucker and macular holes, where prolonged, intense illumination is used near the fovea.[29–32]

Management and Prevention

The only way to manage this problem is through prevention. Because the mechanism of damage involves light, heat, and oxidation, the ways to decrease risk include minimizing operating time (exposure), keeping the light source as far as possible from the retina and using the lowest illumination setting possible, using a filter for short wavelengths, using cool infusion fluids, and minimizing the oxygen delivered to the patient.[27]

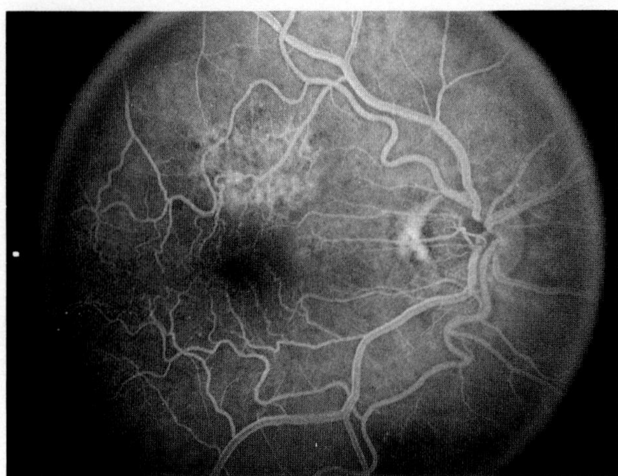

Figure 11-2. Fluorescein angiogram in late laminar flow phase showing mottled hyperfluorescence of a macular phototoxicity lesion. The lesion fades in the latest frames, confirming its nature as a window defect of the retinal pigment epithelium.

Intraocular Hemorrhage

Complications

Intraoperative bleeding is the only major complication that has become more frequent despite improvements in vitreous surgical instrumentation and technique.[9] This is probably due to the changing indications for surgery, especially in diabetic retinopathy, where eyes with extensive, active neovascularization may require significant epiretinal tissue dissection. Less than 1% of cases involve hemorrhage severe enough to cause premature termination of surgery.[9] In nondiabetic eyes, the incidence of hemorrhage varies from 0.4% in vitrectomy for epiretinal membrane removal to 6% in cases of recurrent retinal detachment from proliferative vitreoretinopathy (PVR).[12,13,33] In diabetic eyes, the rate can be as high as 75%.[9] Bleeding most often comes from the retina or from posterior segment neovascular tissue as either is cut or as traction is exerted on vitreoretinal attachments during removal of vitreous or fibrovascular membranes from the retinal surface.

Management

Methods to control intraoperative hemorrhage include elevating the ocular infusion pressure, using endodiathermy or bipolar cautery, and infusing thrombin. Most bleeding will respond to intraocular pressure elevation and diathermy. If the bleeding site cannot be visualized due to rapid hemorrhage into the vitreous cavity, the infusion pressure should be elevated to tamponade the bleeding. After 60 to 90 seconds, the hemorrhage can generally be cleared with an extrusion cannula to allow visualization for application of endodiathermy.

Thrombin may be added to the infusate at a concentration of 100 units/mL to control hemorrhaging that does not respond to conventional measures.[34] Other measures to control significant hemorrhaging include performing fluid–air exchange[35] or injecting silicone oil or sodium hyaluronate; these mechanically confine the hemorrhaging to allow coagulation but need to be removed before surgery can continue.[36]

Prevention

The risk of intraoperative hemorrhage can be reduced by several means. Active neovascularization should be suppressed before surgery if possible by panretinal photocoagulation or peripheral cryotherapy in diabetic eyes. In trauma cases, waiting for 2 weeks before vitrectomy not only lowers the risk of intraoperative hemorrhage but also allows for spontaneous separation of the posterior hyaloid from the retina, making surgery less technically demanding. This waiting period is impossible in the presence of an intraocular foreign body (IOFB) or traumatic endophthalmitis. Bleeding is less likely when scissors are used instead of traction to remove vitreoretinal attachments, especially in diabetic eyes. The amount of hemorrhage can also be minimized by the use of endodiathermy or photocoagulation before or immediately after vascularized tissue is cut or removed.[9]

Hypotony

Complications

Intraoperative hypotony can lead to significant complications that can hinder the normal progress of a procedure. Most notably, blood can reflux into the Schlemm canal and into the anterior chamber, causing deposition of red blood cells and fibrin on the anterior surface of the crystalline lens or intraocular lens; this can significantly limit visualization of the posterior segment. Prolonged hypotony can lead to the development of serous choroidal detachments intraoperatively. If these persist during the procedure and then resolve postoperatively, the eye can be left with a significant underfill of either gas or silicone oil and may require further management if tamponade is inadequate. Hypotony is most often the result of inadequate infusion pressure from pump malfunction or incorrect bottle height. It may also result from sclerotomies that are too large to provide a closed-pressure system.

Management

The first step in management is to secure an adequate intraocular pressure to limit further problems. This requires checking sclerotomies for leaks and examining the infusion system for defects. If blood is in the anterior chamber, paracentesis-style incisions must be made to perform an adequate washout to restore visualization to the posterior pole. This usually leads to significant pupillary miosis, requiring pharmacologic treatment. If choroidal detachments have formed, restoring a normal intraocular pressure often stops their progression, and elevating the pressure above normal levels at interrupted intervals can lead to moderate intraoperative resolution. Immediate drainage is not generally recommended because there is the risk of suprachoroidal hemorrhage, and further hypotony may aggravate the problem.

Prevention

Preventing these problems means preventing intraoperative hypotony. This requires the presence of highly skilled operating room personnel who remain cognizant of the status of the infusion system during the procedure. The surgeon must also take responsibility for the accurate set-up and operation of the equipment. Back-up systems must be available should infusion pressure fall due to defective equipment. The surgeon must also periodically check for oversized or stretched sclerotomies and minimize the time during which a sclerotomy is not plugged or in use. Early detection of hypotony by the presence of excessive corneal striae or a change in the turgor of the globe should lead to prompt action to normalize intraocular pressure.

Intraocular Hypertension

Complications

It is often necessary during vitreoretinal surgery to elevate the infusion pressure to supranormal levels. This is usually done to control or prevent significant intraocular hemorrhaging, but it may also be used during air–fluid exchanges and to treat or limit the development of serous or hemorrhagic choroidal detachments. Although not usually detrimental to the eye, it can occasionally lead to central retinal artery occlusion, which may not be recognized until the early postoperative period. Patients at highest risk include those with proliferative diabetic retinopathy or significant hypertensive retinopathy, and those with systemic hypercoagulable or hyperviscosity states.

Management and Prevention

Recognition of the problem may not occur until many hours after the occlusion, so prevention is the best approach. The surgeon should always be aware of the perfusion status of the retina, especially during hypertensive intervals of the procedure. Some of the newer infusion systems have automatic alarms that alert the operating team that intraocular pressure elevation has been maintained for a preset duration (often 1–2 minutes maximum). With or without these, the surgeon must remain aware of elevated pressure and minimize its use and duration, especially when operating on high-risk patients.

GENERAL POSTOPERATIVE COMPLICATIONS

Corneal Abnormalities

Postoperative nonhealing or slowly healing epithelial defects are most common in diabetic eyes. Several reports of vitrectomy for complications of diabetic retinopathy estimate the incidence of this problem at 3% to 9%.[5,20,37] Risk is further increased by pars plana lensectomy or a history of previous vitreous surgery.[6] Management begins with treating intraocular hypertension, along with simple antibiotic ointments and patching. If this is unsuccessful, hypertonic saline for persistent epithelial edema may be useful. Bandage contact lenses or anterior stromal micropuncture may be required to achieve long-term epithelial adhesion in rare cases.

Management

Postoperative corneal edema is most commonly seen with persistently elevated intraocular pressure. Edema was seen after 6% of vitrectomies for removal of dislocated posterior chamber intraocular lenses in one series.[38] It can also be a manifestation of a persistently detached macula, because in eyes with this complication, stromal edema and keratopathy were more prevalent, with an incidence of 55% to 60%.[39] In eyes with the potential for functional vision that have persistent stromal edema after intraocular pressure and inflammation have been treated, penetrating keratoplasty may be the only treatment option.

Prevention

Band keratopathy is a significant problem in aphakic eyes that have undergone vitrectomy with silicone oil injection. This problem is universal by 6 months in the presence of silicone-endothelial touch; therefore, overfilling with silicone oil must be avoided, and inadequate or secondarily closed inferior iridotomies must be opened.[40–42] Removal of silicone oil has been associated with clearing of keratopathy, the development of postremoval corneal dystrophy requiring penetrating keratoplasty, and the development of keratopathy in previously clear corneas when removal was performed prophylactically.[43] Despite this, the general recommendation is still to remove silicone oil after 3 to 4 months of stable retinal reattachment in an effort to prevent secondary corneal and lenticular complications (see Silicone Oil).

Cataract

Complications

The development or progression of cataract is the most common long-term complication following vitrectomy in phakic eyes. The incidence depends on the patient's age at surgery and the length of follow-up.[44] Regardless of concurrent ocular disease, vitrectomy itself appears to be cataractogenic, causing this in up to 75% of eyes followed for 10 or more years. The most common type of cataract developing or progressing after surgery is nuclear sclerosis.[5,11–15,18,20,37,45–49] Posterior subcapsular cataract development or progression appears to occur most commonly with long-term intraocular gas tamponade, especially after repeat air–fluid exchange following postoperative diabetic vitreous hemorrhage, where the incidence has been reported to be 59% at a mean follow-up period of 78 weeks.[50]

After vitrectomy for complications of proliferative diabetic retinopathy, development or progression of significant cataracts occurs in 1% to 37% of eyes,[5,18,20,37,44,47,48,51] with an average time between surgery and diagnosis of 13 months.[47] The development or progression of nuclear sclerotic cataracts is well known after vitrectomy for macular pucker: the incidence is between 32% and 80%, depending on the patient's age and the length of follow-up.[11–14,44–46] In one series, 32% of nuclear sclerotic cataracts progressed, versus 8% of the posterior subcapsular type, after macular pucker surgery.[15] When compared with fellow eyes, operated eyes were more than three times as likely to develop significant nuclear sclerosis after macular pucker surgery during a mean follow-up period of 29 months.[44] Data on macular hole surgery is not as extensive, but figures appear comparable.[49,52]

Management

Removal of cataracts by extracapsular techniques appears to be safe and effective in improving vision after vitrectomy, especially in diabetic eyes.[47,53,54] A waiting period of 6 months after vitrectomy is recommended before cataract extraction and intraocular lens implantation to ensure stability of the retinopathy and recovery from vitrectomy.[47] Care should be taken to use a fairly large optic (minimum 6.5 mm) to facilitate long-term clinical surveillance of the peripheral retina and to allow unimpeded delivery of supplemental panretinal photocoagulation in diabetic eyes with continued proliferative disease.

Prevention

The rapid development of posterior subcapsular cataracts after outpatient air–fluid exchange for postoperative diabetic vitreous hemorrhage has prompted recommendations for conservative management. Except in cases of erythroclastic glaucoma, or in dense vitreous hemorrhage cases that need either immediate visual rehabilitation or panretinal photocoagulation, several weeks should be allowed to elapse before performing outpatient air–fluid exchange, because spontaneous clearing may occur.[50,55]

Wound Complications

Problems relating only to the pars plana incisions are infrequent, and their effect on the eye can be either trivial or devastating. Complications can best be categorized into three types: fibrovascular ingrowth, hemorrhage (early, late, or recurrent), and tractional and other effects related to the proximity of the vitreous base to the incision (intraoperative, early, or late).[56] Some degree of fibrous ingrowth must occur in all wounds as part of normal healing, and in the sclerotomy the source of most of the granulation tissue and fibroblasts is the uveal layer.[57] True ingrowth occurs when fibrovascular tissue proliferates excessively at the internal aspect of the sclerotomy and invades the vitreous base; this causes contracture, which may lead to vitreous hemorrhage or peripheral traction retinal detachment. Severe ingrowth can cause traction detachment of the ciliary body epithelium, leading to hypotony and phthisis bulbi.

Postoperative vitreous hemorrhage can occur as a result of abnormal sclerotomy wound healing, especially in diabetic patients, where an additional stimulus for anterior segment neovascularization from chronic ischemia is often present. Many recurrent and late vitreous hemorrhages may be mistakenly attributed to persistent retinal neovascularization or presumed to be "idiopathic."[55] Because the postoperative vitreous hemorrhage rate in diabetic patients varies (27% to 60%), accurate diagnosis is imperative.[37,55] Early postoperative vitreous hemorrhage is most likely to originate from persistent bleeding from the lacerated uveal tissue or from "shake out" of red blood cells from the vitreous skirt after vitrectomy for a nonclearing vitreous hemorrhage. However, bleeding from early granulation tissue in the wound has been seen as early as 1 week postoperatively.[56] More characteristic of a wound-related hemorrhage is that seen several weeks to months after the initial vitrectomy. Characteristic clinical evidence is a wedge of hemorrhage found behind the crystalline lens, which localizes the source of bleeding to the Berger space (between the pars plicata and the anterior hyaloid face).[56–58] Because most sclerotomies are made in or just anterior to the anterior vitreous base, blood can easily track along the anterior hyaloid face and present behind the lens. This is not physically possible if the blood originates from the posterior retinal surface, because the intact vitreous base and anterior hyaloid act as a barrier. Hemorrhaging as a result of anterior hyaloidal fibrovascular proliferation (AHFP) can also present with blood in the Berger space, but neovascular fronds crossing the ora serrata and coursing along the anterior hyaloid are signs that distinguish this entity from wound neovascularization.[48,56]

Tractional effects of wound healing can bring about changes similar to those found with anterior PVR. The contraction phase of scarring in the vitreous base region can exert anterior and circumferential traction on the peripheral retina, leading to late peripheral retinal breaks and traction detachments.[56]

Management

Vitreous hemorrhage that is recurrent or renders the patient legally blind requires surgical intervention. Although the vascular component to the scar tissue eventually regresses, this may take years, and recurrent bleeding can plague the patient and increase the risk of cataract, erythroclastic glaucoma, and traction retinal detachment. Traction or rhegmatogenous retinal detachment or hypotony from fibrous ingrowth or mechanical distortion from wound healing also requires surgical intervention. For recurrent hemorrhages, pars plana lensectomy with removal of the lens capsule is required for adequate visualization of the internal aspect of the sclerotomies. The new sclerotomies should be placed at new locations to allow access to the old ones. Using deep scleral depression and external illumination, the sclerotomies can be visualized. The vitreous cutter or vertical scissors can then be used to isolate the stalk of wound tissue from the nearby vitreous base as much as possible. Diathermy should be used to cauterize the remaining stump of fibrovascular tissue until it appears fully blanched. The vertical scissors can then be used to further relieve any remaining anteroposterior or circumferential vitreous base traction on the peripheral retina. If not all the traction can be removed internally, a circumferential scleral buckle is required.[59–61] If a posterior chamber intraocular lens is present, removal along with the lens capsule using 1:5000 alpha-chymotrypsin is recommended for visualization.[56,62]

Intraocular Fibrin Deposition

Complications

The breakdown of the blood–ocular barrier inherent to the postoperative inflammatory response varies greatly in severity, depending on such factors as the length of surgery, the tissues involved, and the procedures performed. Signs of intraocular inflammation are mild after a relatively short procedure involving only excision of abnormal vitreous gel. Severe inflammation with formation of fibrin membranes on all intraocular surfaces is most often seen after prolonged dissection of fibrovascular membranes and lensectomy in a diabetic eye followed by extensive laser or cryotherapy and the use of an intraocular gas bubble. Fibrin deposition can lead to surgical failure either through recurrent retinal detachment from traction or from ciliary body detachment from epiciliary traction with secondary hypotony.[60,63–65] Visual failure can also occur secondary to cataract formation.[66] The risk factors for development of significant postoperative fibrin include preoperative aphakia, operative scatter endophotocoagulation, silicone oil injection, and lensectomy.[67] Overall, the incidence of postvitrectomy fibrin formation ranges from 5% to 22%; it is most commonly seen after surgery on diabetic eyes.[48,66,67] The signs of fibrin formation include a fibrin clot in the anterior chamber or an occlusive pupillary membrane, and they can be seen as early as the first postoperative day.[68] These anterior segment findings are manifestations of similar deposition of fibrin along the surfaces of the retina and ciliary body.

Management

Tissue plasminogen activator (tPA) injection is the treatment of choice for postvitrectomy fibrin formation severe enough to require intervention.[63–65,69–71] It acts by enzymatically converting plasminogen to plasmin, which then lyses fibrin into fibrin degradation products. Before the introduction of tPA, topical and systemic corticosteroids were only partially successful in reducing the incidence of secondary complications. Experimental work has revealed that doses of tPA as low as 25 μg may be toxic to the retina and that a dose as small as 3 μg was found to be 100% safe and effective if given within 10 days after vitrectomy.[71] The range of time between surgery and injection of tPA has varied in the literature from 24 hours to 15 days.[65] However, some fibrin deposition may be later in onset: Dabbs and associates identified membrane formation to occur between 16 and 64 days after vitrectomy in diabetic eyes.[66] Early injections may carry a risk of intraocular hemorrhage, but late injections may be less effective due to maturation of membranes with incorporation of a significant fibrous and fibroglial component.[66]

The injection is usually done using a 30-gauge needle on a 1-mL syringe through the limbus in aphakic and pseudophakic eyes and through the pars plana in phakic eyes to lyse posterior segment fibrin. Postinjection patient positioning may be helpful to direct the greatest concentration of tPA to the intraocular site most involved. Dissolution of fibrin pupillary membranes can be expected as soon as 1 hour after injection.[66] Fibrin degradation products may be toxic to the retina and vascular endothelial cells, which can lead to further fibrin release from damaged vessels, so a washout or fluid–gas exchange may be necessary after tPA injection to prevent this.[66] Hemorrhagic complications of tPA injection usually seen within 24 hours and at doses of 12 μg or more include hyphema and progressive subretinal and suprachoroidal hemorrhage.[66]

Prevention

Prevention of acute postvitrectomy fibrin formation involves minimizing the controllable risk factors mentioned earlier. Iverson and associates used an intraoperative infusion of 5 IU/mL of low-molecular-weight heparin in rabbit eyes to reduce greatly the incidence and severity of postoperative fibrin formation after vitrectomy and lensectomy.[72] In this case, the low-molecular-weight heparin activates antithrombin III, which inhibits the formation of thrombin, which reduces the amount of fibrinogen being converted to fibrin. Intraoperative hemorrhage was not encountered in the rabbit eyes studied, but because experience with human eyes is limited, its routine use cannot be recommended.

Periretinal Proliferation

Complications

Periretinal proliferation is a general term referring to the detrimental result of the proliferative phase of the ocular inflammatory response after surgery. The initial phases include breakdown of the blood–ocular barrier, with release of fibrin and inflammatory cells. The subacute phase of proliferation yields fibrin and fibrocellular membranes that adhere to and distort or detach intraocular tissue such as the retina and ciliary body. This can yield the postoperative problems better known as chronic hypotony, epiretinal and subretinal traction band formation, and macular pucker.

The ocular inflammatory response is a necessary and unavoidable part of the healing process. However, when the stimulus for inflammation is great, the response can be difficult to control and lead to significant periretinal proliferation. This stimulus is greatest in vitreoretinal surgery when heavy cryotherapy is applied to areas of bare RPE, when total operating time is prolonged, and when a retinectomy or retinotomy with extensive intraocular diathermy is required to release retinal traction.[2,73,74] When the location of the periretinal proliferation is mainly posterior and mild, it can lead to macular pucker. When more extensive, it can detach the retina with traction exerted posteriorly, anteriorly, or both.[2,59,68] When the proliferation is mostly anterior, it can distort or detach the nonpigmented ciliary body epithelium to cause chronic hypotony[2,59,68,75] (Fig. 11-3).

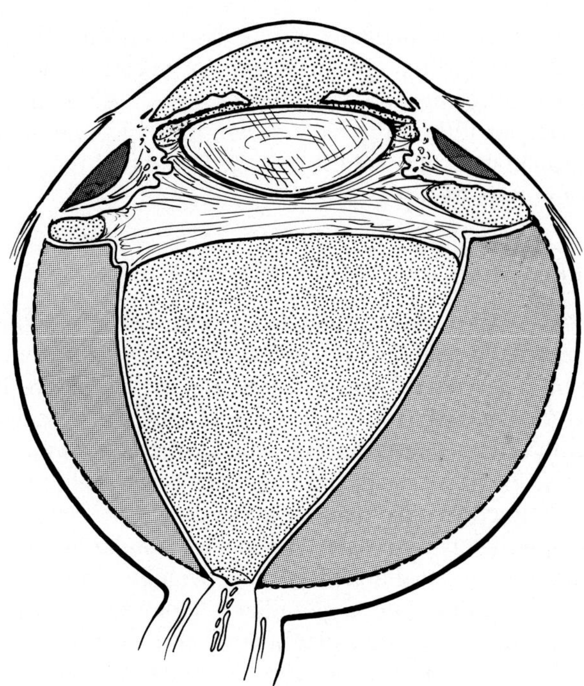

Figure 11-3. Anterior proliferative vitreoretinopathy with anterior and perpendicular traction causing detachment of the ciliary body, which leads to hypotony.

Management

If excessive postoperative inflammation leads to fibrin membrane formation, it should be managed as discussed in the earlier section on intraocular fibrin deposition. Once the results of periretinal proliferation have been recognized, further surgical intervention is often necessary if vision or ocular integrity is significantly compromised. The techniques for removing the posterior epiretinal membranes of macular pucker have been described.[11–13,15,16,76] The approach to treating chronic hypotony with direct dissection of epiciliary fibrous tissue has also been described, with promising results for what were previously unsalvageable prephthisical eyes.[75] Anterior or posterior PVR is the most severe form of periretinal proliferation and is best managed by direct removal of fibrous traction.[2,59,68,77,78]

Prevention

Because of the potentially substantial morbidity caused by epiretinal proliferative disease, its prevention is a topic of intense ongoing research. Most work is focusing on reducing mitosis of proliferative cells with various antimetabolites and growth factor inhibitors, interfering with the attachment of proliferative cells to collagen structures, and reducing the reactive inflammatory process that stimulates cellular proliferation.[2,79] As mentioned earlier, avoiding excessive cryoretinopexy and large radial retinotomies and using meticulous intraocular hemostasis can reduce the risk of subsequent surgical failure from postoperative PVR.[2,73,74]

Retinal Detachment

Complications

The incidence of postoperative retinal detachment after vitrectomy varies depending on the underlying disease and the complexity of the procedure. After vitrectomy for macular pucker, retinal detachment has been reported in 3% of eyes with extramacular iatrogenic breaks, versus 6% for peripheral iatrogenic breaks.[15] Others have also found a general incidence of between 4% and 7% for postoperative rhegmatogenous retinal detachment in this setting.[12,13,45] The incidence is slightly lower (2%) after vitrectomy for impending macular holes.[52] After vitrectomy for progressive proliferative diabetic retinopathy unresponsive to photocoagulation or cryotherapy, the incidence has been reported at 3%.[18] Rhegmatogenous retinal detachment after vitrectomy for nonclearing diabetic vitreous hemorrhage occurs in 10% to 12% of eyes followed for up to 2 years.[3,5] As many as 4% of eyes may develop inoperable traction retinal detachments within 6 months after vitrectomy for nonclearing diabetic vitreous hemorrhage.[51] In more severe cases of traction retinal detachment of the macula with or without a rhegmatogenous component in diabetic eyes, eyes with severe PVR, eyes with GRTs, and after penetrating trauma, the incidence of postoperative retinal detachment varies between 14% and 36%.[10,20,37,74,80] In simpler cases, the most common type of postoperative retinal detachment is rhegmatogenous and is due to undetected iatrogenic retinal breaks. In more complex cases, inflammation with fibrin membrane deposition and recurrent PVR leading to traction retinal detachment are the most common mechanisms for anatomic failure.

Management

Postoperative rhegmatogenous retinal detachment can be managed in several ways. If the break is in the superior two thirds of the fundus, cryoretinopexy followed by pneumatic retinopexy with postoperative positioning suffices. For breaks elsewhere or when positioning may be difficult, traditional scleral buckling is more appropriate. External drainage of a bullous detachment in a vitrectomized eye can lead to significant entry of vitreous cavity fluid through the break into the subretinal space, leading to ineffective removal of subretinal fluid. When this occurs, pneumatic techniques must be used to achieve nearly simultaneous subretinal fluid drainage and retinal break tamponade. This applies to rhegmatogenous retinal detachments occurring both intraoperatively and postoperatively when formed vitreous has already been removed. Management of postoperative traction retinal detachments from severe fibrin deposition or PVR should be approached using techniques outlined elsewhere; a full discussion is beyond the scope of this chapter.[2,59,68,77]

Prevention

Precautions for preventing postoperative rhegmatogenous retinal detachments have been discussed (see Iatrogenic Retinal Breaks and Dialyses). Risk factors for the development of redetachment from PVR have been studied, but reports differ. They are increased use of cryotherapy; excessive or uncontrollable intraoperative vitreous hemorrhage; inadequate removal of posterior proliferative tissue; new iatrogenic retinal breaks; use of long-acting intraocular gas tamponade; use of retinal tacks; large, inferotemporal circumferential retinotomies and radial retinotomies; and younger patient age.[2,68,73,74,81,82] To minimize redetachment, the surgeon must minimize trauma to tissues both posteriorly and near the sclerotomies, meticulously control intraocular hemorrhage, minimize the use of cryotherapy, and use certain adjunctive techniques such as retinal tacks and relaxing incisions only as a last resort.

Choroidal Detachment

Complications

Postoperative choroidal detachments are common after vitreoretinal surgery but typically have little impact on anatomic or visual outcome. They are more often seen when scleral buckling is used in conjunction with vitreous surgery, leading to reduction of episcleral venous outflow and choroidal congestion (Fig. 11-4). Prolonged hypotony during or after surgery increases the risk of developing choroidal detachments. The more common occurrence of intraocular hypertension postoperatively, especially when gas tamponade is used, reduces both the incidence and severity of choroidal detachments. An association between postoperative choroidal detachments and subsequent development of PVR has been reported.[73] This is most likely a result of the association between severe postoperative inflammation and hypotony rather than a direct correlation between choroidal detachments and PVR.

Management

Most choroidal detachments are small and resolve spontaneously. However, significant intraocular inflammation often accompanies them, so increased frequency of topical corticosteroids may be indicated. With larger or anteriorly located detachments that lead to secondary angle-closure glaucoma, systemic corticosteroids (if not medically contraindicated) should be given, as well as aggressive medical management of intraocular pressure. If pressure can be maintained at a level where vascular perfusion is not compromised, ciliary body edema and rotation usually resolve within 24 to 48 hours, with a subsequent reduction in intraocular pressure. If vascular perfusion is compromised, choroidal drainage may be necessary.

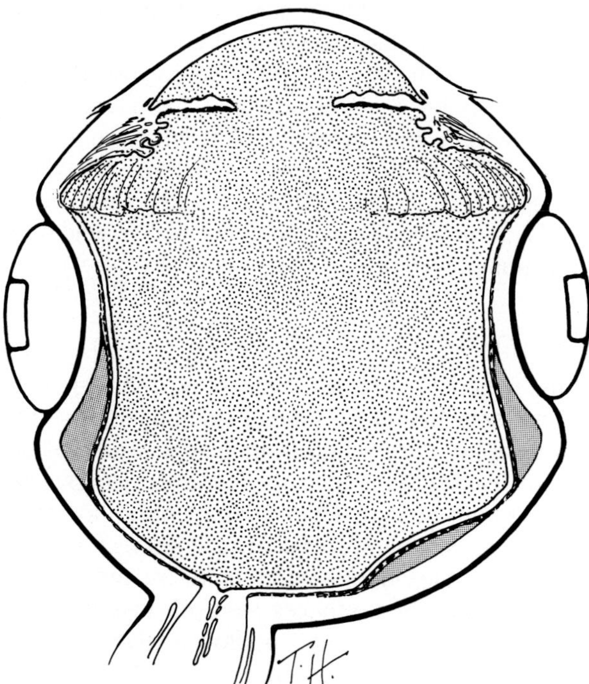

Figure 11-4. High scleral buckle associated with compression of scleral emissary venules, which leads to chronic serous choroidal detachments.

Intraocular Hypertension

Complications

Postoperative elevation of intraocular pressure has many possible causes, including obstruction of trabecular outflow channels by residual inflammatory or red blood cells; damage to the trabecular meshwork endothelium by irrigating fluids; primary angle-closure glaucoma from inflammatory or neovascular tissue; open-angle glaucoma from intraocular inflammation, prolonged use of corticosteroids, or ciliary body edema; and secondary angle closure from pupillary block caused by an expanding gas bubble, silicone oil, or occlusion pupillae from intraocular fibrin.

The risk of developing postoperative intraocular hypertension varies depending on the primary indication for vitrectomy, the success of surgery, and any materials left in the eye, such as gas or silicone oil. A review of 222 cases by Han and associates found that the average intraocular pressure (IOP) elevation in the early postoperative period in all eyes (diabetics, PVR, endophthalmitis, and so forth) was 10.6 mmHg.[83] They found that significant and severe IOP elevation was most common with PVR cases (54%) and least common in surgery for macular pucker (9.5%). Angle closure from expanding gas occurs in about 1% of macular pucker cases,[11] and an open-angle mechanism accounts for significant IOP elevation in from 8% to 35% of eyes operated on for complications of diabetic retinopathy.[5,8,20,37] Neovascular glaucoma occurs in from 2% to 13% of eyes after vitrectomy for diabetic complications, but the incidence is much higher (83%–92%) in the presence of a postoperative retinal detachment.[5,18,20,37,48,51,80] Although erythroclastic outflow obstruction may give rise to transient IOP elevation in as many as one third of eyes following vitrectomy for diabetic vitreous hemorrhage, persistent medically uncontrolled erythroclastic glaucoma requiring reoperation is relatively uncommon (1.4%).[55] Finally, significant IOP elevation has been reported in 9% of eyes receiving C_3F_8 gas versus 13% receiving silicone oil for internal retinal tamponade at the conclusion of surgery for PVR.[84]

Management

Management of postoperative intraocular hypertension depends on its pathophysiology. Persistent erythroclastic glaucoma requires reoperation (washout) because a simple air–fluid exchange may not effectively remove erythroclasts from the anterior chamber angle. In addition, fluid–air exchange has been associated with a 10% incidence of acute IOP elevation when performed on diabetic eyes with postoperative vitreous hemorrhage.[50] Inflammatory glaucoma should be treated with topical corticosteroids and ocular antihypertensives. Fibrin pupillary block glaucoma may respond to argon or YAG laser disruption of the membrane[85] or to injection of tPA to lyse the fibrin (see Intraocular Fibrin Deposition).[66] Pressure rise secondary to an expanding gas bubble may respond to anterior chamber paracentesis, but this may cause or aggravate secondary angle closure. Therefore, decompressing the gas using a trans-pars plana approach with a small-gauge needle is preferred over paracentesis in this setting. Silicone oil-associated IOP elevation may be due to occlusion of the inferior iridectomy by fibrin in aphakic and pseudophakic eyes.[39,86] This should be reopened with the YAG laser if the IOP rise is severe; otherwise, topical corticosteroids with or without tPA injection can lead to fibrinolysis and resolution of normal aqueous flow. If ciliary body edema is the suspected mechanism for the IOP rise, topical steroids with the addition of systemic corticosteroids (if not medically contraindicated) and cycloplegics with or without argon laser iridoplasty may be beneficial.[83] Iridocorneal apposition may cause significant IOP elevation in aphakic gas-filled eyes. This can be remedied by instilling 1 mL of sodium hyaluronate between the iris and cornea to reform the anterior chamber angle and prevent chronic anterior synechiae.[87]

Prevention

Perioperative factors that correlate with the risk of postoperative intraocular hypertension include intraoperative or previous placement of a scleral buckle, intraoperative scatter photocoagulation, use of expansile intraocular gas, intraoperative lensectomy, and postoperative fibrin formation.[83] Preexisting glaucoma is also a significant preoperative risk factor. These intraoperative procedures can seldom be avoided out of concern over the postoperative intraocular pressure, so prevention is difficult. The risk factors are useful mainly for preoperative counseling and identification of patients who need close postoperative pressure monitoring. Significant rises in postoperative IOP have not been found to influence short-term (6-week) visual acuity results significantly.[83]

Intraocular Hemorrhage

Complications

The incidence of postoperative vitreous hemorrhage for all cases is about 6%.[38,51] This figure is understandably higher in eyes that have undergone vitrectomy for complications of proliferative diabetic retinopathy, where reports vary between 11% and 60%.[3,5,18,20,37,55,56,88,89] The highest incidence of postoperative diabetic vitreous hemorrhage occurs in a bimodal temporal distribution—during the first week, and then between the first and sixth months after vitrectomy.[55] The earlier events may be due to inadequate hemostasis during surgery, dispersion of red blood cells from the remaining vitreous skirt, or acute retinal tear with avulsion of a retinal vessel. The later events may be due to inadequate panretinal photocoagulation with progression of proliferative diabetic retinopathy, traction on residual posterior fibrovascular epicenters, acute retinal tear with retinal vessel avulsion, or wound complications (see Wound Complications).

Management

If the patient is not functionally blind and there is no retinal detachment by clinical examination or ultrasonography, observation is indicated, with typically rapid clearing in the absence of formed vitreous gel. Further management depends on identification of the source of the hemorrhage. Dispersion of residual blood from the vitreous skirt requires no further treatment. Wound hemorrhages were discussed earlier. Supplemental panretinal photocoagulation is required for persistent posterior proliferative bleeding sites, and hemorrhagic retinal tears require retinopexy.

Prevention

Preventive measures include meticulous intraocular hemostasis, maximal preoperative and intraoperative panretinal photocoagulation in diabetic eyes, careful removal of prolapsed vitreous gel before sclerotomy closure, and delamination instead of segmentation of epiretinal fibrovascular tissue whenever possible.

Hypotony and Phthisis Bulbi

Complications

Hypotony with or without the development of phthisis bulbi is most often secondary to one or all of four complications seen after vitreous surgery in the absence of a known wound leak:

1. Persistent or recurrent retinal detachment (especially involving the macula).[39]
2. Untreated or newly developed anterior PVR with tractional detachment of the anterior retina and ciliary body.[2,59,61,68]
3. Profound and permanent breakdown of the blood–ocular barrier, leading to massive hemorrhage or fibrin deposition in the region of the ciliary body.[60,63,64,70,74]
4. The development of AHFP in diabetic eyes.[48]

After vitrectomy for complications of proliferative diabetic retinopathy, the incidence of hypotony is between 4% and 11%.[5,20,90,91] This increases for repeat vitrectomy to 20% or more.[84,92] In PVR, the incidence varies between 10% to 39%, depending on the severity of the case and the use of gas versus silicone oil tamponade.[81,84] In a series of complex traction retinal detachments where many eyes required repeat or multiple vitreoretinal procedures for PVR, GRTs with PVR, diabetic traction retinal detachments, and penetrating trauma, the incidence was higher still: 43%.[74] A 16% incidence of hypotony after removal of silicone oil in successfully reattached retinas has been reported.[24] Finally, hypotony is common (25%) after vitrectomy for traction retinal detachments due to the acute retinal necrosis syndrome.[93]

Management

The approach to management depends on the probable cause. In persistent or recurrent retinal detachment, further surgery to reattach the retina is required. With anterior PVR and ciliary body detachment, removal of all anterior vitreous and proliferative tissue (as described in the section on PVR) should be done. With severe inflammation and fibrin deposition, injection of tPA can be effective in dissolving fibrin membranes that adhere to and detach or distort the ciliary body epithelium.[66] For AHFP, confluent photocoagulation to the peripheral retina and pars plana can cause regression of proliferative tissue if the media allows.[48] Otherwise, repeat vitrectomy with diathermy to neovascular tissue and release of all anterior traction followed by photocoagulation to the peripheral retina is required to salvage the eye.[48] A moderate degree of hypotony does not exclude the possibility of continued visual function.[74,81]

Endophthalmitis

Complications

According to reports from the Endophthalmitis Vitrectomy Study, 70% of all endophthalmitis occurs as a complication of intraocular surgery; 88% of these cases occur within 6 weeks after surgery.[94] The overall incidence is still low, in the range of 0.1% to 0.4%.[94] Most cases of endophthalmitis occurring in the setting of vitreoretinal surgery are iatrogenic or a consequence of penetrating trauma for which the vitrectomy is performed.

A large-series report on the incidence of endophthalmitis after vitrectomy estimates that this complication occurs in 0.051% of cases.[95] This represents an improvement over previous reports of 0.2% for all vitrectomies.[9] Smaller series reports are not as reliable, but they remind us of the real possibility of this devastating complication. Examples include a 1.2% incidence after vitrectomy for macular pucker cases,[12,13] a 2% incidence after vitrectomy for nonclearing diabetic vitreous hemorrhage,[51] a 2.3% incidence after repair of macular hole-related retinal detachments,[96] and various case reports, such as late endophthalmitis after transscleral suture-fixation of posterior chamber intraocular lenses.[97] Following penetrating ocular trauma with retained IOFBs, the incidence of endophthalmitis is estimated to be between 7% and 13%.[98,99]

The organisms most often cultured from eyes in posttraumatic endophthalmitis differ significantly from those in postoperative endophthalmitis. *Staphylococcus epidermidis* is by far the most common iatrogenic pathogen, followed by *Staphylococcus aureus*, streptococcal species, and *Propionibacterium acnes*.[95,100,101] A wide variety of organisms is the rule after penetrating trauma with retained IOFBs. Typically seen are *Bacillus* sp; group D *Streptococcus*; coagulase-negative *Staphylococcus* sp; fungi, including *Fusarium* and *Candida* sp. and many varieties of fermenting and nonfermenting gram-negative rods.[98,100] In general, the more indolent organisms such as *P acnes* and the fungi present as late endophthalmitis (beyond 4–6 weeks postoperatively), but some bacteria such as *S epidermidis* can present either early or late (Table 11-1).

Management

Because treatment must be urgently implemented and because only 25% to 30% of cultures are positive, broad-spectrum antibiotics are the initial treatment in all cases and are maintained until a specific organism can be isolated. Immediate management as used by the Endophthalmitis Vitrectomy Study Group consists of immediate cultures of the anterior chamber and vitreous cavity followed by intravitreal injection of amikacin, 400 μg, and vancomycin, 1 mg, and subconjunctival injection of vancomycin, 25 mg, and ceftazidime, 100 mg, with topical cycloplegics.[94] Topical, periocular, and systemic corticosteroids are also used.[94] The role of vitrectomy versus simple vitreous tap or biopsy is being evaluated by this multicenter, prospective, randomized, controlled clinical trial. Other investigators have supported the role of intravitreal antibiotics,[100,101] and the clinician must be prepared to repeat the injections along with the cultures in culture-positive cases that do not rapidly respond to treatment.[101] In cases of penetrating trauma with retained IOFBs, early intervention with vitrectomy, removal of the IOFB, and injection of intravitreal antibiotics with topical and systemic broad-spectrum coverage has been shown to reduce the development of clinical endophthalmitis with serious visual loss even when the removed material is culture-positive.[98]

Sympathetic Ophthalmia

Complications

The development of sympathetic ophthalmia is uncommon after pars plana vitrectomy. Very few articles involving vitrectomy as the primary surgical procedure report on its occurrence. One study involving 41 patients with complicated retinal detachments reported a 0.3% to 1% incidence of sympathetic ophthalmia after vitrectomy with use of retinal tacks.[102] The generally accepted high-risk eyes are those whose fellow eye sustained trauma with loss or prolapse of uvea or vitreous; older studies report the incidence in this setting to be 0.19%.[9] The incidence is much lower (0.007%) after anterior segment procedures such as cataract extraction and trabeculectomy.[9]

Management

Treatment generally consists of systemic corticosteroids at an initial dose of 1 mg/kg until control is achieved, followed by a very gradual taper to a level where inactivity is maintained at the minimum possi-

Table 11-1
Organisms Presenting in Postoperative Endophthalmitis

ORGANISM	EARLY POSTOPERATIVE PERIOD	LATE POSTOPERATIVE PERIOD	TOTAL
Staphylococcus epidermidis	9	1	10
Staphylococcus aureus	0	1	1
Streptococcus pneumoniae	0	1	1
Alpha-hemolytic streptococcus	1	1	2
Group D streptococcus	1	1	2
Propionibacterium acnes	0	1	1
Pseudomonas aeruginosa	1	0	1
Proteus mirabilis	1	0	1
Culture negative	5	2	7

(Adapted from Stern GA, Engel HM, Driebe WT Jr. The treatment of postoperative endophthalmitis: results of differing approaches to treatment. Ophthalmology 1989;96:64)

ble dose. Topical corticosteroids have no impact, and repeated periocular corticosteroids are impractical and uncomfortable for the patient in this potentially long-term disease.

Surgical Complications of Specific Diseases

Proliferative Vitreoretinopathy

Complications

In this section, we will discuss the type and incidence of complications that occur when PVR is the *indication* for surgery, in contrast to the earlier section on periretinal proliferation as a *complication* of surgery.

The most common complications in surgery for PVR are postoperative; their common pathogenetic mechanism is fibrin and scar tissue reproliferation (Fig. 11-5). Indeed, the main cause for anatomic failure after surgery for PVR is new or recurrent anterior PVR leading to retinal redetachment or hypotony.[2,59–61,68,103] Redetachment rates vary depending on the initial cause for the detachment and the severity of the PVR. In mild to moderately complicated cases (with little to no anterior component), redetachment from recurrent PVR occurs in 30% to 40% of eyes,[24,91,104] but the figure may be as high as 60% after surgery for severe PVR with pronounced anterior reproliferation.[81,103–105] Recurrent PVR causes purely tractional or combined tractional and rhegmatogenous retinal detachments by creating new or reopening old retinal breaks. These are the primary reasons for the nearly 30% reoperation rate after vitrectomy for PVR.[1] Anatomic success is therefore usually defined as a final result (after all surgeries) and ranges between 70% and 90% for posterior PVR[1,2,61,84] and 57% for anterior PVR,[2] although the direct approach to removal of anterior traction may result in an anatomic success rate exceeding 70%.[60,68]

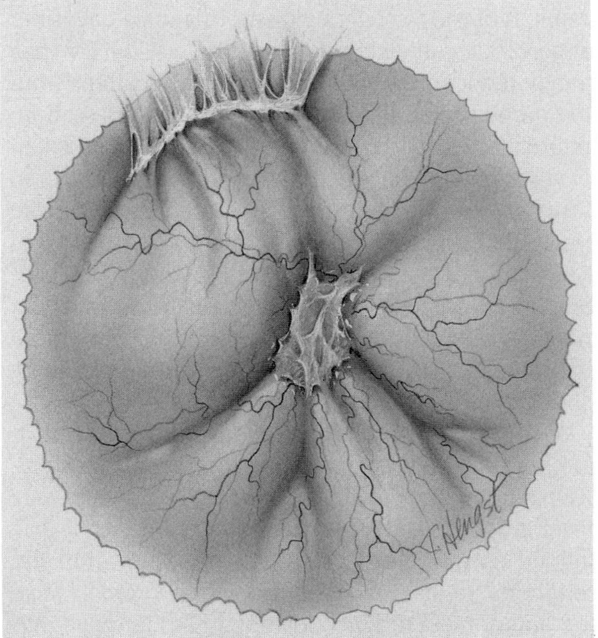

Figure 11-5. Proliferative vitreoretinopathy with both anterior (top) and posterior (center) traction membranes.

The material selected for postoperative retinal tamponade may affect the likelihood of retinal redetachment, as demonstrated in the reports from the Silicone Oil Study Group. The redetachment rate after one operation was 65% when sulfur hexafluoride (SF_6) was used, compared with 54% and 55% for perfluoropropane (C_3F_8) and silicone oil, respectively.[39,84] The distinction between C_3F_8 and silicone oil was small regarding visual and anatomic outcome variables.[84] However, hypotony at 2 years postoperatively was present in 30% of eyes receiving C_3F_8, compared with 16% of eyes receiving silicone oil for tamponade. The incidence of hypotony was highest in eyes in which the macula was detached, regardless of the method of tamponade used. Hypotony with loss of ocular integrity is the main cause of functional failure after vitreoretinal surgery for severe PVR when the retina remains attached.[68] This is most likely a result of anterior reproliferation with distortion or detachment of nonpigmented ciliary epithelium.[2,68,75] Functional outcome is also affected by the development of postoperative macular pucker, estimated to occur in 30% of eyes reattached at 6 months, but this is much less often a reason for reoperation.[1]

Management

The approach to recurrent PVR after primary vitrectomy depends on its configuration. Treatment of anterior PVR is most often the dominant surgical task in this setting. The direct approach to removal of anterior tractional forces has been shown to be the most successful.[59,68] When PFLs are not used, anterior traction should be released first, then posterior traction. When PFLs are used, posterior traction is released, PFL is injected to flatten and immobilize the posterior retina, then anterior traction is released.[68] Relaxing retinotomies are required in only 2% of vitrectomies for initial PVR, but they may be required in up to 27% of cases with anterior and recurrent PVR to release traction fully.[60,61,68] Anatomic success in cases requiring these measures varies between 40% and 64%, reflecting the severe nature of the PVR (see Relaxing Retinotomies and Retinectomies).[74,81,105] When subretinal membranes are present, they should be removed after anterior and posterior epiretinal membrane dissection.

Hypotony as a result of anterior proliferative tissue is best managed using a direct approach with lensectomy and epiciliary tissue dissection and deep scleral depression for visualization.[75] This may lead to an increase in IOP postoperatively but is more effective when performed within 3 months of the diagnosis.[68]

Prevention

Because the overwhelming majority of complications from surgery for PVR result from reproliferation, measures to prevent or limit this are of utmost importance. These measures include minimizing the use of endolaser and cryoretinopexy, especially in areas of exposed RPE; avoiding large, radial retinotomies; avoiding lensectomy;[67] and ensuring meticulous intraoperative hemostasis.[2,73,74] Careful inspection of the retinal periphery for breaks before closure clearly leads to prevention of some postoperative rhegmatogenous detachments, and use of tPA for postoperative fibrin deposition may prevent or limit the severity of further reproliferation.[5,64,66,69,70]

Diabetic Retinopathy

Complications

Complications more likely to occur after vitreoretinal surgery in diabetic eyes compared with nondiabetic eyes include rubeosis iridis, neovascular glaucoma, new or recurrent vitreous hemorrhage, postvitrectomy fibrin deposition, retinal detachment, and AHFP.

The incidence of postvitrectomy rubeosis iridis with about 2 years of follow-up data is between 22% and 24%.[5,20,37] Performing a lensectomy at the time of the vitrectomy increases the risk of rubeosis.[80] This risk may be further increased by the occurrence of iatrogenic breaks,[37] retinal detachment,[18,80] and the use of postoperative tPA.[66] The use of silicone oil has not been definitively linked to the development of rubeosis iridis.[91]

The incidence of neovascular glaucoma is between 2% and 13%. As with rubeosis iridis, its incidence is higher (40%) in the presence of a retinal detachment and higher still (92%) in the presence of both a retinal detachment and aphakia.[80]

New or recurrent vitreous hemorrhage is the most common visually significant complication following vitrectomy for complications of diabetic retinopathy (for intraoperative hemorrhages, see the related sections under General Intraoperative Complications).[55] Its incidence varies between 11% and 60%.[3,5,18,20,37,48,55,56,88,89] Only 22% require repeat vitrectomy for nonclearance, but 15% require reoperation for development of traction or rhegmatogenous retinal detachment.[55] Postoperative vitreous hemorrhage has been reported to be more frequent and to clear more slowly in phakic eyes compared with aphakic eyes.[50,55] (Its pathogenesis and management have been discussed—see Intraocular Hemorrhage.) The most common cause of late-onset postvitrectomy vitreous hemorrhage in the absence of recurrent posterior neovascularization is most likely diabetic wound neovascularization.[56]

Postoperative fibrin deposition is fairly common after vitreoretinal surgery in diabetic eyes.[66] This may be a result of a severe breakdown in the blood–ocular barrier, already compromised by the eye's ischemic status. It usually occurs between 16 and 64 days after surgery but can occur earlier. The use of tPA has greatly reduced the incidence of complications from this problem. (For discussion, see previous section, Intraocular Fibrin Deposition.) Retinal detachment after vitrectomy in diabetic eyes is estimated to occur in from 5% to 31% of eyes.[20,48,91,104] The iatrogenic breaks that lead to them occur in from 18% to 44% of eyes and adversely affect visual outcome.[5,10,18,20,37] The often avascular, atrophic state of the retina in many cases may be why iatrogenic breaks are more common in diabetic eyes than in eyes undergoing vitrectomy for other conditions.[19]

AHFP is the most common severe postoperative complication of vitrectomy for complications of diabetic retinopathy.[48] Thirteen percent of patients may develop it within the first year after surgery.[10,48] It is defined as neovascularization that occurs from the peripheral retina onto and along the vitreous base and anterior hyaloid face leading to hemorrhage into the vitreous cavity or the Berger space. Neovascular capillaries may be seen on the posterior lens surface and pars plicata. As fibrosis occurs, traction retinal detachment of the anterior retina or ciliary body can occur, producing recurrent retinal detachment or hypotony.[48,106] Risk factors for the development of AHFP include young males with severe proliferative disease and extensive retinal ischemia; traction retinal detachment as the indication for surgery; placement of a scleral buckle; postoperative rubeosis; recurrent vitreous hemorrhage or retinal detachment; and multiple surgeries.[48] The first signs of AHFP are late postoperative vitreous hemorrhage in the vitreous cavity or between the anterior hyaloid and posterior lens capsule. It usually develops between the third and eighth week after the initial vitrectomy.[48]

Management

The most common intraoperative complications in vitreous surgery for complications of diabetic retinopathy are iatrogenic retinal breaks and intraocular hemorrhage. Management of these problems was covered earlier. Postoperatively, the most common indication for reoperation is new or recurrent retinal detachment, which is responsible for up to 90% of reoperations.[20,37] Because 20% of postoperative vitreous hemorrhages clear spontaneously,[51] they are less often the indication for reoperation.[20,50] In addition, outpatient air–fluid exchange can effectively remove recurrent vitreous hemorrhage, thereby obviating the need for reoperation.[50] Fluid–gas exchange has also been used to treat postoperative rhegmatogenous retinal detachment without evidence of traction.[10] Postoperative retinal detachments with evidence of traction must be managed with repeat vitrectomy and removal of epiretinal traction, often followed with air–fluid exchange and endolaser photocoagulation.

In general, the recommendation for postoperative vitreous hemorrhage includes watchful waiting for resolution unless the following conditions exist: persistence of vitreous hemorrhage for 4 months, florid rubeosis, ultrasonic evidence of a retinal detachment, erythroclastic glaucoma unresponsive to medical management, and a hemorrhage that occurred in the only sighted eye (only 2 months should be allowed for clearance).[55]

The treatment of postoperative fibrin deposition varies depending on its severity. Mild cases generally resolve spontaneously; moderate cases may respond to topical or retroseptal corticosteroids. Corticosteroids have not been shown to alter the course in severe cases,[2] which do respond to intraocular tPA (see Intraocular Fibrin Deposition).[63–65,69–71]

Postoperative rubeosis iridis is a manifestation of persistent, untreated peripheral retinal ischemia or significant retinal detachment. If no detachment exists and the media are clear, panretinal photocoagulation should be used until regression of rubeosis is seen. If the media are opaque due to vitreous hemorrhage, consideration should be given to peripheral cryotherapy if the patient is not a good medical candidate for surgery. Otherwise, repeat vitrectomy with endolaser photocoagulation should be performed. Air–fluid exchange can clear the media, but panretinal photocoagulation can be difficult through the liquid–air interface.

Neovascular glaucoma is difficult to manage. If it is recent in onset, if may respond to peripheral laser retinal photocoagulation or cryotherapy. This can lead to regression of angle vessels and reopening of normal outflow channels. Otherwise, surgical intervention with a seton for IOP control is necessary because failure rates for other approaches are so high.

Early recognition of AHFP is important in preserving eyes affected by it. Aggressive treatment with heavy confluent laser photocoagulation to the peripheral retina and pars plana in eyes with clear media, and lensectomy, resection of the anterior and peripheral vitreous, membrane dissection, and extensive and confluent laser treatment in eyes with either media opacities or peripheral traction detachments is likely to improve the visual prognosis of patients with this serious condition.[48]

Prevention

The most important and effective step to take in preventing intraoperative and postoperative vitreous hemorrhages in the diabetic eye is to perform adequate preoperative and intraoperative panretinal laser photocoagulation.[5,18] This may also reduce the incidence of de novo iris neovascularization, which has become less common since the widespread use of this technique.[5] Attention to preserving the crystalline lens whenever possible may also be contributing to the lower incidence of rubeosis iridis.[5] Meticulous intraoperative endodiathermy and endolaser to neovascular tissues may reduce the incidence of postoperative vitreous hemorrhage, which also decreases the amount of fibrinogen released into the eye.[55] The risk of developing AHFP may be reduced by avoiding the use of a scleral buckle whenever possible. This further underscores the importance of relieving epiretinal traction by direct dissection rather than using scleral buckling and extensive laser retinopexy.[48]

Trauma

Complications

Vitreoretinal surgery for ocular trauma is a complex topic because of the wide variability of causative factors and their resulting injuries. In this section our goal is simply to cover the most common situations encountered and the complications that can occur during their management.

Penetrating injuries with or without retained IOFBs are one of the more common types of trauma encountered by the vitreoretinal surgeon. Of all ocular perforations, IOFBs occur in about 40%; between 70% and 90% are composed of magnetic metals.[107] If the composition of the foreign body is known to be toxic to ocular tissues, immediate intervention is necessary.[108] Surgical complications related to the removal of posterior segment IOFBs are related to technique and location of the foreign body and can include retinal or lens damage secondary to movement of a metallic IOFB during use of magnets; retinal detachment due to removal of an IOFB that has penetrated the retina but not the posterior sclera; and intraocular hemorrhage on disturbing recently traumatized tissues. Complications seen following surgery include endophthalmitis, seen in 13% of eyes (*Bacillus* sp and *S epidermidis* are the most common pathogens); severe PVR with retinal detachment; vitreous hemorrhage; cataract; corneal opacity; and macular pucker.[99] Anatomic success with perforating injuries is relatively poor, a reported 27% compared with 57% on average for retinal detachments due to severe PVR, proliferative diabetic retinopathy with traction retinal detachment, or GRTs with PVR.[92] The success rate in treating endophthalmitis after penetrating trauma varies between 17% and 83% depending on multiple factors, including the severity of the initial trauma, the time interval between trauma and treatment, and the virulence of the infecting organisms.[100] The incidence of iatrogenic breaks incurred during epiretinal membrane removal for PVR after penetrating trauma is 12.5%.[109]

Management

Most of the complications mentioned can be managed using the general guidelines given earlier, such as for treating retinal breaks or achieving intraoperative hemostasis. Incarceration of retina can occur as a result of trauma or during the repair, especially on attempted removal of IOFBs with electromagnets.[107,108] Traction from anterior incarceration sites may be minimized by cryotherapy and scleral buckle placement. Posterior or large incarcerations may require direct treatment. A retinotomy coupled with endodiathermy to ensure hemostasis will result in the release of tractional forces.[81,108,110] This may be evidenced by mild retraction of adjacent retinal tissue from the incarceration site. An air–fluid–gas exchange followed by several rows of endolaser photocoagulation at retinotomy borders will help ensure retinal attachment. If retained metallic IOFBs are not deeply embedded in the posterior sclera, we prefer to mobilize them with intraocular micromagnets and remove them with IOFB forceps.

Prevention

The highest-risk complications in posterior segment trauma surgery are intraocular hemorrhage and endophthalmitis, both of which are preventable. Methods to minimize intraocular hemorrhage include raising the IOP; using intraocular diathermy; performing fluid–air exchange; using a different irrigating solution (BSS has citric acid, an anticoagulant; BSS Plus does not); adding thrombin to a separate infusion system, 100 IU/mL; using endolaser; using silicone oil injection; and using sodium hyaluronate, 0.5 to 0.75 cc, which causes mechanical confinement of the hemorrhage.[36] Prompt surgical intervention, the use of intravitreal antibiotics in high-risk injuries, and the possible use of vitrectomy surgery may reduce the incidence and severity of endophthalmitis.[98]

Retinopathy of Prematurity

Complications

Vitreoretinal surgery in retinopathy of prematurity (ROP) has generally been reserved for stage 4 and 5 disease. An estimated one fifth of eyes still progress beyond stage 3-plus disease despite therapy.[111] Peripheral traction detachments can proceed to total retinal detachment within a day, and complete detachments can form funnels within a week.[112] Scleral buckling may be appropriate in repairing stage 4 through early stage 5 disease, and anatomic results have been reported in 50% to 100% of patients[112–114]

(Fig. 11-6). Most authorities agree that vitrectomy should be performed for stage 5 disease with a significant tractional component.[112,114–117] Anatomic reattachment of the retina can be achieved in an apparently unsalvageable eye by meticulous removal of proliferative membranes during vitreous surgery.[112,114–117] Despite macular reattachment rates for stage 5 disease as high as 93%,[118] functional visual acuity achievement lags behind, at between 4% and 30%.[112,116,118–124] Phthisis bulbi is eventually reached by 6% of all eyes.[112] The best correlate with anatomic and visual outcome is funnel shape, the more open type doing the best.[113,116,124]

Some complications can be attributed to surgical approach. Proponents of the open-sky approach to stage 5 disease claim better access to retrolental structures, but this technique leads to prolonged hypotony with increased risk of choroidal detachment, corneal clouding, and generally prolonged operating time due to the more complex closure, compared with the simpler closure of the closed vitrectomy approach.[112–114,117] With either technique, intraoperative bleeding is common, occurring in 70% to 80% of cases.[125] This may be due to the fact that 30% of eyes have major vascular connections between the retina and the retrolental membrane.[115] Bleeding also may be a major contributor to the high percentage of recurrent proliferation of scar tissue in these patients.[125] A unique source of hemorrhage can be from a persistent hyaloid artery.[112]

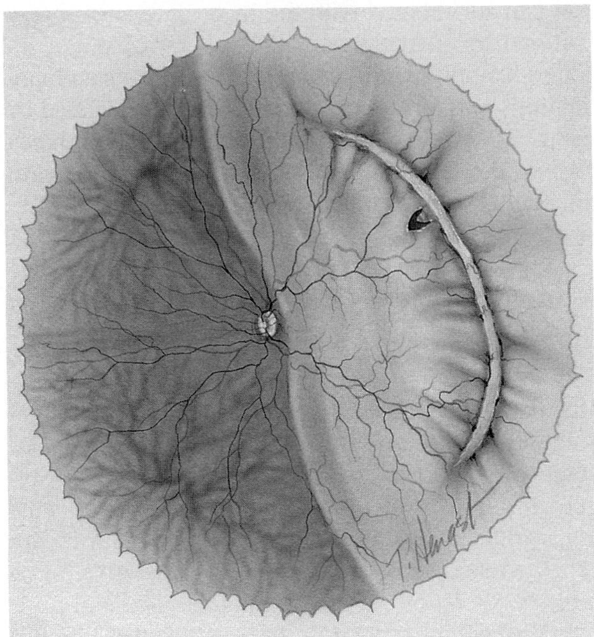

Figure 11-6. Stage 4b retinopathy of prematurity with retinal flap tear associated with contracting fibrous tissue along the fibrovascular ridge. Surgical treatment could be approached with scleral buckling alone or vitreoretinal techniques.

Other complications seen in vitrectomy for ROP include iatrogenic retinal breaks. These occur most often in the periphery but also occur more posteriorly during dissection into the funnel. Their incidence is estimated at 8%, and their presence strongly correlates with anatomic failure postoperatively.[116,122,126] Also correlating with recurrent detachment is the occurrence of reproliferation with vitreoretinal traction.[125,127] With the closed vitrectomy approach, subretinal infusion of irrigating solution may occur if care is not taken to create very anterior sclerotomies or to perform the lensectomy under hand-held anterior infusion with release of circumferential traction before placement of the mounted infusion cannula near the limbus.

Management

The surgical approach to stage 5 ROP may vary (closed versus open-sky), but the goals remain the same: regression of active vascular disease, release of vitreous traction, avoidance of iatrogenic retinal breaks and hemorrhage, and subsequent resorption of subretinal fluid.[121] Active, stage 3-type vascular disease may either spontaneously regress or require preoperative peripheral cryotherapy followed 3 weeks later by lensectomy, vitrectomy, and membrane peeling.[114,121,122,128] Because the adequate release of traction is of paramount importance in these eyes, aggressive anterior dissection is often necessary, especially in the region of the peripheral trough.[117]

Management of intraocular hemorrhage should proceed according to the guidelines previously discussed. The occurrence of iatrogenic peripheral retinal breaks requires the placement of a scleral buckle in most cases where an already foreshortened retina needs support to close breaks.[122] Some authors advocate scleral buckle placement with intraocular gas tamponade and external subretinal fluid drainage.[116] If reproliferation leads to redetachment, reoperation offers a 22% chance for anatomic success.[116] If subretinal infusion occurs during closed vitrectomy because of a closed anterior funnel configuration, the infusion must be stopped, and a separate hand-held infusion introduced through the limbus or peripheral cornea is essential for successfully approaching the anterior circumferential traction.

Prevention

Some authors recommend the infusion of thrombin (100 IU/mL) intraoperatively to help prevent bleeding.[125] These authors did not observe postoperative vitritis or sterile hypopyon in any of their series cases, because they were careful to irrigate the eye well to remove it before closure. Others argue that relaxing iris sphincterotomies are a major cause of reactive reproliferation and that the use of iris hooks or retractors to obtain adequate mydriasis can prevent this.[114] Breaks can be minimized during dissection in the funnel by making repeated injections of small amounts of sodium hyaluronate to help separate tissue planes before sharp dissection.[126] This latter technique is best suited for the open-sky approach.

Dislocated Crystalline and Intraocular Lenses

Complications

When crystalline lenses dislocate into the vitreous cavity and interfere with vision, cause uveitis or glaucoma, or are associated with a retinal detachment, they should be removed, and methods to accomplish this have been described.[129–132] However, these can be associated with significant intraocular complications, particularly retinal damage caused by hard lens fragments falling on the retina during intravitreal lens fragmentation. The incidence of iatrogenic retinal break formation is estimated at 11% during such maneuvers.[17] Similarly, several approaches to the management of dislocated intraocular lenses have been reported.[38,90,97,133–139] However, these techniques can be associated with significant intraoperative or postoperative complications, such as retinal break formation, retinal detachment, intraocular hemorrhage, erosion of the iris or iris root (especially with sutured posterior chamber lenses), chronic uveitis, cystoid macular edema (29%),[38] endophthalmitis, unpredictable centration of the lens, and recurrent dislocation of the lens. With the application of PFLs to the management of dislocated crystalline and intraocular lenses, many of the intraoperative complications have been reduced.[17,140–142]

Management

When retinal detachment complicates the removal of a lens, use of PFLs is especially recommended both to reattach the retina and to bring the lens into the anterior vitreous cavity, where it can be removed safely by either lens loop extraction or ultrasonic fragmentation.[140] First, a complete vitrectomy is performed, with removal of as much basal vitreous gel as possible. Then a PFL is injected over the optic nerve head to float the dislocated lens off the retina and into the anterior vitreous cavity. Simultaneously, the PFL displaces the subretinal fluid through the anterior retinal break into the vitreous cavity and reattaches the retina. If the lens is hard, it may be cryoextracted or removed with a lens loop.[140,141]

Prevention

The use of PFLs has provided an effective means to avoid many complications of lens dislocation surgery, such as problems with visibility, hypotony, postoperative pressure elevation, and retinal, iris, or endothelial damage, which can occur with other techniques.[141] Removal of as much basal vitreous gel as possible before PFL instillation prevents peripheral retinal breaks that might occur if the lens were later ultrasonically fragmented on top of the PFL bubble, where fragments could glide under the iris and become trapped in excess basal vitreous gel.[140] Cryoextraction of hard lenses through a limbal incision reduces operating time and the endothelial damage that can be inflicted with the high ultrasonic energy required to fragment hard lenses.[140] Problems with suture-fixation of intraocular lenses, such as endophthalmitis and lens decentration, can be prevented by using intraocular lenses with four positioning holes for four-point fixation and mini-scleral flaps to guard the suture sites from access by bacteria.[138,143]

Macular Pucker

Complications

Macular pucker, a well-known entity to vitreoretinal surgeons, has many causes, including prior ocular surgery or inflammation; it can be idiopathic.[15] Surgery to remove adherent epiretinal membranes causing significant macular pucker is successful in improving visual acuity in 80% to 90% of patients.[15] In a large-series report, the total intraoperative and postoperative complication rate was estimated at 13%.[12,13] This would include specific complications such as:

1. Development or progression of nuclear sclerotic cataract (the most common complication, seen in up to 60%)[11,14,15,45]

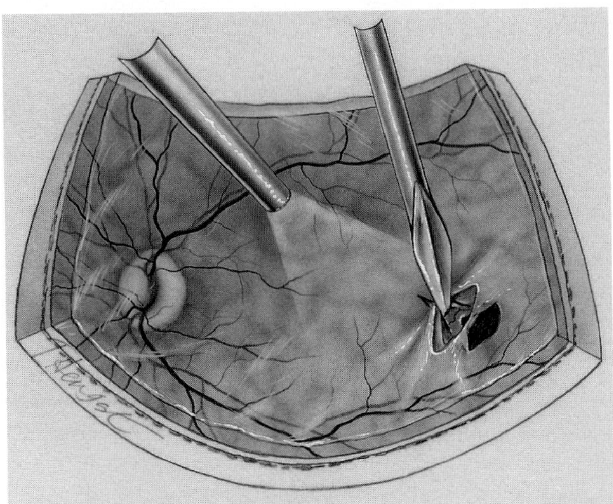

Figure 11-7. An iatrogenic macular retinal break during epiretinal membrane dissection for the treatment of macular pucker.

2. Posterior, extramacular iatrogenic retinal breaks (1%–5% of eyes)[11–15,45] (Fig. 11-7)
3. Peripheral retinal breaks (1%–6% of eyes)[11–15,45]
4. Postoperative rhegmatogenous retinal detachment (3%–7% of eyes)[12–15,45]
5. Macular phototoxicity (2.3% of eyes)[30]
6. Recurrence of epiretinal membranes causing decreased vision (2%–7% of eyes)[12–15,45]
7. Macular hole formation, vitreous hemorrhage, and endophthalmitis (each in less than 1% of eyes).[12,13,15,76]

Eyes whose initial macular pucker was associated with previous retinal detachment surgery were more likely to have iatrogenic retinal breaks and recurrent epiretinal membrane formation than those originally classified as idiopathic.[12–14]

Management

For the most part, management of these complications was discussed in previous sections. Briefly, posterior retinal breaks are treated with endolaser and fluid–gas exchange.[12,13] Peripheral retinal breaks are treated with external cryotherapy.[12,13] Retinal detachments are treated with scleral buckle with or without fluid–gas exchange.[11–13,45] Macular hole and significant recurrent macular pucker are approached with appropriate surgical intervention.

Prevention

The most important complication to avoid is the creation of retinal breaks. A significant difference was found in the 2- to 3-year postoperative visual acuity measurements between eyes that did versus eyes that did not suffer this complication.[12,13] Therefore, standard precautions such as the careful placement of surgical instruments through sclerotomy incisions and delicate tissue dissection may be critical to long-term visual outcome.[27] The sclerotomy sites should be examined internally with indirect ophthalmoscopy before closure in every case to detect iatrogenic peripheral retinal breaks; if present, they can be treated immediately, thereby preventing postoperative retinal detachment.

Macular Holes

Complications

The most common complication associated with vitreoretinal surgery for macular holes is the development or progression of nuclear sclerotic cataracts, seen in 16% to 36% of eyes.[32,49,52,144] Increased age at surgery is a risk factor, and the incidence rises with increasing length of follow-up.[32,46] This is most likely a result of prolonged gas tamponade.

The removal of posterior hyaloid from the retinal surface is thought to be necessary for the successful release of tangential traction around the hole and therefore long-term flattening of the hole.[31,145–148] However, work using transforming growth factor–beta-2 (TGF-β_2) suggests that even this step is not essential.[144] Usually, a silicone-tipped extrusion cannula is used to engage the posterior hyaloid or other epiretinal membrane to elevate it from the retinal surface. This can require prolonged close-up work over the macular region with bright illumination, and macular phototoxicity has been reported.[32] Damage to the RPE in and around the hole and enlargement of the macular hole from accidental engagement by the extrusion cannula have been reported in 14% and 3% of eyes, respectively.[32,148]

Failure of the macular hole to flatten appears to occur in 25% to 42% of eyes.[31,32,148] This rate may be lower with the use of TGF-β_2.[144] The risk of posterior retinal breaks is low, and peripheral retinal breaks posterior to sclerotomy sites occur in 7% of eyes.[49] Postoperative retinal detachments have been reported in 2% of cases.[52]

Management

If the posterior hyaloid cannot be removed during surgery and the hole does not flatten or remain flat after surgery, repeat pars plana vitrectomy with removal of the cortical vitreous may be repeated and may be more successful on the second attempt.[144] If the posterior hyaloid was removed but the hole does not flatten and no epiretinal membranes are found, it is possible that gas tamponade did not last long enough, and a simple gas–fluid exchange will increase the duration of mechanical flattening.

Prevention

To avoid damage to the parafoveal retina, the use of suction should be avoided over the fovea when looking for the cortical vitreous.[32] The retinal periphery should be examined thoroughly toward the close of the case to detect iatrogenic retinal breaks, which can be treated with cryotherapy.[32]

Although about 10% of full-thickness macular holes are bilateral, vitrectomy for impending macular holes is not recommended: this does not reliably prevent macular hole formation in all patients, even when histopathologically proven removal of posterior cortical vitreous has been achieved, and some of these impending holes resolve spontaneously without surgery.[49,52,149] A multicenter, randomized, controlled clinical trial of vitrectomy for prevention of macular hole formation in fellow eyes is underway and includes a control group to address natural history issues. Some authors have found a 20% rate of full-thickness macular hole development after surgery to *prevent* macular holes.[49]

Submacular Hemorrhages and Neovascular Membranes

Complications

During the past few years, increasing attention has been given to applying vitreoretinal surgical techniques to problems in the subretinal space.[150–155] Submacular choroidal neovascular membranes and hemorrhages that are idiopathic or secondary to age-related macular degeneration (ARMD) or the presumed ocular histoplasmosis syndrome have been removed with either forceps or submacular irrigation with tPA.[156] Unfortunately, results for ARMD have been disappointing, with no cases yielding better than 20/200 visual acuity and 48% achieving counting fingers or worse vision.[156]

Complications in this kind of surgery include disciform scars (50%), cataract (36%), retinal detachment with PVR (28.5%), recurrent subretinal hemorrhage (19%), inadvertent retinectomy (5%) (Fig. 11-8), and peripheral retinal breaks (7%).[150,152,153,156,157] In cases with large retinotomies, the postoperative PVR incidence has been reported at 50%; the risk may be proportional to the size of the retinotomy.[154,157] Enlargement of initially small retinotomies has also been reported when fibrotic, subretinal membranes are removed.[152] Removal of RPE along with the clot or membrane is also common, occurring in up to 82% of eyes operated on for hemorrhagic complications of ARMD.[154]

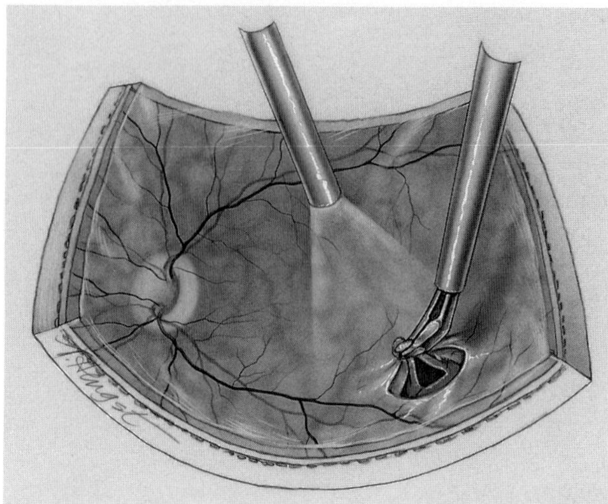

Figure 11-8. Inadvertent retinectomy during forceps removal of a submacular choroidal neovascular membrane. Note forceps accidentally engaging edge of retinotomy.

Management

Intraoperative complications in submacular surgery that require an immediate response include choroidal bleeding and retinotomy problems. If raising the infusion pressure to the eye is not sufficient to stop choroidal bleeding, direct cautery to the hemorrhage site may be necessary, using endophotocoagulation or diathermy.[154,158] Further manipulation in the subretinal space thereafter should be minimized or avoided.

If the best site for a drainage retinotomy places it in the inferior macula, serious consideration should be given to the use of silicone oil for tamponade.[152] Because of this problem with inferior tamponade, we recommend that drainage retinotomies be made in a superior location whenever possible. Management of the other complications listed above was covered earlier in the chapter.

Prevention

The problem of enlarging a retinotomy by delivering a large clot through it can be avoided by using subretinal tPA injection.[159,160] This lyses the clot and allows irrigation rather than forceps delivery as a means of removal. The problem of tearing and inadvertently removing RPE along with a clot or membrane, as well as damage to the outer retina by the same shearing mechanism, may be avoided by injecting tPA, 25 μg, subretinally and allowing it 45 minutes to lyse fibrin clots, which can loosen the clot from the RPE and outer retinal surfaces and facilitate less traumatic removal.[161–163] This dose appears to be safe for the retina. If any clot remains after gentle irrigation and aspiration, it should not be removed to prevent outer retinal or RPE damage.[156] Because blood in the subretinal space has been associated with irreversible retinal damage within a day of hemorrhage, early intervention may limit the degree of subsequent retinal dysfunction.[162,163]

Giant Retinal Tears

Complications

The complications most often encountered during or after vitreoretinal surgery for GRTs include:

1. Cataract formation or progression (6%–9%)[164,165]
2. Macular pucker (up to 34%)[34,165,166]
3. Recurrent retinal detachment by means of extension of the tear or formation of new breaks (9%–22%)[34,24,165]
4. PVR (10%–25%)[4,164]
5. Subretinal migration of air or PFL, depending on the material used to reattach the retina. If PFL is injected too rapidly, it can form "fish eggs" that can pass through existing retinal breaks.[34] In addition, slippage of the posterior edge of the GRT can occur during air–fluid or air–PFL exchange because of the anterior-to-posterior movement of the air bubble.[4] This can leave large folds posteriorly or move the edge of the tear into an unsupported area when a scleral buckle is placed.

Management

There is controversy over whether scleral buckles are useful in primary repair of GRTs *without* PVR, but there is general agreement on their utility in repairing GRTs *with* PVR and in treating recurrent retinal detachments following GRT repair.[164,165] For patients who have developed advanced grade C PVR (new classification),[167] pars plana lensectomy with aggressive removal of anterior traction is essential for achieving long-term reattachment.[164] Subretinal PFLs can be removed by aspiration with a flexible-tipped extrusion cannula passed subretinally or stroked anteriorly by brushing the flexible tip of the cannula gently over the retinal surface.[4] If posterior retinal slippage occurs, reinjection of fluid or PFL may be necessary to restore it to the correct position. Under fluid, this may require mechanical advancement using intraocular forceps.

Prevention

The extension of a GRT occurs because of inadequate release of the tractional forces that contributed to the creation of the original tear. Therefore, a complete dissection of the peripheral vitreous or the use of a broad scleral buckle is necessary to meet this surgical objective.[164] PFLs help minimize complications in several ways. They may reduce the incidence of PVR postoperatively by reducing the amount of manipulation of the posterior flap, which reduces breaks, hemorrhage, and retinal trauma, all of which can lead to PVR.[165] Dispersion of RPE cells during cryotherapy is minimized if PFLs are used to hold the posterior flap of the GRT in place.[164] Finally, to prevent slippage of the posterior flap, a slow and deliberate fluid–air exchange is necessary, stopping frequently to allow the edges of the flap to dry as much as possible. When the edge of the posterior flap is within the air bubble and relatively dry, it will not slip posteriorly.[4]

Nonrhegmatogenous Retinal Detachments

Complications

Relatively little is to be found in the literature regarding surgical complications in this category. Most traction retinal detachments are caused by complications of proliferative diabetic retinopathy or PVR; these were discussed earlier in this chapter. Traction retinal detachment from complications of proliferative sickle retinopathy (PSR) has received some attention. Because the neovascular fronds occur mostly in the retinal periphery, the rate of iatrogenic retinal breaks is higher than that seen for diseases requiring more pos-

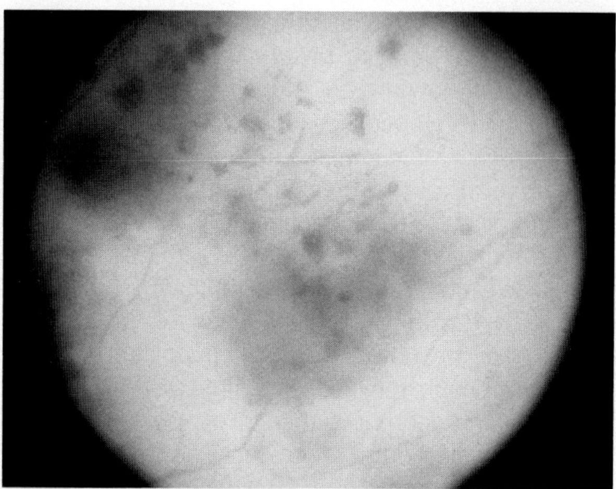

Figure 11-9. Fundus photograph of the characteristic telangiectatic retinal vessels seen in Coats disease with an underlying exudative retinal detachment. (See color plate after page xvi.)

terior dissection. This rate has been reported to be between 18% and 50%.[168,169]

Most serous and exudative retinal detachments do not require surgery unless there is a significant tractional component as well. One exception would be Coats disease, where subretinal exudation can be so severe that a total retinal detachment can lead to rubeosis iridis and a blind, painful eye for a young child (Fig. 11-9). Vitrectomy with endodiathermy to abnormal retinal vessels can allow retinal reattachment by stopping the exudation of fluid, but extensive diathermy may be required, which can cause significant retinal shrinkage.[170]

Management

Because of the increased risk of anterior segment ischemia from encircling scleral buckles in patients with PSR, retinal breaks should be treated with minimal cryotherapy and soft, segmental exoplants for support.[168,169] Significant retinal shrinkage after vascular ablation in Coats disease may require a relaxing retinotomy to allow retinal reattachment, but the prognosis is guarded because the risk of severe PVR is high in this setting.

Prevention

For patients requiring surgery for complications of PSR, it is important to reduce the risk of thrombosis. This may be done through adequate preoperative hydration, local anesthesia without the use of epinephrine, good perioperative oxygenation, avoidance of excessive cryoretinopexy, avoidance of extraocular muscle removal intraoperatively, and avoidance of carbonic anhydrase inhibitors and osmotic agents. In addition, broad and high encircling scleral buckles should be avoided to prevent anterior segment ischemia.[169]

Retinal Detachments From Inflammatory and Infectious Diseases

Complications

In this category, the diseases most often encountered by the vitreoretinal surgeon are the acute retinal necrosis syndrome (ARN) and cytomegalovirus retinitis (CMV-R).[93,171,172] The incidence of retinal detachment in ARN may be as high as 85% and generally is associated with the extent of peripheral retinal involvement and the degree of vitritis.[171] Nearly 11% of eyes with ARN-related retinal detachments have anterior PVR on presentation; this correlates unfavorably with reattachment prognosis.[93,171] Because of the severe degree of preoperative arteritis and intraocular inflammation already present, eyes undergoing scleral buckling for retinal detachment in ARN may be at increased risk for ischemic and inflammatory complications, including fibrin response (12.5% incidence) and choroidal detachment (37.5% incidence).[93] Most complications related to surgical repair of CMV-related retinal detachments involve cataract formation from silicone oil and vision loss due to macular or optic nerve involvement.[172]

Management

The best approach to managing a severe fibrin response is injection of tPA with or without fluid–gas exchange, depending on the attachment status of the retina (see Intraocular Fibrin Deposition for general guidelines).

During attempted repair of CMV-related retinal detachment, it is best to perform a fluid–air exchange before endolaser photocoagulation and injection of silicone oil. If the retina will not reattach or if air enters the subretinal space, retinotomy or retinectomy should be performed.[172]

Prevention

Most preventive measures discussed in the literature refer to ARN. In general, the performance of primary lensectomy, vitrectomy, fluid–gas exchange, and endolaser photocoagulation without scleral buckle is recommended in patients with necrosis involving more than one quadrant.[93] Use of scleral buckles has been discouraged to reduce the incidence of severe fibrin reactions, choroidal detachments, and associated elevation of IOP from secondary angle closure.[93] Lensectomy is advocated to allow aggressive anterior vitreous base dissection to prevent the anterior contraction so prone to develop in eyes after vitrectomy for ARN-related traction retinal detachments, which can lead to redetachment.[171] The development of ARN in the fellow eye may be prevented by giving acyclovir as part of initial therapy. The dose is 1500 mg/m²/day intravenously for 7 to 10 days, followed by 800 mg orally five times a day for 2 to 4 weeks.[173] This appears to reduce the risk of developing bilateral disease from 65% to 25% over the first 2 years.[173] Some authors have proposed that argon laser photodemarcation of necrotic lesions has a protective effect for reducing the risk of retinal detachment in ARN.[174,175] Others have not found this to be beneficial, with retinal detachments occurring right through areas of laser demarcation.[171]

COMPLICATIONS SPECIFIC FOR INTRAOPERATIVE MATERIALS AND TECHNIQUES

Intraocular Gases

Complications

Several problems are unique to the use of intraocular gases. First, gases have a significant expansile capacity, which can be influenced by several factors. If general anesthesia is used with nitrous oxide, partial pressure equilibration of the gas bubble with the nitrogen in the blood causes significant bubble expansion and a rise in IOP (Fig. 11-10). The concentration of the gas also determines its degree of postinjection expansion. Atmospheric pressure reduction can also cause significant expansion. The IOP can increase by as much as 42 mmHg with intraocular air volumes as small as 0.25 cc during simulated air travel in an altitude chamber.[2]

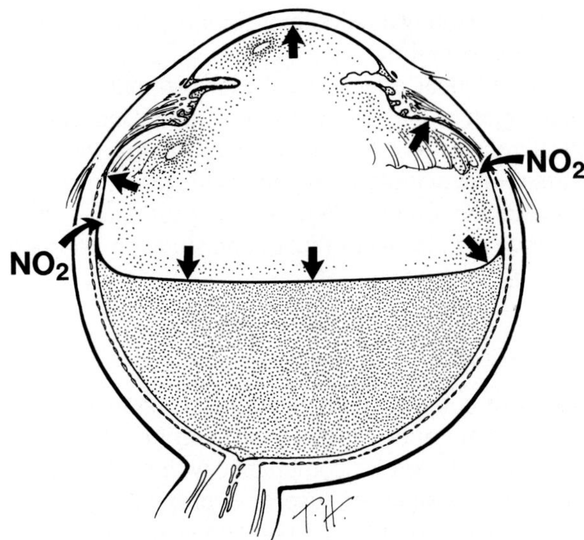

Figure 11-10. Aphakic eye illustrating the expansile effect on an intraocular gas bubble as nitrous oxide from the blood equilibrates with the gas during anesthesia.

Toxicity of the currently used gases has also been reported. Perfluoropropane (C_3F_8) may have a greater capacity to produce intravitreal inflammation than sulfur hexafluoride (SF_6), an effect directly related to its longer existence inside the eye (4–5 weeks).[96] The movement of gas bubbles in the vitreous cavity can create vitreous traction and irritation, which may cause retinal breaks and increase the risk of PVR after pneumatic retinopexy.[96] Others have attributed the RPE lesions seen after vitrectomy and fluid–gas exchange for stage 3 macular holes to retinal toxicity from intraocular gas.[31]

As mentioned in other sections, migration of air or gas subretinally during air–fluid or gas–fluid exchange can occur when residual periretinal traction prevents the retina in the area of a break from being reapposed to the eye wall. The risk is increased when the size of the break is large enough to overcome the surface tension of the air or gas bubble.[68]

Management

When air or gas migrates subretinally, additional periretinal membrane dissection is required to release all traction. If subretinal air or gas remains after complete release of traction, PFLs can be used to push the air into the vitreous cavity through the preexisting retinal breaks.[68] Using PFLs is a better alternative than creating a retinotomy for the sole purpose of removing subretinal air or gas.

The medical and surgical management of acute postoperative IOP elevation was discussed earlier. Measurement of IOP in a gas-filled eye may be inaccurate with Schiøtz and pneumatic tonometry. Applanation tonometry (Perkins type) yields the most accurate results, according to one study on eye bank eyes.[176]

Prevention

The most common complications of intraocular gas use (cataract and IOP elevation) can be avoided by stressing the need for compliance with postoperative face-down positioning; use of appropriate gas concentrations (expansile versus nonexpansile); vigilance about monitoring postoperative IOP; and patient education about the purpose and risks of intraocular gas.

Silicone Oil

Complications

Although silicone oil has been used for over 30 years in the treatment of complex retinal detachments, reports still differ as to its possible retinal toxicity and safety.[2,33,91,177,178] The advantages of silicone oil include the following: it is easier to use than gas (it can be used in children who cannot position postoperatively), its optical qualities allow a clear view of the fundus, and it provides extended or permanent tamponade.[33]

Anterior segment complications associated with silicone oil include keratopathy, cataract, glaucoma, and hyperoleon or emulsification. Corneal decompensation occurs as a consequence of contact between silicone oil and the cornea. A 40% reduction in endothelial cell density can occur within 6 days after silicone oil makes contact.[2] The incidence of keratopathy is about 6% and is most common in aphakic eyes after surgery for complications related to ocular trauma.[104] It is one of the most common causes for early postoperative visual loss after vitrectomy with silicone oil injection.[104]

The development or progression of cataract is common after silicone oil injection. It is seen in all eyes with long-term follow-up. It is seen in 60% of eyes after silicone oil removal, with an 85% progression rate of preexisting opacities.[43] The first opacity to develop is in the posterior subcapsular region.

Glaucoma after silicone oil injection is reported in between 3% and 16% of eyes.[41–43,91,92,104,179] The highest incidence is seen in aphakic eyes and in cases where vitreoretinal surgery was performed for complications of ocular trauma.[104] In aphakic and pseudophakic eyes, a prophylactic inferior iridectomy is performed to prevent silicone-pupillary block glaucoma.[39,86] Despite this, closure of the iridectomy can occur from fibrin membranes in 6% to 14% of cases, leading to pupillary block glaucoma in 3%.[41,104]

Silicone oil can emulsify in the eye, leading to reduced vision and media opacity.[41,104] Biomicroscopically detectable emulsification occurs in only 0.7% of eyes.[104] However, by 6 months, 85% of eyes may show emulsification.[41] Increased purity of silicone oil has been associated with a reduced incidence of this complication.[104] The migration of emulsified silicone oil into the anterior chamber can cause the clinical appearance of an inverted (superior) hypopyon because of its creamy-white color; this has been called a *hyperoleon*.

Posterior segment complications include perisilicone oil proliferation (PSP) with or without retinal redetachment and redetachment of the retina after removal of silicone oil. The retinal redetachment rate from PSP has been reported to be as high as 49% after vitrectomy for severe PVR and GRTs.[33] The development of PSP without regard to retinal attachment status was 61% in this series.[33] The mean time to PSP development was 5 weeks (range, 2–12 weeks).[33] Redetachment of the retina after removal of silicone oil is common. The incidence varies between 21% and 25% and appears to be independent of the amount of time the silicone was left in the eye postoperatively.[24,166] It occurs most often as a result of loss of tamponade of persistent retinal breaks.

Management

Most complications in the anterior segment can be managed with removal of silicone oil if doing so will not jeopardize the status of the retina. Keratopathy is either improved or unchanged after silicone oil removal and does not appear to cause new glaucoma or keratopathy.[43] Simultaneous glaucoma surgery at the time of oil removal appears to be successful if needed, because over 90% can be controlled in this fashion.[43] For silicone oil in the anterior chamber, injection of sodium hyaluronate into the anterior chamber through a limbal incision can be performed while evacuating silicone oil through a second paracentesis site opposite the first.[104,180]

For PSP, membranes have been found to be easier to remove during repeat vitrectomy when they have had some time to mature (more than 6–10 weeks).[33] Recurrent retinal detachments after removal of silicone oil often require repeat vitrectomy, lensectomy, and anterior vitreous dissection to release all anterior traction, followed by scleral buckle placement or revision, if necessary, and laser photocoagulation for retinopexy.[33]

Prevention

The use of high-purity and high-viscosity silicone oil has been associated with better long-term anatomic and visual results.[41,104,177] This is partially due to the lower rate of emulsification of the higher-grade oil.

Silicone oil should not be injected into the eye with great force: doing so can cause zonular lysis with migration of silicone oil into the anterior chamber.[104] This complication is also seen less frequently in eyes that have an air–fluid exchange before injection of silicone oil.[104]

The ideal time to remove silicone oil has not been clearly determined, but reports indicate that between 2 and 6 months is recommended to allow for retinal reattachment while minimizing the risks of long-term complications.[33,41,43,91,179] The timing of removal must be tailored to the patient's situation, taking into account the risk of silicone-related complications and the risk of retinal redetachment after silicone oil removal.

Perfluorocarbon Liquids

Complications

Perfluorocarbon liquids are a significant addition to the vitreoretinal surgeon's armamentarium against complex retinal detachments. They are being used for repair of GRTs, complicated retinal detachments associated with PVR,[181] complicated diabetic traction retinal detachments, and retinal detachments associated with trauma,[182] and for removing and repositioning posteriorly dislocated lenses.[17,140–142] Their most significant feature is a higher specific gravity than water, ranging from 1.76 to 2.03.[183] Because the boiling point of PFLs is higher than saline, laser can be applied through them.[184]

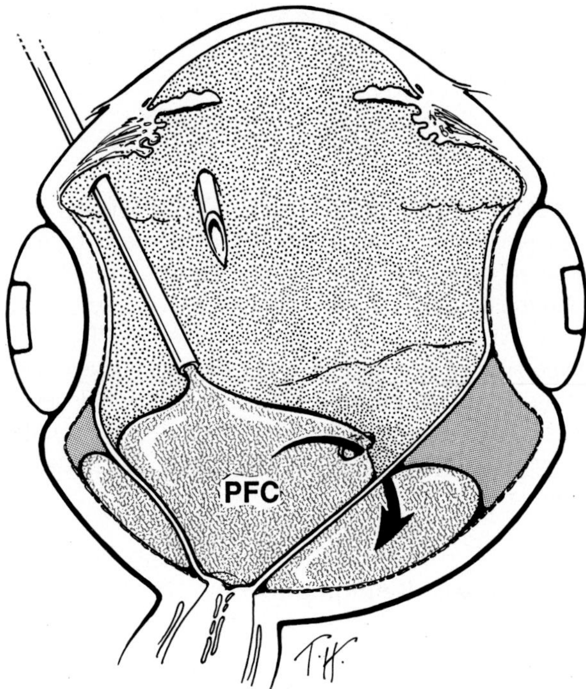

Figure 11-11. Perfluorocarbon liquid entering the subretinal space through a retinal break. The tractional forces for retinal detachment in the area of the break cannot be overcome by the flattening force of the heavy liquid, and the size of the break is sufficient to allow the liquid to pass (overcoming surface tension).

The main complications specifically associated with PFL use include subretinal migration of PFL (22% incidence)[181,182] (Fig. 11-11), slippage of the posterior edge of a GRT on PFL–air exchange,[183] and dispersion of PFL into "fish eggs" from the force of the infusion fluid, causing reduced visibility to the posterior segment.[4,68] No evidence has been found for increased postoperative inflammation and its associated complications due to the use of PFLs.[4]

Management

Small bubbles of subretinal PFL have been well tolerated by the eye.[183] However, larger bubbles, which may interfere with retinal reattachment, should be removed with a soft-tipped extrusion cannula or flute needle.[181,182] Residual epiretinal PFL droplets vaporize (perfluoro-n-octane) after PFL–air exchange.[183] The use of silicone oil–PFL exchange directly can prevent GRT slippage because as a liquid, silicone oil is relatively incompressible and the incoming oil meniscus engages the edge of the tear as the PFL is removed.[183]

Prevention

Migration of PFL into the subretinal space can be prevented by relieving significant traction around any elevated breaks before elevating the level of PFL beyond the break and by avoiding excessive traction on the retina near a break already apposed by PFL.[181,182] Dispersion of PFL into "fish eggs" can be prevented by reducing the infusion pressure as the PFL level rises close to the tip of the mounted infusion cannula or by keeping the level of PFL below the infusion cannula tip.[68]

Endodrainage Retinotomies

Complications

Two significant complications relate specifically to endodrainage retinotomies. The first is undesirable placement in an inferior retinal quadrant. Because tamponade of the retinotomy is preferable in addition to retinopexy, they are best made in a superior quadrant, where either gas or silicone oil can provide this tamponading effect (Fig. 11-12). The second is fibrovascular proliferation in or around the retinotomy site secondary to RPE or choroidal damage from trauma induced by the extrusion cannula during drainage.[185] Both choroidal neovascular membranes and disciform scars have been reported after traumatic drainage procedures.[185] The fibrosis that ensues can be exuberant enough to cause elevation and reopening of the retinotomy, causing a recurrent retinal detachment.[185]

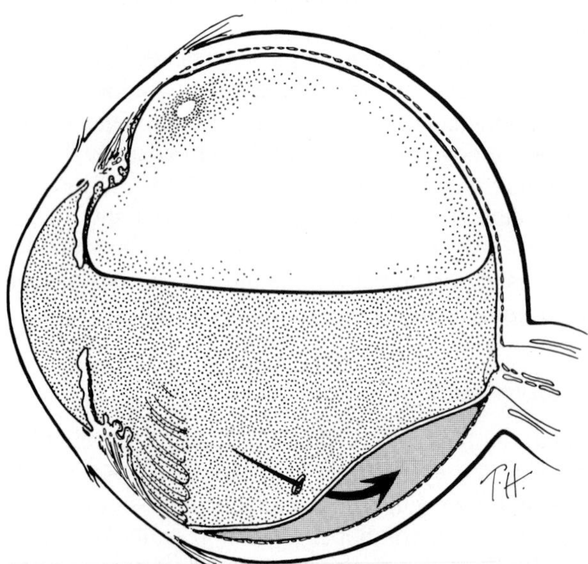

Figure 11-12. Inferior drainage retinotomy. Note that the retinotomy is not supported by the gas bubble when the patient's eye is in primary position, which can lead to early retinal redetachment.

Management

Any active hemorrhage at a retinotomy site should be treated with infusion pressure elevation and endodiathermy. Rhegmatogenous retinal detachments from a retinotomy site may require scleral buckling alone, or if the retinotomy is too posterior to reach with a buckle, repeat epiretinal dissection to release traction from the retinotomy site with repeat retinal tamponade may be necessary.[185]

Prevention

Trauma to the endodrainage site must be minimized by attempting to avoid direct touching of the RPE and by draining only enough subretinal fluid to obtain light laser takes when applied. The drainage instrument should be blunt in design (preferably with a flexible tip) and should be kept just above or at the plane of the retinotomy during the last stages of the air–fluid exchange.[185] PFLs can also be used to flatten the retina while extruding subretinal fluid through preexisting peripheral retinal breaks, thereby avoiding the use of a suction device on or near the RPE.[68]

Relaxing Retinotomies and Retinectomies

Complications

Relaxing retinotomies and retinectomies are helpful surgical techniques in the treatment of severe cases of retinal detachment with incarcerated retinas, retinal shrinkage caused by PVR, proliferative vasculopathies, and trauma after failure of membrane removal and scleral buckling to reattach the retina. They should be used as a last resort. Complications related to the procedure include persistent traction because of inadequate retinotomy size and late reproliferation along the retinotomy site, which can cause redetachment, especially in cases where hemorrhage occurs along the incision.[105] Redetachment rates vary between 24% and 36%, depending on the severity of the original problem.[2,81,186]

Management

Because many retinotomies and retinectomies are made as a last resort to enable anatomic reattachment of the retina, recurrent retinal detachment is a grave prognostic sign for the eye. If more surgery can be tolerated, repeat dissection of periretinal traction should be performed to enable lasting reattachment. In the case of hemorrhage from the retinotomy site during incision, infusion pressure elevation and diathermy to the cut edge usually secures hemostasis.[81]

Prevention

If a large relaxing incision is needed to enable retinal reattachment, a circumferential, superonasal retinectomy is preferred for several reasons. First, poorer functional outcome has been associated with large, inferior, and temporal retinotomies, as well as with radial retinotomies.[2,74,81] Secondly, if the retina anterior to a circumferential retinotomy is not removed, it can contract postoperatively and exert traction on the ciliary body, thus causing or contributing to the development of hypotony. Also, the anterior retina is ischemic and can lead to postoperative iris neovascularization.[74] Bleeding during the incision can be minimized or prevented by placing two confluent rows of endodiathermy on both sides of the proposed incision line before making the incision.[68] If the retinotomy is made in an area of shallow detachment, the vertical scissors used to make the incision should first lift the retina slightly from the surface of the RPE to avoid causing choroidal hemorrhaging.[105] Making a clean, smooth edge may reduce the degree of periretinal proliferation postoperatively, but this has not been strictly evaluated.

Retinal Tacks

Complications

Retinal tacks can be used as an adjunctive tool in vitreoretinal surgery to help prevent retinal slippage during air–fluid exchange after the creation of a circumferential retinotomy or during repair of a GRT. The most common complication with their use is perforation of the retina by the collar of the tack, leading to loss of its effectiveness[102] (Fig. 11-13). Other complications include choroidal bleeding on insertion,[102] intrusion of the tack into the vitreous cavity due to inadequate placement or poor tack design,[187] retinal contusions from dropping tacks inside the eye,[102] periretinal proliferation causing recurrent retinal detachment, and dislocation of the tack into the subretinal space.[187]

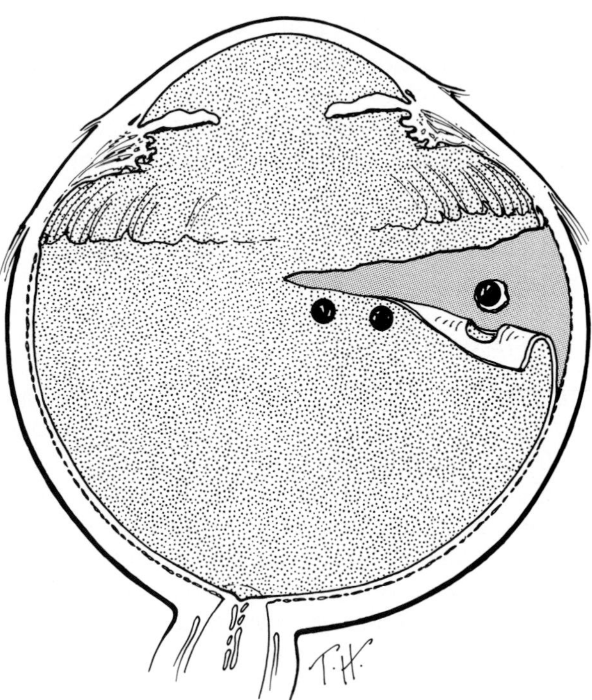

Figure 11-13. Retinal tacks used to support posterior edge of a giant retinal tear. Note that the tack to the right has perforated the retina and thereby lost its effect. This most commonly occurs when placement of the tack is too deep.

Management

Bleeding on insertion may stop from direct tamponade from the tack; otherwise, endodiathermy should be used. If the bleeding is too great, fluid infusion should be used and hemorrhage should be aspirated through a new or used retinotomy site to allow visualization of the bleeding site.[102] Dislocated tacks may require no intervention if they are not jeopardizing ocular integrity or vision.

Prevention

The infusion pressure to the eye should be increased just before insertion and removal of retinal tacks to minimize bleeding.[102] If the sclerotomies for the vitrectomy are made near the horizontal meridians, it is easier to achieve orthogonal placement of the tacks, which reduces their risk of dislocation or intrusion.[102] Otherwise, the applicator can be bent to allow perpendicular placement.[188]

Retinal Glue

Complications

The first clinical reports on the use of tissue glue for retinopexy were by Faulborn and colleagues in the 1970s. At that time, no obvious toxic effects were seen other than a mild foreign-body reaction. More recently, cyanoacrylate retinopexy has been used on a series of 25 eyes undergoing pars plana vitrectomy for complicated retinal detachments, and no evidence of retinal toxicity was seen when minute amounts of the adhesive were delivered in air-filled eyes[189] (Fig. 11-14). On more detailed examination, however, focal and circumscribed areas of coagulative necrosis of the retina and RPE layers were noted on histologic examination 7 days after application in the animal model.[190] The intensity of this effect appears to depend on the amount of adhesive used. The authors thought that the cause of the necrosis was heat released by the polymerization reaction or microimpurities in the adhesive itself.[190] Other than these possibly toxic effects and the pigmented scar seen around the glue site 1 month after application, no other complications specific to retinal glue have been reported.[190]

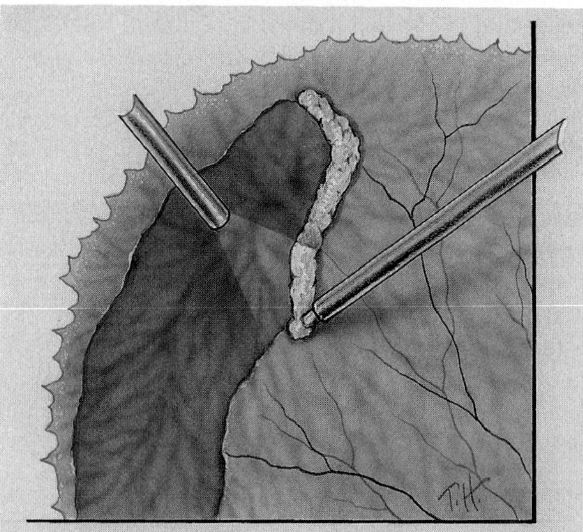

Figure 11-14. The use of tissue adhesive (glue) to treat the edge of a giant retinal tear. Small amounts precisely placed give the best results.

Prevention

The delivery of glue to the area requiring retinopexy requires good visualization. Early studies involved application of the adhesive while the eye was air-filled. Because of its superior optics intraoperatively, silicone oil has been used as the medium through which glue is delivered. It does not interfere with the polymerization reaction and it provides for more precise placement.[191] The adhesive strength and speed of adhesion appear to be superior to transscleral cryoretinopexy, but more study is needed to elucidate its utility and risks fully.

SUMMARY

The multitude of complications to be anticipated in vitreoretinal surgery is clearly sobering, as evidenced by the comprehensiveness of the preceding discussion. The surgeon, the patient, the underlying disease, and the surgical tools all interact in ways that can produce improvement or morbidity. In nearly every case, complications that are common to vitreoretinal surgery in general should be anticipated and prevented whenever possible, and the means to manage them must be mastered to minimize their impact on the anatomic and functional outcome of the eye. Likewise, the pitfalls unique to or characteristic of vitreoretinal surgery for specific disease entities and with certain tools and techniques can be avoided if the surgeon remains aware of them and takes the appropriate steps to minimize risk. Although avoiding all complications of all surgical challenges is an unrealistic expectation for anyone, we think that an understanding of the potential problems and the means with which to manage them can help the vitreoretinal surgeon to minimize their overall effect on patients.

References

1. Lopez R, Chang S. Long-term results of vitrectomy and perfluorocarbon gas for the treatment of severe proliferative vitreoretinopathy. Am J Ophthalmol 1992;113:424–428.

2. Aaberg TM. Management of anterior and posterior proliferative vitreoretinopathy. XLV Edward Jackson Memorial Lecture. Am J Ophthalmol 1988;106:519–532.
3. Diabetic Retinopathy Vitrectomy Study Group. Early vitrectomy for severe vitreous hemorrhage in diabetic retinopathy: 2-year results of a randomized trial. DRVS Study Report II. Arch Ophthalmol 1985;103:1644–1652.
4. Glaser BM, Carter JB, Kuppermann BD, Michels RG. Perfluorooctane in the treatment of giant retinal tears with proliferative vitreoretinopathy. Int Ophthalmol Clin 1992;32(2):1–14.
5. Thompson JT, de Bustros S, Michels RG, Rice TA. Results and prognostic factors in vitrectomy for diabetic vitreous hemorrhage [published erratum appears in Arch Ophthalmol 1987;105:496]. Arch Ophthalmol 1987;105:191–195.
6. Chung H, Tolentino FI, Cajita VN, Acosta J, Refojo MF. Reevaluation of corneal complications after closed vitrectomy. Arch Ophthalmol 1988;106:916–919.
7. Mittl RN, Koester CJ, Kates MR, Wilkes E. Endothelial cell counts following pars plana vitrectomy in pseudophakic and aphakic eyes. Ophthalmic Surg 1989;20:13–16.
8. Stern WH. Complications of vitrectomy. Int Ophthalmol Clin 1992;32:205–212.
9. Michels RG, Wilkinson CP, Rice TA. Vitreous surgery: complications. In: Michels RG, Wilkinson CP, Rice TA. Retinal detachment. St. Louis, CV Mosby, 1990:858–878.
10. Abrams GW, Williams GA. En bloc excision of diabetic membranes. Am J Ophthalmol 1987;103:302–308.
11. de Bustros S, Thompson JT, Michels RG, Rice TA, Glaser BM. Vitrectomy for idiopathic epiretinal membranes causing macular pucker. Br J Ophthalmol 1988;72:692–695.
12. Pesin SR, Olk J, Grand MG, et al. Vitrectomy for premacular fibroplasia. Ophthalmology 1991;98:1109–1114.
13. Pesin SR, Olk RJ. Incidence and management of complications associated with pars plana vitrectomy for premacular fibroplasia. Int Ophthalmol Clin 1992;32:95–104.
14. Poliner LS, Olk J, Grand MG, Escoffery RF, Okun E, Boniuk I. Surgical management of premacular fibroplasia. Arch Ophthalmol 1988;106:761–764.
15. Rice TA, de Bustros S, Michels RG, Thompson JT, Debanne SM, Rowland DY. Prognostic factors in vitrectomy for epiretinal membranes of the macula. Ophthalmology 1986;93:602–610.
16. Smiddy WE, Michels RG, Gilbert HD, Green WR. Clinicopathologic study of idiopathic macular pucker in children and young adults. Retina 1992;12:232–236.
17. Wallace RT, McNamara JA, Brown G, et al. The use of perfluorophenanthrene in the removal of intravitreal lens fragments. Am J Ophthalmol 1993;116:196–200.
18. de Bustros S, Thompson JT, Michels RG, Rice TA. Vitrectomy for progressive proliferative diabetic retinopathy. Arch Ophthalmol 1987;105:196–199.
19. Carter JB, Michels RG, Glaser BM, de Bustros S. Iatrogenic retinal breaks complicating pars plana vitrectomy. Ophthalmology 1990;97:848–853.
20. Thompson JT, de Bustros S, Michels RG, Rice TA. Results and prognostic factors in vitrectomy for diabetic traction retinal detachment of the macula. Arch Ophthalmol 1987;105:497–502.
21. Piper JG, Han DP, Abrams GW, Mieler WF. Perioperative choroidal hemorrhage at pars plana vitrectomy: a case-control study. Ophthalmology 1993;100:699–704.
22. Speaker MG, Guerriero PN, Met JA, et al. A case-control study of risk factors for intraoperative suprachoroidal expulsive hemorrhage. Ophthalmology 1991;98:202–210.
23. Lambrou FH Jr, Meredith TA, Kaplan HJ. Secondary surgical management of expulsive choroidal hemorrhage. Arch Ophthalmol 1987;105:1195–1198.
24. Casswell AG, Gregor ZJ. Silicone oil removal. II. Operative and postoperative complications. Br J Ophthalmol 1987;71:898–902.
25. Lakhanpal V, Schocket SS, Elman MJ, Dogra MR. Intraoperative massive suprachoroidal hemorrhage during pars plana vitrectomy. Ophthalmology 1991;97:1114–1119.
26. Lakhanpal V, Schocket SS, Elman MJ, Nirankari VS. A new modified vitreoretinal surgical approach in the management of massive suprachoroidal hemorrhage. Ophthalmology 1989;96:793–800.
27. Michels M, Sternberg P Jr. Operating microscope–induced retinal phototoxicity: pathophysiology, clinical manifestations and prevention. Surv Ophthalmol 1990;34:237–252.
28. McDonald HR, Harris MJ. Operating microscope–induced retinal phototoxicity during pars plana vitrectomy. Arch Ophthalmol 1988;106:521.
29. Kuhn F, Morris R, Massey M. Photic retinal injury from endoillumination during vitrectomy. Am J Ophthalmol 1991;111:42.
30. Michels M, Lewis H, Abrams GW, Han DP, Mieler WF, Neitz J. Macular phototoxicity caused by fiberoptic endoillumination during pars plana vitrectomy. Am J Ophthalmol 1992;114:287–296.
31. Poliner LS, Tornambe PE. Retinal pigment epitheliopathy after macular hole surgery. Ophthalmology 1992;99:1671–1677.
32. de Bustros S, Wendel RT. Vitrectomy for impending and full-thickness macular holes. Int Ophthalmol Clin 1992;32:139–152.

33. Lewis H, Burke JM, Abrams GW, Aaberg TM. Perisilicone proliferation after vitrectomy for proliferative vitreoretinopathy. Ophthalmology 1988;95:583–591.
34. Maxwell DP Jr, Orlick ME, Diamond JG. Intermittent intraocular thrombin as an adjunct to vitrectomy. Ophthalmic Surg 1989;20:108–111.
35. Joondeph BC, Blankenship GW. Hemostatic effects of air versus fluid in diabetic vitrectomy. Ophthalmology 1989;96:1701–1706.
36. de Bustros S. Intraoperative control of hemorrhage in penetrating ocular injuries. Retina 1990;10(suppl 1):S55–S58.
37. Thompson JT, de Bustros S, Michels RG, Rice TA. Results and prognostic factors in vitrectomy for diabetic traction-rhegmatogenous retinal detachment. Arch Ophthalmol 1987;105:503–507.
38. Campo RV, Chung KD, Oyakawa RT. Pars plana vitrectomy in the management of dislocated posterior chamber lenses. Am J Ophthalmol 1989; 108:529–534.
39. The Silicone Study Group. Vitrectomy with silicone oil or sulfur hexafluoride gas in eyes with severe proliferative vitreoretinopathy: results of a randomized clinical trial. Arch Ophthalmol 1992;110:770–779.
40. Federman JL, Eagle RC Jr. Extensive peripheral retinectomy combined with posterior 360-degree retinotomy for retinal reattachment in advanced proliferative vitreoretinopathy cases. Ophthalmology 1990;97:1305–1320.
41. Federman JL, Schubert HD. Complications associated with the use of silicone oil in 150 eyes after retina–vitreous surgery. Ophthalmology 1988;95: 870–876.
42. Lemmen KD, Dimopoulos S, Kirchhof B, Heimann K. Keratopathy following pars plana vitrectomy with silicone oil filling. Dev Ophthalmol 1987;13:88.
43. Casswell AG, Gregor ZJ. Silicone oil removal. I. The effect on the complications of silicone oil. Br J Ophthalmol 1987;71:893–897.
44. Cherfan GM, Michels RG, de Bustros S, Enger C, Glaser BM. Nuclear sclerotic cataract after vitrectomy for idiopathic epiretinal membranes causing macular pucker. Am J Ophthalmol 1991;111:434–438.
45. de Bustros S, Rice TA, Michels RG, Thompson JT, Marcus S, Glaser BM. Vitrectomy for macular pucker: use after treatment of retinal tears or retinal detachment. Arch Ophthalmol 1988;106:758–760.
46. de Bustros S, Thompson JT, Michels RG, Enger C, Rice TA, Glaser BM. Nuclear sclerosis after vitrectomy for idiopathic epiretinal membranes. Am J Ophthalmol 1988;105:160–164.
47. Hutton WL, Pesicka GA, Fuller DG. Cataract extraction in the diabetic eye after vitrectomy. Am J Ophthalmol 1987;104:1–4.
48. Lewis H, Abrams GW, Williams GA. Anterior hyaloidal fibrovascular proliferation after diabetic vitrectomy. Am J Ophthalmol 1987;104:607–613.
49. Smiddy WE, Michels RG, Glaser BM, de Bustros S. Vitrectomy for impending idiopathic macular holes. Am J Ophthalmol 1988;105:371–376.
50. Han DP, Murphy ML, Mieler WF, Abrams GW. Outpatient fluid–air exchange for severe postvitrectomy diabetic vitreous hemorrhage: long-term results and complications. Retina 1991;11:309–314.
51. Benson WE, Brown GC, Tasman W, McNamara JA. Complications of vitrectomy for non-clearing vitreous hemorrhage in diabetic patients. Ophthalmic Surg 1988;19:862–864.
52. Margherio RR, Trese MT, Margherio AR, Cartright K. Surgical management of vitreomacular traction syndromes. Ophthalmology 1989;96:1437–1445.
53. Blankenship GW, Flynn HW Jr, Kokame GT. Posterior chamber intraocular lens insertion during pars plana lensectomy and vitrectomy for complications of proliferative diabetic retinopathy. Am J Ophthalmol 1989;108:1–5.
54. Blankenship GW. Posterior chamber intraocular lens implantation during pars plana lensectomy and vitrectomy for diabetic complications. Graefes Arch Clin Exp Ophthalmol 1989;227:136–138.
55. Tolentino FL, Cajita VN, Gancayco T, Skates S. Vitreous hemorrhage after closed vitrectomy for proliferative diabetic retinopathy. Ophthalmology 1989;96: 1495–1500.
56. Kreiger AE. Wound complications in pars plana vitrectomy. Retina 1993;113:335–344.
57. Kreiger AE. The pars plana incision: experimental studies, pathologic observations, and clinical experience. Trans Am Ophthalmol Soc 1991;89:549–621.
58. Kreiger AE. Wound complications following pars plana vitrectomy. Trans Pac Coast Otoophthalmol Soc 1987;68:124–125.
59. Lewis H, Aaberg TM. Anterior proliferative vitreoretinal. Am J Ophthalmol 1988;105:277–284.
60. Lewis H, Aaberg TM. Causes of failure after repeat vitreoretinal surgery for recurrent proliferative vitreoretinopathy. Am J Ophthalmol 1991;111:15–19.
61. Lewis H, Aaberg TM, Abrams GW. Causes of failure after initial vitreoretinal surgery for severe proliferative vitreoretinopathy. Am J Ophthalmol 1991;111: 8–14.
62. Lewis H, Aaberg TM, Abrams GW, Han DP, Kreiger AE. Management of the lens capsule during pars plana lensectomy. Am J Ophthalmol 1987;103:109–110.
63. Jaffe GJ, Abrams GW, Williams GA, Han DP. Tissue plasminogen activator for postvitrectomy fibrin formation. Ophthalmology 1990;97:184–189.
64. Snyder WR, Lambrou FH, Williams GA. Intraocular

fibrinolysis with recombinant human tissue plasminogen activator. Arch Ophthalmol 1987;105:1277–1280.

65. Williams DF, Bennet SR, Abrams GW, et al. Low-dose tissue plasminogen activator for treatment of post-vitrectomy fibrin formation. Am J Ophthalmol 1990;109:606–607.
66. Dabbs CK, Aaberg TM, Aguilar HE, Sternberg P, Meredith TA, Ward AR. Complications of tissue plasminogen activator therapy after vitrectomy for diabetes. Am J Ophthalmol 1990;110:354–360.
67. Han DP, Jaffe GJ, Schwartz DM, et al. Risk factors for postvitrectomy fibrin formation. ARVO Abstracts. Invest Ophthalmol Vis Sci 1989;30(suppl):272.
68. Management of severe proliferative vitreoretinopathy. In: Lewis H, Ryan SJ, eds. Medical and surgical retina: advances, controversies, and management. St. Louis, Mosby–Year Book, 1994:115–145.
69. Jaffe GJ, Lewis H, Han DP, Williams GA, Abrams GW. Treatment of postvitrectomy fibrin pupillary block with tissue plasminogen activator. Am J Ophthalmol 1989;108:170–175.
70. Williams GA, Lambrou FH, Jaffe GA, et al. Treatment of postvitrectomy fibrin formation with intraocular tissue plasminogen activator. Arch Ophthalmol 1988;106:1055.
71. Boldt HC, Abrams GW, Murray TG, Han DP, Mieler WF. The lowest effective dose of tissue plasminogen activator for fibrinolysis of postvitrectomy fibrin. Retina 1992;12(suppl 3):575–579.
72. Iverson DA, Katsura H, Hartzer MR, Blumenkranz MS. Inhibition of intraocular fibrin formation following infusion of low-molecular-weight heparin during vitrectomy. Arch Ophthalmol 1991;109:405–409.
73. Cowley M, Conway BP, Campochiaro PA, et al. Case-control study of clinical risk factors for proliferative vitreoretinopathy. Invest Ophthalmol Vis Sci 1989;30:108.
74. Morse LS, McCuen BW II, Machemer R. Relaxing retinotomies: analysis of anatomic and visual results. Ophthalmology 1990;97:642–648.
75. Zarbin MA, Michels RG, Green WR. Dissection of epiciliary tissue to treat chronic hypotony after surgery for retinal detachment with proliferative vitreoretinopathy. Retina 1991;11:208.
76. Smiddy WE. Atypical presentations of macular holes. Arch Ophthalmol 1993;111:626–631.
77. Lewis H, Aaberg TM, Abrams GW, McDonald HR, Williams GA, Mieler WF. Subretinal membranes in proliferative vitreoretinopathy. Ophthalmology 1989;96:1403–1415.
78. Murray TG, Boldt C, Lewis H, Abrams GW, Mieler WF, Han DP. A technique for facilitated visualization and dissection of the vitreous base, pars plana and pars plicata. Arch Ophthalmol 1991;109:1458–1459.
79. Glaser BM, Cardin A, Biscoe B. Proliferative vitreoretinopathy: the mechanism of development of vitreoretinal traction. Ophthalmology 1987;94:327.
80. Wand M, Madigan JC, Gaudio AR, Sorokanich S. Neovascular glaucoma following pars plana vitrectomy for complications of diabetic retinopathy. Ophthalmic Surg 1990;21:113–118.
81. Han DP, Lewis MT, Kuhn EM, et al. Relaxing retinotomies and retinectomies: surgical results and predictors of visual outcome. Arch Ophthalmol 1990;108:694–697.
82. Machemer R. Proliferative vitreoretinopathy: a personal account of its pathogenesis and treatment. Invest Ophthalmol Vis Sci 1988;29:1771.
83. Han DP, Lewis H, Lambrou FH Jr, Mieler WF, Hartz A. Mechanisms of intraocular pressure elevation after pars plana vitrectomy. Ophthalmology 1989;96:1357–1362.
84. The Silicone Study Group. Vitrectomy with silicone oil or perfluoropropane gas in eyes with severe proliferative vitreoretinopathy: results of a randomized clinical trial. Arch Ophthalmol 1992;110:780–792.
85. Lewis H, Han D, Williams GA. Management of fibrin pupillary-block glaucoma after pars plana vitrectomy with intravitreal gas injection. Am J Ophthalmol 1987;103:180–182.
86. Beekhuis WH, Ando F, Zivojnovic R, Mertens DAE, Peperkamp E. Basal iridectomy at 6 o'clock in the aphakic eye treated with silicone oil: prevention of keratopathy and secondary glaucoma. Br J Ophthalmol 1987;71:197–200.
87. Han DP, Lewis H, Williams GA. Management of complete iridocorneal apposition after vitrectomy. Am J Ophthalmol 1987;103:108–109.
88. The Diabetic Retinopathy Vitrectomy Study Group. Early vitrectomy for severe proliferative diabetic retinopathy in eyes with useful vision: results of a randomized trial. DRVS Report III. Ophthalmology 1988;95:1307–1320.
89. Oldendorp J, Spitznas M. Factors influencing the results of vitreous surgery in diabetic retinopathy. I: Iris neovascularization and/or active neovascularization at the fundus. Graefes Arch Clin Exp Ophthalmol 1989;277:1–8.
90. Smiddy WE. Dislocated posterior chamber intraocular lens: a new technique of management. Arch Ophthalmol 1989;107:1678–1680.
91. Yeo JH, Glaser BM, Michels RG. Silicone oil in the treatment of complicated retinal detachments. Ophthalmology 1987;94:1109–1113.
92. Punnonen E, Laatikainen L, Ruusuvaara P, Setälä K. Silicone oil in retinal detachment surgery—results and complications. Acta Ophthalmologica 1989;67:30–36.
93. Blumenkranz M, Clarkson J, Culbertson WW, Flynn

HW Jr, Lewis ML, Young GM. Visual results and complications after retinal reattachment in the acute retinal necrosis syndrome. Retina 1989;9:170–174.

94. Doft BH. The endophthalmitis vitrectomy study. Arch Ophthalmol 1991;109:487–489.
95. Kattan HM, Flynn HW Jr, Pflugfelder SC, Robertson C, Forster RK. Nosocomial endophthalmitis survey—current incidence of infection after intraocular surgery. Ophthalmology 1991;98:227–238.
96. Garcia-Arumi J, Correa CA, Corcostegui B. Comparative study of different techniques of intraocular gas tamponade in the treatment of retinal detachment due to macular hole. Ophthalmologica 1990; 201(2):83–91.
97. Heilskov T, Joondeph BC, Olsen DR, Blankenship GW. Late endophthalmitis after transscleral fixation of a posterior chamber intraocular lens (letter). Arch Ophthalmol 1989;107:1427.
98. Mieler WF, Ellis MK, Williams DF, Han DP. Retained intraocular foreign bodies and endophthalmitis. Ophthalmology 1990;97:1532–1538.
99. Williams DF, Mieler WF, Abrams GW, Lewis H. Results and prognostic factors in penetrating ocular injuries with retained intraocular foreign bodies. Ophthalmology 1988;95:911–916.
100. Nobe JR, Gomez DS, Liggett P, Smith RE, Robin JB. Posttraumatic and postoperative endophthalmitis: a comparison of visual outcomes. Br J Ophthalmol 1987;71:614–617.
101. Stern GA, Engel HM, Driebe WT Jr. The treatment of postoperative endophthalmitis—results of differing approaches to treatment. Ophthalmology 1989; 96:62–67.
102. de Juan E Jr, McCuen BW II, Machemer R. The use of retinal tacks in the repair of complicated retinal detachments. Am J Ophthalmol 1986;102:20–24.
103. Hanneken AM, Michels RG. Vitrectomy and scleral buckling methods for proliferative vitreoretinopathy. Ophthalmology 1988;95:865–869.
104. Riedel KG, Gabel V, Neubauer L, Kampik A, Lund O. Intravitreal silicone oil injection: complications and treatment of 415 consecutive patients. Graefes Arch Clin Exp Ophthalmol 1990;228:19–23.
105. Machemer R, McCuen BW II, de Juan E Jr. Relaxing retinotomies and retinectomies. Am J Ophthalmol 1986;102:7–12.
106. Lewis H, Abrams GW, Foos RY. Clinicopathologic findings in anterior hyaloidal fibrovascular proliferation after diabetic vitrectomy. Am J Ophthalmol 1987;104:614–618.
107. Coleman DJ, Lucas BC, Rondeau MJ, Chang S. Management of intraocular foreign bodies. Ophthalmology 1987;94:1647–1653.
108. Koster HR, Kenyon KR. Complications of surgery associated with ocular trauma. Int Ophthalmol Clin 1992;32(4):157–178.
109. Isernhagen RD, Smiddy WE, Michels RG, Glaser BM, de Bustros S. Vitrectomy for nondiabetic vitreous hemorrhage not associated with vascular disease. Retina 1988;8:81–87.
110. Han DP, Mieler WF, Abrams GW, Williams GA. Vitrectomy for traumatic retinal incarceration. Arch Ophthalmol 1988;106:640–645.
111. Cryotherapy for Retinopathy of Prematurity Cooperative Group. Multicenter trial of cryotherapy for retinopathy of prematurity: preliminary results. Arch Ophthalmol 1988;106:471–479.
112. Hunter DG, Mukai S. Retinopathy of prematurity: pathogenesis, diagnosis, and treatment. Int Ophthalmol Clin 1992;32(1):163–184.
113. Hirose T, Katsumi O, Mehta MC, Schepens CL. Vision in stage 5 retinopathy of prematurity after retinal reattachment by open-sky vitrectomy. Arch Ophthalmol 1993;111:345–349.
114. Machemer R. Retinopathy of prematurity: approaches to surgical therapy. Aust N Z J Ophthalmol 1990;18(1):47–56.
115. Jabbour NM, Eller AE, Hirose T, Schepens CL, Liberfarb R. Stage 5 retinopathy of prematurity. Ophthalmology 1987;94:1640–1645.
116. Zilis JD, de Juan E, Machemer R. Advanced retinopathy of prematurity: the anatomic and visual results of vitreous surgery. Ophthalmology 1990; 97:821–826.
117. de Juan Jr E, Machemer R. Retinopathy of prematurity: surgical technique. Retina 1987;7:63–69.
118. Noorily SW, Small K, de Juan E Jr, Machemer R. Scleral buckling surgery for stage 4B retinopathy of prematurity. Ophthalmology 1992;99:263–268.
119. Bradford JD, Trese MT. Management of advanced retinopathy of prematurity in the older patient. Ophthalmology 1991;98:1105–1108.
120. Kalina RE. Treatment of retinal detachment due to retinopathy of prematurity: documented disappointment. Ophthalmology 1991;98:3–4.
121. Quinn GE, Dobson V, Barr CC, et al. Visual acuity in infants after vitrectomy for severe retinopathy of prematurity. Ophthalmology 1991;98:5–13.
122. Trese MT. Surgical therapy for stage 5 retinopathy of prematurity: a two-step approach. Graefes Arch Clin Exp Ophthalmol 1987;225:266–268.
123. Machemer R, de Juan Jr. E. Retinopathy of prematurity: approaches to surgical therapy. Aust N Z J Ophthalmol 1990;18:47–56.
124. Hirose T, Schepens CL, Katsumi O, Mehta M. Open-sky vitrectomy in severe retinal detachment caused by advanced retinopathy of prematurity. In: Flynn JT, Tasman W, eds. Retinopathy of prematurity. New York, Springer-Verlag, 1992:95–114.

125. Blacharski PA, Charles ST. Thrombin infusion to control bleeding during vitrectomy for stage 5 retinopathy of prematurity. Arch Ophthalmol 1987; 105:203–205.
126. Tasman W, Borrone RN, Bolling J. Open-sky vitrectomy for total retinal detachment in retinopathy of prematurity. Ophthalmology 1987;94:449–452.
127. Sneed SR, Pulido JS, Blodi CR, Clarkson JG, Flynn HW Jr, Mieler WF. Surgical management of late-onset retinal detachments associated with regressed retinopathy of prematurity. Ophthalmology 1990; 97:179–183.
128. Sira IB, Nissenkorn I, Kremer I. Retinopathy of prematurity. Surv Ophthalmol 1988;33(1):1–16.
129. Urrets-Zavalia A. Displacement of the crystalline lens. In: Draeger J, Winter R, eds. New microsurgical concepts: II. Cornea, posterior segment, and external microsurgery. Dev Ophthalmol, 1989:59–65.
130. Laqua H. Intravitreal phacoemulsification for luxated lenses. In: Draeger J, Winter R, eds. New microsurgical concepts: II. Cornea, posterior segment, and external microsurgery. Dev Ophthalmol, 1989:18:66–68.
131. Haymet BT. Removal of a dislocated hypermature lens from the posterior vitreous. Aust N Z J Ophthalmol 1990;18:103.
132. Girard LJ, Canizales R, Esnaola N, Rand WJ. Subluxated (ectopic) lenses in adults: long-term results of pars plana lensectomy–vitrectomy by ultrasonic fragmentation with and without phacoprosthesis. Ophthalmology 1990;97:462–465.
133. Flynn HW Jr. Management and repositioning of posteriorly dislocated intraocular lenses. In: Stark WJ, Terry A, Maumenee AE, eds. Anterior segment surgery: intraocular lenses, lasers, and refractive keratoplasty. Baltimore, Williams & Wilkins, 1987:321–329.
134. Flynn HW Jr. Pars plana vitrectomy in the management of subluxated and posteriorly dislocated intraocular lenses. Graefes Arch Clin Exp Ophthalmol 1987;225:169–172.
135. Smith JG, Lindstrom RL. Intraocular lens: complications and their management. Thorofare, NJ, Slack, 1988:135–141.
136. Insler MS, Mani H, Peyman GA. A new surgical technique for dislocated posterior chamber intraocular lenses. Ophthalmic Surg 1988;19:480–481.
137. Flynn HW Jr, Buus D, Culbertson WW. Management of subluxated and posteriorly dislocated intraocular lenses using pars plana vitrectomy instrumentation. J Cataract Refract Surg 1990;16:51–56.
138. Friedberg MA, Pilkerton AR. A new technique for repositioning and fixating a dislocated intraocular lens. Arch Ophthalmol 1992;110:413–415.
139. Chan CK. An improved technique for management of dislocated posterior chamber implants. Ophthalmology 1992;99:51–57.
140. Lewis H, Blumenkranz MS, Chang S. Treatment of dislocated crystalline lens and retinal detachment with perfluorocarbon liquids. Retina 1992;12:299–304.
141. Shapiro MJ, Resnick KI, Kim SH, Weinberg A. Management of the dislocated crystalline lens with a perfluorocarbon liquid. Am J Ophthalmol 1991; 112:401–405.
142. Liu R, Peyman GA, Chen M, Chang K. Use of high-density vitreous substitute in the removal of posteriorly dislocated lenses or intraocular lenses. Ophthalmic Surg 1991;22:503–507.
143. Lewis H, Sanchez G. The use of perfluorocarbon liquids in the repositioning of posteriorly dislocated intraocular lenses. Ophthalmology 1993;100:1055–1059.
144. Lansing MB, Glaser BM, Liss H, et al. The effect of pars plana vitrectomy and transforming growth factor–beta 2 without epiretinal membrane peeling on full-thickness macular holes. Ophthalmology 1993; 100:868–871.
145. Campochiaro PA, Van Niel E, Vinores SA. Immunocytochemical labeling of cells in cortical vitreous from patients with premacular hole lesions. Arch Ophthalmol 1992;110:371–377.
146. Funata M, Wendel RT, de la Cruz Z, Green WR. Clinicopathologic study of bilateral macular holes treated with pars plana vitrectomy and gas tamponade. Retina 1992;12:289–298.
147. Glaser BM, Michels RG, Kuppermann BD, Sjaarda RN, Pena RA. Transforming growth factor–β_2 for the treatment of full-thickness macular holes. Ophthalmology 1992;99:1162–1173.
148. Kelly NE, Wendel RT. Vitreous surgery for idiopathic macular holes. Arch Ophthalmol 1991;109:654–659.
149. Smiddy WE, Michels RG, de Bustros S, de la Cruz Z, Green WR. Histopathology of tissue removed during vitrectomy for impending idiopathic macular holes. Am J Ophthalmol 1989;108:360–364.
150. Bennett SR, Folk JC, Blodi CF, Klugman M. Factors prognostic of visual outcome in patients with subretinal hemorrhage. Am J Ophthalmol 1990;109: 33–37.
151. Slusher MM. Evacuation of submacular hemorrhage: technique and timing. In. Vitreoretinal surgery and technology. Thorofare, NJ, Slack, 1989;1:2–3.
152. Vander JF, Federman JL, Greven C, Slusher MM, Gabel VP. Surgical removal of massive subretinal hemorrhage associated with age-related macular degeneration. Ophthalmology 1991;98:23–27.
153. Wade EC, Flynn HW Jr, Olsen KR, Blumenkranz MS, Nicholson DH. Subretinal hemorrhage management

by pars plana vitrectomy and internal drainage. Arch Ophthalmol 1990;108:973–978.

154. Thomas MA, Williams DF, Grand MG. Surgical removal of submacular hemorrhage and subfoveal choroidal neovascular membranes. Int Ophthalmol Clin 1992;32:173–188.
155. Hanscom TA, Diddie KR. Early surgical drainage of macular subretinal hemorrhage. Arch Ophthalmol 1987;105:1722–1723.
156. Lewis H. Management of submacular hemorrhage. In: Lewis H, Ryan SJ, eds. Medical and surgical retina: advances, controversies, and management. St. Louis, Mosby–Year Book, 1994:54–62.
157. de Juan E Jr, Machemer R. Vitreous surgery for hemorrhagic and fibrous complications of age-related macular degeneration. Am J Ophthalmol 1988; 105:25–29.
158. Thomas MA, Halperin LS. Subretinal endolaser treatment of a choroidal bleeding site (letter). Am J Ophthalmol 1990;109:742–744.
159. Peyman GA, Nelson NC, Alturki W, et al. Tissue plasminogen activator factor–assisted removal of subretinal hemorrhage. Ophthalmic Surg 1991;22: 575–582.
160. Vander JF. Tissue plasminogen activator irrigation to facilitate removal of subretinal hemorrhage during vitrectomy. Ophthalmic Surg 1992;23:361–363.
161. Lewis H, Jaffe GJ, Blumenkranz MS. Management of submacular hemorrhage with vitreoretinal surgery and subretinal injection of tissue plasminogen activator (abstract). Invest Ophthalmol Vis Sci 1992;33:898.
162. Lewis H, Resnick SC, Flannery JG, Straatsma BR. Tissue plasminogen activator treatment of experimental subretinal hemorrhage. Am J Ophthalmol 1991; 111:197–204.
163. Toth CA, Morse LS, Hjelmeland LM, Landers MB. Fibrin directs early retinal damage after experimental subretinal hemorrhage. Arch Ophthalmol 1991; 109:723–729.
164. Chang S, Lincoff H, Zimmerman NJ, Fuchs W. Giant retinal tears: surgical techniques and results using perfluorocarbon liquids. Arch Ophthalmol 1989; 107:761–766.
165. Kreiger AE, Lewis H. Management of giant retinal tears without scleral buckling—use of radical dissection of the vitreous base and perfluorooctane and intraocular tamponade. Ophthalmology 1992;99: 491–497.
166. Leaver PK, Billington BM. Vitrectomy and fluid/silicone oil exchange for giant retinal tears: 5-year follow-up. Graefes Arch Clin Exp Ophthalmol 1989;227:323–327.
167. Machemer R, Aaberg TM, Freeman HM, Irvine AR, Lean JS, Michels RG. An updated classification of retinal detachment with proliferative vitreoretinopathy. Am J Ophthalmol 1991;112:159–165.
168. Morgan CM, D'Amico DJ. Vitrectomy surgery in proliferative sickle retinopathy. Am J Ophthalmol 1987;104:133–138.
169. Pulido JS, Flynn HW Jr, Clarkson JG, Blankenship GW. Pars plana vitrectomy in the management of complications of proliferative sickle retinopathy. Arch Ophthalmol 1988;106:1553–1557.
170. Machemer R, Williams JM Sr. Pathogenesis and therapy of traction detachment in various retinal vascular diseases. Am J Ophthalmol 1988;105:170–181.
171. McDonald HR, Lewis H, Kreiger AE, Sidikaro Y, Heckenlively J. Surgical management of retinal detachment associated with the acute retinal necrosis syndrome. Br J Ophthalmol 1991;75:455–458.
172. Kreiger AE. Management of combined inflammatory and rhegmatogenous retinal detachments (ARN and AIDS). In: Ryan SJ, ed. Retina. St. Louis, CV Mosby, 1989:591–598.
173. Palay DA, Sternberg P Jr, Davis J, et al. Decrease in the risk of bilateral acute retinal necrosis by acyclovir therapy. Am J Ophthalmol 1991;112:250–255.
174. Han DP, Lewis H, Williams GA, Mieler WF, Abrams GW, Aaberg TM. Laser photocoagulation in the acute retinal necrosis syndrome. Arch Ophthalmol 1987;105:1051–1054.
175. Sternberg P Jr, Han DP, Yeo JH, et al. Photocoagulation to prevent retinal detachment in acute retinal necrosis. Ophthalmology 1988;95:1389–1393.
176. Poliner LS, Schoch LH. Intraocular pressure assessment in gas-filled eyes following vitrectomy. Arch Ophthalmol 1987;105:200–202.
177. Crisp A, de Juan E, Tiedeman J. Effect of silicone oil viscosity on emulsification. Arch Ophthalmol 1987;105:546–550.
178. Lambrou FH, Burke JM, Aaberg TM. Effect of silicone oil on experimental traction retinal detachment. Arch Ophthalmol 1987;105:1269–1272.
179. Sell C, McCuen BW II, Landers MB, Machemer R. Long-term results of successful vitrectomy with silicone oil for advanced proliferative vitreoretinopathy. Am J Ophthalmol 1987;103:24–28.
180. Kirkby GR, Gregor ZJ. The removal of silicone oil from the anterior chamber in phakic eyes. Arch Ophthalmol 1987;105:1592.
181. Chang S, Ozmert E, Zimmerman NJ. Intraoperative perfluorocarbon liquids in the management of proliferative vitreoretinopathy. Am J Ophthalmol 1988;106:668–674.
182. Chang S, Reppucci V, Zimmerman NJ, Heinemann MH, Coleman DJ. Perfluorocarbon liquids in the management of traumatic retinal detachments. Ophthalmology 1989;96:785–791.

183. Chang S. Perfluorocarbon liquids in vitreoretinal surgery. Int Ophthalmol Clin 1992;32:153–163.
184. Chang S. Low-viscosity liquid fluorochemicals in vitreous surgery. Am J Ophthalmol 1987;103:38–43.
185. McDonald HR, Lewis H, Aaberg TM, Abrams GW. Complications of endodrainage retinotomies created during vitreous surgery for complicated retinal detachment. Ophthalmology 1989;96:358–363.
186. Iverson DA, Ward TG, Blumenkranz MS. Indications and results of relaxing retinotomies. Ophthalmology 1990;97:128.
187. Lewis H, Aaberg TM, Packo KH, Richmond PP, Blumenkranz MS, Blankenship GW. Intrusion of retinal tacks. Am J Ophthalmol 1987;103:672–680.
188. Abrams GW, Williams GA, Neuwirth J, McDonald HR. Clinical results of titanium retinal tacks with pneumatic insertion. Am J Ophthalmol 1986;102:13–19.
189. McCuen BW II, Hida T, Sheta SM. Transvitreal cyanoacrylate retinopexy in the management of complicated retinal detachment. Am J Ophthalmol 1987;104:127–132.
190. Hida T, Sheta SM, Proia AD, McCuen BW II. Retinal toxicity of cyanoacrylate tissue adhesive in the rabbit. Retina 1988;8:148–153.
191. Sheta SM, Hida T, McCuen BW II. Experimental transvitreal cyanoacrylate retinopexy through silicone oil. Am J Ophthalmol 1986;102:717–722.

Ophthalmic Surgery Complications: Prevention and Management,
edited by Judie F. Charlton and George W. Weinstein.
J. B. Lippincott Company, Philadelphia © 1995.

12

Terry L. Schwartz

Complications of Strabismus Surgery

Like any other surgical procedure, strabismus correction has its share of complications. Some are transient and inconsequential, whereas others, like the death of a child from malignant hyperthermia, are tragic. Most problems are preventable or at least predictable. Anticipating potential sources of complications can help minimize unwanted results.

PARTICIPATION IN ANESTHETIC CARE

Because strabismus surgery is often performed on children, careful monitoring of anesthesia care throughout the preoperative, intraoperative, and postoperative periods is especially important. This is the responsibility not only of the anesthesiologist but also of the surgeon.

Preoperative Discomfort

The issue of anesthetic care first emerges in the preoperative period for the child experiencing discomfort. Preoperative discomfort is usually a result of hunger or thirst, and anxiety. Because of the fast rate of gastric emptying, children can be offered clear liquids up to 3 hours before their scheduled operation.

In young children, to allay fears and allow easier separation from parents, premedication with midazolam can be administered either orally[1] or nasally.[2] The nasal route requires no patient cooperation, but causes a severe burning sensation. It can be mixed with cherry syrup and given sublingually or orally, 0.5 to 0.8 mg/kg. The sublingual route has the same pharmacokinetic curve as the intravenous (IV) route, and even brief contact with the buccal mucosa will ensure significant absorption. The average mean time to sedation is 6 to 8 minutes. Older children are often frightened by mask anesthesia. If intravenous access is available, they can be sedated before transfer to the operating room. Children as young as 7 years of age can be premedicated with a topical anesthetic cream to facilitate IV placement. Eutectic mixture of local anesthetic, a 50:50 mixture of lidocaine and prilocaine, is applied to the back of the hand under an occlusive dressing.[3] It numbs to the fascia after 1 hour of skin contact. Anesthetic effect increases for up to 4 hours of contact.

An induction room adjacent to the preoperative "holding" area is appropriate for some children. Sleep is induced with the child seated on a parent's lap. The parents leave, and the child is intubated and transported to the operating suite.

INTRAOPERATIVE COMPLICATIONS

Possible intraoperative complications of strabismus surgery include perforation of the globe, lost or slipped muscles, bleeding, and complications associated with anesthesia. Fortunately, the most serious of these, perforation of the globe and malignant hyperthermia, are rare. Nevertheless, an awareness of possible intraoperative complications, the patients most prone to them, and the techniques with which they are most often associated can be important in their prevention.

Perforation of the Globe

Perforation of the globe is one of the rare vision-threatening complications of strabismus surgery. Although endophthalmitis and retinal detachment are possible sequelae, both are rare, and most perforations go unnoticed. Perforation should be suspected in the presence of unexplained posterior chamber hemorrhage or hyphemas in aphakic patients.[4,5] The incidence of unrecognized perforation was as high as 9% to 12% of all strabismus cases and 16% of Faden procedures during the 1960s and 1970s. More recent estimates are significantly lower. Several prospective studies demonstrated a 1% to 3% incidence in routine cases and a 7% incidence with the technically more difficult Faden procedure.[6–8] This decrease is likely due to modification of surgical technique and instrumentation.

As one would expect, scleral perforation most commonly occurs while suturing the detached muscle onto the globe. However, perforation can and does occur at many points throughout the strabismus procedure, including muscle disinsertion, passage of the traction suture beneath the lateral rectus during inferior oblique procedures, suture preplacement in the muscle before muscle disinsertion, undue pressure from calipers, and careless passes of the muscle hook.[9]

Anticipating the patients and procedures associated with a higher risk for perforation is the first step in prevention. Highly myopic patients and patients with connective tissue abnormalities have thin sclera, and tissue should be handled with extreme care. Reoperation and procedures such as placement of posterior fixation sutures carry a greater risk of perforation. Scarring found during reoperation may obscure normal anatomy. Excessive dissection through areas where scar and sclera are not easily separated can result in inadvertent entry into the eye. Greater frequency of holes in the globe are reported with Faden procedures. In these cases, the scleral pass is posterior, often with suboptimal exposure and awkward hand position. An unfamiliar operation, or one infrequently performed, can also result in a greater tendency to perforate. Experience decreases the incidence of perforations. The surgeon should be particularly vigilant with novice residents and operating room personnel.[8]

Modifying surgical technique can also decrease the likelihood of perforation. Spatulate needles, which cut only at the tip and sides (with no inferior cutting edge), are superior for scleral passes. The needle should be held parallel to sclera with the tip visible at all times during the scleral pass. Silk traction sutures passed beneath the lateral rectus muscle should be passed on an atraumatic needle with the tip pointing away from the globe. Alternatively, extra time can be taken to expose the entire lateral rectus insertion and pass the needle under direct visualization. For large recessions, "hang-back" sutures can be used. Reattachment of the muscle is through the thicker sclera at the insertion, where exposure is greatest. The muscle is suspended posteriorly as is done with adjustable sutures. Adequately sharpened scissors should be used; dull blades will grab tissue, tenting the sclera into the path of the scissors' cutting edge. Making multiple small snips while disinserting the muscle allows better control. Although this may not prevent scleral incision, it will ensure a smaller rent that can be sutured primarily. Large scleral lacerations must be sutured. Nylon, polyglactin 910, or Mersilene are among the sutures that can be used.

If perforation is suspected, careful indirect ophthalmoscopy should be performed. Routine instillation of 2.5% phenylephrine hydrochloride (Neo-Synephrine) at the start of surgery provides adequate pupil dilation by the end of the operation and has the added benefit of improved intraoperative hemostasis. Often, a hemorrhage is initially present at the perforation site, and it can break through to the vitreous (Fig. 12-1). Within 1 to 2 days, sclera is visible surrounded by residual hemorrhage and light pigmentation.[10] Although retinal detachment is rare, it can and does occur. Detachments are more common during the immediate postoperative period but have been reported as late as 3 years after perforation.[11] At one time, prophylactic cryotherapy was widely practiced. Its routine use is now controversial. Mittelman and Bakos[12] demonstrated similar frequency of retinal detachment after either a single application of cryotherapy or no cryotherapy after experimental perforation. Heavily applied cryotherapy resulted in more detachments than in the other condition. This study supports reserving treatment for patients with abnormal vitreous (ie, aphakes, high myopes, or patients with connective disorders), or massive vitreous hemorrhage, in whom retinal detachment is more likely. When the view is not obscured by blood, diode indirect laser is an alternative option for prophylaxis.

Other possible sequelae of scleral perforation include endophthalmitis, ectopia lentis, intraocular hemorrhage, and cataract. Because of the potentially

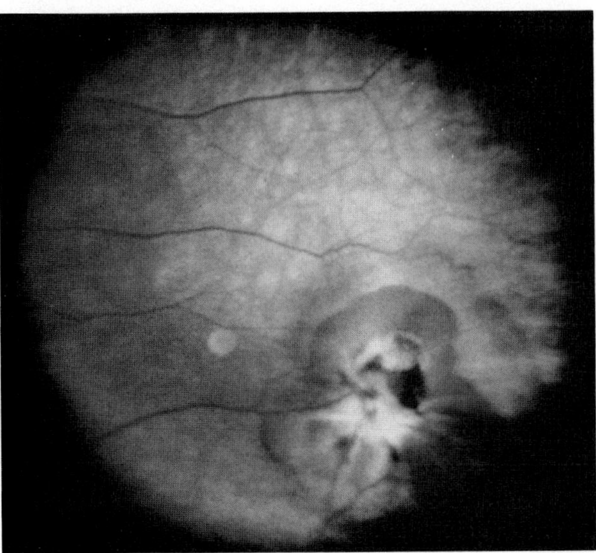

Figure 12-1. Recent scleral perforation is seen with centrally exposed sclera and surrounding intraretinal hemorrhage. (Courtesy of M. Edward Wilson, Jr, MD, Storm Eye Institute, Charleston, SC)

blinding, albeit rare, complications of perforation, the patient or the family should be informed as soon as the perforation is discovered. Refusal on the surgeon's part to acknowledge and admit an error is the greatest blunder. Because of the risk of late detachment, frequent examinations should be performed both during the immediate postoperative period and every 6 to 12 months for several years after surgery.

Lost Muscle

Losing a muscle intraoperatively (or postoperatively) is an infrequent occurrence. More common is the muscle that has "slipped" postoperatively. The lost muscle is one that has retracted beyond the area where it penetrates the Tenon capsule. It has completely detached from the globe and therefore is extremely difficult to retrieve despite early recognition. The slipped muscle is still attached to the sclera by its capsule or by fibrous tissue to its intended insertion, but it has retracted posteriorly within the capsule. The capsule acts as a pseudotendon, excessively lengthening (and weakening) the muscle.[13–16]

Although the lost muscle is usually recognized during surgery, the slipped muscle is not. Eye alignment may appear adequate until postoperative recovery of muscle function, which causes the muscle to retract within the capsule. Symptoms can present hours to weeks postoperatively. With both lost and slipped muscle, the muscle appears paretic. In other words, eye movement is significantly limited in the field of action of the affected muscle (Fig. 12-2). With a lost muscle, the eyeball cannot move beyond midline or greater than 10 degrees away from midline.[16] Smaller limitations can be seen following "slipping." If a recessed muscle is the culprit, there is an overcorrection. Slipped or lost resected muscles result in unexpected undercorrections. Another sign is widening of the palpebral fissure, which is especially noticeable with gaze toward the muscle's field of action.

To confirm a suspected diagnosis, additional assessment can include forced generations, saccadic velocities, and measurement of intraocular pressure changes with different gaze positions.[16] Computed tomographic (CT) scan is useful both for making a diagnosis and locating the muscle before attempting to retrieve it during surgical repair. Locating a lost muscle is often difficult and, in the case of the medial rectus, often hopeless.

Prevention of lost muscle is largely through careful surgical technique and anticipating the points during

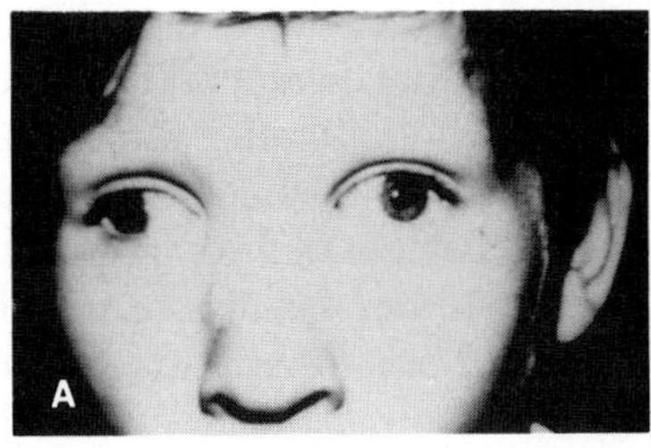

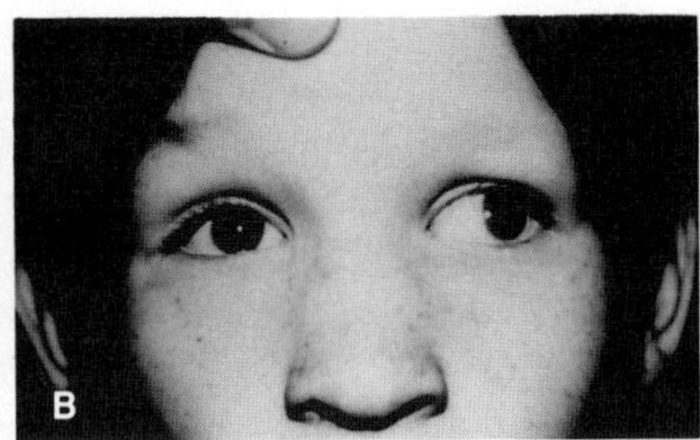

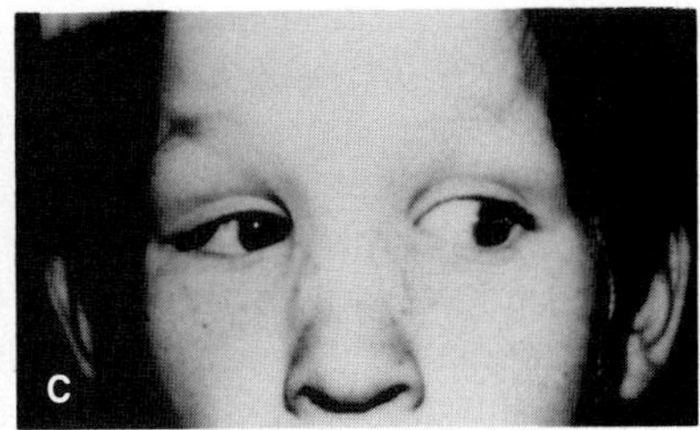

Figure 12-2. In a patient with a lost left medial rectus muscle, large angle exotropia (**B**) is demonstrated. On attempted right gaze (**A**), there is no adduction beyond midline. Full ductions are seen on left gaze (**C**) with a widened palpebral fissure. (Courtesy of M. Edward Wilson, Jr, MD, Storm Eye Institute, Charleston, SC)

the procedure where it is more likely to occur. During muscle disinsertion, the unintentional cutting of the preplaced suture can result in muscle loss. A series of small snips instead of one grand cut can preserve at least one site of suture attachment. Muscles can snap in half while on the muscle hook. Although one might expect that excessive force is responsible, this is not always so. A snapped muscle is especially likely during reoperation of a muscle with a tenuous connection to the globe. Previously operated muscles are also susceptible to disinsertion during the attempt to identify and expose it. During dissection of previously operated muscles, the tissues must be handled gently, and nothing should be snipped that has not been identified.[17] Unknowingly cutting a rectus muscle during myectomy or tenotomy of the adjacent oblique muscle has also been reported. Painstaking identification of oblique muscles with adequate exposure of the adjacent rectus is necessary. Scleral tunnels with the suture passing only through episclera may be inadequate.

The slipped muscle can be avoided with attention to the preplaced sutures. The anterior Tenon capsule should be meticulously cleaned so that the lock bite clearly includes both muscle capsule and either tendon or muscle. Dissection of the muscle posteriorly, in particular the intramuscular septum, should be minimized to limit the extent of possible posterior slippage and to increase the chance of finding the muscle.[16] This modification has been shown to have no adverse effect on surgical outcome.[18]

When a muscle is lost during surgery, the search should begin immediately. The conjunctival incision should be enlarged to provide adequate exposure. A supplemental light source, such as a head light or the operating microscope, can be helpful. Special care should be taken not to rotate the eye away from the muscle because this might cause further retraction of the muscle within the capsule.

The muscular capsule should be identified. Toothed forceps are used in a hand-over-hand technique to advance the muscle within the capsule. Sometimes, irrigation with saline may reveal the white cut edge of the retracted tendon.[13] Remember that the muscle capsule of the medial rectus is parallel to the medial orbital wall. Searching posteriorly, adjacent to the globe, one is more likely to find and damage the optic nerve than the medial rectus muscle.

Often the loss or slippage of a muscle is not recognized until after surgery. Correction should be undertaken as soon as possible. Delay can result in further retraction of the muscle as well as contraction of its antagonist. This contracture adds a restrictive component to the repair. CT scan or MRI can be used to identify the muscle preoperatively.

Operative technique to repair a lost muscle includes adequate exposure, lighting, and hemostasis. If the previous surgery was recent, more bleeding than usual should be anticipated. Proximity to oblique muscles can be used to find most rectus muscles because of the significant intramuscular connections between them. Specifically, the superior rectus is connected to the superior oblique, and the inferior and lateral rectus to the inferior oblique. Unfortunately, the medial rectus has no such attachment, which makes it especially difficult, if not impossible, to find. The oculocardiac reflex[19] can be a useful sign that one has located and grabbed rectus muscle tissue. However, this is not effective in the patient premedicated with a parasympatholytic agent (eg, atropine).[19] Other possibly helpful measures include intraoperative electromyographic stimulation[13] and ultrasound. Neosynephrine can be used to cause blanching of tissue surrounding the muscle. If anything appears "muscular," it should be secured with suture before further exploration is undertaken.

The success rates for repair of the "slipped" muscle as compared with a lost muscle are much greater.[16] The medial rectus is most commonly involved[16] and is the most difficult muscle to find. In the best of circumstances, the inferior, superior, and lateral rectus can be identified in 50% to 75% of cases. However, the medial rectus is retrieved only 10% of the time.[16] Surgical judgment should be guided by several principles. The most important is not to cause extensive tissue disruption while searching for the muscle. Resultant bleeding and fat prolapse impairs identification of the muscle, and can result in excessive postoperative scarring or the adhesive syndrome.

If the muscle is identified, remember that both the slipped muscle and its antagonist can contract, causing restriction. Therefore, intraoperative forced ductions can be used to guide muscle placement on the globe. In particular, advancement of the slipped muscle to its intended insertion may result in a overcorrection postoperatively. Whenever possible, adjustable suture surgery can help avoid postoperative surprises.

If the muscle cannot be located during the initial surgery, adjacent muscle fascia can be attached to the globe in combination with a large recession of the antagonist muscle. If this is unsuccessful, little tissue has been disturbed, and a reoperation can be attempted without much scarring.[20] If significant limitation remains, a transposition procedure (eg, moving the medial and lateral rectus superiorly for a lost superior rectus muscle) can improve ductions and alignment. In a series of lost medial rectus muscles, this approach resulted in modest improvement in alignment with no overcorrections. However, overcorrections are possible when compensating for vertical muscle deficiencies.[16,21] Despite the surgeon's best efforts, most patients with irretrievable muscles are left with some deficient range of motion.

Hemostasis

Bleeding during surgery is, for the most part, an annoyance. It obscures the surgical field, particularly during reoperation, but is easily controlled with bipolar cautery. Although retrobulbar hemorrhage is a possible consequence, it is an extremely rare one. Bleeding can be avoided at several steps throughout the procedure. Conjunctival vessels can be constricted with 2.5% phenylephrine. One drop is instilled before and after prepping the face and conjunctiva.

Prophylactic cauterization of the anterior ciliary arteries at the muscle insertion can control bleeding following disinsertion. In resections, hemostasis is augmented by the placement of a hemostat just anterior to the preplaced sutures. The resected edge of muscle is usually cauterized before its release from the clamp. Inferior oblique weakening procedures also employ the use of a hemostat followed by cautery. Despite careful inspection of the cut muscle edge, additional bleeding in the immediate postoperative period can result in periocular ecchymosis. Drying the inferior temporal quadrant with a cotton applicator and irrigation with saline can help identify occult bleeding before wound closure. The proximity of the vortex vein to the oblique makes it an easy target to snag while passing the muscle hook. For this reason, the hook should be passed under direct visualization. The same precaution should be taken with the other vertical muscles. Particular care should be taken with dissection required to place sutures for a Faden procedure of the inferior rectus. The vortex veins are usually found adjacent to the muscle, 14 to 15 mm posterior to the insertion, which is the optimal location for suture placement. If the vortex is violated, bleeding can be managed with cautery.

Complications Associated With Anesthesia

Of all anesthesia-related complications, the most dreaded are those that result in the unexpected death of a child during elective surgery. Therefore, discussion of anesthetic complications must include malignant hyperthermia, oculocardiac reflex, and prolonged neuromuscular blockade.

Malignant Hyperthermia

Malignant hyperthermia (MH) is no longer the anesthesiologist's nightmare it once was. Mortality rates have dropped from 80% to less than 10% during the past 20 years.[22] However, deaths *still* occur despite optimal care.

MH morbidity can be decreased in several ways. MH-susceptible patients can often be identified through careful family and anesthetic histories. There is an increased frequency of MH in patients with myopathies, in particular, central core disease; however, the commonly assumed link with strabismus is tenuous.[23] MH is transmitted in an autosomal dominant fashion. Clinically, however, it may skip generations. Preoperative diagnosis is possible with the halothane-caffeine contracture test, which involves muscle biopsy, and is offered at a few centers throughout the country. There are no reliable noninvasive tests, but if one suspects MH, it is easy to avoid potential triggers, such as succinylcholine and inhalational drugs.

The surgeon should be familiar enough with the signs and symptoms of MH to help identify it and initiate treatment in a timely manner. Morbidity is directly correlated with the duration of the symptoms. The full-blown syndrome is rarely seen (1:60,000–200,000).[24] The milder abortive forms are more common and more frequently seen in children (1:4500). Extreme rigidity of the masseter muscle (ie, the mouth cannot be opened) following succinylcholine administration may be the earliest symptom. Fifty percent of these patients have biopsy-proven MH.[25–27] Although the disease usually presents intraoperatively, symptoms can present up to 4 hours after surgery.

MH is a hypermetabolic state of skeletal muscle. Because of a genetic predisposition, on exposure to a triggering agent, calcium is released from the sarcoplasmic reticulum. Intracellular calcium rises, and the cell dies, releasing its contents. Symptoms are reminiscent of heavy aerobic exercise. There is excessive oxygen consumption (venous desaturation), followed by carbon dioxide (hypercarbia) and lactic acid buildup. The patient's heart rate increases (tachycardia), and the patient breathes rapidly (tachypnea) and becomes overheated (fever). Metabolic and respiratory acidosis follows.

The initial treatment is directed at stopping the hypermetabolic state. The triggering agents should be discontinued and the ventilation circuit changed. Intravenous dantrolene is administered as an intravenous bolus. Dantrolene stops the calcium release from the sarcoplasmic reticulum. The initial dose is 2.5 mg/kg IV, which is repeated, up to 20 mg/kg, until the symptoms abate.

Next, the respiratory acidosis should be corrected with hyperventilation. This increases oxygenation and blows off CO_2. Then, treat the metabolic acidosis, fever, and arrhythmias. Untreated metabolic acidosis results in cardiovascular instability, arrhythmia, and death early in the course of the disease. Dantrolene is continued for up to 12 hours intravenously and up to 28 hours orally, 1 mg/kg every 6 hours, with aggressive monitoring for recrudescence.

Time is of the essence in recognizing and treating MH. Morbidity is directly associated with symptom duration. Questions about diagnosis, treatment and preoperative diagnosis can be answered by a 24-hour MH hotline* operated by the Malignant Hyperthermia Association of the United States.

Oculocardiac Reflex

Bradycardia following traction on an extraocular muscle is a familiar experience, with a reported incidence from 32% to 90%.[28] But many surgeons are unaware that the oculocardiac reflex (OCR) and resultant arrhythmias, including sinus bradycardia, bigeminy, nodal rhythms, and ventricular fibrillation, have been responsible for more than 60 reported deaths.

This trigeminovagal reflex is precipitated most commonly by acute traction on the extraocular muscle; however, it can be caused by pressure on the globe, intraorbital injection or hematoma, acute glaucoma, and stretching of the eyelid muscles.

Slow, gradual traction on extraocular muscles is the best prevention; if the oculocardiac reflex is triggered, it is less intense.[28] At the onset of symptoms, pull on the muscle should be released immediately. Repeated gentle traction can be used to fatigue the reflex.

Anticholinergics, in particular atropine, 0.01 to 0.02 mg/kg, and glycopyrrolate, 0.005 to 0.01 mg/kg, are the mainstay of pharmacologic treatment. In the recommended doses, they do not completely block the vagal reflex, and OCR can still be produced with excessive tugging. In fact, arrhythmias that occur after drug treatment may be more long-lasting and difficult to treat.[29,30]

Glycopyrrolate has been touted because it is longer acting and has fewer associated arrhythmias in contradistinction to atropine, which more often results in tachycardia.[31] However, both have been shown to produce sinus tachycardia and prevent intraoperative bradycardia in children when administered before surgical stimulation.[31] In older patients, neither drug reliably decreases the incidence of bradycardia.

All bradycardias and arrhythmias are not caused by the oculocardiac reflex. If there is no resolution after traction is discontinued, hypoxia, hypercapnia, acidosis, and electrolyte imbalance may be the culprits. Arterial blood gases and electrolytes should be monitored, and the adequacy of the airway assured.

Prolonged Neuromuscular Blockade

Prolonged neuromuscular blockade resulting in respiratory paralysis is another serious but preventable problem. It is seen after administration of succinylcholine in patients with low pseudocholinesterase levels. A common strabismus-related cause of low pseudocholinesterase is the administration of phospholine iodide drops preoperatively. This drug should be discontinued 2 to 3 weeks before surgery.

POSTOPERATIVE COMPLICATIONS

Complications Associated With Anesthesia

Vomiting

Of all unmedicated strabismus patients, 41% to 85% have at least one episode of vomiting after surgery.[32] Often occurring in the immediate postoperative period, it can persist or present hours after surgery and hospital discharge. The reflex is probably centrally mediated and has been attributed to changes in vi-

** The 24-hour telephone MH hotline number of the Malignant Hyperthermia Association of the United States is 209-634-4917.*

sual perception, vestibuloocular disturbance, or proprioceptive changes after muscle repositioning.

It occurs less frequently in children under the age of 2 years and more often in females.[32] There is no relation to the number of muscles operated, type of ventilation used, duration of anesthesia, or surgeon.[33] Similar frequencies are noted for both general anesthesia and local (retrobulbar) anesthesia,[34] and there is no improvement by patching the surgical eye in monocular cases.[33] Forcing liquids in the immediate postoperative period probably increases vomiting.[33,35] Neither acupressure[36] or acupuncture[33] have been shown to reduce emesis.

Droperidol, a dopamine antagonist, has been the most common antiemetic used for prophylaxis. The most efficacious dose is 0.075 mg/kg given intravenously. Smaller doses, 0.025 and .05 mg/kg, do not prevent vomiting as well and can still produce prolonged postoperative sedation, which is the main disadvantage of droperidol.[37–39] Dosing during induction might produce superior results, compared with intraoperative or postoperative administration,[37] but this has not been adequately substantiated. Oral droperidol has also been shown to be effective when given preoperatively.[40]

Other drugs have been demonstrated to have comparable antiemetic properties with possibly less sedation. These include intravenous metoclopramide, 0.25 mg/kg,[41,42] and scopolamine patches.[43,44] The patches are placed the evening before surgery and removed the day after. However, appropriate scopolamine dosages for children have yet to be determined.

The use of propofol, an intravenous hypnotic agent, has been shown to diminish postoperative vomiting and sedation, if halothane is avoided. It has the added benefit of earlier ambulation and hospital discharge with a faster, clearer-headed recovery and little hangover.[45,46]

Postoperative vomiting seems unavoidable, but the frequency and severity can be diminished with pharmacologic intervention.

Postoperative Sedation

To diminish postoperative sedation, one might substitute another antiemetic instead of droperidol, or choose topical or retrobulbar anesthesia instead of general. If general is required or desired by the patient, opt for propofol in combination with a short-acting narcotic.

Pain Management

Postoperative pain is usually minimal. Most of the time it is adequately managed with acetaminophen, although opiates are standard at some institutions. The origin of the pain is in great part conjunctival and is diminished with topical tetracaine.[47] This is particularly useful for diminishing discomfort in adjustable suture patients. However, corneal toxicity precludes repeated use. Newer nonsteroidal antiinflammatory drugs with potent analgesic properties may further decrease postoperative discomfort without the side effects of sedation and nausea produced by opiate administration. The challenge remains to find an anesthetic technique that allows rapid recovery with a minimum of pain, sedation, and vomiting. However, careful preoperative planning and surgeon participation in anesthetic management can decrease surgical morbidity and mortality, and improve the quality of the experience for both patients and their families.

Infections

Bacterial infection following strabismus surgery is rare. Orbital cellulitis is the most common, although endophthalmitis, usually from globe perforation, and keratitis from dellen have also been reported.

Orbital Cellulitis

Postoperative orbital infection is a serious but infrequent occurrence. Fewer than one dozen cases of orbital cellulitis have been reported in the literature.[48–51] The incidence of cellulitis is estimated to be approximately 1:1900.[49] There is no difference in infection rates with the use of routine prophylactic antibiotics (topical, oral, or intravenous) before or after surgery.[49] Although povidone-iodine (Betadine) solution reduces conjunctival colony counts, there is no significant effect on infection rate.[49,52]

Symptoms typically appear on the second or third postoperative day (Fig. 12-3). Preseptal infection can be differentiated from orbital involvement in the presence of limited extraocular motility, proptosis, decreased visual acuity, and signs of postseptal infection. Chemosis, pain, lid edema, and fever can be seen in both conditions.

Laboratory studies should include a complete blood count with differential, and blood and conjunctival cultures. Neither culture is particularly useful

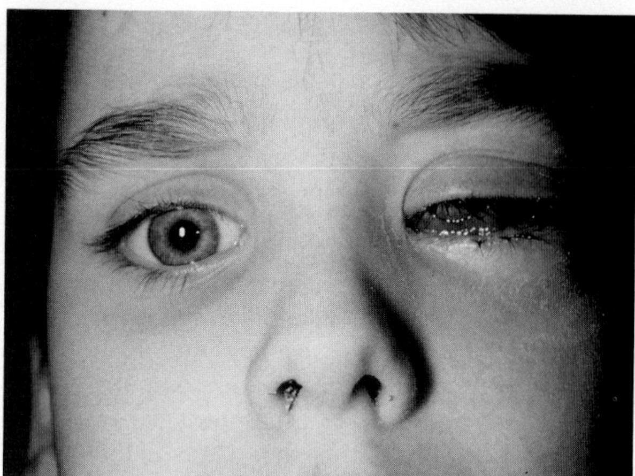

Figure 12-3. Orbital cellulitis several days after inferior oblique surgery. Marked limitations of ocular rotations were present.

clinically, however. The blood cultures rarely grow bacteria, and the conjunctiva has been sterilized by postoperative antibiotics or contains a mixture of normal flora.

Treatment includes prompt hospitalization for intravenous antibiotics. Broad-spectrum coverage is appropriate until a responsible organism has been identified. For patients between 6 months and 3 years of age, antibiotics should include coverage for *Haemophilus influenzae* in addition to *Staphylococcus* and *Streptococcus* spp. No improvement during the initial 24 hours of therapy should prompt an orbital imaging (eg, CT scan) study to rule out abscess formation. Abscesses require incision and drainage.

Early detection and treatment can prevent vision loss. Patient education is essential for early detection. Parents and patients should be instructed to call immediately when the symptoms or signs of infection occur. Specifically, they should be alert for prominent swelling of the lids or conjunctiva, fever greater than 101°F, limitation of eye movements, decreased vision, or persistent or excessive pain.[48]

A topical steroid-antibiotic combination is routinely administered prophylactically for days to weeks during the immediate postoperative period. Theoretically, this decreases the risk of both infection and postoperative inflammation. Because the risk of postoperative infection is minimal, another rationale for its use is primarily to minimize postoperative inflammation. However, controlled studies have failed to show that either topical[53] or subconjunctival[54] application significantly decreases postoperative inflammation. These combination drugs are not benign, and allergic conjunctivitis is a frequent side effect. Allergic stigmata of burning, itching, conjunctival chemosis and hyperemia, epiphora, and lid edema can be confused with early infection. One distinguishing characteristic is that allergic symptoms and signs are worse immediately after drop instillation, and improve until the next drop is administered. Avoid drops to which the patient has a known allergy as well as those with a reputation to be sensitizing (ie, neomycin).

Endophthalmitis

Endophthalmitis after strabismus surgery is extremely rare, with an incidence between 1:3500 to 1:8000 cases.[9] This complication almost always arises from recognized or occult scleral perforation but can rarely be caused by a contiguous orbital infection.

Suspect intraocular infection if the patient complains of increasing pain and diminished visual acuity. Examination may reveal conjunctival hyperemia and chemosis, corneal edema, hypopyon, and eyelid swelling. Endophthalmitis commonly presents during the first 72 hours following surgery.[20,55,56] Prompt vitrectomy should be performed with administration of intravitreal, subconjunctival, and topical antibiotics. Intravenous antibiotics with good ocular penetration are also appropriate. Although *Staphylococcus epidermidis* is the organism most commonly reported, initial coverage should be broad spectrum. The choice of medication should be modified based on the results of the vitreous culture.

Anterior Segment Complications

Anterior segment complications are annoyingly commonplace. The most serious of these is anterior segment ischemia. Fortunately, most others are minor, transient problems that can often be avoided.

Anterior Segment Ischemia

Ischemia of the anterior segment (ASI) occurs in approximately 1:13,000 cases.[57] Mild forms of the disease occur with greater frequency than previously suspected.[58] Although the pathogenesis has not been entirely elucidated, it is clearly associated with severing of the anterior ciliary arteries. ASI has been reported in association with almost every strabismus procedure with the exception of single rectus muscle surgery.[57] At greatest risk are procedures involving detachment of three and four rectus muscles.[57–60]

Surgery on vertical rectus muscles results in greater reduction of anterior segment blood supply as demonstrated by filling delay on iris angiography.[58] Clinically, almost 25% of patients who undergo surgery on only one vertical muscle or one vertical in combination with two horizontal muscles develop only subclinical pupillary dysfunction or iris filling defects.[59] Primary surgical procedures on two vertical recti with or without a horizontal rectus demonstrate up to a 50% incidence of mild ASI with minimal long-term complications.[59–61]

Adults are more susceptible than children.[57] Children usually tolerate recession of three and four muscles without a problem.[57,60] However, one child with cicatricial retinopathy of prematurity developed ischemia after a recess-resect procedure of only two horizontal muscles.[62] At a greater risk are older patients. Systemic disease, in particular atherosclerosis, has been implicated as a risk factor. However, this is not a consistent association.[57] ASI is described more commonly in patients with abducens palsy; however, this is most likely explained by the corrective transposition procedure, which involves multiple muscles and not the palsy. An alternative is to transpose the vertical muscles and inject the medial rectus with botulinum toxin, decreasing but not eliminating the risk of ischemia.[63]

ASI can present within 1 to 7 days of surgery but is most often seen during the first 24 to 48 hours.[57,59] The duration of symptoms varies with the severity of the disease. Milder forms of ASI, consisting of only anterior chamber cell and flare with filling defects on iris fluorescein angiography[59] tend to resolve without treatment in 1 to 2 days. Moderate changes may persist for 2 to 3 weeks[59] with severer changes lasting as long as 9 weeks[60] and sometimes resulting in permanent sequelae. Moderate and severe cases present with anterior uveitis and keratitis,[64] striate keratopathy, chemosis, lid edema, and visual loss. Pupils may become dilated, fixed, or irregularly shaped with posterior synechiae. Intraocular pressure decreases because of inflammation.[57,59] Severe forms of ASI include permanent corneal opacification, iris atrophy, peripheral anterior synechiae, neovascularization of the cornea and iris, cataract, hypotony, and phthisis.[59] Severe forms of ASI can be confused with endophthalmitis. In these cases, iris fluorescein angiography is a useful tool to demonstrate both filling defects and vessel leakage, both signs of anterior segment ischemia.[59]

To avoid ASI, identify high-risk patients and procedures. Unfortunately, iris angiography is not predictive of ASI risk.[65] If surgery on three or four rectus muscles in one eye is required, the surgery can be performed in stages. A wait of 2 to 5 months will allow recovery of blood flow to the anterior segment and uvea.[57,59–61,66] Recovery of blood circulation may be complete as early as 2 to 4 weeks.[65] Fornix incision may preserve the perilimbal conjunctival–Tenon capsule circulation better than limbal conjunctival incision.[67] Alternative surgical plans can be formed. The correction can be divided among muscles in both eyes. For transposition procedures, partial muscle transfer can be substituted for complete muscle displacement (ie, Jensen procedure). The surgeon can preserve at least one bundle of anterior ciliary artery in each vertical muscle.[66] In some cases, botulinum toxin might be substituted for muscle recession.

If high-risk surgery is unavoidable, preservation of the anterior ciliary vessels can be accomplished with microdissection as described by McKeown.[68] Monkey models clearly show that this technique can prevent anterior segment ischemia.[69] However, preservation of these vessels is not as successful as it may appear intraoperatively. Inadvertent occlusion from compression or excessive stretch is not uncommon. Sometimes only the fibrous bundle is included in the dissection without the vessel.[69] Other disadvantages include the need for an operating microscope and increased operating time (about 1 hour per muscle).

Fortunately, ASI is infrequent, and when it does occur, it is often mild with no significant sequelae. Treatment usually includes topical or intravenous steroids.[57] Hyperbaric oxygen has been used successfully in one patient in whom steroids were contraindicated.[70] Recovery without any intervention is also well documented.[57]

Dellen

Dellen are small areas of limbal corneal thinning with intact overlying epithelium that present 1 to 2 weeks after surgery as a result of postoperative conjunctival swelling near the limbus (Fig. 12-4). Tear film breakup is disturbed, which leads to desiccation of the cornea. Resection procedures are implicated more often than recessions[71] and limbal incisions more often than fornix incisions.[13,71] Although dellen tend to resolve spontaneously within 2 to 4 weeks of

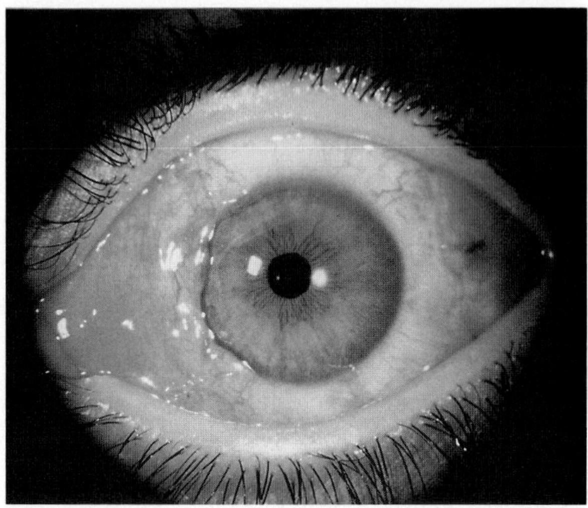

Figure 12-4. Dellen at inferonasal limbus after large medial rectus resection. Note edematous conjunctiva with override of the cornea. (See color plate after page xvi.)

surgery, epithelial defects and corneal infection can result, with permanent vascularization and scarring of the cornea.[72]

Bunching of the conjunctiva at the limbus should be minimized. Fornix incisions are particularly useful, especially in conjunction with large muscle resections. Conjunctiva can be recessed and attached to the sclera posterior to the limbus with an absorbable suture. The bare sclera will reepithelialize rapidly.

Supplemental artificial tears solution or ointment should be applied frequently to help alleviate corneal drying. A pressure patch can be applied for 1 to 2 days, which usually results in resolution. Topical steroids can be applied to diminish conjunctival swelling,[14] although the lesions must be examined repeatedly to check for the development of secondary infection.[71]

Suture-Related Complications

Occasionally, granuloma formation is noted over the site of muscle attachment (Fig. 12-5). Previously caused by chromic catgut suture, now associated with more commonly used Vicryl (polyglactin 910; Ethicon, Somerville, NJ), granulomas appear 2 to 3 weeks after surgery.[73] They are localized, hyperemic nodules that are more unsightly than uncomfortable. Spontaneous regression within 4 to 6 weeks is the usual course; however, some do persist.[73] Topical steroids administered two to three times daily for 7 to 10 days can be effective treatment for most granulomas.[74] Larger lesions may require surgical excision.

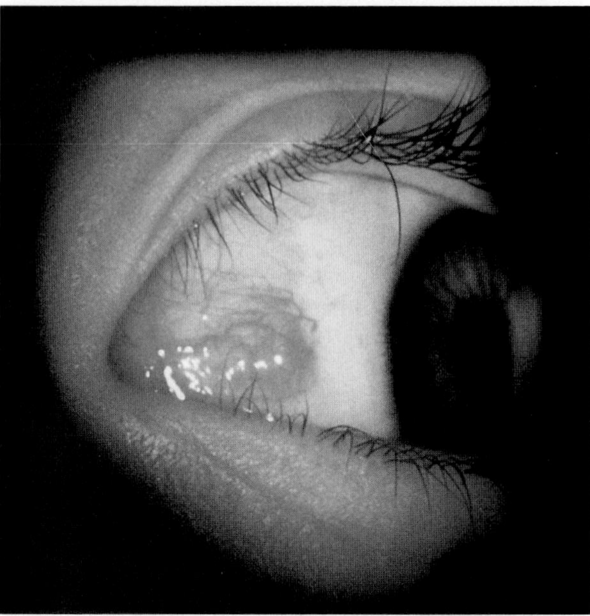

Figure 12-5. Hyperemia and granuloma over site of muscle insertion. (See color plate after page xvi.)

Suture abscesses have rarely been reported, usually in association with nonabsorbable sutures (ie, Mersilene).[13] Noted within the first week after surgery, they appear as yellow fluctuant elevations over the suture site. Treatment consists of incision and drainage with suture removal. Topical antibiotics should be started after culture.

Suture allergy is another complication more commonly associated with the use of chromic catgut. Although allergic reactions can still be seen with the use of Vicryl, they occur in less than 1% of patients. Itching and irritation present 1 to 7 days postoperatively.[75] The area over the suture becomes injected and chemotic. Epiphora and lid edema are sometimes noted. The condition is usually self-limited. Symptoms subside over several weeks but may be ameliorated with topical steroids and cool compresses. Occasionally, the suture must be removed.

Conjunctival Scarring and Symblepharon

Not only is excessive postoperative scarring unsightly, but shortening or contracture of the conjunctiva can result in incomitant ocular misalignment from restriction. This is especially common with reoperation in which subconjunctival fibrosis is a problem.

To avoid conjunctival scarring, careful handling of tissue with appropriate forceps is essential. Incision placement (ie, fornix incision versus limbal incision) can also improve cosmetic appearance postoperatively. The fornix incision decreases conjunctival reaction and limits visible scarring within the palpebral fissure. Avoid incisions near the caruncle and plica semilunaris. Tissue disruption in this area is particularly noticeable. Conjunctival closure should be performed carefully, with dissection and excision of excessive fibrotic tissue. Contracted conjunctiva can be recessed and the sclera left bare to reepithelialize. Sclera reepithelializes promptly, within several days postoperatively.[24] The redness disappears given time.

Conjunctival Cysts

Cysts within the conjunctiva following strabismus surgery fortunately are rare; however, once present, they can be difficult to treat surgically. Most cysts are epithelial and filled with clear fluid. Pseudosebaceous cysts have also been reported. There is a tendency to confuse these with abscesses when the milky fluid they contain is mistaken for purulence.[76] Cyst development has been ascribed to incarceration of conjunctival epithelium within the wound. More recently, Kushner[76] has theorized that the conjunctiva or Tenon capsule is caught on the suture, and dragged into the scleral tunnel.

Lesions appear as single or multiple translucent masses beneath the conjunctiva (Fig. 12-6), within several weeks to months after strabismus surgery but have been reported 2 to 35 years later.[76] When surgical repair is attempted, the lesions are often found to be larger than they appeared at preoperative examination. Although some are isolated lesions within conjunctiva or more rarely the muscle,[77] attachment to the muscle by way of a pseudotendon is often found. Careless dissection can result in inadvertent disinsertion and loss of the muscle.[76]

Surgical management consists of complete excision, or marsupialization. Simply draining is not effective because the fluid recollects promptly. Every attempt should be made to excise the cyst without rupturing it. To avoid piercing the cyst with toothed forceps, it can be stabilized with a cryoprobe.[78] Cysts adherent to sclera may need to be shaved with a surgical blade to ensure no cyst wall remains. If extraocular muscle is adherent to the cyst wall, suture should be preplaced in anticipation of inadvertent disinsertion during dissection. Extensive cysts, which in the surgeon's judgment extend too far posteriorly for complete removal, can be marsupialized.

Tenon Capsule Prolapse

Prolapse of Tenon capsule through the conjunctival incision is seen in the immediate postoperative period (Fig. 12-7). The Tenon capsule appears as a bright-white mass and is often mistaken for mucus discharge. The parents report attempting to wipe this "mucus" from the eye. The Tenon capsule prolapse is the result of incomplete conjunctival closure and can result in chronic inflammation, preventing adequate healing of the conjunctival incision. Avoidance is simply achieved with meticulous closure. Excessive

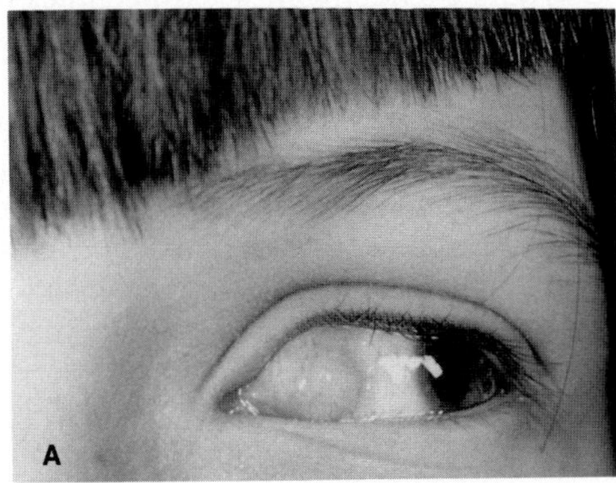

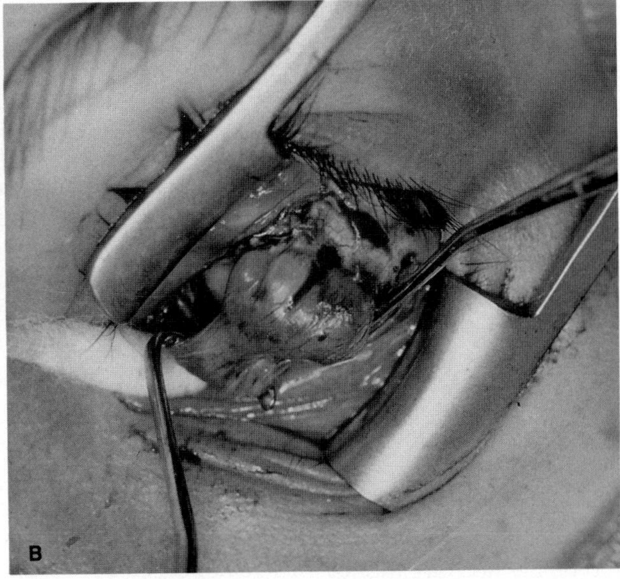

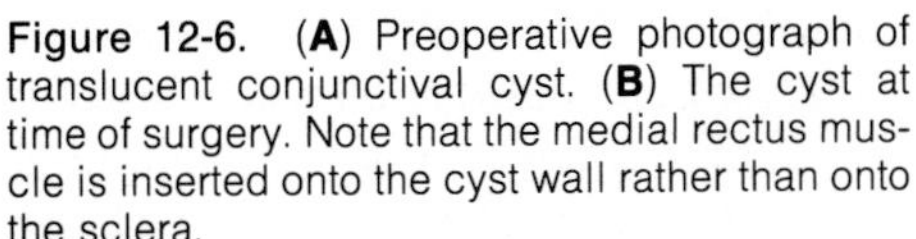

Figure 12-6. (**A**) Preoperative photograph of translucent conjunctival cyst. (**B**) The cyst at time of surgery. Note that the medial rectus muscle is inserted onto the cyst wall rather than onto the sclera.

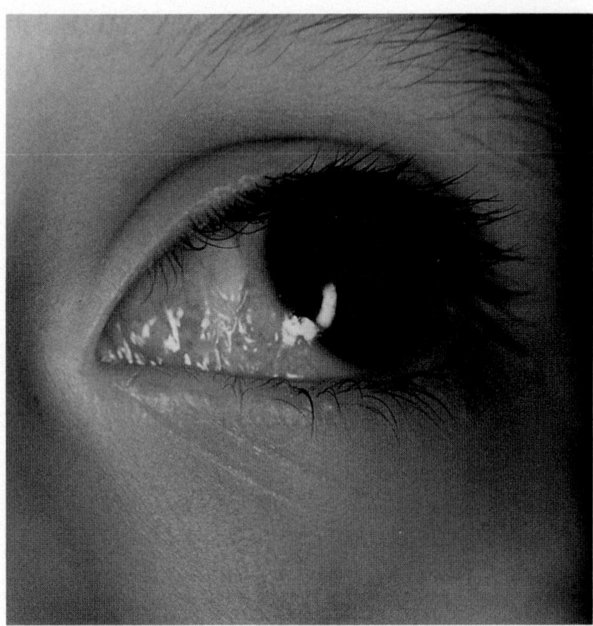

Figure 12-7. Tenon capsule prolapsed from conjunctival incision. (See color plate after page xvi.)

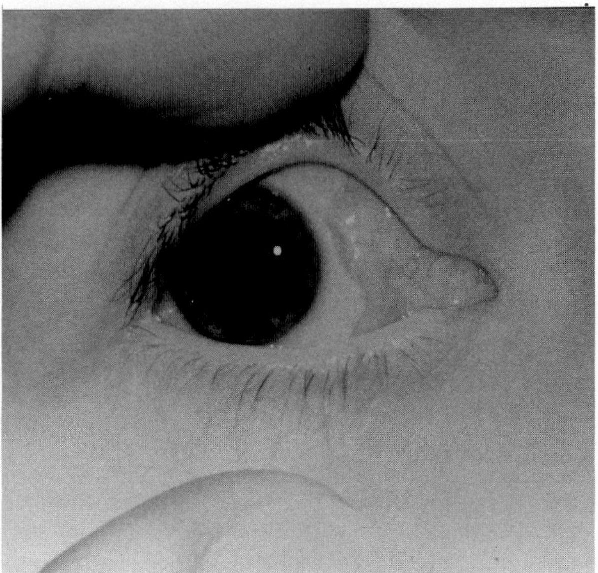

Figure 12-8. Prolapsed fat following surgery. (Courtesy of Linda M. Christmann, MD, Richland Memorial Hospital, West Columbia, SC, Lexington Medical Center, West Columbia, SC, Baptist Medical Center, Columbia, SC) (See color plate after page xvi.)

irrigation should be avoided to prevent ballooning of the Tenon capsule.[75] Observation is usually all that is required. The protrusion resolves spontaneously by retracting within the incision. If persistent and unsightly, excision may be required.

Fat Prolapse

Prolapse of orbital fat occurs occasionally after violation of the Tenon capsule (Fig. 12-8). This is most common during posterior dissection and reoperation. It appears as a yellow mass or bulge under the conjunctiva.

To prevent rents in the posterior Tenon capsule, Parks[79] advises that one avoid "deep dipping" with the muscle hook. Deep or careless passes of the hook posteriorly along the globe can rupture the Tenon capsule, allowing fat to pop through this newly created opening.[79] The dehiscence can be repaired at the initial surgery or during a subsequent operation with absorbable suture. Protruding fat should be excised by clamping it with a hemostat, excising the unwanted fat, and cauterizing the stump before releasing the clamp.

Scleritis

Scleritis is a more significant complication of strabismus surgery but is rarely seen. Postoperative scleritis tends to be the necrotic variety.[80] There appear to be two clinical presentations. In one group, symptoms begin shortly after surgery (mean, 10 weeks). These patients tend to have had multiple ocular procedures that need not be limited to strabismus surgery.[80] The other group has a later onset, from 6 to 40 years postoperatively (mean, 22 years), and are usually female.[80] After investigation, most are found to have a coexisting autoimmune disease.

Patients complain of deep boring pain and on examination have a tender, diffusely hyperemic eye. Occasionally, there are conjunctival elevations with a granulomatous appearance.[81] The lateral rectus tends to be involved, even when the medial rectus in the same eye has also been operated. Most cases respond rapidly to high-dose systemic steroids or cytotoxic drugs. Nonsteroidal antiinflammatory drugs are ineffective for the most part.[80] Low-dose maintenance therapy may be required for months to years after initial treatment.

Changes in the Lid Fissure

Lid fissure changes are among the expected postoperative problems. More common with vertical muscle surgery, they can be associated with horizontal muscles as well. In particular, unacceptable fissure narrowing can be produced by resection of the lateral rectus in Duane syndrome. After multiple recessions in one eye, the globe can become proptotic, causing fissure widening. Not only a cosmetic concern, lid retraction can lead to significant exposure problems, especially when compounded by proptosis as found in patients with thyroid eye disease.

The superior rectus is associated with the levator palpebrae superioris by the Tenon capsule and other fibrous connections. Whitnall ligament, the fibrous condensation in which levator muscle becomes aponeurosis, reflects onto trochlea, superior oblique tendon, and superior rectus fascia. The inferior rectus has more direct connections to the lower lid from the capsulopalpebral fascia (CPF), which arises from the muscle itself. The CPF is the analogous structure to the levator muscle of the upper lid. It condenses to become the capsulopalpebral head and can be identified intraoperatively as a white, thick fibrous mass adherent to the inferior surface of the inferior rectus beginning 5 mm posterior to the insertion.

As a result of these fascial connections, muscle resection can result in lid advancement and recession in retraction of the lids. Changes after inferior rectus (IR) procedures are the most common.[82] IR recessions as small as 1 mm produce lid retraction in 94% of patients. The degree of retraction directly correlates with the amount of muscle recession. Advancement of the lid is found in virtually all patients undergoing IR resection. Changes in contour (ie, flattening) have also been noted.[82]

Changes in the upper lid height, usually associated with superior rectus (SR) surgery, are less frequent and less significant. Lid elevation is more likely to result from unusually large recessions, such as those performed for dissociated vertical deviations (Fig. 12-9). Some authors suggest that at least 10 mm of recession is necessary before lid changes are noted.[74] However, Pacheco and associates[82] demonstrated retraction in 90% of patients undergoing 3- to 12-mm superior rectus recessions. Unlike surgery on the inferior rectus, there was no correlation between the amount of recession and the amount of upper lid retraction.[82] Ptosis of the upper lid can result from SR resection and inadvertent disinsertion of Whitnall ligament after blindly passing the muscle hook into the superonasal quadrant.

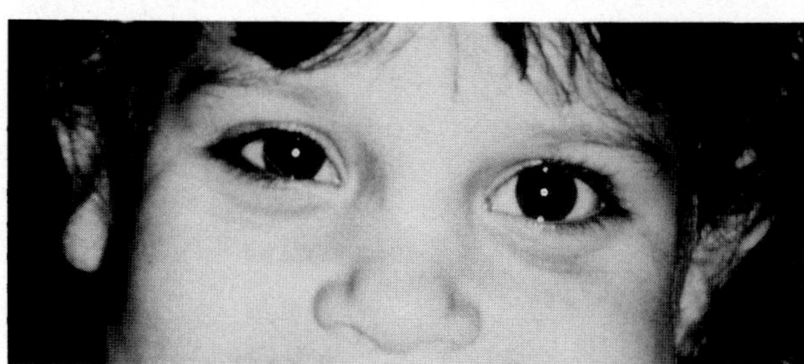

Figure 12-9. Upper lid retraction following large superior rectus recession for dissociated vertical deviation. (Courtesy of Richard A. Saunders, MD, Charleston, SC)

Despite attempts to sever connections between the inferior rectus and the lower lid, or to limit the amount of muscle surgery, some change in lid position seems unavoidable. Two promising procedures have been described for surgery on the inferior rectus; however, neither procedure completely eliminates lid changes. Lid changes in thyroid patients are not addressed by either study. Kushner[83] recommends disinsertion of the capsulopalpebral head with reattachment to the IR 15 mm posterior to the limbus. Lid position is generally improved with this procedure, except with adjustable suture surgery. In these patients, increasing IR recession during adjustment increases lower lid retraction at least 1 mm. It is also causes increased discomfort and edema of the lower eyelid, complicating the adjustment.

Pacheco and associates recommend extensive IR dissection at least 25 mm posterior to the limbus.[82] The capsulopalpebral head is identified and placed on suture that is passed through the sclera anterior to the IR insertion. Lid height is adjusted postoperatively by repositioning the suture after adjustment of the inferior rectus. Despite a reduction of lid retraction in all patients, there is a persistent effect of muscle surgery on lower lid height proportional to the amount of IR recession.

If, despite the surgeon's best effort, exposure or unacceptable cosmesis results, oculoplastic corrective procedures of the lid may be necessary. Adequate preoperative patient education is paramount to avoid disappointment after surgery. Patients need to understand that changes in lid position may be unavoidable, especially after vertical muscle surgery.

Changes in Refractive Error

Changes in refractive error, although minor, are not infrequent after strabismus surgery, especially horizontal rectus recess-resect procedures.[84,85] Most commonly "with the rule" astigmatism is induced.[85,86] Up to 40% of patients experience increased cylinder of 0.50 to 1.00 diopter. Ten percent can expect to have changes of 1 D or greater. Conversely, changes are infrequent when only one horizontal rectus muscle or oblique muscle has been operated per eye. When produced, alterations are small and transient.[84]

More dramatic differences are likely following correction of restrictive strabismus, such as fibrosis syndrome or thyroid eye disease. In these cases, the restricted muscles may be responsible for a significant amount of preoperative astigmatism, which is relieved by surgery.[87,88] Although change in refractive error is unavoidable, patients should be educated to expect small changes in refractive error, which may require spectacle change after surgery.

Restriction After "Uneventful" Strabismus Surgery

The appearance of unexpected restriction and new muscle imbalances after initial strabismus procedures is disappointing and often perplexing. Postoperative restrictions are found more frequently after surgery on the oblique muscles but are also seen after routine horizontal muscle cases. More common causes include contracted conjunctiva, excessive muscle resection, large superior oblique tucks, and adhesions.

Iatrogenic Brown syndrome presents as limitation of elevation in adduction after superior oblique tuck. The restriction can be assessed intraoperatively with forced duction testing. After the tendon has been tucked, the suture is secured temporarily with a bow tie. Surgical instruments are removed from the eye and passive ductions are performed. The amount of tuck can be modified to limit restriction. Alternatively, the amount of tuck can be limited empirically or a 6- to 8-mm tendon resection can be performed.[24]

Inadvertent inclusion of the inferior oblique muscle during procedures on the lateral rectus muscle is another cause of postoperative restriction. It can be hooked on deep passes of the muscle hook and included in the muscle clamp or sutured to the lateral rectus during resections.[89,90] Incomplete dissection of fascial attachments between the lateral and inferior oblique muscles can cause it to be pulled forward during the resection. To avoid this complication, the lateral rectus should be hooked immediately posterior to its insertion. After disinsertion, the underbelly and inferior border should be examined and dissection of the attachments between the two muscles completed. Finally, direct visualization is essential during placement of suture and muscle clamps.[89]

Poor surgical technique, including rough or sloppy surgery, excessive bleeding or cautery, and violation of the posterior Tenon capsule, all contribute to the development of adhesions.[91–94] The fat adherence syndrome as described by Parks[95] is the most extreme example. In this syndrome, the Tenon capsule is inadvertently violated 10 mm posterior to the limbus. Extraconal fat comes in contact with globe or extraocular muscle. Trauma to the fat induces fibrosis, adhesion, and scarring, which extends through the fat septa to the periorbita. The septa lose their elasticity, becoming restrictive bands.[93] Extraocular muscle becomes adherent to the scarred Tenon capsule as it penetrates, causing restriction.[7,90,93] Incomitant horizontal or vertical deviations with positive forced ductions result.

To prevent this postoperative disaster, the muscle should be hooked immediately posterior to its insertion. Blind hooking of the muscle or "deep dipping" should be avoided, especially in the inferotemporal quadrant. Excessive dissection adjacent to the posterior Tenon capsule is not advisable. It is particularly easy to expose fat during reoperation.

Attempts at surgical repair are disappointing. In a "good" result, the eye is in primary position, but severe limitation of movement persists. Although initial postsurgical alignment can look promising, recurrence and contracture of the scar result in changes in the eye alignment up to 6 months postoperatively.[93]

Restriction can also follow excessive dissection. The Tenon capsule acts as a "purse string," pulling the muscle on top of itself to create redundant muscle. The effect of the recession is negated.[90] Minimal dissection of check ligaments and intramuscular septum is an acceptable alternative. It has been shown to have no adverse effect on surgical outcome in recessions for infantile esotropia.[18] A balance between overly zealous dissection and a more modest severing of the Tenon capsule needs to be achieved.

Pharmacologic and mechanical attempts to limit scar tissue following muscle surgery have been, for the most part, unsuccessful. These include polyglactin meshes surrounding the muscle,[91] synthetic polypeptide sleeves,[96] and sodium hyaluronate.[94,97] Preservation of the Tenon capsule with minimal dissection, control of bleeding with judicious use of cautery, and avoidance of orbital fat are still the best approaches to avoid the consequences of adhesions.

Complications Associated With Thyroid Eye Disease

Surgical treatment of thyroid eye disease remains unpredictable and fraught with complications. Unstable postoperative alignment, torsional diplopia, and lid retraction are just some of the problems.

Although adjustable suture surgery has improved the odds of obtaining acceptable ocular alignment after one surgical correction,[98] it is not infallible. Surgical timing is crucial. Operating in the presence of smoldering inflammatory disease can provoke a dramatic inflammatory response that will adversely alter postoperative eye position. Conjunctival injection and chemosis suggest active disease.[99] A wait of 3 to 6 months is recommended after stabilization of ocular alignment to avoid triggering a flare.[98]

Excessive recession of the inferior rectus, although necessary for correction of large deviations in some patients, can cause torsional diplopia, A-pattern exotropia, late overcorrections, and hypertropia in downgaze. Postoperative overcorrections can be minimized by leaving some limitation of elevation or empirically limiting recessions to 4 to 5 mm.[100,101] Avoid simultaneous weakening procedures of the inferior oblique for correction of excyclotorsion. The inferior oblique is rarely involved in thyroid eye disease, and this combination produces postoperative incyclotropia.[100] Superior oblique weakening can be used to correct torsional diplopia and medial displacement of the inferior rectus for A-pattern exotropia.[100,101]

Late overcorrections of hypotropia can occur weeks to months after surgery. Patients at risk can often be identified preoperatively. Overcorrections are more likely in proptotic eyes and in eyes with unilateral enlargement of the superior rectus,[102] eyes with hypotropia greater in primary position than in downgaze, and eyes with positive forced ductions of the superior rectus.[101] These patients should have conservative surgery. Smaller bilateral inferior rectus recessions on adjustable suture can be performed as an alternative to a single large recession in asymmetric disease. Early postoperative inflammatory changes in eye alignment may be arrested with a brief course of rapidly tapered oral steroids.

Changes in refractive error[87] and lid position, necrotizing scleritis,[81] and dellen formation from conjunctival inflammation are more common in patients with thyroid eye disease.

Adjustable Suture Complications

Widely used in adults and older children, adjustable sutures increase the predictability of most strabismus repairs and reduce the reoperation rate to between 4% to 11%.[103,104] This technique is especially useful in reoperation, paralytic or restrictive disease, and vertical deviations. In patients with combined horizontal and vertical deviations, postoperative position of more than one muscle can be altered. For cases in which this procedure is used, adjustment of muscle position is required in 35% to 50% of cases.[103,104] Preoperative and intraoperative planning can assure smooth adjustments with a minimum of complications. Patient cooperation during adjustment is essential; therefore, patient selection is an important consideration. The lower age limit of patient tolerance is about 12 to 13 years. Appropriate patients can be identified during clinical examination by assessing responses to measurement of applanation pressure[104] or manipulation of nonanesthetized conjunctiva with a cotton swab.[105] If these procedures are well tolerated, then one can be reasonably certain that adjustment will be too.

The next concern is limiting the effect of anesthesia after surgery. The procedure can be performed under general or local anesthesia. To improve patient alertness and cooperation after general anesthesia, propofol infusion in combination with a short-acting narcotic are superior to standard inhalational agents.[106,107]

Lidocaine (2%) without epinephrine is an appropriately short-acting drug choice for local anesthesia. Hyaluronidase is added to promote tissue penetration. Ninety percent of preoperative muscle function returns between 5 to 6 hours after injection.[108] Bupivacaine should be avoided as this causes akinesia for up to 12 hours.

Postoperative muscle adjustment is optimally performed the day of or the morning after surgery to minimize tissue adhesion and avoid tissue edema. Surgery should be scheduled for early in the morning if one intends to perform the adjustment that afternoon; if early morning surgery is not an option, plan adjustment for the next morning. Postoperatively, sedating drugs (ie, promethazine hydrochloride [Phenergan] or narcotics) should be avoided. Elevating the patient's head and using ice packs decrease patient discomfort and tissue edema, contributing to an easier adjustment.[103,104]

There are two basic adjustable suture techniques: the bow-tie and the sliding knot. Both require that the suture be securely attached to the muscle with generous lock bites. At least 25% of the muscle should be incorporated[104] to secure tissue adequately at the time of adjustment. Scleral passes, which are made through the original insertion, should be substantial. To ease the pass of the suture through sclera during adjustment, the track can be enlarged with a "see-saw" movement of the suture.[104] This movement will also help determine whether the depth was adequate or too shallow.

With the bow-tie technique, the double-throw must be laid out flat. Having the needles exit about 2 mm apart facilitates this. The throw should be free of the Tenon capsule. Therefore, the insertion site should be cleaned carefully. Otherwise, the suture cannot be easily loosened, and the muscle position cannot be changed.

When using a sliding knot, the "slider" must demonstrate some friction with attempted movement. Otherwise, the immediate postoperative muscle position cannot be maintained. With restrictive disease, especially thyroid myopathy, the sliding knot may not hold. The excessive pull of the contracted muscle causes it to slip posteriorly before or during adjustment. In this case, the knot can be slid to the end of the suture and removed. The surgeon can then convert to the bow-tie technique.

It is often convenient to stabilize the globe during postoperative adjustment. A "bucket handle" can be placed in sclera 2 to 3 mm posterior to the limbus with either 6-0 Vicryl or 5-0 nylon. Suture is passed through sclera, and three or more square knots are tied over smooth forceps or muscle hook to create a loop for grasping.[104] For easy access, the loop should be placed inferior to the muscle for horizontal rectus adjustments, and temporal to the muscle for vertical rectus and superior oblique surgery. If the suture tears loose from the sclera, or was not placed during surgery, the insertion site can be grasped painlessly with toothed forceps. In contrast, attempts to grasp the conjunctiva without adequate topical anesthesia is painful and poorly tolerated. Often, tetracaine drops must be augmented with lidocaine 4% on a cotton swab.

Adequate knot exposure is crucial for the adjustment procedure. However, for patient comfort, it is equally important to bury the knot under conjunctiva once the manipulation is concluded. Exposed suture knots can cause significant foreign body reaction. A modification of the standard conjunctival closure may be useful. One end of the conjunctival flap can be tied to conjunctiva in the routine fashion, while leaving the other end tied with a loop that can be removed for the adjustment and easily retied afterward.[104] If the knot cannot be covered with conjunctiva at the end of the adjustment, it can be removed in the office at the 1-week postoperative visit without destabilizing the muscle position.[105] Granulomas are more common with the sliding-knot technique[109]; however, they usually resolve spontaneously or following topical steroids.

Intraoperative muscle positioning can also facilitate adjustment. Overrecession of muscles is preferred because it is far easier to pull a muscle up than to slide it posteriorly. For adjustable resections, an extra 2 to 3 mm should be resected and the muscle recessed the same amount.[104] In this way, the muscle can be advanced to strengthen the surgical effect or recessed to weaken it.

Occasionally, patients have bradycardia from the oculocardiac reflex during adjustment. Fortunately, this is a rare occurrence and usually produces no serious or permanent sequela.[110] It is helpful to perform the adjustment in a chair that can recline, so that patients who become faint or have a syncopal episode can easily be reclined with the feet elevated. The episode usually resolves quickly. Patients usually are comforted by a cool, wet wash cloth on the back of the neck or the forehead. The adjustment procedure can then be resumed with minimal delay.

Other, more common complications during adjustment include suture breakage, unraveling, or eroding the scleral tunnel; minor bleeding; or an uncooperative patient. With the exception of the latter, these problems can be managed by having appropriate instruments and suture on hand. In addition to a lid speculum, needle holders, toothed forceps and scissors, the adjustment tray should include smooth forceps for direct manipulation of the muscle, and cotton-tipped applicators. A caliper is handy for assessing location of the muscle as well as untangling or loosening knotted suture. The room should be stocked with additional suture for the unexpected, and a battery-powered cautery for hemostasis. Almost any complication can be managed with topical anesthesia; however, a lost muscle will necessitate a return to the operating room.

The frightened or squeamish patient requires reassurance and a gentle touch. An assistant providing lid traction can be substituted for a lid speculum. Exposure is usually adequate. Intravenous access should be maintained by heparin lock for mild sedation if the patient is unwilling to cooperate.

Postoperative alignment is the final important consideration. Most surgeons suggest that esotropic and hypertrophic patients should be left orthophoric at the time of adjustment.[103,104,111] A small amount of overcorrection for hypertropia is acceptable with superior rectus recessions, because the superior rectus demonstrates some recovery of function after surgery.[105,111] However, the weakened inferior rectus usually does not recover and may show additional loss of function, resulting in overcorrection.[105,111]

Postoperative Misalignment and Diplopia

Overcorrection and Undercorrection

It is beyond the scope of this chapter to cover the broad range of unexpected outcomes of alignment following strabismus surgery. So, discussion is limited to the most common conditions: congenital esotropia, intermittent exotropia, and diplopia.

The general principles of avoiding overcorrections and undercorrections, or unwanted ocular misalignments after surgery are to obtain multiple preoperative measurements and to avoid operating on patients with a variable alignment, inadequately treated amblyopia, and refractive errors. Forced ductions in surgery help identify patients with restrictive disease. In adults, adjustable suture technique has eliminated problems with overcorrection and undercorrection in most cases. One should try to uncover an accommodative component of esodeviations and provide an adequate trial of antiaccommodative therapy. Despite our best efforts, however, there is still unpredictability in strabismus surgery results. This should be communicated clearly to parents and patients preoperatively so that expectations of surgical outcome are realistic. Do not suggest that only one procedure is needed, and warn adult patients about the possibility of postoperative diplopia.

CONGENITAL ESOTROPIA. Secondary exotropia following surgery for congenital esotropia is disappointing to the parents and often an embarrassment to the surgeon. It is seen in more than 20% of congenital esotropes. There seem to be two different presentations. In the first, exotropia appears soon after the initial surgery, within weeks to months. A slipped or overweakened medial rectus muscle may be responsible. On examination, adduction is limited, with an incomitant horizontal deviation. Limited adduction in the early postoperative period is a poor prognostic sign for the development of secondary exotropia.[112,113] For most secondary exotropes, a slipped muscle is not usually the cause.[113,114]

The second group of secondary exotropes has a later onset. The appearance of new exotropia up to 8 years after the initial operation underscores the instability of ocular alignment in congenital esotropes.[112,114] The cause has not been elucidated; however, the absence of binocular function may play a role.[113] The incidence decreases between the ages of 8 to 10 years, which may be a function of the decreased convergence associated with that age group.[114]

Generally speaking, patients at risk are those with large medial rectus recessions, underestimated accommodative components to their deviation,[113] A and V patterns, poor binocular function, and a history of multiple operations. Amblyopia or poor visual acuity in an eye increases the risk of overcorrection.[112,114] However, small differences between eyes are probably not significant.[113] The cause in most cases is indeterminant. The age at surgery appears unrelated.[114] The longer congenital esotropes are followed postoperatively, the greater the incidence of exotropia.

An initial small to moderate overcorrection in the immediate postoperative period has been advocated, after which the eyes drift toward orthophoria.[115] Overcorrections greater than 15 prism diopters that persist beyond 6 to 8 weeks following surgery generally need additional management. Accommodative therapy with −2.00-D spectacles is one option. Also, occlusion for significant amblyopia should be instituted. If nonsurgical attempts at correcting the deviation fail, surgical correction is appropriate for consistent deviations. Cooper's dictum should be followed,[116] or the deviation should be managed as if it were occurring in a new patient (ie, perform bilateral rectus recessions as if initially treating an exotropia). However, if limitations of adduction are present, a slipped muscle should be suspected and the medial rectus advanced. Advancement of one medial rectus muscle to the original insertion can correct a mean of 23 PD of exotropia at distance, and 30 PD at near. Bilateral medial rectus advancement offers no advantage for distance deviation; however, it can decrease near deviation by 40 PD. Additionally, advancement of the medial rectus normalizes adduction deficiency in most patients.[117]

Congenital esotropia is corrected with the initial operation in only 80% of patients at best. Undercorrections are common and usually present by 2 months after surgery. Undercorrections less than 15 PD may respond to simple observation[114] or correction of hypermetropia greater than +1.50 D. An accommodative component develops in 50% of patients 3 months to 5 years after surgical realignment[118] and cannot be predicted preoperatively. Greater than +3.00 D of hyperopia should be corrected if a 15-PD reduction in the esotropia is seen with antiaccommodative treatment. In lieu of spectacles, phospholine iodide 0.125% can be used diagnostically to uncover an accommodative component to the esotropia. After 2 to 3 weeks of daily drop administration, ocular alignment is reassessed. If deviation greater than 15 PD persists, a second operation is required. Either bilateral rectus muscle resection or unilateral recession and resection may be performed, depending on which operation was performed initially. Re-recession of the medial rectus muscles often results in unacceptably high rates of consecutive exotropia and is discouraged.[119]

INTERMITTENT EXOTROPIA. Initial overcorrection after surgical correction of intermittent exotropia has been advocated[120] to counteract the outward drift of the eyes postoperatively. Persistence of an esodeviation causes intractable diplopia. Children risk the loss of stereopsis and development of amblyopia. Fortunately, in actual practice, this is rare.[120] After initial overcorrection, there is usually a drift toward orthophoria during the first 6 to 8 weeks after surgery. However, there is a greater tendency for the esodeviation to persist in adults. Medical management for reducing diplopia includes fresnel prisms and occlusion. As with overcorrections after esotropia surgery, if there are no limitations of ocular rotations, the patient should be treated as a "new patient." Bimedial rectus recessions or unilateral recession/resection procedures are appropriate.

For persistent exodeviations following surgery, medical management includes overminusing with −2.00-D spectacles or part-time occlusion 4 to 6 hours per day for 4 to 6 weeks. The dominant eye is usually patched. If there is no preferred eye, patching may be alternated between eyes. Surgical interventions for significant deviations are usually bimedial rectus resections or unilateral procedures on the "untouched" eye.

Diplopia

Diplopia in the immediately postoperative period is neither an unexpected nor an infrequent complication of strabismus surgery. The patient should expect that transient diplopia is a normal consequence of strabismus surgery. Persistent diplopia is a problem. Patients with incomitant deviations from restrictions or paralysis need a full preoperative explanation that there may be some residual postoperative diplopia in some gazes.

The most dreaded sensory disturbance is central disruption of fusion producing intractable diplopia. Although rare, it is more common in adults with longstanding deviations. Susceptible patients can sometimes be identified preoperatively. When a neutralizing prism fails to resolve preoperative double vision (or induces it) in either free space or with red filter testing, postoperative sensory problems may be more frequent. Another approach is to apply fresnel prism over the patient's spectacle correction. These are worn for a 1- to 2-week trial period and may provide information about the patient's ability to fuse the image after correction of the eye misalignment.

Adjustable stitch surgery can prevent many of the unexpected overcorrections and undercorrections responsible for diplopia. Fortunately, most postoperative diplopia regresses spontaneously. Double vision can be treated temporarily with patching, frosting of the glasses, or fresnel prism. The patient's own ability to suppress the second image is a frequent and helpful adaptation.

Treatment postoperatively can involve fresnel or permanent prism. In patients for whom images remain diplopic, eliminating one image through patching, opaque contact lens, or frosting of the glasses, or eliminating correction of refractive error over one eye are helpful solutions. Most patients learn to suppress the second image over time.

Role of Botulinum Toxin

Botulinum toxin can be used to augment the surgical effect or to eliminate secondary deviations.[121] It is particularly useful for resolving diplopia in adults with small undercorrected or overcorrected horizontal deviations. An initial dose of 2.5 units can be administered under local anesthesia as an office procedure.

Botulinum is unlikely to correct a deviation because of an underacting extraocular muscle. Therefore, if limited ocular rotation or lateral gaze incomitance is present, surgical intervention is indicated. At the time of this publication, it has not yet received Food and Drug Administration approval for unrestricted use in children younger than 16 years of age.

References

1. Weldon BC, Watcha MF, White PF. Oral midazolam in children: effect of time and adjunctive therapy. Anesth Analg 1992;75:51.
2. Wilton NC, Leigh J, Rosen DR, Pandit UA. Preanesthetic sedation of preschool children using intranasal midazolam. Anesthesiology 1988;69:972.
3. Soliman IE, Broadman LM, Hannallah RS, McGill WA. Comparison of the analgesic effects of EMLA (eutectic mixture of local anesthetics) to intradermal lidocaine infiltration before venous cannulation in unpremedicated children. Anesthesiology 1988; 68:804.
4. Greenberg DR, Ellenhorn NL, Chapman LI, et al. Posterior chamber hemorrhage during strabismus surgery. Am J Ophthalmol 1988;106:634.
5. Keszei VA, Helveston EM. Hyphema as a complication of strabismus surgery in an aphakic eye. Arch Ophthalmol 1986;104:637.
6. Lyons CJ, Fells P, Lee JP, McIntyre A. Chorioretinal scarring following the Faden operation: a retrospective study of 100 procedures. Eye 1989;3:401.
7. Morris RJ, Rose PH, Fells P. Incidence of inadvertent globe perforation during strabismus surgery. Br J Ophthalmol 1990;74:490.
8. Cibis GW. Incidence of inadvertent perforation in strabismus surgery. Ophthalmic Surg 1992;23:360.
9. Simon JW, Lininger LL, Scheraga JL. Recognized scleral perforation during eye muscle surgery: incidence and sequelae. J Pediatr Ophthalmol Strabismus 1992;29:273.
10. McLean JM, Galin MA, Baras I. Retinal perforation during strabismus surgery. Am J Ophthalmol 1960;50:1167.
11. Basmadjian G, Labelle P, Dumas J. Retinal detachment after strabismus surgery. Am J Ophthalmol 1975;79:305.
12. Mittelman D, Bakos I. The role of retinal cryopexy in the management of experimental perforation of the eye during strabismus surgery. J Pediatr Ophthalmol Strabismus 1984;21:186.
13. Helveston EM. Complications in strabismus surgery, ed 4. St. Louis, CV Mosby, 1993.
14. Del Monte MA, Archer SM. Complications of strabismus surgery. Atlas of pediatric ophthalmology and strabismus surgery. New York, Churchill Livingstone, 1993.
15. Dunlap WD. Complications in strabismus surgery. Int Ophthalmol Clin 1966;6:609.
16. Plager DA, Parks MM. Recognition and repair of the lost rectus muscle. Ophthalmology 1990;97:131.
17. MacEwen CJ, Lee JP, Fells P. Aetiology and management of the detached rectus muscle. Br J Ophthalmol 1992;76:131.
18. Friendly DS, Parelhoff ES, McKeown CA. Effect of severing the check ligaments and intermuscular membranes on medial rectus recessions in infantile esotropia. Ophthalmology 1993;100:945.
19. Apt L, Isenberg SJ. The oculocardiac reflex as a surgical aid in identifying a slipped or lost extraocular muscle. Br J Ophthalmol 1980;64:1980.
20. McNeer KW. Three complications of strabismus surgery. Ann Ophthalmol 1975;7:441.
21. Plager DA, Parks MM. Recognition and repair of the slipped rectus muscle. J Pediatr Ophthalmol Strabismus 1988;25:270.
22. Kaplan RF. Hypothermia/hyperthermia. In: Gravenstein N, ed. Manual of complications during anesthesia. Philadelphia, JB Lippincott, 1991:121.
23. Brownell AKW. Malignant hyperthermia: relationship to other diseases. Br J Anaesth 1988;60:303.
24. Helveston EM. Complications of strabismus surgery: pediatric ophthalmology and strabismus. Trans New Orleans Acad Ophthalmol 1986;34:61.
25. Kaplan RF. Malignant hyperthermia. In: Annual Refresher Course Lectures. American Society of Anesthesiologists, San Francisco, 1991.
26. Relton JES. Muscle biopsy for malignant hyperthermia. In: Stehling LC, ed. Common problems in pediatric anesthesia. Chicago, Year Book Medical, 1982.
27. Cody JR. Muscle rigidity following administration of succinylcholine. Anesthesiology 1986;29:159.
28. Blanc VF, Hardy JF, Milot J, Jacob JL. The oculocardiac reflex: a graphic and statistical analysis in infants and children. Can Anaesth Soc J 1983;30:360.
29. Gold RS, Pollard Z, Buchwald IP. Asystole due to the oculocardiac reflex during strabismus surgery: a report of two cases. Ann Ophthalmol 1988;20:473.
30. Hunsley JE, Bush GH, Jones CJ. A study of glycopyrrolate and atropine in the suppression of the oculocardiac reflex during strabismus surgery in children. Br J Anaesth 1982;54:459.
31. Meyers EF, Tomeldan SA. Glycopyrrolate compared with atropine in prevention of the oculocardiac reflex during eye-muscle surgery. Anesthesiology 1979;51:350.
32. Kaufmann H. Complications in eye muscle surgery. Dev Ophthalmol 1987;13:113.
33. Lerman J. Surgical and patient factors involved in postoperative nausea and vomiting. Br J Anaesth 1992;69:24S.
34. Cheng KP, Larson CE, Biglan AW, D'Antonio JA. A prospective, randomized, controlled comparison of retrobulbar and general anesthesia for strabismus surgery. Ophthalmic Surg 1992;23:585.
35. Schreiner MS, Nicolson SC, Martin T, Whitney L. Should children drink before discharge from day surgery? Anesthesiology 1992;76:528.
36. Lewis IH, Pryn SJ, Reynolds PI, et al. Effect of P6

acupressure on postoperative vomiting in children undergoing outpatient strabismus correction. Br J Anaesth 1991;67:73.
37. Eustis S, Lerman J, Smith DR. Effect of droperidol pretreatment on post-anesthetic vomiting in children undergoing strabismus surgery: the minimum effective dose. J Pediatr Ophthalmol Strabismus 1987; 24:165.
38. Abramowitz MD, Elder PT, Friendly DS, et al. Antiemetic effectiveness of intraoperatively administered droperidol in pediatric strabismus outpatient surgery: a preliminary report of a controlled study. J Pediatr Ophthalmol Strabismus 1981;18:22.
39. Hardy JF, Charest J, Girouard G, Lepage Y. Nausea and vomiting after strabismus surgery in preschool children. Can Anaesth Soc J 1986;33:57.
40. Nicolson SC, Kaya KM, Betts EK. The effect of preoperative oral droperidol on the incidence of postoperative emesis after paediatric strabismus surgery. Can J Anaesth 1988;35:364.
41. Lin DM, Furst SR, Rodarte A. A double-blinded comparison of metoclopramide and droperidol for prevention of emesis following strabismus surgery. Anesthesiology 1991;76:357.
42. Broadman LM, Ceruzzi W, Patane PS, et al. Metoclopramide reduces the incidence of vomiting following strabismus surgery in children. Anesthesiology 1990;72:245.
43. Horimoto Y, Tomie H, Hanzawa K, Nishida Y. Scopolamine patch reduces postoperative emesis in paediatric patients following strabismus surgery. Can J Anaesth 1991;38:441.
44. Horimoto Y, Naide M. Transdermal scopolamine patches reduce postoperative emesis in pediatric patients undergoing strabismus surgery. Can J Anaesth 1990;37:S94.
45. Watcha MF, Simeon RN, White PF, Stevens JL. Effect of propofol on the incidence of postoperative vomiting after strabismus surgery in pediatric outpatients. Anesthesiology 1991;75:204.
46. Weir PM, Munro HM, Reynolds RI, et al. Propofol infusion and the incidence of emesis in pediatric outpatient strabismus surgery. Anesth Analg 1993;76:760.
47. Watson DM. Topical amethocaine in strabismus surgery. Anaesthesia 1991;46:368.
48. Von Noorden GK. Orbital cellulitis following extraocular muscle surgery. Am J Ophthalmol 1972;74:627.
49. Ing MR. Infection following strabismus surgery. Ophthalmic Surg 1991;22:41.
50. Wilson ME, Paul TO. Orbital cellulitis following strabismus surgery. Ophthalmic Surg 1987;18:92.
51. Weakley DR. Orbital cellulitis complicating strabismus surgery: a case report and review of the literature. Ann Ophthalmol 1991;23:454.
52. Apt L, Isenberg SJ, Yoshimori R, Spierer A. Outpatient topical use of povidone-iodine in preparing the eye for surgery. Ophthalmology 1989;96:289.
53. Wortham E, Anandakrisshnan I, Kraft SP, Smith D, Morin JD. Are antibiotic-steroid drops necessary following strabismus surgery: a prospective, randomized, masked trial. J Pediatr Ophthalmol Strabismus 1990;27:205.
54. Choy AE, Weiss S, Chow C, Kato D, Cacace L. Dexamethasone sodium phosphate (Decadron) versus saline placebo injections in strabismus surgery. J Pediatr Ophthalmol Strabismus 1982;19:140.
55. Salamon SM, Friberg TR, Luxenberg MN. Endophthalmitis after strabismus surgery. Am J Ophthalmol 1982;93:39.
56. Uniat LM, Olk RJ, Kenneally CZ, Windsor CE. Endophthalmitis after strabismus surgery with a good visual result. Ophthalmic Surg 1991;19:42.
57. France TD, Simon JW. Anterior segment ischemia syndrome following muscle surgery: the AAPO&S experience. J Pediatr Ophthalmol Strabismus 1986; 23:87.
58. Hayreh SS, Scott WE. Fluorescein iris angiography. Arch Ophthalmol 1978;96:1390.
59. Virdi PS, Hayreh SS. Anterior segment ischemia after recession of various recti. Ophthalmology 1987; 94:1258.
60. Saunders RA, Phillips MS. Anterior segment ischemia after three rectus muscle surgery. Ophthalmology 1988;95:533.
61. Simon JW, Price EC, Krohel GB, et al. Anterior segment ischemia following strabismus surgery. J Pediatr Ophthalmol Strabismus 1984;21:179.
62. Elsas FJ, Witherspoon CD. Anterior segment ischemia after strabismus surgery. Am J Ophthalmol 1987;103:833.
63. Rosenbaum Al, Kushner BJ, Kirschen D. Vertical rectus muscle transposition and botulinum toxin (Oculinum) to medial rectus for abducens palsy. Arch Ophthalmol 1989;107:820.
64. Krupin T, Johnson MF, Becker B. Anterior segment ischemia after cyclocryotherapy. Am J Ophthalmol 1977;84:426.
65. Olver JM, Lee JP. Recovery of anterior segment circulation after strabismus surgery in adult patients. Ophthalmology 1992;99:305.
66. Von Noorden GK. Anterior segment ischemia following the Jensen procedure. Arch Ophthalmol 1976; 94:845.
67. Fishman PH, Repka MX, Green WR, et al. A primate model of anterior segment ischemia after strabismus surgery: the role of the conjunctival circulation. Ophthalmology 1990;97:456.
68. McKeown CA, Lambert HM, Shore JW. Preservation of the anterior ciliary vessels during extraocular muscle surgery. Ophthalmology 1989;96:498.

69. Lavin CW, McKeown CA, Chaturvedi N, et al. Preservation of the anterior ciliary vessels during strabismus surgery in a primate model of anterior segment. Invest Ophthalmol Vis Sci 1993;34:709.
70. de Smet MD, Carruthers J, Lepawsky M. Anterior segment ischemia treated with hyperbaric oxygen. Can J Ophthalmol 1987;22:381.
71. Tessler HH, Urist MJ. Corneal dellen in the limbal approach to rectus muscle surgery. Br J Ophthalmol 1975;59:377.
72. Pedersen LR. Corneal changes following operation for strabismus surgery (rectus surgery) with special reference to occurrence of dellen. Acta Ophthalmol 1972;50:771.
73. Elkington A. Granulomas following squint surgery. Trans Ophthalmol Soc U K 1971;91:543.
74. de Sa L, Hoyt CS, Good WV. Complications of pediatric ophthalmic surgery. Int Ophthalmol Clin 1992; 32:31.
75. Wagner RS, Nelson LB. Complications following strabismus surgery. Int Ophthalmol Clin 1985;25: 171.
76. Kushner BJ. Subconjunctival cysts as a complication of strabismus surgery. Arch Ophthalmol 1992; 110:1243.
77. Cibis GW, Waeltermann JM. Muscle inclusion cyst as a complication of strabismus surgery. Am J Ophthalmol 1985;99:740.
78. Illif CE, Illif WJ, Illif NT. Tumors of the ocular adnexa. In: Oculoplastic surgery. Philadelphia, WB Saunders, 1979:272.
79. Parks MS. The weakening surgical procedures for eliminating overaction of the inferior oblique muscle. Am J Ophthalmol 1972;73:107.
80. O'Donoghue E, Lightman S, Tuft S, Watson P. Surgically induced necrotizing sclerokeratitis (SINS): precipitating factors and response to treatment. Br J Ophthalmol 1992;76:17.
81. Kaufman LM, Folk ER, Miller MT, Tessler HH. Necrotizing scleritis following strabismus surgery for thyroid ophthalmopathy. J Pediatr Ophthalmol Strabismus 1989;26:236.
82. Pacheco EM, Guyton DL, Repka MX. Changes in eyelid position accompanying vertical rectus muscle surgery and prevention of lower lid retraction with adjustable surgery. J Pediatr Ophthalmol Strabismus 1992;29:265.
83. Kushner BJ. A surgical procedure to minimize lower-eyelid retraction with inferior rectus recession. Arch Ophthalmol 1992;110:1011.
84. Thompson WE, Reinecke RD. The changes in refractive status following routine strabismus surgery. J Pediatr Ophthalmol Strabismus 1980;17:372.
85. Fix A, Baker JD. Refractive changes following strabismus surgery. Am Orthoptic J 1985;35:59.
86. Preslan MW, Cioffi G, Min Y. Refractive error changes following strabismus surgery. J Pediatr Ophthalmol Strabismus 1992;29:300.
87. Switko S, Feldon S, McDonnell PJ. Corneal topographic changes following strabismus surgery in Graves' disease. Cornea 1992;11:36.
88. Reynolds RD, Nelson LB, Greenwald M. Large refractive changes after strabismus surgery. Am J Ophthalmol 1991;111:371.
89. Helveston EM, Alcorn DM, Ellis FD. Inferior oblique inclusion after lateral rectus surgery. Graefe's Arch Clin Exp Ophthalmol 1988;226:102.
90. Price RL. Role of Tenon capsule in postoperative restrictions. Int Ophthalmol Clin 1976;16:197.
91. Sondhi N, Ellis FD, Hamed LM, Helveston EM. Evaluation of an absorbable muscle sleeve to limit postoperative adhesions in strabismus surgery. Ophthalmic Surg 1987;18:441.
92. Dunlap EA. Surgery of muscle adhesions and effects of multiple operations. Br J Ophthalmol 1974;58:307.
93. Wright KW. The fat adherence syndrome and strabismus after surgery. Ophthalmology 1986;93:411.
94. Yaacobi Y, Hamed LM, Kaul KS, Fanous MM. Reduction of postoperative adhesions secondary to strabismus surgery in rabbits. Ophthalmic Surg 1992; 23:123.
95. Parks MM. The overacting inferior oblique muscle. Am J Ophthalmol 1974;77:787.
96. Elsas FJ, Gowda DC, Urry DW. Synthetic polypeptide sleeve for strabismus surgery. J Pediatr Ophthalmol Strabismus 1992;29:284.
97. Searl SS, Metz HS, Lindahl KJ. The use of sodium hyaluronate as a biologic sleeve in strabismus surgery. Ann Ophthalmol 1987;19:259.
98. Kramar P. Management of eye changes of Graves' disease. Surv Ophthalmol 1974;18:369.
99. Metz HS. Complications following surgery for thyroid ophthalmopathy. J Pediatr Ophthalmol Strabismus 1984;21:220.
100. Kushner B. Torsional diplopia after transantral orbital decompression and extraocular muscle surgery associated with Graves' orbitopathy. (Letter) Am J Ophthalmol 1992;114:239.
101. Lueder GT, Scott WE, Kutschke P, Keech RV. Long-term results of adjustable suture surgery for strabismus surgery secondary to thyroid ophthalmopathy. Ophthalmology 1992;99:993.
102. Hudson HL, Feldon SE. Late overcorrection of hypotropia in Graves' ophthalmopathy: predictive factors. Ophthalmology 1992;99:356.
103. Keech RV, Scott WE, Christensen LE. Adjustable suture strabismus surgery. J Pediatr Ophthalmol Strabismus 1987;24:97.
104. Kraft SP, Jacobson ME. Techniques of adjustable suture strabismus surgery. Ophthalmic Surg 1990;21:633.
105. Wright KW. Practical aspects of the adjustable suture

technique for strabismus surgery. Int Ophthalmol Clin 1989;29:10.

106. Sebel PS, Lowdon JD. Propofol: a new intravenous anesthetic. Anesthesiology 1989;71:260.
107. Korttila K, Ostman E, Faure E, et al. Randomized comparison of recovery after propofol-nitrous oxide versus Thiopentone-isoflurane-nitrous oxide anaesthesia in patients undergoing ambulatory surgery. Acta Anaesthesiol Scand 1990;34:400.
108. Brown DR, Pacheco EM, Repka MX. Recovery of extraocular muscle function after adjustable suture strabismus surgery under local anesthesia. J Pediatr Ophthalmol Strabismus 1992;29:16.
109. Eustis HP, Hesse RJ. Conjunctival reaction using adjustable sutures: a comparison of the cinch and bow knot methods. J Pediatr Ophthalmol Strabismus 1993;30:149.
110. Vrabec MP, Preslan MW, Kushner BJ. Oculocardiac reflex during manipulation of adjustable sutures after strabismus surgery. Am J Ophthalmol 1987; 104:61.
111. Weston B, Enzemauer R, Kraft SP, Gayowsky GR. Stability of the postoperative alignment in adjustable suture strabismus surgery. J Pediatr Ophthalmol Strabismus 1991;28:206.
112. Folk ER, Miller MT, Chapman L. Consecutive exotropia following surgery. Br J Ophthalmol 1983;67:546.
113. Bradbury JA, Doran RML. Secondary exotropia: a retrospective analysis of matched cases. J Pediatr Ophthalmol Strabismus 1993;30:163.
114. Yazawa K. Postoperative exotropia. J Pediatr Ophthalmol Strabismus 1981;18:58.
115. Scott EW. Temporary surgical overcorrection of infantile esotropia. Trans New Orleans Acad Ophthalmol 1976;81:399.
116. Cooper EL. The surgical management of secondary exotropia. Trans Am Acad Ophthalmol Otolaryngol 1961;65:595.
117. Ohtsuki H, Hasebe S, Tadokoro Y, et al. Advancement of medial rectus muscle to the original insertion for consecutive esotropia. J Pediatr Ophthalmol Strabismus 1993;30:301.
118. Baker JD, DeYoung-Smith M. Accommodative esotropia following surgical correction of congenital esotropia: frequency and characteristics. Graefes Arch Clin Exp Ophthalmol 1988;226:175.
119. King RA, Calhoun JH, Nelson LB. Reoperations for esotropia. J Pediatr Ophthalmol Strabismus 1987; 24:136.
120. Keech RV, Stewart SA. The surgical overcorrection of intermittent exotropia. J Pediatr Ophthalmol Strabismus 1990;27:218.
121. McNeer KW. An investigation of the clinical use of botulinum toxin A as a postoperative adjustment procedure in the therapy of strabismus. J Pediatr Ophthalmol Strabismus 1990;27:3.

Ophthalmic Surgery Complications: Prevention and Management,
edited by Judie F. Charlton and George W. Weinstein.
J. B. Lippincott Company, Philadelphia © 1995.

13

Dale R. Meyer

Complications of Oculoplastic and Orbital Surgery

Oculoplastic and orbital surgery is generally highly successful. However, as with other ophthalmic subspecialties, complications can occur, and those related to these procedures have their own special causes and treatment. Surgery involving the eyelids, lacrimal system, and orbit is decidedly different from most forms of intraocular surgery. The variety of oculoplastic and orbital surgical procedures is also diverse. In fact, there are more than 100 procedures specified in the current procedural terminology that fall into these categories. These "certified procedures" do not begin to describe the many subtle variations in technique employed and described by creative surgeons. As an example, for a relatively common problem such as entropion, the surgeon may choose from numerous variations of procedures for entropion repair. Conversely, certain ophthalmic diseases, such as orbital tumors, are of such rarity that the average ophthalmologist may not attain "technical proficiency" for the surgical management of such lesions, without additional fellowship training.

Faced with this great diversity and range of surgical difficulty, this chapter on prevention and treatment of complications of oculoplastic and orbital surgery must, by necessity, be selective. This chapter is organized into sections on eyelid, lacrimal, and orbital surgery. At the start of each section a general discussion of complications common to procedures in that section is given, followed by a more detailed discussion of selected procedures. The procedures selected for discussion are those either commonly performed or those important for the perspective of the section. This chapter is intended primarily for the general ophthalmologist and residents-in-training, and not all ophthalmic surgeons necessarily perform all of these procedures. The procedures chosen reflect to some degree the author's bias. The references are correspondingly selective but representative of available publications. Several excellent textbooks (some encompassing two volumes and more than 1000 pages) dealing exclusively with oculoplastic and orbital surgery have been published, and readers can refer to such resources if they are interested in more details on specific surgical techniques. This chapter, therefore, is intended to supplement such reading and fill the void, which nevertheless exists pertaining to detailed prevention and management of related complications.

Good training, thorough knowledge of eyelid, lacrimal, and orbital anatomy, proper patient selection, evaluation, and proper surgical technique keep complications to a minimum. It is incumbent on the surgeon performing any procedure to have a thorough knowledge of associated complications and know how to manage them accordingly. It is also important that patients have a realistic idea of the complications and their relative frequency so that they can make a well-informed decision as to the merits (benefits) of surgery versus the risks.

COMPLICATIONS OF EYELID SURGERY

Eyelid surgery is among the most rewarding and commonly performed procedures involving the ocular adnexa. The eyelids are crucial to the health of the eye,

Table 13-1
Potential Complications of Eyelid Surgery

Blindness/orbital hemorrhage
Hematoma
Direct ocular injury (iatrogenic)
Anxiety
Eyelid edema
Conjunctival chemosis
Incision complications
Infection
Lid malpositions
Exposure keratopathy
Blepharoptosis
Diplopia/ocular motility disturbances

serving to distribute tears (lubricate) and otherwise protect the eye properly. Blepharoptosis, ectropion, entropion, eyelid malignancies, and eyelid trauma are conditions that may be associated with visual consequences. Dermatochalasis of the eyelids is a common condition that may be aesthetically displeasing to patients and in advanced cases may be associated with visual impairment. The prevention or treatment of complications associated with surgical repair of these conditions is the focus of this section. Table 13-1 lists complications common to many types of eyelid surgery. Additional complications related to specific procedures are detailed later in the text. In general, apart from other factors, the severity and frequency of complications are related to surgical complexity.

Blindness/Orbital Hemorrhage

Blindness from extensive orbital hemorrhage, although rare, is possible with eyelid procedures that involve opening of the orbital system or manipulation of orbital fat.[1–4] From a technical aspect, when the orbital septum is opened and the orbit is entered, the procedure can be considered an anterior orbitotomy. For blepharoplasty, the statistical risk of extensive orbital hemorrhage causing blindness has been estimated to be on the order of 0.04% (ie, 1/2500). With such a low incidence, most ophthalmic surgeons are fortunately unlikely to encounter a single case in their careers. The mechanism of blindness in such cases is thought to be compression of the orbital portion of the optic nerve, resulting in ischemic optic neuropathy or less likely central retinal artery occlusion. Other types of eyelid surgeries, such as ptosis repair (external levator resection) or ectropion/entropion repair, may include "blepharoplasty-type" approaches, incorporating a transverse eyelid incision and opening of the orbital septum. Orbital fat manipulation in the latter cases is usually less than that done for primary blepharoplasty, and although exact figures for risk of blindness after these procedures are less readily available, one would reasonably expect this risk, while present, to be lower. To minimize the risk of serious bleeding, the preoperative evaluation of all patients undergoing eyelid surgery should include inquiry as to any history of bleeding problems as well as use of aspirin or more potent anticoagulants such as dipyridamole or warfarin (Coumadin). Such agents should be stopped at least 1 week (2 weeks for aspirin) before surgery if the medical risk of discontinuing anticoagulation is acceptable. Patients are advised to check with their primary care physician beforehand. In most cases, a letter sent to the primary physician explaining the nature of surgery and its indications is helpful. It is prudent to include the risk of blindness, even though it is rare, as part of the informed consent for most eyelid procedures. Most patients are willing to accept this remote risk when weighing the benefits of the proposed surgery. Occasionally, however, a monocularly sighted patient may consider this small risk unacceptable enough to decline surgery, even though it may mean living with some degree of ophthalmic deficit.

Intraoperative Hemostasis

Intraoperatively, meticulous hemostasis is recommended for all forms of eyelid surgery. Local anesthetics containing 1/100,000 or 1/200,000 epinephrine may be used for local anesthesia or in general anesthesia cases for the hemostatic effect. Dissection should proceed deliberately, with care to control bleeding at more superficial levels before proceeding with deeper dissection. The dissection itself can be performed with the aid of thermal cautery or electrocautery devices to minimize bleeding. Care must be taken to protect the cornea and ocular surface from collateral thermal damage when these modalities are used extensively, however. Hemostatic agents such as thrombin and Gelfoam (The Upjohn Company, Kalamazoo, MI) may occasionally be useful for control of diffuse oozing. Local small vessel bleeding is stopped by direct isolation and cauterization or ligation. Manually applied pressure to control bleeding must be used cautiously so as not to unduly increase orbital pressure if orbit hemorrhage has occurred. If bleeding is only anterior, pressure applied for up to 5 minutes (while periodically monitoring the eye) is appropriate. In some cases in which bleeding or oozing seems excessive during the initial dissection, the better part of valor may be to obtain control of the superficial bleeding and close the incision. A hematologic work-up following such cases is appropriate, to rule out an unusual bleeding abnormality, before rescheduling the case.

Deeper eyelid dissection, extending posterior to the orbital septum should proceed cautiously. The orbital fat pads should be handled gently, avoiding excessive anterior traction. Koorneef[4] has shown that the "orbital fat" is actually composed of an intricate interconnected fibroadipose connective tissue system. Blood vessels course through and are supported by the fibroadipose connective tissue. Traction of the "orbital fat" can, therefore, rupture more posteriorly located blood vessels. Any "fat excision" is done best under direct visualization followed by cauterization. The technique of clamping ("cross-clamping") the fat with a small hemostat before excision may be of additional benefit; however, as previously emphasized, excessive anterior traction by the clamp should be avoided.

Postoperative Oribital Hemorrhage

Postoperatively, pressure patches after most eyelid surgeries are avoided (allowing the patient to detect a problem if it develops). Ice is used postoperatively to reduce ecchymosis and relieve pain. All patients are given instructions to call immediately if any sign of severe pain, external bleeding, proptosis, or decreased vision is noted. Generally in the setting of severe postoperative orbital hemorrhage these signs occur together. If orbital hemorrhage occurs, it is a true emergency requiring prompt medical and surgical care to minimize or prevent loss of vision. Initial management of orbital hemorrhage must be understood by all surgeons who perform eyelid surgery. The general management principle is relief of increased orbital and secondary ocular pressure (tension). Before instituting treatment, the severity of orbital hemorrhage and ocular compromise should be quickly assessed. Visual acuity, pupil examination, and possibly confrontation visual field and undilated fundus examinations provide an approximate measure of the visual impairment. Proptosis and eyelid ecchymosis are usually obvious with significant hemorrhage. Palpation reveals a "tense orbit." When a patient presents with obvious proptosis and profound visual loss based on the preceding initial assessment, acute intervention is warranted. If visual function is good, further evaluation may include measurement of intraocular pressure and dilated fundus evaluation. (*Note:* It is best to avoid dilation of both eyes if pupil examination needs to be repeated to detect an afferent pupillary defect.) This more complete examination should also be performed on all patients at the earliest reasonable time after emergency measures have been instituted. Computed tomographic (CT) scanning may also be helpful in some cases to delineate extent of hemorrhage.

In the setting of postoperative orbital hemorrhage, management is directed at opening the surgical wounds (including the septum) to relieve orbital pressure and evacuate blood. Lateral cantholysis (of both the superior and inferior crus) may also be helpful to further reduce orbital pressure. Medical treatment can be primarily useful for lowering secondary raised intraocular pressure, and includes topical hypotensive eye drops (β-blockers) and systemic agents, such as diuretics (acetazolamide) and osmotic agents (mannitol). In generally, these pharmacologic agents take time to work and are limited in their overall effectiveness. They are generally used alone only in mild cases of orbital hemorrhage when surgical management is not acutely needed. Use of high-dose intravenous corticosteroids may be considered; however, their efficiency remains to be determined in the setting of orbital hemorrhage. In the worst-case scenario, in which visual compromise and increased orbital pressure persist, orbital bony decompression is required. Orbital decompression involves removal or outfracture of one to three orbital walls. The various approaches to orbital decompression are well described in the literature dealing with surgical management of Graves orbitopathy, the details of which are beyond the scope of this discussion. Emergency consultation with a surgeon skilled in orbital surgery may be indicated in such cases.

Postoperative Hematomas

Hematomas (ie, a localized collection of blood) may occur after eyelid surgery, usually confined to the anterior portion of the eyelid presenting as a purplish mass, which usually is painless. Small hematomas can be managed by having the patient use warm compresses. Warm water in a sealable plastic bag wrapped with a warm cloth works well. Care should be taken to avoid excessively hot water, which can burn the skin. Large hematomas must usually be drained, as they may pose a risk for infection. Postoperative hematomas can usually be drained via the incision. Within 1 to 2 weeks after surgery, the edges of the incision can usually be separated bluntly with cotton-tipped applicators, after removing one or more sutures. The congealed blood that generally has a gelatinous quality can then be directly removed by applying gentle pressure around the hematoma directed toward the opened incision. Alternatively, direct aspiration of the hematoma can be attempted with a large-bore needle. However, unless the hematoma is fresh, it may be difficult to aspirate the thickened blood.

Direct Ocular Injury (Iatrogenic)

Iatrogenic direct penetrating or thermal injury to the eye during surgery is, it is hoped, an uncommon event. One must remember that the eyelids are quite thin and in some places (eg, near the upper eyelid crease) immediately adjacent to the globe. Many incisions are made at the eyelid crease where the anteroposterior thickness of the eyelid is only a millimeter or so. Local anesthetic injections of the eyelids can also pose a risk to the eye if not performed properly. Angling the needle transversely across the eyelid and thus tangential to the globe avoids the chance of ocular penetration when infiltrating anesthetic subcutaneously. Because the globe and overlying eyelid is curved and the needle is straight, two or three "stepped" injections across the lid may be safer than attempting to infiltrate the entire eyelid from one lateral injection site. It is also advisable to rest the ulnar side of the hand (holding the syringe) on the patient's cheek (zygoma) while injecting. This way, if the patient moves suddenly during injection, the needle and syringe move *with* the patient and *not* deeper *into* the patient.

Penetrating injury to the eye may potentially occur by the scalpel during incision. Avoiding undue downward pressure on the scalpel when cutting ("letting the scalpel do the work") and keeping the ulnar aspect of the hand close to the face when cutting prevents this possibility. Penetration of the eye may also occur during suturing of the eyelid. This is more likely when posterior eyelid structures (eg, levator, tarsus, and conjunctiva) are being sutured. In most cases, the eyelid can be pulled away from the eye and suturing performed at a more comfortable working distance. Thermal injury may occur by overzealous or misdirected use of thermal or electrocautery devices. Small local thermal burns of the cornea (or conjunctiva) generally heal without sequelae and can be treated with topical antibiotic or antibiotic-steroid ointment. Observance of these principles significantly reduces the risk of ocular penetration. As an additional precaution, a scleral shell may be placed on the eye if the surgeon desires. Should ocular penetration (ie, scleral or corneal perforation) occur, appropriate evaluation and management guidelines should be followed, although the chance of endophthalmitis developing after a simple needle stick under aseptic conditions would be expected to be exceedingly small.

Pain

Adequate intraoperative anesthesia is a prerequisite for surgery. The choice of anesthetic is based on the expected duration of the surgical procedure. Most eyelid procedures can be performed in less than 2 hours; therefore, 2% lidocaine with 1/200,000 or 1/100,000 epinephrine is usually adequate. Longer-acting anesthetics, such as bupivacaine (Marcaine), are also useful. Subcutaneous infiltration of the immediate operative site is usually sufficient for most cases. Regional nerve blocks can also be used. Before beginning the procedure, the extent of anesthesia is tested by pinching the skin with toothed forceps. Local anesthetic should be available (drawn up) to supplement the initial anesthesia during the case if necessary.

Postoperative discomfort is expected to some degree after eyelid surgery. Pain is a subjective phenomenon, and different patients have different pain thresholds. In general, however, most patients do not experience more then a moderate "ache," which usually responds to acetaminophen (Tylenol). Aspirin should be avoided. Ice is also helpful, to relieve discomfort, and is applied as tolerated for 12 to 24 hours after surgery. Interestingly, transverse (lid crease) incisions extending below the orbicularis muscle frequently cause prolonged anesthesia or numbness distal to the sensory nerves transected. Sensation usually returns in several months. Severe pain after eyelid surgery is uncommon, and any patient complaining of severe pain, particularly if accompanied by complaints of decreased vision, proptosis, or bleeding should be seen immediately to exclude orbital hemorrhage.

Anxiety

Anxiety is included in this discussion, not because it is a complication per se, but because the anxious patient may present a problem at the time of surgery. Most eyelid procedures on adults can be performed under local anesthesia without the need for sedation. Anxiety-prone patients can usually be identified during the initial consultation by their reactions to the physician's description of the procedure. Responses such as "I don't think I could do that" (be awake during surgery) or "I'm very sensitive to pain," or "I'm deathly afraid of needles" (anesthetic injection) should alert the physician to the possible need for adjunctive sedation before or during the operation. In extreme cases, general anesthesia may be indicated. Immediately before surgery, it is helpful to reassure patients that aside from the brief discomfort initially associated with the local anesthetic, they will be comfortable thereafter. Communication with patients during the surgery is also helpful for reassurance and continual monitoring of the patient's well-being. "Open-face" draping for oculoplastic procedures is also valuable, particularly for patients prone to "claustrophobia."

Infection

Postoperative eyelid infections are uncommon due, in part, to excellent vascularity of the eyelids. Preseptal or orbital cellulitis is rare but has been reported after eyelid surgery.[5,6] Immunocompromised patients may be at higher risk. Preventative measures include aseptic technique and proper instrument sterilization. Prophylactic systemic antibiotics are not generally used, although topical antibiotic ointment is applied postoperatively and continued for several days to a week. In the immediate postoperative period, the physician should be careful to make a distinction between tissue reaction to surgery (or sutures) and frank infection. Both conditions may show erythema, edema, warmth, and tenderness. The index of suspicion for preseptal cellulitis should be increased if purulent discharge is present accompanied possibly by fever. Orbital cellulitis should not be difficult to diagnose as proptosis; ocular motility limitation is usually apparent and, when severe, may be associated with optic neuropathy (positive afferent pupillary defect and decreased visual acuity).

Treatment regimens for preseptal and orbital cellulitis are well described. For mild preseptal cellulitis without ocular compromise, treatment with an oral antibiotic is appropriate if close follow-up can be arranged. Culture of purulent discharge should be performed. Empiric antibiotics should cover staphylococcus, streptococcus, and, in children, *Haemophilus influenzae.* Cephalexin for adults and ampicillin for children are good choices, although several other antibiotics are appropriate.

Patients with orbital cellulitis should be admitted to the hospital for intravenous antibiotic treatment and close ophthalmic evaluation. CT imaging to delineate the extent of infection is recommended. Drainage of frank orbital abscess is required.

Eyelid Edema/Conjunctival Chemosis

Eyelid edema can be expected to various degrees after surgery and is directly related to the degree of tissue disruption (Fig. 13-1). Conjunctival edema (chemosis) sometimes occurs after eyelid surgery, and is more likely if surgery involves direct conjunctival manipulation or surgery is in close proximity to the conjunctiva. Thermal cautery close to or directly involving the conjunctiva appears to be particularly "inciting." Prevention, therefore, entails keeping such

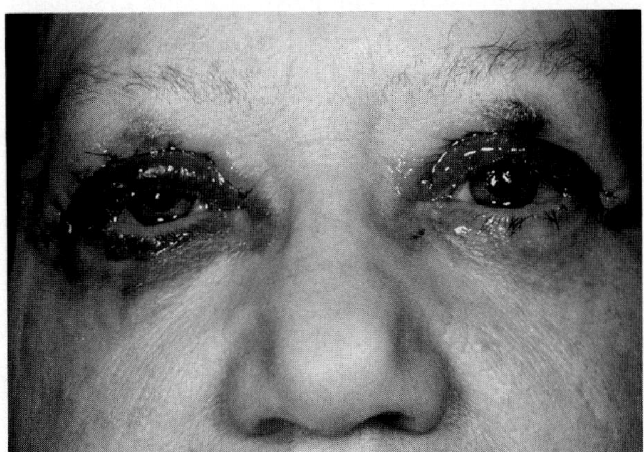

Figure 13-1. Patient with moderate eyelid edema and ecchymosis of both eyes 1 day after bilateral upper lid blepharoplasty. Note the slight mechanical ptosis created by the eyelid edema. These signs generally resolve within approximately 2 weeks.

conjunctival manipulation to a minimum. Patients with predisposing inflammatory conditions, such as Graves ophthalmopathy, may manifest more pronounced chemosis and eyelid edema after surgery. In most cases, eyelid edema and chemosis are self-limited. Cold compresses in the first 12 to 24 hours after surgery help reduce swelling. Some surgeons also advocate warm compresses after the second or third postoperative day. Edema largely subsides within 2 weeks. A trace amount of edema may occasionally persist for several weeks or even months after procedures that involve lateral eyelid dissection, which is likely a result of lymphatic disruption. Patients who have had local radiation therapy may have more of a protracted course.

Occasionally chemosis may be sufficient to cause conjunctiva prolapse. Management of conjunctival prolapse focuses on keeping the conjunctiva well lubricated to avoid drying by frequent (hourly if necessary) application of a bland ophthalmic lubricating ointment (eg, Lacri-Lube or Refresh PM). Moisture preserving measures, such as plastic-wrap dressings or patching at bedtime, may also be required. Topical corticosteroid ointment or drops may also be beneficial. The preceding conservative measures are generally effective. Rarely is surgical repositioning or conjunctival excision required.

Incision Complications (Abscesses, Granulomas, Cysts, and Scars)

Postoperative complications, such as suture abscesses, granulomas, epithelial inclusion cysts, and prominent scarring involving eyelid incisions, are usually minimal. However, because of their obvious location and the thin nature of eyelid skin, these complications may be disproportionately distressing to the patient. All suture material incites some degree of inflammatory response by the tissues. Monofilament synthetic sutures (ie, nylon) are the least reactive and braided natural sutures (ie, silk) are among the most reactive. Acute focal reaction to suture material may result in a small suture abscess. In some cases, a small granuloma may develop. Such reactions may be minimized by using less reactive suture material or removing sutures by 5 days postoperatively. Epithelial inclusion cysts can occur when epithelial cells are buried during closure or "implanted" by the needle. The former situation is avoidable by making sure the thin eyelid skin is not "rolled under" at the edges of the incision and slightly everting the wound edges. Absorbable sutures that "dissolve" within 1 week (ie, plain gut or fast-absorbing gut) work surprisingly well for eyelid incision closure, provided they are kept well lubricated with ointment to ensure timely disappearance.

Small suture abscesses or cysts can be treated by simply opening them with a sharp 25-gauge needle or a no. 11 blade. In most cases, no anesthesia is necessary. Granulomas usually "respond to time," although massage with a mild corticosteroid or vitamin E ointment may be helpful. Simple excision may be performed for granulomas not responding to more conservative measures.

Prominent, unsightly scarring of eyelid incisions is fortunately rare. Keloid formation does not occur on the eyelids (perhaps because of the thin dermis) even in patients who are prone to keloids elsewhere. Hypertrophic scarring can occur in some individuals and may be more likely if the wound is closed under tension or the wound edges are traumatized. Careful positioning of incisions along natural skin tension lines minimizes scar visibility and provides optional camouflage. One must be particularly careful with incisions involving the medial canthal area to avoid linear contraction of the scar ("bowstringing") or webbing in this multicontoured area. Initial treatment of hypertrophic scars are similar to that described for granulomas, namely, time and massage. Scar maturation occurs over several months. In most cases, at least 6 months should be allowed before scar revision is considered. In this interim, injection of the scar with corticosteroid (triamcinolone) may be helpful. If associated lid malposition (ectropion or retraction) is present, then the eye may require lubrication to prevent exposure keratopathy. Scar revisions may involve simple linear scar excision or Z-plasties to relieve webbing or excessive tension.

Lid Malpositions

Lid malpositions that can occur after eyelid surgery include ectropion, entropion, and eyelid retraction. The lower eyelids are typically more at risk for postoperative lid malposition than the upper eyelid. Blepharoptosis may also be considered a lid malposition, but will be considered separately. Lid malpositions are best understood by considering the multidirectional vector forces operating on the eyelid margin. It is also helpful to think of the eyelids as being composed of two lamellae; the anterior lamella is the skin and orbicularis muscle, and the posterior lamella is the tarsus and conjunctiva. (The orbital septum is frequently considered the intermediate lamella.) In the natural state the eyelids are well apposed to the globe. Horizontal laxity may cause instability of the eyelid margin, allowing involutional ectropion or less commonly entropion to develop. Loss of tissue, shortening, or contracture of the anterior lamellae may cause cicatricial ectropion, whereas similar involvement of the posterior lamella may produce entropion. In some cases, these forces may cause retraction of the eyelid, with "scleral show," but without rotation of the eyelid margin. Shortening or contracture of the orbital septum or the "eyelid retractors" may also lead to frank eyelid retraction. Significant retraction may be associated with lagophthalmos (ie, inability to fully close the eyelids), which may further cause drying of the cornea (exposure keratopathy). With entropion, the eyelashes may also directly abrade the cornea. Corneal ulcer may develop as a complication, which can occasionally result in frank ocular perforation or corneal scarring, with permanent loss of vision. With such dire consequences possible, it is incumbent on the surgeon performing eyelid surgery to understand these risks, take every measure to prevent such complications, and know how to handle such problems should they occur.

Prevention is the first line of defense. Preoperatively, any preexistent horizontal lower eyelid laxity should be noted. If the proposed lower eyelid surgery involves excision of anterior lamellar tissue (such as blepharoplasty), then consideration should be given to shortening the lower eyelid horizontally. Two tests are useful preoperatively for assessing horizontal lower eyelid laxity. The "eyelid distraction" test can be performed by simply pulling the eyelid away from the globe. A separation of 7 to 8 mm from the globe suggests horizontal laxity. The "snap-back" test can be performed by pulling the eyelid inferiorly, with the patient looking straight ahead. The eyelid should snap back against the globe with the next blink; failure to do so indicates lid laxity. Horizontal eyelid laxity is usually due to stretching (attenuation) of the canthal tendons. The lateral canthal tendon is more frequently affected. Several procedures have been described to treat horizontal lid laxity. One of the most useful is the "lateral tarsal-strip" procedure.[7] In this procedure, the lower lid is detached from the orbital rim (via lateral canthotomy and cantholysis), and the lateral tarsus is fully exposed to create a tarsal strip (Fig. 13-2). The eyelid is then advanced laterally and plicated to the inner aspect of the lateral orbital rim periosteum. Alternatively, a pentagonal ("block") resection of full-thickness eyelid can be performed near the lateral canthus to tighten the lid. Occasionally, medial canthal tendon laxity may be more prominent than lateral canthal tendon laxity. This can be determined preoperatively by manually advancing the eyelid laterally to simulate the effect of horizontal tightening. The punctum normally moves laterally only 1 mm or so with this maneuver. If the punctum can be moved significantly past the nasal corneal limbus, tightening of the medial canthal tendon may also be beneficial.

Intraoperatively, any maneuver that may potentially increase vertical tension on the upper or lower eyelid should be carefully assessed. This includes anterior lamellar (skin/muscle) excision (eg, blepharoplasty, ptosis repair, tumor excision, and others), which may cause ectropion or retraction, as well as posterior lamellar (tarsus and conjunctiva) excision (eg, lid reconstruction, conjunctival surgery, and so forth), which may cause entropion or retraction. The orbital septum should never be vertically shortened; suturing of the septum should be avoided, and care taken not to catch or include the septum in the closure of the incision.

In general, the lower eyelid is "less forgiving" than the upper eyelid. Even when these principles are observed, lower lid retraction may occasionally be seen following transverse skin incisions alone (ie, without

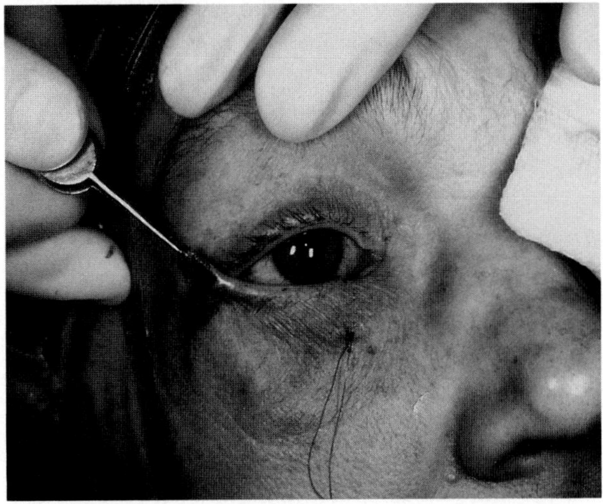

Figure 13-2. Creation of lateral tarsal strip, which is plicated to the lateral orbital rim to tighten the lower lid horizontally.

skin removal). This phenomenon is not completely understood, but contracture/scarring of the orbital septum has been implicated.[8] The treatment of eyelid malpositions and their sequelae is detailed in the section on blepharoplasty. However, the general principles apply to other surgeries in which eyelid malpositions may occur.

Blepharoptosis

Ptosis ("droop") of the upper eyelid may be a complication of a number of ocular and oculoplastic surgeries. Ptosis can occur despite any obvious violation of the eyelid itself and has been reported after both cataract surgery and keratorefractive procedures. The origin appears to be indirect or direct levator aponeurosis injury, causing dehiscence or disinsertion. Although indirect levator aponeurosis injury from eyelid manipulation or edema may cause ptosis, this discussion focuses primarily on direct injury to the levator aponeurosis associated with eyelid surgery.[9] Preoperatively, it is obviously important to note and document any preexistent ptosis, as sometimes after surgery, the patient or physician may attribute such a finding to the surgery itself. Preoperative photographs thereby become a valuable part of the record.

Any procedure involving deep dissection of the supratarsal eyelid (blepharoplasty, tumor excision, and others) must be performed with utmost regard for the levator aponeurosis. Unfortunately, the various connective tissue planes of the upper eyelid may not appear as well defined during surgical dissection as they appear in textbooks. The levator aponeurosis can be identified by proceeding in a stepwise subcutaneous or submuscular dissection to the more superior portion of the eyelid where the orbital septum can then be opened to reveal the preaponeurotic fat pads. The levator aponeurosis can then easily be identified by retracting the fat pads. Two points regarding this dissection deserve special mention. First, the area near the eyelid crease is the thinnest part of the eyelid. In most patients, the orbital septum and levator aponeurosis are "fused" together and not separately identifiable at the level of the eyelid crease. Posteriorly directed dissection at the level of the eyelid crease, therefore, carries a risk of levator aponeurosis or full-thickness eyelid injury. Dissection beneath the skin or orbicularis muscle approximately 5 mm superior to the lid crease before opening the septum increases the "margin of safety" and lessens the possibility of levator or full-thickness injury (Fig. 13-3). The second anatomic variable that surgeons need to be aware of is the layer of fibroadipose tissue beneath the orbicularis muscle.[10] Grossly, this tissue appears yellowish like fat but is not well-encapsulated like the preaponeurotic fat pads. This tissue has been called by various names including "suborbicularis fascia," "preseptal fat," and "retroorbicularis oculus fat"[11] among others. The more generic term, "submuscular fibroadipose layer," has been advocated, as this tissue is more complex than simple fat and continues

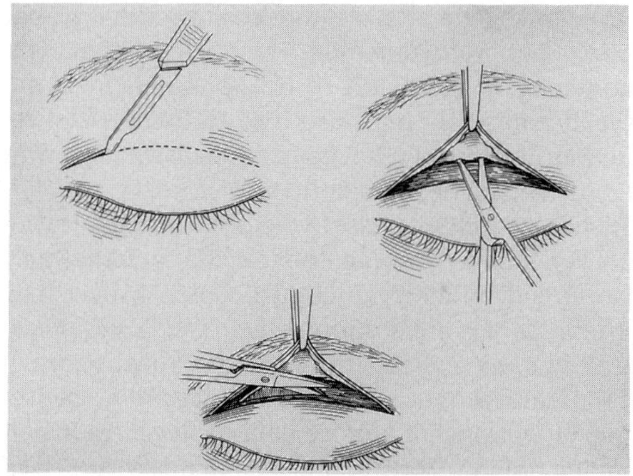

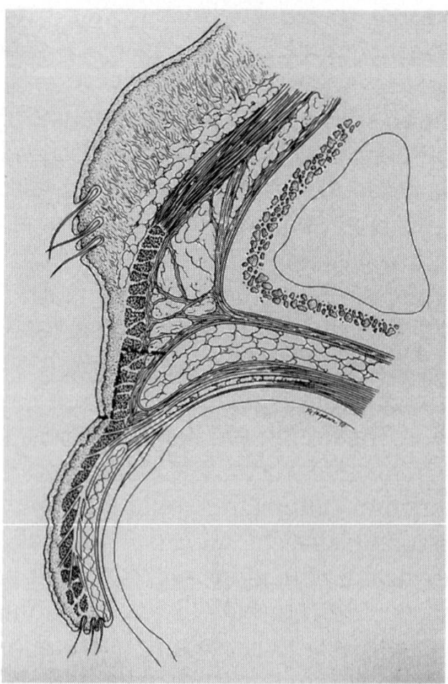

Figure 13-3. Dissection beneath the skin or orbicularis muscle approximately 5 mm superior to the eyelid crease before opening the orbital septum increases the "margin of safety" and lessens the possibility of iatrogenic injury to the levator aponeurosis. The dotted lines on the lower diagram indicate the planes of dissection.

from the eyelid into the eyebrow.[10] In some patients, this submuscular fibroadipose layer is prominent, and the surgeon may mistake it for preaponeurotic fat and consequently mistake the orbital septum for the levator aponeurosis. A good understanding of these anatomic principles should, it is hoped, avoid any intraoperative misadventure.

Postoperatively, if blepharoptosis is noted after eyelid surgery, one should first attempt to determine its cause. Postoperative ptosis may be mechanical (from edema or hemorrhage) or aponeurotic (from direct or indirect injury) in origin. Mechanical ptosis caused by postoperative edema is usually obvious (see Fig. 13-1). The degree of ptosis is usually related to the amount of eyelid swelling and can be profound with extensive edema. In the latter case, the patient may not be able to open the eye, and levator function may appear poor. Cold compresses applied to eyelids immediately after surgery for 12 to 24 hours minimizes edema. Warm compresses after the third postoperative day is advocated by some to speed resolution of edema. In most patients, edema largely subsides in 1 to 2 weeks, at which time eyelid position normalizes. Ptosis resulting from direct or indirect levator injury usually persists at 2 weeks. Levator function is usually good in such cases despite the ptotic appearance of the eyelid. Mild ptosis may resolve spontaneously during 3 to 6 months, and a period of observation may be appropriate. Treatment (ptosis repair) is necessary if ptosis persists past this time. Severe ptosis when present at 2 weeks (in the absence of edema) generally implies a significant injury to the levator aponeurosis, and exploration with early repair should be considered.

Diplopia/Ocular Motility Disturbance

Diplopia after eyelid surgery is fortunately a rare complication.[12,13] Diplopia reported immediately after surgery may be caused by posterior infiltration (diffusion) of anesthetic agents, resulting in various (usually mild) degrees of ophthalmoplegia. A dilated pupil may also be noted if the ciliary ganglion is affected. This may be more likely to occur if the orbital fat is directly injected with anesthesia. This type of diplopia resolves completely, usually within several hours.

Permanent diplopia after eyelid surgery may result from injury or adhesions involving the extraocular oblique muscles. The relatively anterior location of the superior oblique tendon (and trochlea) and the inferior oblique tendon exposes these structures to injury. Realistically, this only occurs with deeper eyelid dissection involving the orbital fat. Awareness of the anatomic location and orientation of these muscles, as well as good surgical exposure, is the key to avoiding this complication. Contusion or laceration of one of these muscles may cause weakness (paresis) most notable in the muscle's primary field of gaze. Adhesions (scarring) of the muscle to surrounding tissues produces restriction and limitation of ocular motility in the opposite field of gaze. The distinction between paresis and restriction can usually be made by forced duction testing. Early intervention, possibly with the assistance of a strabismus specialist, is indicated for restrictive causes to release adhesions. Late intervention (strabismus surgery) is indicated for treatment of muscle paresis that persists without improvement after 6 months. Prisms may be also used as a temporizing or permanent therapy. Young children must be monitored for amblyopia.

SPECIFIC EYELID PROCEDURES

Having reviewed the prevention and management of the general complications of eyelid surgery, attention is given to specific oculoplastic procedures. The following discussion is intended to supplement the preceding section on complications common to many procedures. As noted in the introduction to this chapter, this discussion is, by necessity, selective and addresses those procedures most commonly employed or currently favored. Details of surgical technique are mentioned only to the extent that certain steps may be associated with specific complications. This section should be viewed as an adjunct to traditional surgical atlases and texts.

Blepharoplasty

The term *blepharoplasty* is defined by *Stedman's Medical Dictionary* as "any operation for the correction of a defect of the eyelid." This rather loose definition may apply to virtually any procedure that changes the position or shape of the eyelid. Conventionally, however, the blepharoplasty procedure involves excision of various portions of skin, muscle, or fat for cosmetic or functional reasons. An extensive amount of literature on blepharoplasty exists in multiple disciplines.[14–17] This is, in part, due to the popularity of the procedure and, in part, to a continuous effort to achieve the desired benefit of surgery while minimizing complications. Whether blepharoplasty is performed for primarily cosmetic reasons or not, the final result always has an aesthetic impact. Functionally, the eyelids are essential in protecting the eyes and distributing tears. Results that produce cosmetic deformity accompanied by ocular morbidity are understandably, poorly accepted by patients. The challenge of blepharoplasty is to remove sufficient tissue to achieve a satisfactory cosmetic and functional result while avoiding the complications of brow ptosis, lagophthalmos, lid malposition, and secondary exposure keratopathy (dry eye), which may result from overzealous tissue excision or postoperative cicatrization. Such complications are the focus of this section. (The general complications of eyelid surgery, including the rare risk of blindness from orbital hemorrhage, have already been detailed.)

Preoperative Assessment

Preoperatively, it is important to identify any patient who is at "increased risk" for developing postoperative lagophthalmos, lid malposition, or secondary exposure keratopathy. A patient who has a history of dry eyes is most obviously at greatest risk for aggravating the condition after blepharoplasty. While blepharoplasty is not an absolute contraindication in such patients, it is prudent to make sure that the dry eye condition is adequately controlled (ie, minimal or no corneal staining and symptoms) with topical lubrication before considering surgery. Such patients should be aware of the risk of blepharoplasty aggravating the condition and the need for more intensive treatment (ie, lubrication or perioperative punctal occlusion). The value of preoperative Schirmer testing is somewhat controversial. Schirmer testing is admittedly a crude measure of aqueous tear production and by itself is probably not predictive of patients who have dry eyes. Schirmer testing is best used in conjunction with routine slit-lamp biomicroscopy and corneal examination with rose bengal and fluorescein staining. Basal secretion ("wetting") less than 10 mm is suggestive of impaired tear production. Other patients at risk for developing lagophthalmos are those with "prominent eyes." Prominent eyes occur because of a more anterior position of the globe relative to the orbital margins. Exophthalmos (from Graves disease and other conditions) or large globes (high myopia) are possible causes; however, in most cases, the globe and orbital soft tissues are normal, but the orbits are merely "shallow." In particular, the presence of inferior rim and malar hypoplasia should alert the surgeon to the increased possibility of lower lid retraction and lagophthalmos after lower lid blepharoplasty. These patients not infrequently also have preexistent mild inferior scleral show. Lower lid "tone" should also be assessed when lower lid blepharoplasty is contemplated. The "lid distraction" and "snap-back" tests described earlier are useful for detecting lower lid laxity. If significant lower eyelid laxity is noted, an adjunctive horizontal lower lid tightening (eg, tarsal strip) in conjunction with blepharoplasty is advisable to avoid postoperative lower eyelid malposition and scleral show.

The resting position of the upper eyelids and eyebrow should also be assessed preoperatively. Large degrees of dermatochalasis can create an apparent ptosis if the redundant tissues overhang the true upper eyelid margin. It may be necessary to lift the redundant tissue gently to check the actual eyelid margin position. It is important to determine preoperatively if the patient has significant ptosis attributable to other causes, such as a levator aponeurotic disinsertion or dehiscence, in addition to dermatochalasis. The eyelid margin is normally >2.5 mm above the visual axis (approximated by the corneal light reflex to lid margin height). An upper eyelid (margin) position below this level suggests blepharoptosis. Aponeurotic defects are the most common cause of the ptosis in the adult population. Good levator function (eyelid excursion) and a high or indistinct lid crease are typically associated with an aponeurotic defect. Aponeurotic defects can be repaired in combination with upper lid blepharoplasty. Failure to address eyelid margin ptosis results in a suboptimal result (Fig. 13-4).

The normal position of the eyelid creases should also be noted preoperatively. In general, lid creases are higher in women than in men, and higher in whites than in Asians. (In the latter case, the lid crease may be nonexistent.) It is generally best to maintain a man's lid crease near the preoperative level. Women may prefer "enhancement" of the eyelid crease at or above their preoperative level. Asian blepharoplasty requires special discussion with the patient as to the degree of lid crease formation or enhancement desired.

Finally, the preoperative evaluation should include examination of the resting eyebrow position. Many

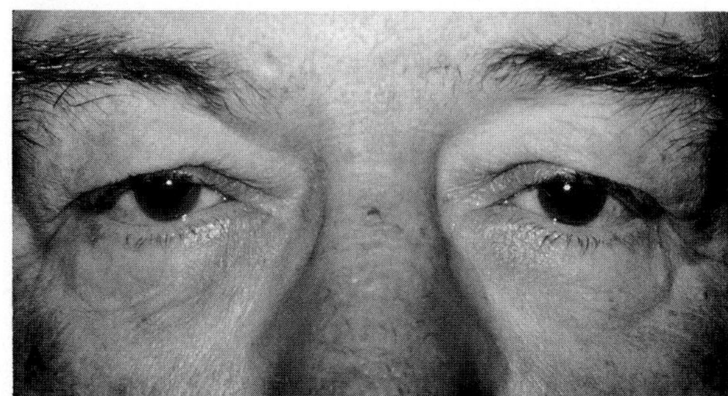

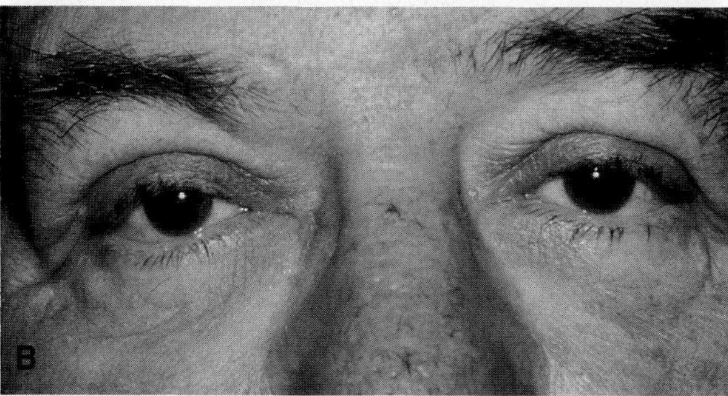

Figure 13-4. (**A**) Patient with prominent dermatochalasis and ptosis of both upper lids. (**B**) Same patient after bilateral upper lid blepharoplasty. Note that the eyelid margins are still ptotic, indicating preexistent levator aponeurosis dehiscence. Ptosis surgery combined with blepharoplasty in such cases generally provides a more optimal result.

patients with severe dermatochalasis or ptosis unconsciously raise their brows, presumably in an attempt to improve their visual field or relieve the "heavy feeling" of the eyelids. It may be necessary to place one hand on the forehead to inhibit frontalis contraction to determine the true resting eyebrow position (and eyelid position). The normal eyebrow is at or just above the superior orbital rim in men, and further above the superior rim in women. Brow ptosis may develop as part of the generalized laxity of the face associated with aging. If significant brow ptosis is present, consideration should be given to brow ptosis repair. Brow ptosis repair should always be performed before blepharoplasty, either as a separate (staged) procedure or along with blepharoplasty in some operative settings. If significant brow ptosis is not addressed first, blepharoplasty can worsen brow ptosis by "pulling the brows into the eyelids." It can be difficult to treat iatrogenically induced brow ptosis, because the postblepharoplasty eyelid skin is tight, and later attempts to lift the eyebrows can lead to severe lagophthalmos. Prevention is, therefore, the key, either by performing brow surgery first or by performing only moderate upper lid blepharoplasty in the setting of mild brow ptosis. Several procedures are available to address ptotic brows.[18–20] For women, particularly if significant forehead wrinkles are present, coronal forehead lift is ideal. Women with high hairlines and men (prone to alopecia) are not good candidates for coronal approaches. Midforehead brow lifts are sometimes acceptable for men and (if meticulously closed) for women with mild forehead creases. Direct brow lifts are certainly the most simple external approach to elevate the brows; however, the incisional scars are cosmetically less acceptable. A useful way to elevate mild or moderately ptotic brows is via an internal brow plication. In this technique, the posterior aspect of the brow is approached via a blepharoplasty incision, after dissection and removal of the submuscular fibroadipose tissue of the eyelids and eyebrows. The brows are then plicated with permanent sutures to the periosteum of the frontal bone in a higher position. Blepharoplasty is then completed if desired. The brow plication procedure is effective for mild to moderate brow ptosis and requires minimal additional operating time to the routine blepharoplasty. Enhancement ("sculpting") of the superior sulcus is an additional benefit of submuscular fibroadipose tissue excision. Care must be taken not to extend dissection too far medially so as to avoid the supraorbital neurovascular bundles. Temporal forehead numbness of a transient nature is nevertheless not uncommon after this procedure.

Intraoperative prevention and management of upper eyelid blepharoplasty and lower eyelid blepharoplasty complications merit separate discussion. In both cases it is wise to remember when excising tissue, "you can always take more, but it's hard to put it back." This is particularly true of skin excision, but also applies to fat and to a lesser extent muscle. Additional tissue can always be taken later in the surgery or as a secondary revision. A second surgery to remove more redundant tissue is certainly better than a second procedure to treat lagophthalmos.

Upper Eyelid Blepluroplasty

With upper lid blepharoplasty, a pinch technique is typically used to determine how much skin (skin/muscle) should be removed above the proposed lid crease. A subtle eversion of the lashes is a safe end-point. The upper margin of the planned skin ellipse is marked and then double-checked by repeating the pinch technique medially, centrally, and laterally. In many cases, a larger amount of tissue can safely be removed laterally.

Many instruments can be used to make the skin incision including cold steel (scalpel and scissors), electrocautery, or various lasers. Each instrument has its advocates; however, the relevant point is to avoid injury to important structures, such as the levator aponeurosis during the incision and subsequent dissection. This is particularly true near the lid crease portion of the upper eyelid incision. Maintaining slight upward and lateral traction on the skin or skin/muscle ellipse of tissue as excision proceeds in a lateral to medial direction is helpful in this regard. When the ellipse is removed it can be wrapped in saline-moistened, sterilized gauze for the rare case in which tissue must be replaced to allow closure without tension. Any bleeding should be controlled at this point before proceeding. Bleeding from the skin edges per se is usually minimal. Most bleeding tends to emanate from the orbicularis muscle or the adjacent blood vessels. Monopolar, bipolar, or hand-held thermal cautery is sufficient with the previous caveat that vital structures must be protected if extensive cautery is necessary. Taking an additional strip of muscle from the undersurface of the thicker upper skin edge is helpful to match the thinner lower skin edge of the incision. The orbital septum is best opened 5 mm or more above the eyelid skin crease. As previously mentioned, the preaponeurotic fat pad is thicker superiorly; therefore, a greater separation exists between the orbital septum and levator aponeurosis at this level. The orbital septum is "tented up," and only a small incision is initially made. The orbital septum has a multilayered quality, and sometimes several sequential snips are required before the septum can be completely opened to reveal the preaponeurotic fat. Moderate excision of fat can be performed directly or after clamping the fat. The lacrimal gland may occasionally be prolapsed temporally. Unlike fat, the lacrimal gland is firm and pinkish-gray, and should not be excised. (A prolapsed lacrimal gland can be sutured back under the rim directly to the periosteum.) Extensive traction of the orbital fat should be avoided so as not to disrupt deeper orbital blood vessels. Excision of too much orbital fat can produce a cachectic look (manifested by an abnormally deep superior sulcus). Some patients with prominent submuscular fibroadipose eyelid tissue (ie, "retroorbicularis oculi fat") additionally benefit from debulking of this tissue. The adequacy of the excision is best checked by having patients open their eyes. Any fine-tuning is completed at this point, and complete hemostasis is achieved before closing. Closure may be done in a simple fashion or with adjunctive lid crease enhancement. In general, lid crease enhancement as previously mentioned is most valuable in women. Lid crease enhancement is performed with supratarsal fixation (of the lid crease skin to the levator aponeurosis) using deep bites of the skin crease closure or with separately placed deep sutures. Supratarsal fixation at distances greater than 2 mm above the superior tarsal border has at times been noted to cause postoperative ptosis, and more modest levels are therefore recommended. In men, supratarsal fixation (lid crease enhancement) is usually avoided.

Postoperative complications of upper eyelid blepharoplasty not already covered include lid crease asymmetry and lagophthalmos. Lid crease asymmetry is most easily handled by raising the lower of the two eyelid creases during the first 2 postoperative weeks. It is generally more difficult to lower a high crease. Lagophthalmos after upper eyelid blepharoplasty is usually due to excessive skin removal but may also be caused by trapping the orbital septum in the incision closure. Mild lagophthalmos immediately in the first few postoperative weeks is not cause for concern and usually resolves during 2 to 3 months. Eyelid massage with bland ointment may be helpful, along with topical ocular lubricants. Significant lagophthalmos can, however, be a serious problem because of corneal exposure and the subsequent increased risk of corneal ulcer. If significant lagophthalmos is noted at the end of the operation, serious consideration may be given to taking down the incision to make sure that the orbital septum is not caught in wound. If the lagophthalmos appears to be due to excess skin excision, then a small strip of the previously excised skin (saved in saline-soaked gauze) can be sutured back in place as an instant autograft. If the area of wound tightness is focal, a few sutures may be removed, allowing the wound to "gape" slightly in this small area and thus heal by secondary intent. Some surgeons store (refrigerate) excised eyelid skin in case autografting is required should postoperative lagophthalmos occur. If this is done, appropriate protocols for tissue handling and storage of banked tissue should be followed. In the case in which severe lagophthalmos is noted postoperatively and upper eyelid skin is not available for grafting, consideration may be given to use of retroauricular skin grafts. Less preferred sites include the supraclavicular area and the inner aspect of the upper arm. Because eyelid skin has a unique character and is the thinnest skin of the body, all of these alternative skin graft sites have a less than ideal final cosmetic result. One edge of the skin graft is placed at the proposed eyelid crease. The bed of the skin graft may extend superiorly (sulcus) or alternatively inferiorly (supratarsally, sparing the lashes). The graft should be large enough to allow the lid to close to the inferior corneal limbus. Postoperatively downward traction is maintained on the upper lid by means of sutures through the lid margin taped to the cheek, with two to three eye pads as a dressing.

Lower Eyelid Blepharoplasty

In comparison with upper lid blepharoplasty, lower lid blepharoplasty carries a greater risk of lid retraction, ectropion, and lagophthalmos. Much literature has been devoted to these complications and their prevention.[14,21–24] Excessive skin excision or cicatrization of the orbital septum are thought to be largely responsible for these complications. It is also said that "gravity works against the lower lid." Transconjunctival lower lid blepharoplasty theoretically lessens the risk of eyelid retraction because only fat is removed, and the orbital septum and skin are not violated. Transconjunctival blepharoplasty, however, has its own complications, which include entropion and more prominent postoperative chemosis.

Prevention of lower eyelid retraction and lagophthalmos includes careful preoperative evaluation, looking for preexisting features, such as lower lid laxity, relative prominence of the eyes, inferior scleral show, and malar hypoplasia as discussed earlier. Patients with these features are at greater risk for complications with transcutaneous lower lid blepharoplasty. Any significant lid laxity should be addressed as a separate procedure before or more typically adjunctively with blepharoplasty. In these particularly "high-risk" individuals, consideration may also be given to transconjunctival blepharoplasty rather than transcutaneous blepharoplasty, or blepharoplasty may be avoided altogether. Intraoperatively, certain measures may be taken to minimize or avoid lagophthalmos and eyelid retraction. First and foremost, it is important not to remove too much skin. After making the infraciliary incision and creating a skin or skin-muscle flap, the patient is advised to look up and open the mouth. The flap is then draped across the incision (without unduly stretching the flap), and only the redundant tissue above the incision line is excised. The initial incision needs only to extend minimally into the lateral canthus (with a mild inferior angulation into a crow's foot), and never goes above the lateral canthal angle. Alternatively, a pinch technique similar to that described for upper eyelid blepharoplasty may be used for lower eyelid skin (skin/muscle) excision. With either technique, it is advisable to leave a strip of pretarsal orbicularis muscle intact. If gross laxity is not present, it may still be helpful to tighten the lower eyelid prophylactically by plicating the lateral canthal tendon (such as is done with a "Webster stitch"). Observance of the preceding measures generally helps avoid or minimize scleral show and lower lid retraction.

Management of lower lid retraction that develops postoperatively can be difficult. Lower lid retraction is typically associated with inferior scleral show and a rounded, inferiorly displaced lateral canthus, particularly if retraction is greatest laterally. This produces both cosmetic (ie, "round, sad eye") and functional (ie, exposure keratopathy) problems. Exposure keratopathy may tend to be worse if the patient had upper lid blepharoplasty as well. Postblepharoplasty lower lid retraction as indicated earlier is thought to result from excessive skin excision or scarring of the orbital septum. "Forced duction" testing of the lower lid may be helpful to determine which component is primarily responsible. Normally, the lower lid can be manually elevated to nearly the superior corneal limbus. Restriction without the development of skin tension lines on manual elevation suggests cicatrization of the orbital septum (middle lamella). Restriction with development of skin tension lines suggests shortening of, at least, the anterior lamellae. In many cases, it may be difficult to differentiate the two causes clinically. Unless there is dramatic shortening of the skin, the point may be moot, as treatment involves elevation of the eyelids without the use of skin grafts whenever possible. The appearance of skin grafts (even from upper eyelid skin) is frequently unacceptable to cosmetically oriented patients. Various techniques have been described for dealing with persistent lower lid retraction, and the choice of technique is based on the severity of lid retraction, time elapsed from original surgery, and the surgeon's preference and experience.[7,21–24] For mild lid retraction with minimal or no symptoms, massage and topical lubricants may be sufficient. Persistent symptomatic eyelid retraction generally requires treatment consisting of two components, namely elevation of the lateral canthus (possibly including the upper cheek) with lysis of the middle lamellar cicatrix. Recession of the lower lid retractors, with or without insertion of a spacer graft (ie, ear cartilage, hard palate mucosa, and so forth) may be helpful in more severe cases. An intentional "overcorrection" of the lateral canthal and vertical eyelid margin height is recommended, and reverse Frost sutures are generally used to maintain upward traction on the lower eyelid postoperatively for 5 to 7 days.

In the severest cases of lid retraction or frank ectropion, clearly resulting from severe anterior lamellar shortening, skin grafting must be performed. Persistent lower lid laxity must be corrected before skin grafting is performed, and only full-thickness skin grafts are recommended. The previous infraciliary incision is reopened and a skin/muscle flap created, lysing any scar tissue. The lower lid is placed on moderate upward traction (to the level of the pupil), and the resulting "defect" is covered with a skin graft trimmed to the same size. Reverse Frost sutures are maintained for 5 to 7 days with a firm dressing.

In summary, a conservative approach to blepharoplasty is recommended to avoid the postoperative cosmetic and functional problems associated with lid retraction and lagophthalmos. Because lower lid blepharoplasty is performed primarily for cosmetic reasons, it is particularly important for patients to understand these considerations before electing surgery.

Blepharoptosis Surgery

On the surface, ptosis surgery might seem rather straightforward. After all, how difficult can it be to raise a droopy eyelid? However, even experienced ptosis surgeons confess that ptosis surgery can be frustrating at times because the eyelid does not always stay where it is put. Ptosis surgery is "a game of millimeters." Ideally the goal of ptosis surgery is to achieve good symmetry (generally considered to be < 1 mm difference between the eyelid fissures) and functional improvement in visual field.[25] Many types of ptosis procedures have been described; however, this section focuses on levator resection and frontalis suspension ("sling"). The surgeon who understands these two procedures and their postoperative management can repair virtually any type of ptosis. Ptosis procedures, such as the Fasanella-Servat and Mueller muscle resection, although valuable, are generally limited to a select subset of "minimal ptosis" patients. However, many of the general principles of this section may nevertheless apply to other types of ptosis procedures. The specific complications of ptosis surgery aside from those common to all eyelid surgeries include overcorrection, undercorrection, contour abnormalities, and lagophthalmos.

Preoperative Evaluation

Preoperative examination must include determination of resting eyelid position (interpalpebral fissures and margin reflex distances) and, most important, levator function. The amount of levator function is the major determinant for the type of surgery required. Poor levator function (ie, < 4 mm eyelid excursion from downgaze to upgaze) generally necessitates a frontalis sling. Good function greater than 8 mm allows levator resection. Intermediate function between 5 to 7 mm is a somewhat "gray area"; however, many surgeons favor large levator resections or "internal slings" (eg, Whitnall ligament suspension) in such cases. Any preexistent lid lag or lagophthalmos should be noted and is more typical in congenital ptosis. Associated disorders that may pose risks for postoperative exposure keratopathy, such as poor eye elevation (eg, third nerve palsy or inferior rectus restriction), poor Bell phenomenon, or preexistent dry eye, should be sought, because a more conservative elevation or no surgery at all may be appropriate. Preoperative evaluation of patients with unilateral ptosis (or bilateral-asymmetric ptosis) should include manual or pharmacologic elevation of the more ptotic eyelid to unmask "latent ptosis" of the contralateral eyelid (Fig. 13-5). Patients with moderate to severe unilateral ptosis frequently have induced elevation (retraction or "pseudoretraction") of the opposite eyelid because of increased innervation to both levators (Hering phenomenon). Manual elevation or application of phenylephrine 2.5% in the (more) ptotic eye are useful tests to detect this phenomenon. A decrease in the resting position of the contralateral eyelid greater than 1 mm has been reported in approximately 20% of ptosis patients.[26] In such situations, the surgeon can decide beforehand if less surgical elevation of the ptotic lid versus bilateral surgery is appropriate. If this phenomenon is not detected before surgery, a drop in the contralateral eyelid can surprise both patient and surgeon after unilateral surgery, with resultant unsatisfactory eyelid asymmetry. Even with this caveat, the patient needs to be informed of the possible need for secondary surgery to achieve symmetry. For acquired ptosis, revision may

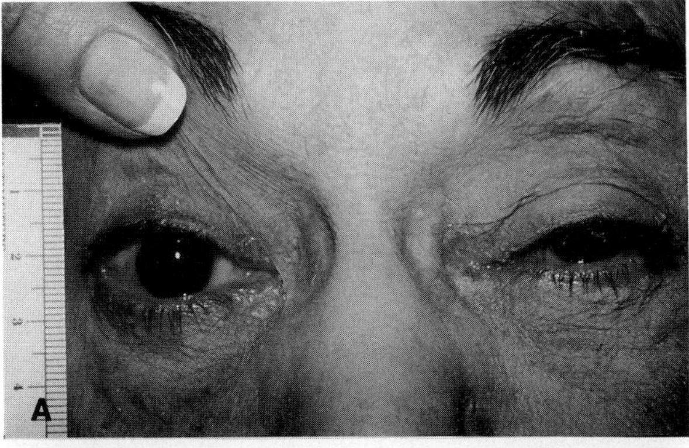

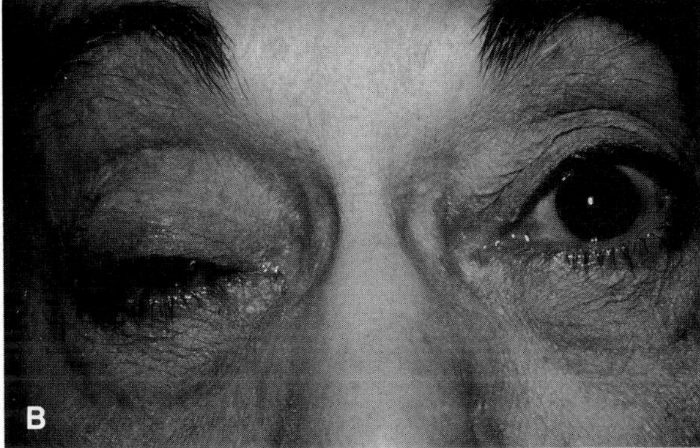

Figure 13-5. (**A**) Patient with apparent right unilateral ptosis. (**B**) A drop in the left upper lid position with manual elevation of the right upper lid reveals that the patient actually has a bilateral, assymetric ptosis, representing masked "pseudoretraction" of the less involved eyelid.

be required 5% to 10% of the time after levator resection under local anesthesia. For congenital ptosis repair performed under general anesthesia, the revision rate is much higher.

Levator Aponeurosis Ptosis Repair

Several points are important when performing anterior levator aponeurosis surgery. First, surgery is more predictable when performed under local anesthesia with full patient cooperation. Second, the surgeon must be thoroughly familiar with the anatomy of the eyelid. As discussed earlier, the anatomic landmarks encountered during surgical dissection are not always as clear as those shown in textbooks. Opening the orbital septum 5 mm above the lid crease (after subcutaneous or submuscular dissection), allows a greater margin of safety compared with posterior dissection continued directly beneath the lid crease. The preaponeurotic fat pad should be seen after incising the septum. The preaponeurotic fat pads are a key landmark, because of their distinct yellow color and encapsulated appearance. The levator aponeurosis can be found directly beneath the preaponeurotic fat pads. If the submuscular fibroadipose layer is prominent, the unwary surgeon may confuse this tissue for the preaponeurotic fat pad and subsequently mistake the orbital septum for the levator aponeurosis.

Two tests helpful for distinguishing the orbital septum from the levator aponeurosis are as follows. First, grasp the tissue in question with forceps and pull downward while palpating just inside the superior orbital rim. If the tissue is orbital septum, it will become taut inside the rim at its insertion (the arcus marginalis). If the patient is awake (local anesthesia), the presumed levator aponeurosis may be grasped, and the patient asked to look up. A distinct tug is felt if the tissue is aponeurosis, and the tissue retracts under the orbital rim. After the aponeurosis is identified, the anterior border of the tarsus is exposed. Care should be taken to avoid the peripheral vascular arcade that runs just above the superior tarsal border anterior to Mueller muscle. This vessel bleeds profusely if lacerated. Only the upper third of the tarsus generally needs to be exposed. Once the tarsus and aponeurosis are exposed, the real challenge of ptosis surgery is at hand, namely, deciding how much aponeurosis to resect. Fortunately, with an awake patient, the surgery is easily "titratable." Double-armed sutures with spatula needles are used to plicate the aponeurosis to the tarsus. The first suture should be placed partial thickness in the upper third of tarsus. Placement too far inferiorly can lead to buckling or kinking of the tarsus postoperatively. The first suture is the most critical and should be centered approximately in line with the nasal aspect of the pupil. The needle is passed through the tarsus much like strabismus sutures are placed in the sclera. A spatula needle significantly lessens the chance of full-thickness penetration of the tarsus. For added safety, the lid can be lifted away from the globe during needle passage. After passing the suture, the conjunctival tarsal surface can be inspected by everting the eyelid to make sure suture is not exposed. The sutures are then passed through the aponeurosis. A temporary bow knot is tied, and patients are asked to open their eyes and look straight ahead (usually in the upright sitting position). Suture adjustment is then performed to achieve the desired lid height. An additional one or two sutures may be used to adjust contour if necessary. A slight (0.5–1 mm) overcorrection is usually performed, as a slight drop in lid position postoperatively is typical. Occasionally, however, a rise in lid position may occur postoperatively. There lies part of the art and mystique of ptosis surgery.

A significant advantage of levator aponeurosis surgery is that the lid position (ie, lid margin height and contour) can be adjusted relatively easily within the immediate 2-week postoperative period if necessary. Within this period, the surgical wound can be opened bluntly, and new sutures can be placed to position the eyelid higher or lower. Lid position at 1 week is generally a good predictor of final lid position, and therefore adjustment is typically performed 1 to 2 weeks postoperatively.[27] Some surgeons advocate adjustment even earlier at 3 to 4 days postoperatively. Lagophthalmos is surprisingly uncommon except with large aponeurosis resections. If unusually significant lagophthalmos is noted postoperatively, one should consider wound exploration to make sure that the orbital septum has not inadvertently been incorporated into the closure. As discussed earlier, any evidence of corneal exposure is treated with topical lubricants. Other postoperative complications specific to levator resection include conjunctival prolapse and superior tarsal kinking. Both conditions occur because of interruption of the surrounding support tissues. Tarsal kinking can be prevented by keeping sutures in the upper third of tarsus. Conjunctival prolapse, if symptomatic, can be treated by repositioning the conjunctiva into the fornix with three double-arm chromic or plain gut sutures passed in a mattress fashion through the fornix and out through the eyelid skin (full thickness). Corneal irritation is minimal provided the sutures are placed well into the superior fornix. Tarsal kinking, if symptomatic, can be treated by repositioning the sutures higher on the tarsus. If the lid margin position is satisfactory, another option is simply to excise the superior aspect of the tarsus from a posterior approach. No suturing is necessary with this latter procedure, and the eye is merely patched for 10 to 15 minutes for hemostasis. Lid position is unaffected because the levator remains attached more inferiorly.

Frontalis Suspension Ptosis Repair

For more severe types of ptosis with poor levator function a frontalis sling is necessary. Repair of poor levator function-ptosis by levator resection is more apt to result in undercorrection. Good preoperative measurements of lid position and levator function are, therefore, important. Various materials can be used for frontalis suspension ptosis repair and include autogenous fascia lata, cadaver ("banked") fascia lata, and a host of synthetic materials including silicone rods, Gore-Tex, and various permanent suture materials. Autogenous fascia lata is thought to be "the best" material because there is no infection risk, and it has shown the best long-term results.[28] However, the fascia of the leg (tensor fascia lata) is not well developed until after age 3, and therefore surgery must be delayed until this time. If amblyopia is present before this age, then another material must be used for frontalis suspension, understanding the compromise involved. For adults at risk for exposure (third cranial nerve palsy, chronic progressive external ophthalmoplegia, and so forth) silicone rods are preferred by some surgeons, because of their elasticity and relative ease of postoperative adjustment. Thus, the choice of suspension material must be individualized.

For bilateral frontalis suspension ptosis repair, there is really no major decision, other than the choice of material and pattern of suspension (to be described). For unilateral cases, the decision must be made to operate on one side or both sides. Advocates of bilateral surgery, in which the levator on the normal side is surgically weakened and frontalis suspension also performed on the "normal side," argue that better symmetry can be obtained with this approach. Advocates of unilateral surgery argue that acceptable function and appearance can be obtained with a unilateral sling while avoiding any risk to the opposite eye (which is a reasonable concern of many parents). Clearly the pros and cons of both approaches need to be discussed preoperatively with patients and their families, so that they may participate in the decision-making process. Those involved must understand that secondary adjustment (revision) may be required with *either* technique to achieve satisfactory results. It is also important that those involved understand that such surgery does not make the eyelids "normal," and that brow elevation is required to elevate the eyelid(s) maximally. Lagophthalmos and secondary corneal exposure are somewhat more likely with frontalis suspension procedures than with most other types of ptosis surgery. A compromise must be struck, therefore, between adequate (functional) elevation and acceptable lagophthalmos. Patients and their families must clearly understand these limitations.

Intraoperatively, the surgeon can choose from a variety of approaches for placement of the frontalis sling material including traditional transcutaneous passage, a transconjunctival approach, or an "open sky" blepharoplasty approach with direct fixation to tarsus.[29–31] The "pattern" of the frontalis sling can also be varied with the choice of either a single- or double-triangle or rhombic pattern. Successful results have been reported with each approach; therefore, the choice is largely based on the surgeon's preference and experience. Complications common to all frontalis suspension procedures include placement of the frontalis sling material too superficially in the eyelid (forming visible cords), and abnormalities of lid height or contour. Ideally, the frontalis sling material should be passed posterior to the orbital septum in the eyelid, exiting anteriorly through the orbital septum just below the superior orbital rim (avoiding periosteum) into the brow incisions. When placed in this manner, the sling material is rarely if ever visible. Achieving proper lid position and contour can be a challenge. If only one triangle or rhomboid configuration is used, there is a greater demand on proper positioning. Ideally, the contour of the eyelid has a gradual arch usually centered over the nasal aspect of the pupil. Lid position (height) is adjusted relative to the superior corneal limbus and is almost always higher "on the table" than postoperatively. In most cases of severe ptosis with poor levator function in which a frontalis sling is needed, the lid is elevated to or just below the superior limbus with the patient under general anesthesia. One must be careful to make sure the eyes themselves are aligned, because during various stages of general anesthesia the horizontal or vertical position of the eyes can shift. In cases in which postoperative exposure keratopathy is a greater risk, a more conservative elevation is undertaken.

Postoperatively, if the lid position is lower than desired or if a contour abnormality exists (Fig. 13-6), two approaches can be used to adjust the eyelid. Additional elevation should only be considered if significant lagophthalmos with exposure is not present. One approach is to reopen the brow incisions, untie the sling material, and retie, thus further elevating the eyelid. This method requires that the original material be tied and fixed in a reversible manner with sufficient material to allow the revision. Alternatively, a lid crease incision can be made (or reopened), and the frontalis sling material can be tightened or plicated in a new position directly on the tarsus with permanent sutures. One must be careful during the dissection not to lyse the original sling material. Overcorrection

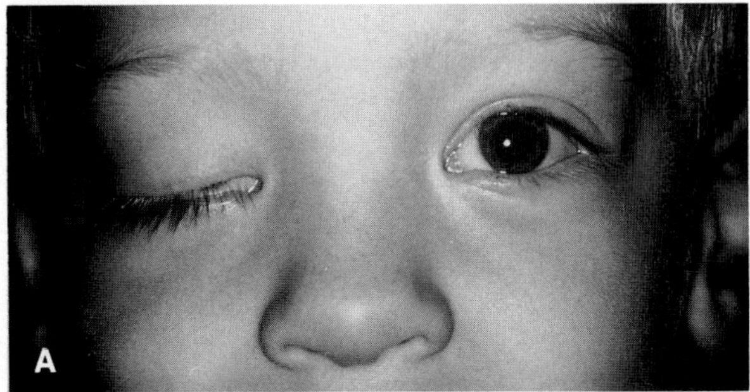

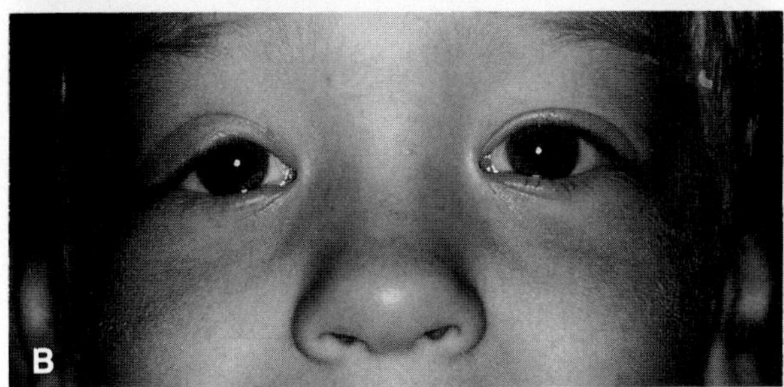

Figure 13-6. (**A**) This young patient has profound right upper lid congenital ptosis and poor levator function. (**B**) Good elevation was achieved with unilateral transconjunctival frontalis suspension; however, the patient had a persistent droop of the lateral aspect of the eyelid.

(ie, lid position too high) is rare. However, some lagophthalmos after frontalis suspension procedures can be expected. Usually the eye tolerates surprising amounts of lagophthalmos well, particularly in younger patients. Significant exposure keratopathy requires medical therapy (lubrication) as previously described. If the exposure problem is refractory to medical management, or such treatment becomes unduly inconvenient, then consideration must be given to "relaxing" the sling. It is wise to leave sufficient material (ends long after original fixation) so that this task can be accomplished; otherwise, fresh material may be required.

Ectropion/Entropion

Numerous procedures have been described for repair of ectropion and entropion.[7,32,33] Although this section cannot cover in detail all possible variations, some general points regarding surgery to correct lid malpositions are provided. Preoperatively, the primary diagnostic consideration when evaluating ectropion or entropion is to determine if the lid malposition is due to an involutional (laxity) or cicatricial process. This is important because the repair is different for severe cicatricial lid malpositions compared with that for laxity related processes. Lid laxity is a much more common cause of acquired lid malpositions and the techniques for repair, which usually involve horizontal eyelid tightening are therefore more well known and frequently used.[7] Unfortunately, most of these techniques are not sufficient alone to correct severe or even moderate cicatricial lid malpositions and are likely to result in failure. Severe cicatrization generally requires grafting to replace the deficient lamella. Some milder cases of cicatricial entropion can be repaired with transverse tarsotomy or blepharotomy, combined with lid rotation sutures.[32]

For repair of involution ectropion or entropion, the lateral tarsal strip procedure alone or in combination with other adjunctive measures (eg, medial spindle for prominent medial ectropion or lower lid retractor plication and orbicularis muscle excision for entropion) has great utility (see Fig. 13-2). Preoperatively, the effect of the lateral tarsal strip procedure can be estimated by manually advancing the lateral aspect of the eyelid laterally and slightly superiorly with a fingertip. Failure of the lid margin to reposition normally over most of its width should raise suspicion for a cicatricial process with the following exception. Occasionally, the lower punctum (with ectropion) does not fully appose the globe with this maneuver, even though the rest of the lid margin is satisfactorily positioned. Usually, this focal malposition merely implies that a medial spindle excision is required along with horizontal tightening. One additional caveat regarding ectropion is worth noting. Patients with longstanding involutional ectropion may rub their eyes because of associated epiphora. Chronic rubbing may cause a secondary dermatitis and mild cicatrization. The involved skin of the eyelids becomes erythematous and thickened, and patients usually readily admit that they chronically rub their eyes. A 2- to 3-week trial of corticosteroid ointment (ie, dexamethasone) massaged into the involved skin usually produces remarkable softening and relief of cicatrization if due to this type of self-induced dermatitis. Ectropion repair (lid tightening) to reposition the puncta usually relieves epiphora, and no further treatment is usually required.

Undercorrection and Overcorrection

In addition to complications common to all types of eyelid surgery, the two primary complications related to ectropion or entropion repair are undercorrection and overcorrection. In general, an undercorrection implies that "too little" surgery was done initially to correct the problem. In laxity (involutional) cases, this may be a function of insufficient horizontal tissue excision or inadequate rotation effect from adjunctive measures such as rotation sutures or retractor plication (ie, entropion). Conversely, in cicatricial cases, failure to diagnose cicatrization as the underlying process followed by a procedure designed only to correct laxity results in undercorrection. Undercorrection may also occur in severe cicatricial malpositions if diagnosed correctly, insufficient graft material is used, or graft contracture occurs postoperatively. Graft contraction is more common with split-thickness skin grafts, and thus full-thickness grafts are usually recommended for repair of cicatricial ectropion. If undercorrection is noted in the immediate postoperative period, and the initial diagnosis and surgery were correct, then more of the same surgery is usually needed. Although intervention for repair of an undercorrection may not necessarily be urgent, there is no advantage to waiting for spontaneous improvement, and early revision while the surgical wounds are still fresh is recommended. In the long term, any active or recurrent cicatrizing skin or conjunctival disease can progress, leading to recurrence of lid malposition, and patients should be aware of the possible need for additional treatment.

Management of overcorrection in the immediate postoperative period (ie, entropion that is now ectropion and vice versa) is not as straightforward. An early mild overcorrection is acceptable and even desirable, as relaxation in the direction of the previous malposition may occur. Ocular lubrication should be maintained until lid position normalizes. Gross overcorrection generally implies that "too much" surgery was performed. Overcorrections can be more common in procedures in which sutures are used to rotate the lid margin. Overcorrection may be caused by overtightening of lid rotation sutures (or lid retractor plication) and is more prone to occur if horizontal tightening was not performed (when laxity was present). Overcorrection is generally uncommon after repair of cicatricial lid malpositions using grafts. For gross overcorrections not likely to revolve with conservative measures, early revision is appropriate. The goal in such cases is to "relax" the overcorrection by removing or replacing previous rotation sutures and addressing any coexistent horizontal laxity in the same setting.

LACRIMAL SURGERY

Surgery involving the lacrimal drainage system is indicated primarily for the relief of obstructed tear flow causing epiphora. Lacrimal obstruction may be congenital or acquired, and may occur at any portion of the lacrimal drainage system from the eyelid puncta to the nasal ostium of the nasolacrimal duct. The aim of lacrimal surgery is to relieve obstruction and restore the normal tear flow necessary for the health and comfort of the eye. An adequate understanding of the anatomy, physiology, and pathology of the lacrimal drainage system is essential to the surgical management of obstructive lacrimal disorders. Nasolacrimal duct obstruction is much more common than obstruction of other portions of the lacrimal drainage system. Prevention and management of complications related to procedures performed for nasolacrimal duct obstruction are the focus of this section. The treatment of congenital and acquired nasolacrimal duct obstruction is different due, in part, to different pathophysiologic mechanisms. Congenital nasolacrimal duct obstruction is most commonly due to focal membranous obstruction of the nasolacrimal duct near the nasal ostium. Acquired nasolacrimal duct obstruction, conversely, is most commonly due to diffuse narrowing of the nasolacrimal duct caused by chronic inflammation and fibrosis that are usually idiopathic in origin.[34] Thus, congenital nasolacrimal duct obstruction is usually amenable to treatment by simple probing or probing with temporary stent placement. Treatment of acquired nasolacrimal duct obstruction by such measures has limited utility; therefore, dacryocystorhinostomy is the surgery of choice with modern success rates greater than 95%.

Preoperative Evaluation

Success in lacrimal surgery means relief of symptomatic epiphora (and secondary sequelae of lacrimal obstruction, such as conjunctivitis or dacryozcystitis). Failure to relieve epiphora (ie, establish adequate tear drainage) may be considered the most common "complication" of lacrimal surgery. Prevention of this relative complication begins with the preoperative evaluation of the patient presenting with epiphora. When evaluating a "tearing patient," one must distinguish between a tearing caused by true lacrimal outflow obstruction and tearing resulting from nonobstructive causes, such as reflux tearing resulting from hypersecretion or ocular surface disease (such as dry eye syndrome) and physiologic lacrimal pump failure (eyelid malpositions). The term *epiphora* is used specifically to describe overflow of tears onto the cheek, and epiphora usually results from a relative imbalance between tear production and tear drainage (a small portion of the aqueous tear film is also lost through evaporation). Many authors reserve the term *epiphora* to describe tearing specifically caused by lacrimal outflow obstruction, and they typically use the term *pseudoepiphora* to describe tearing from nonobstructive causes.

History

Evaluation of the tearing patient begins with a directed history and proceeds with appropriate examination to determine whether tearing is from a nonobstructive or obstructive cause. Furthermore, if the cause of tearing is from outflow obstruction, the location of obstruction must be determined to guide surgical management. The history of present illness should include a determination of the onset and severity of tearing. Patients should be specifically asked whether they experience tears overflowing onto the cheek or are bothered only by a "watery eye." Environmental factors may also influence tearing, such as wind, sun, cold, allergies, or occupational exposure. Patients may complain of itching, which when prominent usually suggests an allergic cause. Use of topical eye medications that may be directly irritating to the eye, particularly those containing preservatives, should be assessed. Hemorrhage, either in the form of "bloody tears" or epistaxis, should raise the suspicion for underlying malignancy. Past medical history should be explored for the presence of known ocular or periocular disease or surgery. A history of previous Bell palsy may cause weakness of the orbicularis muscle and subsequent impairment of lacrimal pump function, which may cause epiphora. Previous treatment with chemotherapy or cytotoxic agents, such as fluorouracil, is important, because these agents may be a cause of canalicular stenosis. The same is true of any history of radiation therapy involving the midface. Finally, a history of sinus disease, or sinus surgery, or history of midfacial blunt trauma (fractures) or medial canthal trauma (lacerations or burns) may also cause various injuries to the lacrimal outflow system.

Examination

Physical examination is performed after obtaining a full history. Many aspects of the lacrimal examination are included in routine ophthalmic evaluation, whereas some features are specific. The eyelids are examined for evidence of lid malpositions, such as ectropion, entropion, or trichiasis, which may cause reflex tearing from irritation of the ocular surface. Lid retraction or lagophthalmos (incomplete eyelid closure) may also be associated with reflex tearing because of development of exposure keratopathy. The lacrimal puncta are examined for signs of malposition or stenosis, and the medial canthal area is examined for evidence of mass or inflammation. Slit-lamp biomicroscopy is used for further evaluating the eyelid margin, punctal abnormalities, conjunctival disease, and the cornea. Rose bengal and fluorescein stains are helpful for highlighting corneal defects; however, the use of fluorescein should be in conjunction with subsequent lacrimal drainage dye tests, which are described subsequently. Nasal examination is also an important, frequently overlooked part of the evaluation of the tearing patient, as there are several neoplastic, inflammatory, and structural disorders of the nasal passages, which are potential causes of epiphora.

Lacrimal Tests

Nonobstructive causes of tearing are usually detected with the evaluation described earlier. However, additional diagnostic lacrimal tests may be useful. Tear production can be evaluated by use of Schirmer tests to determine if aqueous tear insufficiency (dry eye) is present. Basal tear secretion (ie, the amount of tear production after a topical anesthetic is applied) should be generally greater than 10 mm. Less than 10 mm of wetting if collaborated by clinical history and other physical findings suggests dry eye. The lacrimal drainage apparatus can be assessed with a series of office tests that include the fluorescein dye disappearance test, the Jones I and II dye tests, and diagnostic lacrimal probing. Used in a sequential logical manner, these tests generally determine whether lacrimal obstruction exists as well as the anatomic location of the obstruction. The fluorescein dye disappearance test is very useful and can be performed in cooperative children as well as adults. A drop of fluorescein 2% ophthalmic solution is placed in each eye after previously anesthetizing the eyes. Patients are asked to blink normally; after 5 minutes, there is generally little or no dye remaining in the normal eye. A delayed dye disappearance may be due to partial or complete lacrimal drainage obstruction at any level or may be due to impaired lacrimal pump function. The presence of lacrimal pump function is usually obvious, however, on physical examination. Thus, when this possibility is eliminated, a positive fluorescein dye disappearance test usually indicates lacrimal outflow obstruction.

The Jones I dye test is a test of functional tear drainage. The test is performed 5 minutes or longer after instillation of fluorescein (after noting the results of fluorescein dye disappearance). A cotton-tipped applicator is inserted under the inferior turbinate in the area near the ostium of the nasolacrimal duct to detect fluorescein in the nose. This test may be simplified somewhat by having patients blow their nose into a tissue to detect the fluorescein.

The secondary Jones dye test (Jones II) is a test of anatomic lacrimal drainage system patency and is performed immediately after the Jones I test. Clear saline is used to irrigate the lacrimal system with a syringe and a 23-gauge lacrimal cannula inserted into the canaliculus. The nature and location of lacrimal drainage obstruction can generally be determined based on the outcome of the Jones II irrigation tests along with the other tests.[35] In the presence of a delay in fluorescein dye disappearance and a "negative" Jones I test (no dye passively in the nose), clear fluid obtained from the nose with Jones II irrigation suggests partial obstruction (stenosis) of the canalicular system. A dye-tinged fluid from the nose suggests a partial nasal lacrimal duct obstruction, which nevertheless allows pooling of fluorescein dye in the lacrimal sac. The inability to irrigate any fluid into the nose indicates a complete anatomic lacrimal obstruction. Complete obstruction at the level of the nasolacrimal duct is frequently accompanied by palpable distention of the lacrimal sac, with or without regurgitation of dye-tinged fluid from the opposite canaliculus when irrigation is attempted. Regurgitation of clear fluid from the opposite canaliculus not accompanied by lacrimal sac distention suggests complete obstruction at the level of the common canaliculus. Finally, regurgitation of clear fluid from the same canaliculus indicates a high-grade obstruction within the same canaliculus lateral to the common canaliculus. In cases in which canalicular obstruction is suspected, further diagnostic probing of the canaliculus system is indicated. The location of the obstruction, measured in millimeters from the lacrimal puncta, should be specifically noted because obstruction close to the common canaliculus may be amendable to direct reconstructive procedures, whereas high-grade obstruction generally requires a conjunctivodacryocystorhinostomy with a Jones tube. In children, the examination is somewhat more limited. Usually, however, the history of tearing from the time since birth, along with variable amounts of crusting and discharge, allows the diagnosis to be made in a relatively straightforward manner. In some cases, however, complete lacrimal evaluation cannot be made until the time of initial lacrimal surgery.

Special Studies

In most cooperative patients, the office evaluation alone is usually sufficient to determine the nature and location of lacrimal dysfunction. Additional tests that are available, however, include dacryoscintigraphy, dacryocystography, CT, and magnetic resonance imaging (MRI). Dacryoscintigraphy is a radionucleotide scan useful for assessing physiologic tear flow. Dacryocystography provides a radiographic image of the internal lumen of the entire lacrimal drainage apparatus after instillation of radiopaque contrast media, thereby revealing any obstruction or mass within the lacrimal drainage passageway. CT and MRI are generally reserved for those cases in which a neoplastic process is suspected. Thus, the history and physical examination along with relatively simple office tests, and occasionally more complex special imaging, usually separate nonobstructive from obstructive lacrimal disorders, allowing the appropriate treatment to be recommended. The surgical procedures to relieve congenital and acquired nasolacrimal duct obstruction are discussed in the next section.

Nasolacrimal Duct Probing

Controversy persists regarding the timing of nasolacrimal duct probing for the treatment of congenital nasolacrimal duct obstruction. One approach advocates early probing (typically by age 6 months) performed in the office while the child is still small enough to handle. The alternative approach is to wait until age 12 to 13 months for spontaneous resolution. In most cases, probing at this later age is typically performed in the operating room under general anesthesia. Each strategy has its own (sometimes strongly opinionated) supporters, and readers can decide for themselves the relative pros and cons of both approaches. Suffice it to say that relatively equivalent success rates have been reported with both approaches in the hands of experienced practitioners.[36] The emphasis on experience cannot be understated with either approach, with avoidance of creating "false passages" essential. A false passage may be created when the probe violates the wall of any portion of the intact lacrimal system. This is most likely in the upper part of the lacrimal drainage system, which includes the delicate canaliculi. Significant scarring of the involved segment may lead to a more complex or "high-grade" lacrimal obstruction, necessitating secondary reconstructive surgery. There is no question that probing requires a "feel" on the part of the surgeon that can only be acquired after performing several procedures. Probing is diagnostic as well as therapeutic, because the position of the obstruction (usually the distal nasolacrimal duct) can be determined. The probe should pass smoothly to the point of obstruction. A gritty sensation usually implies that the probe is in direct contact with bone (ie, bony nasolacrimal canal) outside of the mucosally lined membranous duct.

Operative Steps

The steps of lacrimal probing are simple in principle and well known to most ophthalmologists. After dilating the puncta, the lacrimal probe is passed first into the vertical portion of the canaliculus 1 to 2 mm, and then advanced in the normal anatomic orientation of the individual canaliculus. The lower canaliculus angles upward, and the upper canaliculus angles downward approximately 45 degrees. It is important to maintain lateral traction on the eyelid during this maneuver to prevent "kinking" of the canaliculus, which might lead to a false passage. The probe is advanced until a "hard stop" is encountered. The hard stop confirms that the probe is now within the lacrimal sac, abutting the medial wall of the lacrimal sac, which is supported by bone. Once the probe is in the sac (hard stop palpated), the probe is rotated inferiorly into the nasolacrimal duct. The normal angle of the nasolacrimal duct is slightly posterior and lateral. Using the brow as a guide is helpful to steady and orient the probe during the initial rotation. In most cases, the probe will "drop" into the upper portion of the nasolacrimal duct and continue to slide smoothly until the membranous obstruction is encountered. Only slightly greater pressure is required to overcome this obstruction, and a popping sensation is usually felt as the probe passes into the nose. If unusual resistance is encountered at any time during the initial probing steps, the surgeon is advised to withdraw the probe and repeat the sequence.

Occasionally, the probe does not drop immediately into the nasolacrimal duct. This may be because the angle of the probe is not in alignment with the nasolacrimal duct or because frank obstruction is present at the lacrimal sac–nasolacrimal duct junction. Repeating the probing sequence with only slight variation of the probe angle will usually be successful in either case. Back-and-forth movements of the probe inside the sac ("jabbing") in an attempt to locate the duct should be avoided because the probe may slip out of the sac into the canalicular system, resulting in a false passage. Rarely, a total bony obstruction of the nasolacrimal system is present, which is not amenable to simple probing. In summary, probing should proceed in a deliberate stepwise sequence to avoid traumatizing the lacrimal drainage system. When probing is performed under general anesthesia, patency can be confirmed by irrigation, or direct visualization, or palpation of the probe within the nose by a second metal instrument ("metal to metal contact"). Lacrimal irrigation is usually reserved for intubated patients to avoid the risk of aspiration. Direct visualization or palpation of the probe can be performed in patients receiving mask inhalation anesthesia when the mask is removed momentarily.

Postoperative Complications

Postoperative complications of nasolacrimal duct probing are few. Occasionally, mild epistaxis may occur in the first 24 to 48 hours after surgery but is usually self-limited, requiring no treatment. Failure of probing to relieve epiphora, as previously noted, is the most common relative "complication," and the failure rate is known to increase proportionately with children's age at time of initial probing.[37] Failure may be due to inadequate surgical opening of the obstruction or iatrogenic injury but is most commonly due to closure of the new ostium by the natural healing response. Treatment of failed probings is based on the child's age and severity of obstruction, as noted during the initial procedure. For children under 18 to 24 months of age with mild nasolacrimal obstruction, repeat probing alone is usually appropriate. For older children or those with more complex obstruction, repeat probing with placement of a stent (ie, silicone intubation) has a greater likelihood of ultimate success. In the rare case of bony lacrimal obstruction, a dacryocystorhinostomy (DCR) is required. Some lacrimal surgeons advocate delaying DCR until the child is 3 years of age or even older, provided nasolacrimal duct obstruction is not complicated by significant episodes of acute dacryocystitis.

Silicone Intubation

Nasolacrimal duct probing with placement of a silicone stent ("silicone intubation") is indicated in cases of failed probing and in children older than 18 to 24 months of age in whom primary simple probing may be less successful. Silicone intubation is most useful in treatment of congenital nasolacrimal obstruction and has limited utility in the management of adult-acquired nasolacrimal duct obstructions. Silicone intubation works best in situations in which a focal obstruction is present, which can be opened with a lacrimal probe. The silicone tubing acts as a stent to prevent recurrent obstruction caused by the natural healing response of the surrounding tissues. The procedure includes probing of the nasolacrimal duct, and thus all points described earlier for simple nasolacrimal probing apply. Additionally, the procedure requires retrieval of the probes and tubing from the nose, a maneuver that can be technically challenging because of the relatively small working space within the nose, and the sometimes less familiar anatomic surroundings. Several silicone intubation sets (probe and retrieval units) have been devised to facilitate this procedure. Each has its own merits and shortcomings. The silicone tubing is usually kept in place for 6 weeks or longer, and then removed. The complications of silicone intubation include inability to intubate the lacrimal system (ie, pass or retrieve the probe and tubing), postoperative epistaxis, inadvertent postoperative dislocation of the silicone tubing as well as soft tissue injury or reaction to the silicone tubing, and, finally, failure to relieve lacrimal obstruction (epiphora).[38–45]

Surgical Procedure

Intubation of the lacrimal drainage system requires that the lacrimal probe(s) be passed through the lacrimal drainage system just as for simple probing. Bicanalicular (ie, placement of stents through both canaliculi) is the more commonly used approach, although a planned monocanalicular technique, using silicone tubing flanged onto a punctal plug can also be performed. Occasionally, the surgeon must resort to "unplanned" monocanalicular fixation if intubation of the opposite canaliculus cannot be accomplished. The most commonly used commercially available intubation sets include the Crawford set, which consists of a probe with a dilated "olive tip" and a special hook for retrieval; the Quickert set in which the tubing is flanged onto a tapered probe; and the Guibor set in which the tubing is attached via a smaller diameter connector, allowing the tubing to remain relatively flush with the probe itself. The Crawford probes are perhaps the easiest to retrieve with the special hook, but the bulbous tip sometimes makes passage of the probe through the lacrimal system more difficult. Both the Quickert and Guibor probes are commonly retrieved with a small, straight hemostat. The Quickert probes come in a variety of sizes with the thinner, more malleable probes being easier to retrieve from the nose. Occasionally, however, the silicone tubing can slip off the Quickert probes as they are pulled through the system, which generally causes great frustration. The Guibor probes are relatively thick and less malleable, which makes passage easy but retrieval a bit more difficult. The silicone tubing virtually never comes off the Guibor tubes during retrieval, because of the flush fitting. A device known as a "grooved director" is available for probe retrieval but can be difficult to use in smaller noses of young infants. A newer set that works like a snare is also available, but clinical experience is lacking.

PROBE RETRIEVAL. Some points pertaining to retrieval are common to all techniques and are worth mentioning to minimize complications associated with this portion of the procedure. First, it is important to establish good nasal mucosal decongestion by packing the inferior meatus with pledgets soaked in cocaine 4% or oxymetazolone .05%. The amount of cocaine should not exceed 3 mg/kg. Second, an attempt should be made to visualize the probe within the inferior meatus. A good headlight is essential. Creating a slight curve or bend near the end of the probe, orientated medially, helps direct the probe tip away from the lateral wall of the nose. If this modification of the probe is not done, the probe tip tends to lie directly against the mucosa, making visualization and retrieval difficult. Third, if the inferior meatus is narrow, infracture of the inferior turbinate can be performed using a small Freer elevator against the lateral aspect of the turbinate. Infracture of the inferior turbinate also may have the secondary benefit of relieving any associated nasal obstruction near the nasolacrimal duct ostium. Mild bleeding may occur after this maneuver, and a small flexible no. 8 or no. 10 suction catheter is helpful for evacuating the inferior meatus. If necessary, the initial nasal packing can be replaced for a few minutes. At this point, after hemostasis is achieved, one can usually visualize the probe. Moving the probe backward and forward slightly within the duct and rotating the probe tip medially can be helpful. If a straight hemostat is used to retrieve the probe, the probe should be grasped close to the tip to keep the tip from "digging into" the mucosal floor of the nose when withdrawing the probe. If the probe cannot be directly visualized, it can be grasped after "palpating" its location with the retrieval instrument (ie, hook or hemostat). Each probe is retrieved, and the ends of the silicone tubing are pulled out of the nose.

SILICONE TUBING FIXATION. Several options are available related to positioning of the silicone tubing. The simplest technique is merely to tie the ends of tubing together with a single square knot, check the position of the tubing at the medial canthus to make sure it is not too tight, and then cut the ends of tubing just inside the nose. The tubing must obviously remain long enough inside the nose to stent the nasolacrimal duct ostium. The single square knot technique allows the tubing to be removed from the medial canthus postoperatively in the office with relative ease. The "downside" of this technique is that occasionally the child may dislodge the tubing from the medial canthus, necessitating early removal or repositioning of the tubing. Alternatively, the silicone tubing can be secured to the nose with suture or by attaching larger synthetic material to the tubing within the nose, to prevent early dislocation of the tubing. The downside of these latter techniques is that tissue reaction to the suture or synthetic material may occur, and removal of silicone tubing becomes more complex, sometimes requiring a second trip to the operating room. If a fixation technique is used, care must be taken not to create undue tension by the silicone tubing at the medial canthus, which can cause erosion ("cheese-wiring") of the puncta. Generally, bicanalicular intubation is preferred by most lacrimal surgeons. If only one canaliculus can be intubated, then the options include tying the two ends to form an external loop or alternatively fixing the tubing within or near the single intubated canaliculus.[42,43]

Tubing removal is performed when healing of the ostium is thought to be complete. Six weeks appears to be sufficient for healing, although some surgeons leave the tubing in place for longer periods.[44,45] Complications related to the silicone material itself include granuloma formation (medial canthus and intranasal) and ocular surface irritation (conjunctivitis or keratitis). Such complications appear to be more likely with extended placement of the silicone tubing. Although serious complications are rare, parents should be instructed to return the child for reexamination if a red eye or discomfort is noted. Keratitis with corneal ulcer formation merits prompt topical antibiotic treatment and consideration of tube removal.

Failure of silicone intubation to relieve congenital nasolacrimal duct obstruction is uncommon. A delay in treatment (ie, older child), however, is associated with a greater risk of failure.[45] Failure of silicone intubation suggests recurrent nasolacrimal duct obstruction or diffuse narrowing (stenosis) of the nasolacrimal duct not amenable to silicone intubation (Fig. 13-7). Such failures generally require dacryocystorhinostomy to achieve proper lacrimal drainage. If the patient was relatively asymptomatic with the silicone tubing in place and the silicone tubing was well tolerated, consideration may be given to extended placement of silicone tubing as a repeat attempt at cure, or as a temporizing procedure until dacryocystorhinostomy is performed. Occasionally, high-grade canalicular stenosis is responsible for failures. Such cases require more complex lacrimal reconstructive surgery.

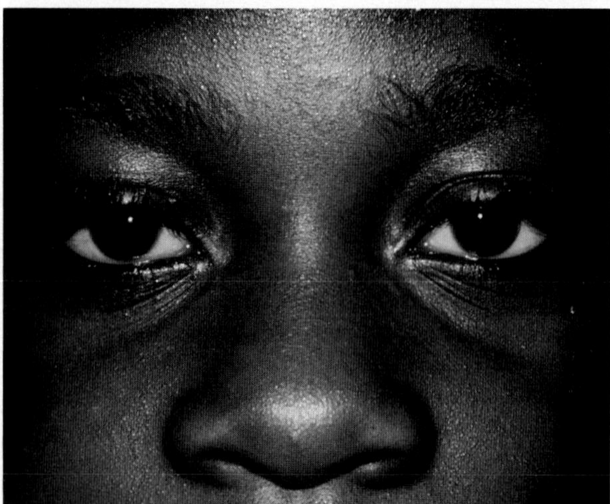

Figure 13-7. Six-year-old girl with persistent epiphora after uncomplicated silicone intubation. Note increased tear meniscus (delay in dye disappearance) bilaterally.

Dacryocystorhinostomy

Dacryocystorhinostomy (DCR) as the name implies, is a procedure to bypass obstruction at the level of the nasolacrimal duct by creating a direct anastomosis between the lacrimal sac and the nasal mucosa. Essentially two approaches are currently available to achieve this goal, namely, external (transcutaneous or transconjunctival) and intranasal. Endoscopic instrumentation and various laser delivery systems have been used to facilitate the intranasal approach.[46,47] DCR is indicated for treatment of symptomatic epiphora and the other sequelae of nasolacrimal duct obstruction (ie, conjunctivitis or dacryocystitis). Historically, the external transcutaneous approach has given the highest success rates (with percentages in the middle to high 90% range). Intranasal approaches (including endoscopic laser assisted) have achieved more modest long-term success rates on the order of 80% or less. The lower success rate with the intranasal approach is likely related to current limitations on the size of the ostium that can be created. The intranasal approach does avoid an external skin incision, and the greater risk of failure may be acceptable to those patients wishing to avoid a small external scar. Future technologic and pharmacologic advances will likely improve the success rate of intranasal DCR. Lower morbidity has been touted as an additional benefit of intranasal DCR; however, there are currently no large comparative studies to support this contention and both procedures can be performed safely on an outpatient basis.[48] Epistaxis is the main complication seen in the immediate postoperative period with either procedure and is discussed in detail later in this section. In centers where intranasal DCR is available, the patient can choose between this procedure and external DCR based on an informed discussion of the merits of each procedure. The option to convert to an external approach must always be available if necessary. In the future, "endocanalicular" DCR may provide an additional alternative but is currently investigational.[49]

Preoperative Evaluation

As discussed earlier, preoperative evaluation is essential for determining those patients with epiphora who are likely to benefit from dacryocystorhinostomy. Pseudoepiphora from dry eye or other ocular surface disease as well as "lacrimal pump" dysfunction from facial palsy or eyelid malposition must be ruled out. Canalicular stenosis requires special attention. "Low-grade" stenosis involving the common canaliculus and more medial portions of the upper or lower canaliculi requires surgery (ie, canaliculoplasty), which can usually be performed as an addition to primary DCR. "High-grade" canalicular stenosis in which most of the canalicular system is obliterated, however, requires a conjunctivodacryocystorhinostomy (CDCR) with the insertion of a Jones (Pyrex glass) tube. High-grade canalicular stenosis is fortunately rare in the general population, and such repair is usually performed by those with particular expertise in complex lacrimal problems.

Acute dacryocystitis that sometimes complicates nasolacrimal duct obstruction should be treated before surgery with appropriate antibiotics and adjunctive measures.[50] Because epistaxis is the primary complication occurring in the immediate postoperative period, special attention should be given to use of aspirin or anticoagulants as well as any history of bleeding disorders. Aspirin and other antiplatelet drugs should be stopped 2 weeks before surgery, if medically acceptable. Warfarin may generally be discontinued 1 week before surgery with approval and close monitoring by the patient's internist. Bleeding disorders require hematologic evaluation and optimal treatment before, during, and immediately after surgery.[51,52] Other medical problems that may have an impact on surgery include destructive granulomatous diseases affecting the midface (such as Wegener granulomatosis), which have a lower DCR success and may require perioperative immunotherapy.

In addition to standard office lacrimal testing, nasal examination should be performed on all patients in whom DCR is contemplated. A deviated nasal septum may limit the "working space" for intranasal DCR. If the nasal septum is deviated, repair by an otolaryngologist may be required beforehand. Hypertrophy or prominence of the anterior aspect of the middle turbinate may also interfere with intranasal DCR and to a lesser degree external DCR. Anterior middle turbinectomy may be necessary in some cases to allow the DCR to be completed, and the surgeon should be prepared for this possibility. Patients who have previously undergone medial maxillectomy for removal of a nasal or sinus tumor may pose a unique challenge if the lacrimal sac was injured or secondary scarring of the lacrimal sac has occurred. Conversely, such patients usually have a cavernous nasal cavity on the involved side with plenty of working space. Lacrimal drainage imaging studies, such as dacryocystogram (DCG), CT, or MRI, are rarely needed unless tumor is suspected preoperatively. DCG may be more helpful before planned intranasal DCR, particularly to rule out the presence of a dacryolith or lacrimal sac cicatrization.[53]

Intraoperative Complications

Both external and intranasal DCR can be performed under general anesthesia or local anesthesia with sedation (ie, monitored anesthesia care). Because intraoperative complications with external and intranasal DCR differ slightly, they are discussed separately. Intraoperative complications with external DCR include bleeding, incomplete exposure and opening of the lacrimal sac, inadequate osteotomy, and, rarely, cerebrospinal fluid (CSF) leak. Bleeding is the most disturbing intraoperative DCR complication and may occur from the angular vessels, which lie approximately 7 to 8 mm from the medial canthal angle, small vessels perforating bone, ethmoidal sinus mucosa, or nasal mucosa. Bleeding from small- and medium-sized arteries and veins in soft tissue can usually be handled with bipolar or monopolar cautery and occasionally direct ligation. Bleeding from bone may be handled by application of bone wax. Not infrequently the anterior ethmoid sinuses lie medial to the lacrimal sac fossa and are encountered during dissection. The mucosa of the ethmoid sinuses is thin and grayish in contrast to the nasal mucosa, which is pink and usually thicker. Bleeding or oozing from "the ethmoids" tends to be self-limited but may interfere with visualization. Temporarily packing the entire ethmoid sinus with a moistened gauze strip or Cottonoid strip is helpful. Topical thrombin or similar hemostatic agents are occasionally helpful. Bleeding from the nasal mucosa may occur when the mucosa is incised to create the rhinostomy. Bleeding from nasal mucosa can be minimized by appropriate use of vasoconstrictors. Oxymetazoline nasal spray is given to the patient immediately preoperatively, usually while the patient is in the holding area. Cottonoid strips soaked with cocaine 4% solution are used to pack the nose (middle meatus) at least 15 minutes before manipulation of the nasal mucosa. Cocaine 10% solution can be used but does not provide much more vasoconstriction. Therefore, the potential for cocaine toxicity can be reduced without significant sacrifice in hemostasis (or local anesthesia) by use of the 4% solution. Additional vasoconstriction of the nasal mucosa can be achieved later by direct injection with local anesthetic containing 1:200,000 or 1:100,000 epinephrine. The anesthesiologist should always be informed before any of the aforementioned vasoconstrictors are used, as some general anesthetics (ie, halothane) may increase cardiosensitivity to these agents.

Inadequate exposure or incomplete opening of the lacrimal sac is also a potential complication of DCR surgery. Dissection is usually carried down to the anterior lacrimal crest with a Freer periosteal elevator. It is important to remember the lacrimal sac fossa is concave, and the plane of dissection must follow this contour posterior to the anterior lacrimal crest to adequately reflect the lacrimal sac laterally (while protected within its periosteal covering). Failure to follow these anatomic boundaries can result in inadvertent laceration of the lacrimal sac. Adequate exposure of the lacrimal sac may necessitate disinsertion of the medial canthal tendon. This is most easily done by reflecting the tendon's attachment (periosteum) off the bone rather than directly transecting the tendon more laterally. Although medial canthal displacement (telecanthus) is a theoretic complication of canthal disinsertion, in practice, it rarely if ever occurs provided the surrounding tissue layers are closed accurately.

After the lacrimal sac is reflected laterally, the osteotomy is performed using a rongeur instrument or a drill. Care must be taken to avoid injury to the underlying nasal mucosa. It is helpful to use a right-angled, blunt instrument, such as a muscle hook, to reflect the mucosa off the bone after the initial opening in the bone is made, before further enlarging the osteotomy. Opinions differ on how large an osteotomy should be created, with some recommending a 15-mm diameter osteotomy or larger. Practically speaking, a 10-mm osteotomy appears to be adequate to ensure a high success rate. Particular care must be taken when removing bone in the superior portion of the osteotomy site, as CSF leaks have been reported during DCR. CSF leaks have been attributed to fracture of the cribriform plate caused by torsional forces during rongeuring.[54] There is generally no need to extend the osteotomy above the medial canthal tendon. When removing the bone, it is wise to "let the rongeur do the work" and use only a gentle back-and-forth motion to remove bone. Fortunately, CSF leak is a rare complication when the preceding guidelines are followed. If CSF leak should occur, neurosurgical consultation may be helpful. Conservative treatment, usually consisting of packing the nose with antibiotic impregnated gauze and placing the patient at bed rest, is usually sufficient to stop any mild CSF leak. Antibiotic prophylaxis (for meningitis) can be considered.

Creation of an anastomosis between the lacrimal sac and nasal mucosa is essential to the DCR procedure. This involves opening the medial aspect of the lacrimal sac and opening the nasal mucosa adjacent to the lacrimal sac (with or without the creation of flaps). The full thickness of the medial lacrimal sac wall must be incised, without injuring the lateral lacrimal sac wall, which contains the common canaliculus. This step can be deceptive because sometimes the periosteum separates from the underlying lacrimal sac wall, creating a space simulating the lacrimal sac lumen. Traditionally, a probe is passed into the lacrimal sac from the canaliculus, and a pointed scalpel is used to initiate the opening of the lacrimal sac, which may be completed with scissors or the scalpel. Various techniques have been described to increase the margin of safety of this step including the injection of viscous or viscoelastic solutions into the lacrimal sac to distend the sac before opening. Organic dyes, such as fluorescein or methylene blue, may also be added to highlight these solutions. After the lacrimal sac is open, it is advisable to inspect its internal lumen directly. The lacrimal sac mucosa has a distinctively smooth appearance and the common canalicular ostium (occasionally two separate ostia) can be visualized laterally by retracting the anterior portion of the lateral lacrimal sac wall. At this point, if any membranous stenosis is present around the canalicular ostium, it can usually be teased open with a blunt instrument, such as a small muscle hook. The absolute necessity of creating nasal and lacrimal sac flaps is somewhat uncertain because relatively good success rates have been reported with "flapless" techniques. One must, therefore, consider the increased surgical time and complexity of flap creation and suturing when deciding on the appropriate technique. Many lacrimal surgeons favor excision of the medial aspect of the lacrimal sac, which also provides a biopsy specimen if desired, and creation of only an anterior-based nasal mucosal flap, which can be easily sutured to the anterior cut edge of the lacrimal sac. Placement of a stent is also not a necessity with DCR; however, many surgeons feel that the success rate is increased by routinely stenting the new surgical ostium with silicone tubing, before suturing the anterior flaps. Complications of the silicone stent itself appear to be few. The stent is removed in 6 to 12 weeks. Intranasal fixation of silicone tubing is not required, as the tubing can easily be visualized intranasally and repositioned if dislodged in the postoperative period. Routine nasal packing after DCR surgery is not required; however, placement of a small piece of collagen hemostat (Instat, Johnson & Johnson) in the middle meatus is helpful to minimize postoperative epistaxis (Fig. 13-8).[55] This material "dissolves" in about 1 week and does not need to be removed.

Intranasal (Endoscopic) Dacryocystorhinostomy

Intranasal DCR has its own set of intraoperative complications. Modern intranasal DCR generally employs endoscopic visualization and various laser delivery systems. When using the laser, appropriate precautions must be observed to protect the patient and operating room personnel. These protocols are well described elsewhere and familiar to most operating room staff. To perform endoscopic laser-assisted intranasal DCR, the surgeon must be skilled in both nasal endoscopy and the use of the chosen laser system. The KTP laser is most popular for this procedure, although it has limited abilities to cut through bone. Endoscopy requires practice and numerous courses are available to improve these skills. Endoscopy can also be used routinely in the office for preoperative and postoperative evaluation. To minimize operative complications and maximize postoperative success, endoscopic laser-assisted DCR is best performed only when these technical skills are mastered. The fundamental intraoperative complications associated with the endoscopic DCR include bleeding (particularly if extensive manipulation of the middle turbinate is done), inadequate working space intranasally because of a deviated septum or hypertrophic turbinates, and inability to complete the DCR intranasally (usually because of difficulty in creating the osteotomy). The surgeon may have to convert to an external approach if anatomic or technical difficulties are encountered with intranasal DCR, and the patient should be advised of this possibility preoperatively. The adequacy of the nasal "working space" should be noted preoperatively; if a deviated septum (toward the ipsilateral, operative side) is noted, repair of the deviated septum by an otolaryngologist may be indicated before DCR. Bleeding can be minimized by use of appropriate topical vasoconstrictors, as described for external DCR. Additionally, direct anesthetic/epinephrine injection of any nasal mucosa to be incised is recommended. Because the position of the DCR ostium tends to be more posterior with the endoscopic laser-assisted intranasal DCR (as currently practiced), excision of the anterior portion of the middle turbinate (anterior turbinectomy) may be required. The turbinates are vascular, and bleeding can be profuse when the mucosa is violated, thus obscuring the operative site. Temporary intraoperative nasal packing may be necessary. Creation of an "adequate" osteotomy is a limiting technical aspect of the intranasal approach. The most commonly employed argon and KTP lasers have good mucosal cutting/coagulation ability, but do not penetrate bone well. In many cases, the thinner lacrimal bone is disrupted primarily using the light pipe to create the osteotomy. To enlarge the osteotomy anteriorly through the thicker maxillary bone, the surgeon can use a microdrill with cutting burr or various (back-biting) rongeurs designed specifically for endoscopic sinus surgery. Newer lasers, such as the "holmium laser," may allow creation of a larger osteotomy by virtue of improved ability to penetrate bone; however, clinical experience is still somewhat limited.

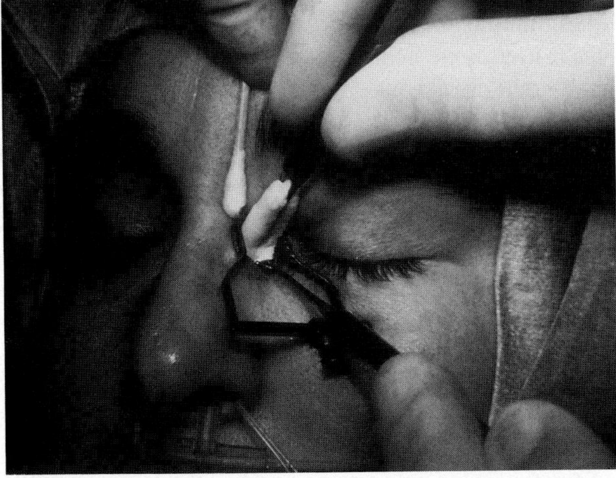

Figure 13-8. A small piece of collagen hemostate (Instat) is placed in the middle meatus to minimize postoperative epistaxis.

Postoperative Complications

Postoperative complications after external or internal DCR include epistaxis and failure of the procedure to relieve lacrimal obstruction. Wound infection or hypertrophic scarring are rare complications with external DCR incision. Some degree of epistaxis after DCR surgery is not uncommon in the first postoperative week. Occasionally, bleeding during this period may be significant enough to require nasal packing, and this contingency must be planned for, by having the necessary equipment and supplies available. In rare cases, blood loss may be sufficient to require hospitalization and, rarely, transfusion. If necessary, packing the nose is relatively straightforward, because the site of bleeding is known (anterior middle meatus-DCR ostium). A continuous length of gauze strip (0.5–1 in. wide) is used. The gauze must be well-coated with antibiotic ointment (eg, bacitracin) to prevent sticking when the packing is removed. Bayonet forceps are used to place the packing in the nose with one hand, whereas the other hand holds the nasal speculum. Direct visualization using a headlight and suction is helpful, but not essential, and the procedure can be performed in the office or at the bedside. The gauze strip is initially packed superiorly and posteriorly within the nose and additional packing is added, working anteriorly and inferiorly until the nose is completely packed. The excess gauze strip is cut, leaving the edge of the packing flush with the nostril. The packing can be removed in 3 days in the office.

Failure of DCR to relieve epiphora can be frustrating for both the patient and the physician. The cause of this complication is best sought by essentially repeating the lacrimal evaluation, which includes office lacrimal tests, ophthalmic and nasal examination, and occasionally special imaging. Statistically, the most common cause of failed DCR is closure of the DCR ostium. Coincident or secondary canalicular stenosis are other causes that should also be considered and evaluated. If evaluation reveals closure of the DCR ostium by soft tissue and the surgeon knows that a large bony osteotomy was previously made, then an intranasal approach for revision is usually adequate (regardless of whether the primary DCR was external or intranasal) to remove soft tissue and reopen the ostium. Silicone tubing is then used to stent the system for 6 to 12 weeks. Intranasal corticosteroid sprays may be used postoperatively, although their efficiency is unclear. In other cases, it may be necessary to enlarge the osteotomy as well as remove soft tissue. This may require an external approach. If canalicular stenosis is determined to be the cause of persistent epiphora, then surgery, such as canaliculoplasty or CDCR to address this type of obstruction, must be considered.

ORBITAL SURGERY

Orbital surgery encompasses a wide variety of procedures to treat an even wider variety of bony or soft tissue neoplastic, traumatic, vascular, or inflammatory problems. Perhaps there is no other place in the body where the concentration and variety of vital tissues is so great. The presence of numerous motor and sensory cranial nerves as well as a rich vascular network within a confined space makes the orbit an imposing place to work. Many ophthalmologists are justifiably reluctant to perform complex orbital procedures, such as lateral orbitotomy, without additional training. Because this chapter is intended primarily for general or comprehensive ophthalmologists, this section is somewhat less in-depth than previous sections; it focuses specifically on enucleation, and, for completeness, orbital blow-out fracture repair, and anterior and lateral orbitotomy.

Enucleation

Enucleation is one of the oldest procedures detailed in ophthalmic surgery. Removal of an eye is indicated for extensive (irreparable) ruptured globe, intraocular malignancies of large size, or those refractory to previous treatment, blind, painful eyes from chronic end-stage ocular disease, and occasionally for control of refractory infection (ie, sclerokeratitis or endophthalmitis) in eyes with no visual potential. Improved diagnostics and treatment have fortunately lessened the need for enucleation in many cases. The loss of an eye can be emotionally challenging for many patients, even if the eye was uncomfortable as well as useless. These patients need appropriate support before and after surgery. Preoperatively, the ophthalmologist must make a determination as to whether enucleation is appropriate. In most cases, the eye is determined to have no useful vision, with no reasonable chance of improvement. Usually the eye has little or no light perception. Even slightly better vision in a recalcitrant, painful eye is not a contraindication to enucleation if all other modalities of treatment have failed, and the other eye has useful vision. In most cases, the underlying disorder and reason for the enucleation is known. Special imaging (CT or MRI) or ultrasound is recommended preoperatively for larger intraocular tumors to rule out gross extrascleral extension, which might merit more aggressive treatment (exenteration). A similar approach is recommended in any eye in which the fundus cannot be viewed directly, and the history is uncertain.

The option of evisceration may be discussed if the underlying eye disease is not a malignancy, and the surgeon thinks this is appropriate. Evisceration is a technically simpler procedure, with inherently less disruption of the surrounding orbital soft tissues and consequently fewer secondary socket complications (eg, ptosis, sunken sulcus, socket contracture, implant migration, eyelid malpositions, and so forth). Postoperative prosthesis motility is generally better after evisceration compared with traditional enucleation (with nonintegrated implant). Newer integrated hydroxyapatite ocular implants, however, allow good to excellent motility even after enucleation. Evisceration unlike enucleation does not completely eliminate the risk of sympathetic ophthalmia. Although this risk is small (< 1:1000), this may be unacceptable to some patients. The discussion of sympathetic ophthalmia should be well documented in the chart of the patient who accepts this risk and elects evisceration.

On the surface, enucleation would seem to be a rather straightforward procedure; however, because the removal of the eye entails dissection and manipulation of the surrounding orbital structures, numerous complications are possible. The primary and most visible intraoperative complication associated with enucleation is bleeding. Postoperative complications include relative ocular/orbital volume deficiency (typically causing a sunken superior sulcus), shallow inferior fornix, contracted socket, eyelid malpositions, blepharoptosis, and implant-related problems including migration within the socket to an eccentric location and frank extrusion.[56–59] Some of these problems are inevitable due to the physiologic changes that occur in the orbit after the eye is removed. Others may be prevented or minimized by attention to a few basic principles during surgery. First and foremost, the surgeon must not remove the wrong eye. Fortunately, enucleation of the wrong eye has only rarely occurred in medicolegal history. Short of operative mortality, this is the worse complication imaginable. Utmost caution to avoid this possibility must be undertaken. Writing out "right eye" and "left eye" is preferred to "OD" and "OS," respectively, on all permits, as misinterpretation is less likely. The patient should be told immediately before surgery which eye will be removed. Placing a mark on the ipsilateral brow and dilating only the affected eye immediately before surgery can be reassuring to the patient, particularly if the eye appears normal externally. For intraocular tumors, a physician is advised to take one more look at the fundus immediately before the surgery begins.

Operative Technique and Intraoperative Complications

Several variations in technique as well as implant options exist for enucleation. The principles to be described are generally well accepted to minimize intraoperative and postoperative complications. After conjunctival peritomy is completed, the rectus muscles are identified. If the muscles are to be attached to the proposed implant or anterior fornix, they are tagged with a double arm suture. If a nonintegrated implant is used, the medial and lateral rectus muscles can be attached to the anterior fornix (Tenon capsule and conjunctiva) near the end of the surgery. This maneuver provides stability to the implant within the muscle cone and can enhance prosthesis mobility. The older technique of imbricating the rectus muscles over the implant is avoided because it limits the maximal size implant that can be used and may be associated with a higher incidence of implant migration. The oblique muscles are simply disinserted from the globe. After the extraocular muscles are detached from the eye, only the optic nerve holds the eye in the socket. A final 360-degree "sweep" around the eye with a cotton-tipped applicator is advised to make sure all other attachments to globe are gone. Most bleeding during enucleation occurs when the optic nerve is cut, although other vascular branches of the ophthalmic artery within the orbit (in addition to the central retinal artery) are also disrupted and contribute to bleeding.

Intraoperative complications (some with postoperative consequences) are most likely to occur when attempts are made to cut the optic nerve. Extensive dissection or manipulation deep in the orbital apex (particularly superiorly) is best avoided as the innervation of the extraocular muscles and levator occurs posteriorly. In particular, damage to the levator muscle or its innervation causes obvious postoperative ptosis. Conversely, one must avoid lacerating the posterior aspect of the globe when attempting to cut the nerve. The use of a slotted retractor, such as those used for retinal surgery, placed against the posteromedial aspect of the globe, can be used to retract the eye laterally while protecting the globe posteriorly. Before cutting the nerve, the optic nerve is palpated with the scissors. Because the nerve angles medially from the globe toward the orbital apex, only minimal inclination of the scissors is necessary to approach the optic nerve. In many cases, the optic nerve can be directly visualized. A clamp may be used to crush the nerve before cutting (for hemostasis); however, the clamp is best removed before cutting the nerve so as not to limit the length of optic nerve obtainable. After the globe is removed, the socket is packed with gauze for at least 5 minutes under moderate pressure to stop any bleeding. Rarely is it necessary to use topical coagulants, such as thrombin. Hemostasis should be achieved before placement of the implant. The choice of implant material is based on several factors including cost, experience, and patient preference. Most nonintegrated spherical implants today are made of silicone or acrylic. The most popular integrated implant is currently hydroxyapatite. Regardless of implant type, the largest implant that can comfortably fit in the orbit without tension should be used. Typically this is a 20-mm diameter implant. (Wrapping in sclera adds approximately 2 mm to the total diameter.) It is important to remember that the volume of the implant increases as a cube of the radius ($3/4\ \pi r^3$). Adequate orbital volume augmentation is essential to minimize secondary complications, such as sunken sulcus, ptosis, and shallow inferior fornix. After the implant is placed in the socket, the surrounding tissues are closed. Secure closure of Tenon capsule is essential in one layer (anterior), or two (anterior and posterior Tenon), with interrupted sutures. The conjunctiva can be closed with a running suture once Tenon layer has been securely closed. A pressure patch is usually applied for 2 to 5 days after surgery.

Postoperative Complications

Complications in the early (1- to 2-week) postoperative period include hemorrhage, infection, and implant extrusion. Significant orbital hemorrhage is rare, and managed by opening the wound and draining the hemorrhage. Postoperative infection is also rare, and managed by culture and appropriate antibiotic therapy. Severe or recalcitrant infection may require removal of the orbital implant. Early implant extrusion may be related to hemorrhage or infection, inadequate wound closure, or poor tissue quality (which prevents sutures from "holding") (Fig. 13-9). Partial exposure of the anterior surface of the implant can frequently be managed by placement of a scleral patch graft. Frank extrusion of the implant requires replacement with another synthetic implant (usually wrapped with sclera) or a dermis-fat graft. Late complications of the anophthalmic socket include implant migration or extrusion, sunken superior sulcus (which is typically associated with an "enophthalmic" appearance of the prosthesis), blepharoptosis and eyelid malpositions, shallow inferior fornix, and contracted socket. In many cases, it is wise to consult the ocularist to determine whether prosthesis modification alone is sufficient to cure the problem. Implant migration to an eccentric position requires replacement only if the implant position prevents successful positioning of the prosthesis. Orbital volume deficiency (producing a sunken superior sulcus and "enophthalmos") may be corrected by placement of a subperiosteal implant or placement (exchange) of a larger implant within the muscle cone. Blepharoptosis and lid malpositions, such as ectropion and entropion can usually be managed using standard procedures. A shallow inferior fornix sometimes develops after enucleation and is thought to be due to an inferior shifting of the orbital soft tissues, in part, because of the loss of structure support provided by the globe and its investing fibroadipose connective tissues.[60] This may prevent successful prosthesis retention. In mild cases, fornix-deeping sutures extending from the inferior fornix to the inferior orbital rim periosteum may be sufficient to hold the prosthesis in

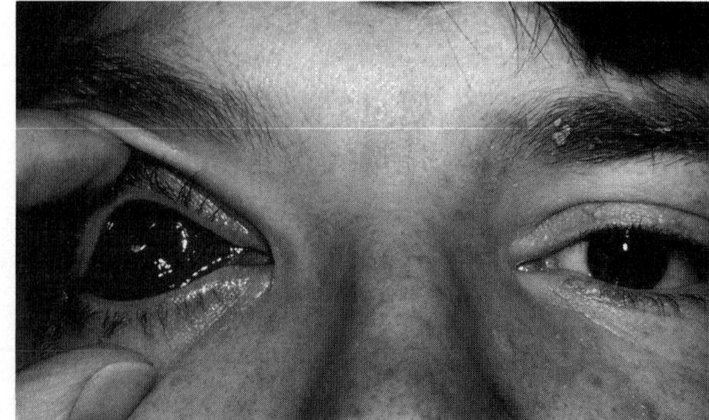

Figure 13-9. Early exposure of silicone implant several weeks after enucleation with placement of a silicone orbital implant.

place. If conjunctival shrinkage (contracture) has also occurred, a mucous membrane graft may be necessary. More extreme contracture involving the entire socket may also occur, particularly in irradiated sockets or those with alkali burns. Repair of severe socket contracture is complex, involving mucous membrane grafting and a rigid stent within the socket as well as eyelid reconstruction. Achieving adequate cosmesis in such situations can be challenging. In extreme situations, the better part of valor may be to consider a "black patch."

Orbital Blow-Out Fracture Repair

The treatment of orbital blow-out fractures has been a somewhat controversial subject during the past two-and-one-half decades. The controversy has focused primarily on what and when blow-out fractures need repair. Another later controversy has focused on the choice of autogenous grafts versus alloplastic materials. Ophthalmic complications may result from blow-out fractures as well as their repair. Long-term sequelae of orbital blow-out fractures include predominantly enophthalmos and persistent diplopia. Minimizing the complications of operative repair, while optimizing the functional and aesthetic results, are the goals of surgery. The widespread availability and use of high-quality axial and coronal CT of the orbits has improved our ability to identify those patients most at risk for developing disfiguring enophthalmos because of expansion of the bony orbital walls. To a lesser extent, CT may identify those patients who have frank entrapment of the extraocular muscles; however, the assessment of restrictive strabismus and its symptoms (diplopia) is still made primarily on clinical grounds. Early orbital edema may cause generalized ocular motility restriction. Frequently, the diplopia noted in the first few days after orbital blow-out fracture does not persist, when the orbital edema subsides. Limitation of motility in a plane 90 degrees from the site of fracture (ie, horizontal motility disturbance with isolated floor fracture) cannot usually be explained by restriction, and is more likely due to edema or neurologic injury. Thus, unless a large fracture or frank extraocular muscle entrapment is noted on CT scanning, waiting 1 to 2 weeks for orbital edema to subside is appropriate, at which time a better measure of ocular motility can be determined. Forced duction testing can be valuable preoperatively to assess restriction, and is always performed at the start and finish of surgery. A caveat here is that intramuscular hemorrhage or contracture may also cause mild to moderate degrees of restriction.

Several approaches are available to expose the orbital floor for repair of blow-out fractures in this location. These include a transcutaneous approach via an infraciliary or orbital rim incision as well as a transconjunctival approach. Each approach has its own advocates and its own complications. Of the cutaneous approaches, incisions placed just below the lashes or within the subtle lower lid crease generally leave a less obvious scar than an incision placed directly over the inferior rim. Occasionally, however, subtle or sometimes significant lid retraction may develop postoperatively, presumably from cicatrix formation near or directly involving the orbital septum. The transconjunctival approach, when combined with a lateral inferior canthotomy/cantholysis, provides equivalent exposure of the inferior orbit and has less risk of permanent lid malposition. This latter technique is currently preferred by many oculoplastic surgeons. Transantral (Caldwell-Luc) approaches to the orbital floor, with placement of a balloon catheter to support the floor have largely been abandoned because rigid fixation with miniplating and microplating systems have become readily available.

Operative Technique and Intraoperative Complications

Once the inferior orbital rim is reached by any of the aforementioned approaches, the procedure is, with the exception of implant selection, essentially the same including the intraoperative and postoperative complications related to this portion of the case. The periosteum is carefully elevated until the anterior edge of the fracture is encountered. If possible, as much of the fracture edge should be directly exposed and visualized before attempting to extract the orbital soft tissues from within the fracture itself. The orbital soft tissue should be handled with blunt dissection and gently removed from within the fracture, by using two elevators or malleable retractors in a "hand-over-hand" technique. If the tissues are prolapsed, removing a small amount of the orbital floor (anterior to the fracture) can allow better "leverage" to retract the tissues. The entire 360-degree perimeter of the fracture should be exposed, and all prolapsed tissue replaced back into the orbit. At this point, an orbital implant, usually bone graft or alloplast, is placed so that the edges of the implant rest on intact bone to support the implant. The choice of orbital implant is generally based on the surgeon's preference. In general, bone grafts have the advantage of having no infection risk, but require a second procedure to harvest the bone graft, which may be associated with graft site morbidity. Bone grafts also may show varying degrees of absorption, decreasing the predictability of repair. Alloplastic implants, conversely, simplify the repair of blow-out fractures, but may become infected or extrude.[61–65] Both bone grafts and alloplastic implants may potentially cause problems, such as optic nerve injury or damage to the lacrimal drainage system apparatus, if they are improperly positioned or migrate. Fixation of the orbital implant to an intact orbital rim can alleviate many of these problems. Newer porous materials, such as porous high-density polyethylene (Medpor, Pyrex Corp.) and hydroxyapatite, which become "integrated" with host tissues appear to have great potential as orbital implants. Perioperative antibiotics are usually recommended when an alloplastic implant is used and are continued for 1 to 2 weeks after surgery. Forced duction testing is repeated after the implant is positioned and inspected. Generally, the periosteum is closed as a separate layer. The skin or conjunctival incision can be closed with a running suture. If a transcutaneous approach with lateral cantholysis has been used, it is important to "reconstitute" the lateral canthus properly by plicating the lateral edge of the eyelid to the periosteum just *inside* the lateral orbital rim to recreate a natural eyelid/canthal contour. If the eyelid is sutured to the more anterior aspect of the orbital rim, a slightly unnatural, acutely angled appearance may result.

Postoperative Complications

Several of the potential postoperative complications related to orbital implants have already been discussed, and include implant migration, extrusion, and infection. In general, when such complications occur, removal of the implant may be required. The implant should not be replaced with another alloplastic implant or bone graft in an acutely infected condition. In many cases, fibrous tissue surrounds the implant after several months, which may allow sufficient support, such that a replacement implant is not required.

Other complications after orbital blow-out fracture repair include loss of vision (due to direct or indirect optic nerve injury), globe malposition (ie, undercorrection with persistent enophthalmos and hypoophthalmos, or overcorrection with exophthalmos), and diplopia. Visual loss after surgery is fortunately rare, but may be caused by intraoperative manipulation of the globe/optic nerve, postoperative orbital hemorrhage, or optic nerve compression by the orbital implant. The mechanism of visual loss in such cases is presumably optic nerve ischemia. Early detection of visual loss is essential; therefore, occlusive dressings are avoided, and the patient is followed closely after surgery. Pupil examination, checking for the presence of an afferent pupillary defect is a reliable, simple way to detect optic neuropathy. Orbital hemorrhage is usually obvious and is treated by drainage, along with other adjunctive measures discussed earlier. Indirect traumatic optic neuropathy may be treated by high-dose intravenous corticosteroids (methylprednisolone [Solu-Medrol], 50 mg/kg load over 1 hour, then 5.4 mg/kg/h for 24–48 hours). Repeat CT scanning is appropriate, provided treatment is not significantly delayed.

Globe malpositions after blow-out fracture repair are usually caused by the failure of surgery to reconstruct the normal rigid boundaries (walls) of the orbit. This may result in enophthalmos or hypoophthalmos if the orbital volume is expanded or exophthalmos if the orbital volume has been constricted. Orbital "fat atrophy" has been also suggested to be a contributing cause of enophthalmos (Figs. 13-10 and 13-11). If significant globe malposition is noted postoperatively, CT scanning is recommended to assess the position of the orbital implant. Enophthalmos may be corrected by repositioning the implant or by adding additional bone grafts or alloplast to augment the orbital volume deficiency. Early exophthalmos may be due to postoperative orbital edema. Persistent exoph-

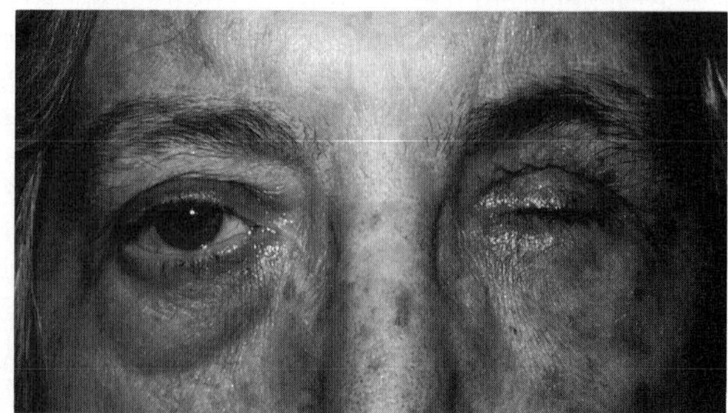

Figure 13-10. Elderly woman with persistent enophthalmos, motility disturbance, and ptosis following extensive blunt injury to the left eye.

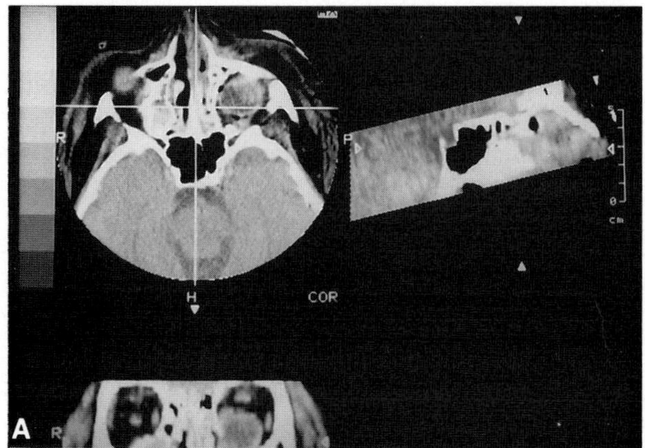

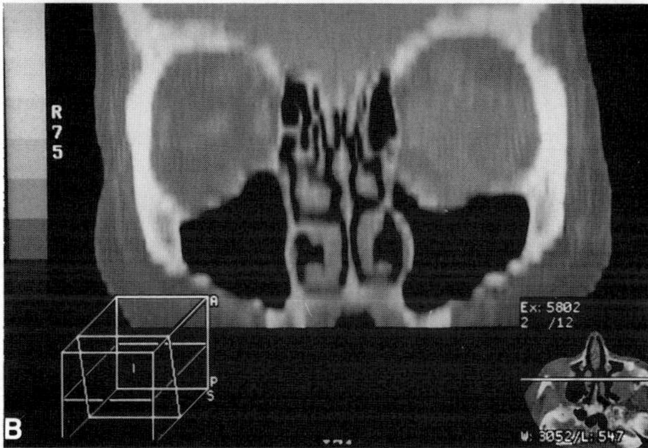

Figure 13-11. Details of preoperative and postoperative computed tomographic (CT) scans. (**A**) Preoperative CT scan shows massive blow-out fracture of the left orbit, with the globe subluxed into the maxillary sinus. (**B**) Postoperative CT scan shows satisfactory reconstruction of the orbital floor. Mild orbital volume expansion is noted; however, the patient's enophthalmos was more marked than would be expected from this finding alone, suggesting some atrophy or cicatrization of the orbital fat. Patient also had extensive cranial neuropathies.

thalmos resulting from implant malposition requires repositioning. Diplopia after orbital blow-out fracture repair may be due to persistent orbital tissue entrapment, but may also be due to direct extraocular muscle injury or scarring or neurologic injury. Most authorities consider blow-out fracture repair successful if diplopia is relieved in functional (30-degree) fields of gaze. Reoperation is usually not indicated if diplopia occurs only in more eccentric fields of gaze, although each case must be individualized. Postoperative orbital edema may also be associated with generalized limitation of ocular motility; therefore, ocular motility is reassessed when the edema resolves (usually in 1–2 weeks). If the clinical examination and CT findings suggest persistent extraocular muscle entrapment in a patient with significant diplopia, then early orbital reexploration is indicated. Persistent ocular motility deficits not amenable to orbital surgery generally require strabismus surgery. Usually 6 months or more is allowed for spontaneous improvement, with serial orthoptic measurements during this time. Diplopia may be symptomatically relieved during this period by the use of prisms or fogging (partial occlusion) of one eye. Young children at risk for amblyopia require close follow-up, and appropriate treatment (patching or optical pharmacologic penalization) should amblyopia develop.

In summary, proper patient selection and adherence to appropriate surgical technique provide the highest likelihood of a good functional and aesthetic result in the management of orbital blow-out fractures. Coincident neurologic or extraocular myopathic injury may be a cause of persistent strabismus in some patients, and it is important to advise patients of this possibility preoperatively.

Orbitotomy

Orbitotomy literally refers to surgical incision of or "opening" the orbit. Technically, some procedures, such as optic nerve sheath fenestration, orbital (bone) decompression, orbital fracture repair, and even portions of some eyelid procedures (which involve dissection posterior to orbital septum), may, by definition, be considered orbitotomies. However, for the purpose of this discussion, orbitotomy refers to those procedures indicated for orbital exploration, incisional or excisional biopsy of orbital tumors, removal of orbital foreign bodies, or drainage of orbital hemorrhage or abscess. Of these indications, orbitotomy is most commonly employed in the diagnosis and management of orbital tumors, and it is in this area that most literature exists. This section focuses primarily on complications of orbitotomy for tumor excision but is also applicable to orbitotomy performed for other reasons. It is beyond the scope of this section to present a comprehensive discussion of the fine points of orbital surgery, however.

Surgical Approaches

The surgical approaches to the orbit can be divided into anterior orbitotomy, lateral orbitotomy, and craniotomy. Craniotomy is performed by a neurosurgeon, followed by unroofing of the orbit and orbital dissection usually by a surgeon with orbital training. Craniotomy is associated with neurosurgical morbidity and mortality, which will not be detailed here, as management is primarily directed by the neurosurgeon. Most orbital space-occupying lesions, however, can be approached by an anterior or lateral orbitotomy.

Intraoperative Complications

Complications of orbitotomy include visual loss (from direct or indirect vascular compromise of the optic nerve or globe), strabismus (due to adhesions [restriction] or direct injury to the extraocular muscle[s] or their innervation), blepharoptosis or eyelid retraction, pupil abnormalities (eg, tonic dilated pupil), neurotrophic keratitis, keratitis sicca, and orbital hemorrhage or hematoma.[66–68] Incomplete tumor removal or recurrence may also be considered a complication, in those cases in which total extirpation and cure was anticipated. Lateral orbitotomy is associated with a higher incidence of complications than anterior orbitotomy. Excision of intraconal lesions has a higher complication rate than that of extraconal lesions.[66] This difference appears to be largely a function of the concentration and close proximity of delicate neurovascular structures within the muscle cone posteriorly. The surgical plan is usually developed based on the clinical and radiologic evaluation. Special orbital imaging, such as CT or MRI, is extremely helpful to document the physical nature and extent of orbital lesions; in most cases, orbital imaging also helps the surgeon "narrow the differential diagnosis," which also impacts on management. In general, well-circumscribed lesions are most amenable to complete surgical excision compared with poorly circumscribed or infiltrative lesions. In the latter case, surgery (short of exenteration or en bloc orbitectomy) is usually performed for incisional biopsy or "debulking." Lacrimal gland fossa lesions deserve special consideration. In particular, incisional biopsy of a suspected benign mixed (pleomorphic adenoma) lacrimal gland tumor is contraindicated, as this increases the likelihood of recurrence. Such tumors can be suspected based on their clinical course (>1 year duration, painless) and absence of bony destructive changes. High-flow vascular tumors or vascular malformations also present additional bleeding risk and may be evaluated using preoperative angiography. Because such lesions carry the potential for significant bleeding with surgical excision, preoperative embolization can be very helpful.

Ultimately, the approach to the orbit is based on suspected tumor type, location within the orbit, and surgical goals (complete excision versus incisional biopsy), and the relative risk-benefit nature of surgery versus other treatment options. The patient, of course, fully participates in the decision-making process. Intraoperatively, the primary challenge of orbital surgery is to obtain adequate exposure while minimizing bleeding and "collateral damage" to vital structures. Proper instrumentation is essential. Blunt dissection is used as much as possible, particularly through orbital fat. Orbital retractors and malleable "ribbon" retractors are used to provide exposure. However, prolonged retraction of the globe is avoided. The extraocular muscles are handled gently, avoiding excessive traction. Encapsulated tumors are "ideal" surgical lesions, because their well-demarcated borders allow a clear plane of dissection. In practice, it can sometimes be difficult to find the exact plane that defines the edge of the tumor, because of a thin rim of fibrous tissue that not infrequently surrounds the tumor itself. Finding the right plane may require a few additional cautious "snips" through this fibrous tissue. Bleeding is controlled by light (intermittent) pressure and topically applied thrombin or other hemostatic agents if necessary. Cautery in the deep orbit is best kept to a minimum, and bipolar is preferred to monopolar or thermal cautery.

Postoperative Complications

Postoperative complications occurring after orbitotomy were listed earlier and are now discussed in more detail. Acute visual loss requires prompt recognition and etiologic diagnosis. Occlusive dressings are avoided if possible, and vision is checked in the immediate postoperative period. Management of indirect traumatic optic neuropathy, central retinal artery occlusion, or orbital hemorrhage is initiated according to established protocols also discussed earlier. A tonic, dilated pupil after surgery is usually the result of injury to the ciliary ganglion or the parasympathetic branches nearby. No treatment, per se, is available, although spontaneous improvement is possible. Neurotrophic keratitis may occur after deep orbital dissection, presumably because of interruption of branches of the ophthalmic nerve (V1) to the cornea. Keratitis sicca (dry eye) may worsen after excision of lacrimal gland tumors. Neurotrophic keratitis and dry eye are managed by intensive topical lubrication. Punctal occlusion, tarsorrhaphy, and conjunctival flap (generally in that order) can be useful when topical therapy is insufficient. Blepharoptosis occurring after orbital surgery may be caused by injury to the superior division of the oculomotor nerve, or direct injury to the levator muscle or aponeurosis. Generally, allowing 6 months or more for spontaneous improvement is appropriate before considering surgical repair. Limitation of ocular motility (with diplopia) after orbital surgery may be caused by extraocular muscle fibrosis or adhesion (restriction), or injury to the corresponding motor nerve (paretic or paralytic). Abduction deficit after lateral orbitotomy is the most frequently described ocular motility disturbance. Forced duction testing and postoperative CT scanning may help differentiate restrictive from paretic causes. Primary early surgical intervention may be attempted to release adhesions; however, the results are frequently disappointing. Definitive strabismus surgery may be performed after waiting 6 or more months for spontaneous improvement in other cases.

SUMMARY

In summary, eyelid, lacrimal, and orbital surgery generally has a high success rate and a high risk–benefit ratio for properly selected patients. Complications may nevertheless occur with even the most seemingly straightforward procedure, and certainly even "the experts" see complications. It is hoped that application of the principles stressed in this chapter will help prevent certain complications by identifying "risk factors" before surgery, aid the surgeon in critical steps during surgery, and guide the management of problems that may nevertheless develop after surgery.

References

1. Goldberg RA, Marmor MF, Shorr N, Christenbury JD. Blindness following blepharoplasty. Ophthalmic Surg 1990;21:85–89.
2. Callahan MA. Prevention of blindness after blepharoplasty. Ophthalmology 1983;90:1047–1051.
3. DeMere M, Wood T, Austin W. Eye complications with blepharoplasty or other eyelid surgery: a national survey. Plast Reconstr Surg 1974;53:634–637.
4. Koorneef L. Orbital septa: anatomy and function. Ophthalmology 1979;86:876.
5. Rees TD, Craig SM, Fisher Y. Orbital abscess following blepharoplasty. Plast Reconstr Surg 1984;73:126–127.
6. Morgan SC. Orbital cellulitis and blindness following a blepharoplasty. Plast Reconstr Surg 1979;64:823–826.
7. Jordan DR, Anderson RL. The lateral tarsal strip revisited. Arch Ophthalmol 1989;107:604–606.
8. Hamako C, Baylis HI. Lower eyelid retraction after blepharoplasty. Am J Ophthalmol 1980:89:517–521.
9. Baylis HI, Sutcliffe T, Fett DR. Levator injury during blepharoplasty. Arch Ophthalmol 1984;102:570–571.
10. Meyer DR, Linberg JV, Wobig JL, McCormack SA. Anatomy of the orbital septum and associated eyelid connective tissues. Ophthalmic Plast Reconstr Surg 1991;7:104.
11. May JW Jr, Fearon J, Zingarelli P. Retro-orbicularis oculus fat (ROOF) resection in aesthetic blepharoplasty: a 6-year study in 63 patients. Plast Reconstr Surg 1990;86:682–689.
12. Jordan DR, Anderson RL, Thiese SM. Photo essay. Avoiding inferior oblique injury during lower blepharoplasty. Arch Ophthalmol 1989;107:1382–1383.
13. Harley RD, Nelson LB, et al. Ocular motility disturbances following blepharoplasty. Arch Ophthalmol 1986;104:542.
14. Baylis HI, Long JA, Groth MJ. Transconjunctival lower eyelid blepharoplasty: technique and complications. Ophthalmology 89;96:1027–1032.
15. Weng CJ, Noordhoff MS. Complications of Oriental blepharoplasty. Plast Reconstr Surg 1989;83:622–628.
16. Lisman RD, Hyde K, Smith B. Complications of blepharoplasty. Clin Plast Surg 1988;15:309–335.
17. Nees TD, LaTrenta GS. The role of the Schirmer's test and orbital morphology in predicting dry-eye syndrome after blepharoplasty. Plast Reconstr Surg 1988;82:619–625.
18. Fett DR, Sutcliffe T, Baylis HI. The coronal brow lift. Am J Ophthalmol 1983;96:751.
19. Cook TA, Brownrigg PJ, Wang TD, Quatela VC. The versatile midforehead browlift. Arch Otolaryngol Head Neck Surg 1989;115:163–168.
20. McCord CD, Doxanos MT, Browplasty and browpexy; an adjunct to blepharoplasty. Plast Reconstr Surg 1990;86:248.
21. Jordan DR, Anderson RL. The tarsal tuck procedure: avoiding eyelid retraction after lower blepharoplasty. Plast Reconstr Surg 1990;85:22–28.
22. Small RG, Scott M. The tight retracted lower eyelid. Arch Ophthalmol 1990;108:438–444.
23. Holds JB, Anderson RL, Thiese SM. Lower eyelid retraction: a minimal incision surgical approach to retractor lysis. Ophthalmic Surg 1990;21:767–771.
24. Shorr N, Falor M. Madam Butterfly procedure: combined check and lateral canthal suspension procedure for post-blepharoplasty "round eye" and lower eyelid retraction. Ophthalmic Plast Reconstr Surg 1985;1:229.
25. Berlin AJ, Vestal KP. Levator aponeurosis surgery: a retrospective review. Ophthalmology 1989;96:1033–1036.

26. Meyer DR, Wobig JL. Detection of contralateral eyelid retraction associated with blepharoptosis. Ophthalmology 1992;99:366.
27. Linberg JV, Vasquez RJ, Chao GM. Aponeurotic ptosis repair under local anesthesia: prediction of results from operative lid height. Ophthalmology 1988; 95:1046.
28. Wilson ME, Johnson RW. Congenital ptosis: long-term results of treatment using lyophilized fascia lata for frontalis suspensions. Ophthalmology 1991;98:1234.
29. Gresley D, Hatt M. Unilateral eyebrow suspension in severe unilateral congenital ptosis. Klin Monatsbl Augenheilkd 1992;200:476–477.
30. Dailey RA, Wilson DJ, Wobig JL. Transconjunctival frontalis suspension (TCFS). Ophthalmic Plast Reconstr Surg 1991;7:289.
31. Malone TJ, Nerad JA. The surgical treatment of blepharoptosis in oculomotor nerve palsy. Am J Ophthalmol 1988;105:57–64.
32. Kersten RC, Kleiner FP, Kulwin DR. Tarsotomy for the treatment of cicatricial entropion with trichiasis. Arch Ophthalmol 1992;110:714–717.
33. Jordan DR. Ectropion following entropion surgery: an unhappy patient and physician. Ophthalmol Plast Reconstr Surg 1992;8:41–46.
34. Linberg JV, McCormack SA. Primary acquired nasolacrimal duct obstruction: a clinicopathologic report and biopsy technique. Ophthalmology 1986;93:1055.
35. Dutton JJ. Diagnostic tests and imaging techniques. In: Linberg SV, ed. Lacrimal surgery. New York, Churchill Livingstone, 1988;19–48.
36. Stager D, Baker JD, et al. Office probing of congenital nasolacrimal duct obstruction. Ophthalmic Surg 1992;23:482.
37. Katowitz JA, Welsh MG. Timing of initial probing and irrigation in congenital nasolacrimal duct obstruction. Ophthalmology 1987;94:698.
38. Leone CR, Van Gemert JV. The success rate of silicone intubation in congenital lacrimal obstruction. Ophthalmic Surg 1990;21:90.
39. Dortzbach RK, France TD, Kushner BJ, Gonnering RS. Silicone intubation for obstruction of the nasolacrimal duct in children. Am J Ophthalmol 1982;94:585.
40. Kraft SP, Crawford JS. Silicone tube intubation in disorders of the lacrimal system in children. Am J Ophthalmol 1982;94:290.
41. Meyer DR, Linberg JV. Modification of lacrimal probe facilitates silicone intubation. Arch Ophthalmol 1989;107:1115.
42. Patrinely JR, Anderson RL. Monocanalicular silicone intubation. Arch Ophthalmol 1988;106:579.
43. Gonnering RS. Simplified monocanalicular silicone intubation. Arch Ophthalmol 1987;105:1024.
44. Migliori ME, Putterman AM. Silicone intubation for the treatment of congenital lacrimal duct obstruction: successful results removing the tubes after 6 weeks. Ophthalmology 1988;95:792.
45. Welsh MG, Katowitz JA. Timing of Silastic tubing removal after intubation for congenital nasolacrimal duct obstruction. Ophthalmic Plast Reconstr Surg 1989;5:43.
46. Massaro BM, Gonnering RS, Harris GJ. Endonasal laser dacryocystorhinostomy: A new approach to nasolacrimal duct obstruction. Arch Ophthalmol 1990; 108:1172.
47. Gonnering RS, Lyon DB, Fisher JC. Endoscopic laser-assisted lacrimal surgery. Am J Ophthalmol 1991; 111:152.
48. Dresner SC, Klussman KG, Meyer DR, Linberg JV. Outpatient dacryocystorhinostomy. Ophthalmic Surg 1991;22:222.
49. Silkiss RZ, Axelrod RN, Iwach AG, et al. Transcanalicular THC:YAG dacryocystorhinostomy. Ophthalmic Surg 1992;23:351.
50. Meyer DR, Linberg JV. Acute dacryocystitis. In: Linberg JV, ed. Oculoplastic and orbital emergencies. Norwalk, CT, Appleton & Lange, 1990, pp 37–46.
51. Jordan DR. Avoiding blood loss in outpatient dacryocystorhinostomy. Ophthalmic Plast Reconstr Surg 1991;7:261.
52. Bartley GB, Nichols WL. Hemorrhage associated with dacryocystorhinostomy and the adjunctive use of Desmopressin in selected patients. Ophthalmology 1991;98:1864.
53. Mannor GE, Milman AL. The prognostic value of preoperative dacryocystography in endoscopic intranasal dacryocystorhinostomy. Am J Ophthalmol 1992; 113:134.
54. Newhaus RW, Baylis HI. Cerebrospinal fluid leakage after dacryocystorhinostomy. Ophthalmology 1983; 90:1091.
55. Daily RA, Wobig JL. Use of collagen absorbable hemostat in dacryocystorhinostomy. Am J Ophthalmol 1988;106:109.
56. Meltzer MA. Complications of enucleation and evisceration: prevention and treatment. Int Ophthalmol Clin 1992;32:213.
57. Perman KI, Baylis HI. Evisceration, enucleation, and exenteration. Otolaryngol Clin North Am 1988;21: 171–182.
58. Oberfeld S, Levine MR. Diagnosis and treatment of complications of enucleation and orbital implant surgery. Adv Ophthalmic Plast Reconstr Surg 1990;8:107–117.
59. Goldberg RA, Holds JB, Ebrahimpour J. Exposed hydroxyapatite orbital implants: report of six cases. Ophthalmology 92;99:831–836.
60. Smith TS, Koorneef L, Zonneveld FW, et al. Computed tomography in the assessment of the postenucleation socket syndrome. Ophthalmology 1990:97:1347.

61. Jordan DR, St Onge P, Anderson RL, et al. Complications associated with alloplastic implants used in orbital fracture repair. Ophthalmology 1992;99:1600.
62. Westfall CT, Shore JW, Nunery WR, Hawes MJ, Yaremchuk MJ. Operative complications of the transconjunctival inferior fornix approach. Ophthalmology 1991;98:1525–1528.
63. Mauriello JA Jr. Complications of orbital trauma surgery. Adv Ophthalmic Plast Reconstr Surg 1987;7:99–115.
64. Hughes SM. Sequelae of orbital fractures. Adv Ophthalmic Plast Reconstr Surg 1987;6:313–341.
65. Dufresne CR, Manson PN, Iliff NT. Early and late complications of orbital fractures. Clin Plast Surg 1988;15:239–253.
66. Purgason PA, Hornblass A. Complications of surgery for orbital tumors. Ophthalmol Plast Reconstr Surg 1992;8:88–93.
67. McCord CD Jr. Complications of orbital surgery. Otolaryngol Clin North Am 1988;21:183–188.
68. Leone CR, Wissinger SP. Surgical approaches to diseases of the orbital apex. Ophthalmology 1988;95:391.

Ophthalmic Surgery Complications: Prevention and Management,
edited by Judie F. Charlton and George W. Weinstein.

14

Nick Mamalis

Inflammation

SURGICALLY INDUCED OCULAR TRAUMA

Inflammation after ocular surgery may have multiple causes. The surgical procedure itself may cause intraoperative trauma that activates a series of inflammatory cascade mechanisms. In addition to intraoperative trauma from the surgical procedure, an infectious origin must also be considered as a cause of a possible postoperative inflammation after ocular surgery. There may be sterile inflammations due to trauma from the surgical procedure itself, mechanical problems related to ocular implants as well as various sterilizing agents or polishing compounds used. Other sources of inflammation include toxic effects from various intraocular fluids, medications, or instruments and tubing used during the cataract surgery. Often the exact cause of inflammation after intraocular surgery is unclear. It is important to attempt to define the exact cause of the inflammation to properly diagnose and treat these patients to prevent the ocular sequelae of inflammation.

COMMON OCULAR RESPONSES TO SURGERY

Inflammation is the most common response to a variety of reactions that occur in the eye after surgery. A common ocular response to these various stimuli often underlie the inflammatory reaction intraocularly. Any inflammation that affects the eye may result in vasodilation and cellular infiltration of ocular tissues because of transient or permanent breakdown of the blood–aqueous barrier.[1] The most common clinical finding after breakdown of the blood–aqueous barrier is the appearance of cells and flare in the anterior chamber. In addition, blood–aqueous barrier breakdown may also be accompanied by miosis, elevated intraocular pressure, and ocular vasodilation.[2]

Inflammation either induced from the surgery or from one of the many intraocular compounds, fluids, or devices used intraoperatively, may lead to chronic inflammatory changes within the eye. These changes may affect both the anterior and the posterior segment of the globe after surgery. The ocular sequelae of postoperative inflammation are protean. Chronic inflammatory changes may affect all segments of the globe. The cornea is especially susceptible to changes of chronic inflammation. Bullous keratopathy with corneal edema, ulceration, and band keratopathy are possible reactions to postoperative inflammation. The anterior chamber may show signs of organized inflammatory membranes as well as a chronic hemorrhage from inflammatory changes and intraocular lens implants. Similarly, the iris may undergo atrophic or fibrotic changes secondary to inflammation with formation of both peripheral anterior synechiae and posterior synechiae. The crystalline lens may undergo cataract formation and opacification with fibrous metaplasia changes from either anterior or posterior segment surgery, which do not directly affect the lens. The ciliary body may react to chronic inflammation by becoming atrophic, which causes chronic hypotony within the eye. In addition, cyclitic membrane formation may occur after severe inflammation.

Posterior segment ocular sequelae of inflammation after ocular surgery may also occur. The vitreous may be affected by forming organized bands or membranes as well as vitreous hemorrhage after an inflammatory insult. The retina and choroid can also respond to inflammation with scarring and atrophy. In addition, cystoid macular edema is commonly seen after both anterior and posterior segment inflammation, and retinal detachment may occur as a result of fibrous membrane formation. Lastly, the optic nerve may undergo atrophic changes secondary to a host of inflammation-related complications including chronic glaucoma.

Uncontrolled or long-standing inflammation may lead to end-stage inflammatory complications in the globe. These include atrophia bulbi and phthisis bulbi with loss of vision as well as function in an eye.

This chapter presents a brief overview of the ocular inflammatory process in general. Specific causes of postoperative inflammation after ocular surgery are then discussed at length. Inflammation after the most commonly performed ocular surgery, cataract extraction with intraocular lens implantation, is covered in detail. However, inflammation after both common anterior and posterior segment surgeries is discussed. Finally, the ocular sequelae of postoperative inflammation is covered. The diagnosis, prevention, and management of the various forms of inflammation after ocular surgery is extremely important to the clinician to ensure optimal postoperative results for the patient.

OVERVIEW OF THE INFLAMMATORY PROCESS

An in-depth review of the inflammatory process after ocular surgery is beyond the scope of this chapter. Inflammatory cell reactions after anterior segment surgery has been relatively thoroughly reviewed by Apple, Mamalis, and coauthors.[3] In addition, Obstbaum[2] in his Binkhorst medal lecture has also provided a brief but thorough summary of the inflammatory cell reaction after cataract surgery with intraocular lens implantation. Finally, Cunha-Vaz[4] has reviewed the various blood–aqueous barriers and their effects on the inflammatory cell reaction after ocular surgery.

Blood–Aqueous Barrier Breakdown

Breakdown of the blood–aqueous barrier is the most common ocular response to surgical trauma and insult by various compounds used during surgery. The breakdown of the blood–aqueous barriers has various ocular sequelae.[4] During this breakdown, the permeability of the capillary walls increases, and the aqueous flow slows within these capillaries. This may lead to infiltration of ocular tissues with various cells, plasma proteins, and fluids, because of the increased permeability of the blood–aqueous barrier.[1] There are also a large amount of inflammatory mediators and toxic substances that are released as a result of ocular inflammation and breakdown of the blood–aqueous barrier.[3]

Tissue Destruction

Inflammation after ocular surgery may release various chemical mediators or start inflammatory cascades, which may lead to direct tissue destruction (Table 14-1). There are many proteolytic enzymes released from the vascular compartment that may directly destroy collagen or elastin.[5] In addition, various inflammatory cells such as neutrophils can release enzymes that can also lead to direct tissue destruction. These enzymes may destroy basement membranes, as well as cellular membranes themselves. Lipolytic enzymes can directly attack lipid-rich cellular membranes, leading to release of fatty acids. Finally, inflammatory cells released from the vascular system can also contain various oxidative metabolites such as hydrogen peroxide and superoxide anions. Release of these oxidative metabolites from the cells may disrupt cellular membranes and promote a free-radical formation.[6]

Inflammatory Mediators

The breakdown of cellular membranes may lead to release of the fatty acid arachidonic acid. It is the metabolism of arachidonic acid through various enzymatic pathways that leads to the production of prostaglandins as well leukotrienes (Fig. 14-1). These materials have multiple and relatively complicated pathways for their production. In addition, these materials act as inflammatory mediators and chemotactic agents, and have direct toxic effects of their own.[3]

Prostaglandins

Since the 1950s, it has been known that mechanical stimulation of the iris in an animal model may lead to release of various inflammatory compounds.

Table 14-1
Examples of Inflammatory Mediators and Toxic Agents

SOURCE	CLASS	EXAMPLE
Plasma	Complement cascade	C3a, C5a, C567
	Clotting cascade	Fibrinopeptides
		Fibrinolysis products
	Kinin system	Bradykinin, kallikrein
Leukocytes	Metabolic burst	H_2O_2, superoxide anion peroxide radicals
	Oxidative agents	
	Proteases	
	Elastases	
Tissues	Vasoactive amines	Histamines, serotonin
	Lysosomal products	Acid and natural proteases, cationic proteins ECF-A
	Lymphokines	Chemotactic factors
	Arachidonic acid cascade	Prostaglandins (PGE_2, $PGF_{2}\alpha$, PGG_2), thromboxanes, HETE, SRS-A, prostacyclins, leukotrienes

(Apple DJ, Mamalis N, Olson RJ, Kincaid MC. Intraocular lenses: Evolution, designs, complications, and pathology. Baltimore, Williams & Wilkins, 1989)

Ambache[6] initially isolated an inflammatory substance from the iris of the rabbit secondary to mechanical stimulation which he called "irin." This same group of investigators later recognized that these inflammatory materials from the rabbit iris were actually prostaglandins E and F, which were released by mechanical stimulation of the iris.[7] Other authors[6,8] then dilineated the role of prostaglandins in the breakdown of the blood–aqueous barrier with subsequent ocular inflammation.

The cascade of events leading to the release of various prostaglandins begins when arachidonic acid is released from cellular membranes by the action of phospholipase A_2. The arachidonic acid is then acted on by the enzyme cyclooxygenase, which culminates in the release of various prostaglandin compounds. Prostaglandins may lead to various inflammatory complications after ocular surgery.[9,10]

Various antiinflammatory medications, including both steroidal and nonsteroidal antiinflammatories, may interfere with prostaglandin synthesis. Corticosteroids work by initially interfering with arachidonic

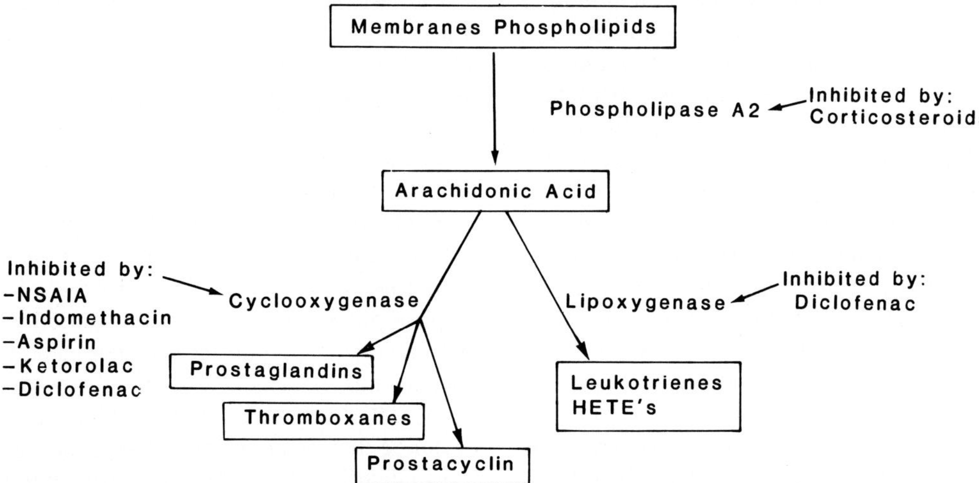

Figure 14-1. Prostaglandin and leukotriene cascade pathways are represented, showing synthesis and inhibitor agents.

acid release by indirectly blocking the action of phospholipase A^2.[11] Nonsteroidal antiinflammatory agents, such as aspirin and indomethacin, have also been shown to interfere with prostaglandin synthesis by blocking the actions of the enzyme cyclooxygenase.[12–17]

Nonsteroidal antiinflammatory agents are thought to decrease postoperative ocular inflammation by inhibiting the action of cyclooxygenase and thus decreasing the production of prostaglandins. In addition to previously studied nonsteroidal antiinflammatory agents, such as aspirin or indomethacin, there are two relatively new agents available for ophthalmic use. Ketorolac tromethamine is one such nonsteroidal antiinflammatory agent that inhibits the action of cyclooxygenase and decreases the production of prostaglandins leading to a decreased inflammation. A second, newer nonsteroidal antiinflammatory agent is diclofenac sodium, which in addition to effecting the cyclooxygenase pathway, has been shown to modulate the lipoxygenase pathway as well. Diclofenac is thought to reduce the intracellular level of free arachidonic acid by enhancing its incorporation into triglycerides, which, in turn, would lead to a reduced rate of formation of lipoxygenase products.

One of the most common findings signifying intraocular inflammation after surgery is a breakdown of the blood–aqueous barrier. Several studies have shown that new nonsteroidal antiinflammatory drops are effective in decreasing the breakdown of the blood–aqueous barrier and reducing postoperative inflammation after cataract surgery. Flach and colleagues[18] have shown that a ketorolac tromethamine solution was more effective than a placebo in suppressing postoperative anterior segment ocular inflammation after extracapsular cataract extraction with implantation of a posterior chamber intraocular lens. In addition to the finding of decreased postoperative inflammation on patient evaluation at the slit lamp, the ketorolac-treated group also showed decrease anterior segment inflammation as measured by fluorophotometry. Fluorophotometry is an effective way of measuring breakdown of the aqueous–aqueous barrier. A further study on the effect of ketorolac tromethamine on postoperative inflammation[19] showed that these drops used before and after cataract surgery decreased the breakdown of the aqueous–aqueous barrier compared with dexamethasone solution when measured by fluorophotometry. In this study, slit-lamp observations of the postoperative ocular inflammation were not different between the two treatment groups. However, ketorolac was more effective than dexamethasone in facilitating reestablishment of the blood–aqueous barrier after surgery, as measured by fluorophotometry.

The nonsteroidal antiinflammatory agent diclofenac sodium has also been evaluated for use after cataract surgery. Diclofenac was shown on fluorophotometry to be more effective than prednisolone sodium phosphate in reducing surgically induced postoperative increase in fluorescein leakage, consistent with reduction in the breakdown of the blood–aqueous barrier after cataract surgery.[20]

Finally, Miyake and coauthors[21] have directly measured the levels of prostaglandin E_2 in the aqueous humor of baboon eyes after phacoemulsification with posterior chamber lens implantation. They found that the use of the nonsteroidal antiinflammatory agent indomethacin, which inhibits cyclooxygenase, significantly reduced the amount of prostaglandin E_2 in the aqueous humor after surgery.

Chronic breakdown of the blood–aqueous barrier with release of prostaglandin-like substances can have effects on all parts of the eye. Obstbaum and Galin[22] described a group of patients with cystoid macular edema and ocular inflammation that they called the "corneo-retinoinflammatory syndrome." They at that time thought that the products of the cyclooxygenase pathway, as well as other pathways including lipoxygenase and complement, might be implicated in this syndrome. They described the common link between increased permeability of vessels in the iris, as well as the perifoveal capillaries leading to cystoid macular edema, as being due to breakdown of the blood–aqueous barriers and release of prostaglandins and other materials. Yannuzzi[15,17] also described at length the relationship between prostaglandin-induced cystoid macular edema (Fig. 14-2) as well as pseudophakic bullous keratopathy. Cystoid macular edema and its treatment will be discussed more extensively further in this chapter.

Although cystoid macular edema has been reported to occur after almost all types of intraocular surgical procedures, it has been studied most closely and occurs most commonly after cataract surgery. Miyake has extensively studied cystoid macular edema after cataract surgery, and has presented good evidence that this condition may occur as a result of prostaglandins that are synthesized intraoperatively in the iris and diffused posteriorly leading to the condition of cystoid macular edema.[16,23] He has found

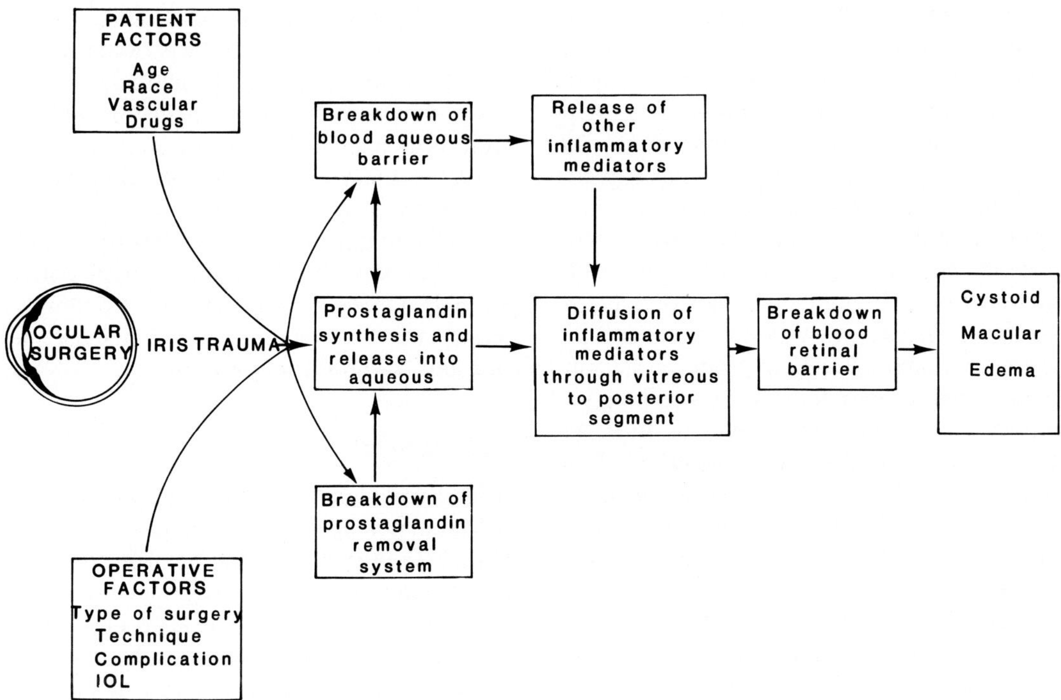

Figure 14-2. Hypothesis for prostaglandin-induced aphakic and pseudophakic cystoid macular edema. (Yannuzzi LA. A prospective on the treatment of aphakic cystoid macular edema. Surv Ophthalmol 1984;28:540–553)

that prostaglandins and other inflammatory substances are synthesized in response to surgical traumas. These substances then result in further disruption of the blood–aqueous and blood–retinal barriers. As a result of the breakdown of the blood–aqueous barrier toxic, immune complexes and other inflammatory mediators may accumulate in the aqueous and may also disrupt the blood–retinal barrier. To effect the posterior part of the eye, these inflammatory mediators must diffuse through the vitreous to the posterior retina. At this point, these mediators may irritate the small capillaries in the area of the macula, as well as the optic disc, and induce leakage of serum that accumulates in the postoperative period.

Inflammatory mediators from the anterior segments, such as prostaglandin, must diffuse to the posterior segment to create the breakdown of the blood–retinal barrier that leads to cystoid macular edema. There have been several studies in the literature that have shown that the incidence of cystoid macular edema is directly related to the type of cataract surgery performed.[24] Several studies were done in the late 1970s and early 1980s to evaluate cystoid macular edema in both aphakic and pseudophakic eyes.[25,26] These studies showed that extracapsular procedures significantly reduced the incidence of the cystoid macular edema compared with intracapsular procedures. Furthermore, there was also a significant decrease in cystoid macular edema occurring when uncomplicated extracapsular procedures were compared with complicated (those in which vitreous loss occurred) ones. A further study by Taylor and coauthors[27] also confirmed that many of the problems associated with intracapsular cataract extraction and iris-supported intraocular lens implantation seemed to be eliminated with the extracapsular cataract extraction/posterior chamber intraocular lens procedure. After analysis of a large amount of data, these authors concluded that the incidence of cystoid macular edema and pseudophakic bullous keratopathy seems to be lower with extracapsular cataract extraction and posterior chamber lens implantation, perhaps because of the presence of an intact capsule. They thought that if the capsule can be left intact, then the low incidence of cystoid macular edema will be maintained.

This so-called barrier function of an intact posterior capsule and extracapsular cataract surgery was studied more closely by Smith and coauthors.[28] These authors studied the distribution of fluorescein between the anterior chamber and anterior vitreous in two groups of patients. One group had undergone extracapsular cataract extraction with an intact capsule and a posterior chamber intraocular lens. The second group had undergone intracapsular cataract extraction with an anterior chamber intraocular lens. The penetration of fluorescein into the anterior vitreous was significantly less in the extracapsular cataract extraction group. The authors concluded that in the extracapsular cataract extraction group versus the intracapsular cataract extraction group, a significantly smaller proportion of fluorescein was found in the anterior vitreous relative to the aqueous after passage through the blood–aqueous barrier. They thought that this suggested a barrier to posterior movement of other molecules that may initially gain access to the eye and the anterior segment after surgery, such as prostaglandins.

A further study of the role of the posterior capsule as a barrier in aphakic and pseudophakic eyes was carried out by Ohrloff and coauthors.[29] They analyzed a group of patients using fluorophotometry to determine if the protective barrier function of an intact posterior capsule breaks down after posterior capsulotomy. These authors found that diffusion of fluorescein into the vitreous postoperatively showed similar values in patients who had undergone intracapsular cataract extraction and those who had undergone extracapsular cataract extraction with intraocular lens implantation and posterior capsulotomy. Furthermore, these values were significantly higher than those obtained in patients after extracapsular cataract extraction and intraocular lens implantation without capsulotomy. These authors concluded that an intact posterior capsule prevents the diffusion of soluble substances, such as prostaglandins or angiogenic factors. These aforementioned studies add further evidence to the observations that an intact posterior capsule between the aqueous and the vitreous may function as a barrier to the diffusion of substances, such as prostaglandins, from the anterior chamber into the vitreous cavity where they can affect the retina.

Leukotrienes

There is a second major inflammatory cell pathway involving arachidonic acid. The enzyme 5-lipoxygenase breaks down arachidonic acid and initiates a cascade of reaction, which leads to the production of the group of compounds called leukotrienes.[30] Obstbaum[2] has reviewed the effects of many of the products from this pathway. Leukotriene B_4 (LTB_4) has been shown to be chemotactic for leukocytes[31] as well as being involved in the release of lysosomal enzymes and the generation of superoxide anions.[32] Unlike cyclooxygenase, lipoxygenase is not blocked by nonsteroidal antiinflammatory drugs, such as aspirin. However, as mentioned previously, corticosteroids may have an effect on this pathway by interfering with arachidonic acid release from the blockage of phospholipase A_2.

Complement System

A final major inflammatory pathway that may be involved in postoperative inflammation in the eye is the complement pathway. The complement system may be activated by antigen–antibody complexes or bacterial endotoxins in the so-called classical pathway. This system may also be activated independent of antibody production by a variety of other stimuli in the so-called alternate pathway.[3] Another important factor involving complements is the possible activation of the alternative pathway by intraocular lenses after cataract surgery.[33–37] Complement products, such as C3a and C5a that are activating components of complement, are anaphylatoxins that can induce mast-cell histamine release.[38] In addition, C5a is also a potent chemotactic agent for neutrophils, eosinophils, and monocytes. Under appropriate circumstances, this may induce neutrophils to aggregate and release lysosomal enzymes that can cause direct tissue damage.[39,40] In addition, fully activated complement with all the components bound together may cause direct cellular damage by producing membrane lysis.

POSTOPERATIVE INFLAMMATION AFTER ANTERIOR SEGMENT SURGERY

Infectious Postoperative Endophthalmitis

Bacterial Endophthalmitis

Bacterial endophthalmitis is a rare but potentially devastating complication following ocular surgery of any kind. Postoperative bacterial endophthalmitis has been thoroughly reviewed by other authors.[41–46]

Generalized infectious endophthalmitis after ocular surgery is a rare complication. Overall, the incidence of postoperative bacterial endophthalmitis has decreased during the past several decades. The Food and Drug Administration report on intraocular lenses found the incidence of pseudophakic bacterial endophthalmitis to be 0.06%.[47] Thus, at the present time, the incidence of postoperative bacterial endophthalmitis is extremely low, probably on the order of 0.05% or lower. The most common cause of postoperative bacterial endophthalmitis is gram-positive bacteria. Driebe and coauthors[41] reported a large series of pseudophakic endophthalmitis including 83 patients. Of those cases with positive cultures, gram-positive bacteria accounted for 76% of the isolates. *Staphylococcus epidermidis* was the most common cause of infection overall (38%). This was followed by *Staphylococcus aureus* (21%) and various streptococcus species (11%). Gram-negative bacteria accounted for only 16% of the isolates in this series.

Adequate diagnosis and treatment of patients with bacterial endophthalmitis require prompt recognition of signs and symptoms (Fig. 14-3). Patients who present with postoperative pain, swelling, chemosis, or hypopyon should undergo taps of both the anterior chamber and the vitreous with aspiration of fluid for culture.[41,42] The treatment of presumed infectious endophthalmitis requires immediate antibiotic therapy with later adjustment of the medication depending on culture results. Intravitreal injection of antibiotics is now the preferred route of antibiotic administration for treatment of this condition.[43,45] Vitrectomy has also become a frequent therapeutic modality in this condition to help remove infectious material and allow better distribution of antibiotics.[44] The exact details on the diagnosis, treatment, and outcome of patients with bacterial endophthalmitis are discussed elsewhere in this book.

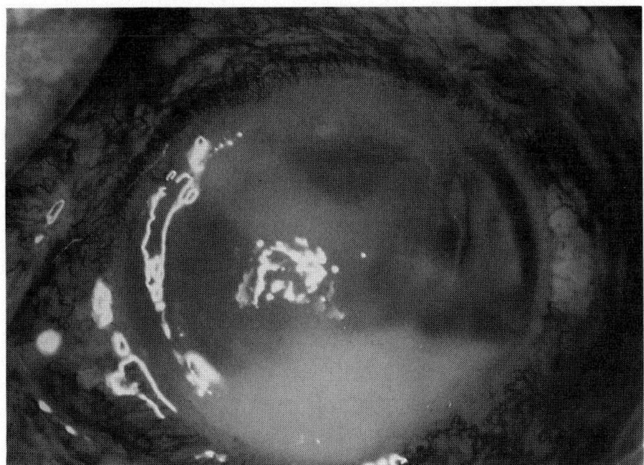

Figure 14-3. Acute postoperative bacterial endophthalmitis following extracapsular cataract extraction with posterior chamber intraocular lens. The conjunctiva shows marked chemosis and injection. The cornea is cloudy with a large hypopyon noted inferiorly. (Mamalis N. Post-cataract inflammation and endophthalmitis: diagnosis, prevention, and management. In: Weinstock FJ, ed. Management and care of the cataract patient. Boston, Blackwell Scientific Pubs., 1992:223)

Fungal Endophthalmitis

The incidence of fungal endophthalmitis is also very low. Mosier and coauthors[48] estimated the incidence of fungal endophthalmitis as 0.062% of postoperative cases at most. The incidence at this time may even be less than that. In general, patients with fungal endophthalmitis tend to have a later onset of symptoms than those with bacterial endophthalmitis, and the course seems to be more indolent.[49] The treatment of patients with suspected fungal endophthalmitis is similar to that of bacterial endophthalmitis with an intravitreal injection of amphotericin B and a vitrectomy.[43,39] Once again, a more thorough discussion of fungal endophthalmitis is included in other chapters of this textbook.

Chronic or Localized Endophthalmitis

Low-grade or late-onset endophthalmitis causing a postoperative inflammation may be due to a bacteria of low virulence. In contrast to acute bacterial endophthalmitis, these patients often have a more indolent or chronic course of inflammation after cataract surgery. Pathogens of low virulence, such as coagulase-negative *S epidermidis,* are common causes of this entity.[50–52] Cases of chronic, low-grade, postoperative inflammation that show an incomplete clinical response to corticosteroids or recurrence of inflammation after decrease of steroid therapy should raise the question of a chronic bacterial endophthalmitis. In this situation, it is important to obtain cultures of the vitreous, as well as the aqueous, to rule out an infectious cause.

Multiple cases of a low-grade, chronic, or localized endophthalmitis resulting from *Propionibacterium acnes* have been well described.[53–58] Patients with *P acnes* endophthalmitis have a relatively indolent course of inflammation that is characterized by chronic iridocyclitis with granulomatous keratic precipitates (Fig. 14-4), as well as the possibility of a

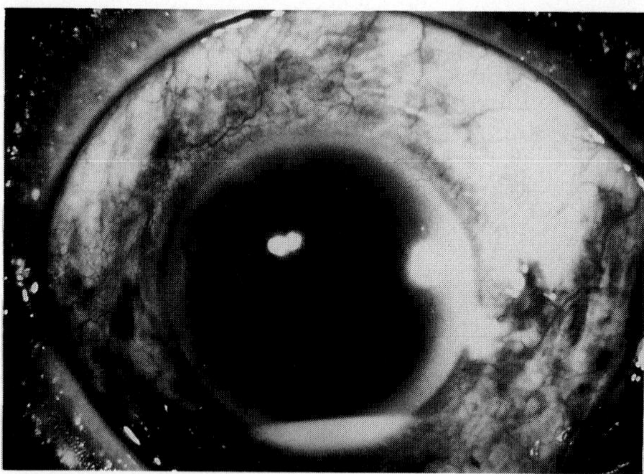

Figure 14-4. Patient who underwent cataract surgery with intraocular lens implantation and was found to have *Propionibacterium acnes* endophthalmitis postoperatively, characterized by keratic precipitates and a hypopyon. (Courtesy of William C. Lloyd, MD, San Antonio, TX)

white plaque on the posterior capsule of the lens.[53,54] Therapy for patients with *P acnes* endophthalmitis consists of a combination of antibiotics and surgical intervention.[53,58,59]

Sterile (Noninfectious) Postoperative Inflammation

Anterior segment inflammation after ocular surgery may have multiple causes. On rare occasions, an otherwise successful cataract extraction with intraocular lens implantation can be complicated by an acute, sterile, inflammatory process (Fig. 14-5). Once an infectious cause has been ruled out, there are multiple factors that may be involved in causing this anterior segment inflammation. These sterile inflammations may be due to trauma from the surgical procedure itself, mechanical problems related to the intraocular lens design or finish, sterilizing agents or polishing compounds, and toxic effects from various intraocular fluids, medications, or instruments and tubing used during the cataract surgery. Often, the exact cause of this acute anterior segment inflammation is unclear. It is important to attempt to define the exact cause of the inflammation to diagnose and treat these patients properly to prevent the ocular sequelae of this inflammation. In addition, the occurrence of inflammation in other patients may be prevented.

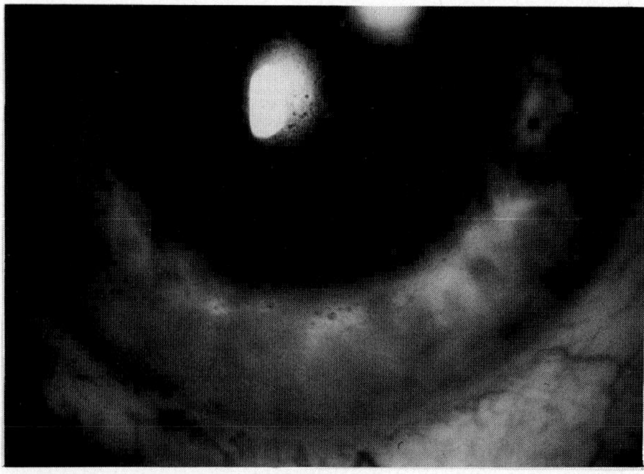

Figure 14-5. Acute sterile (noninfectious) postoperative inflammation following phacoemulsification with posterior chamber intraocular lens.

Sterile Hypopyon or "Toxic Lens Syndrome"

Cataract surgery with intraocular lens implantation may be associated with a sterile postoperative inflammation with a hypopyon and anterior chamber reaction. When initially described, this syndrome was called the toxic lens syndrome.[60,61] Some of the earliest cases of this entity describe a direct ocular toxicity, which was caused by the lens sterilization techniques or various polishing compounds used on the intraocular lenses. Several cases of early postoperative sterile hypopyons or sterile uveitis were reported after cataract surgery with intraocular lens implantation.[62,63] However, at present, the anterior segment inflammation associated with this syndrome is often not related to the intraocular lens itself. Thus, the terms *sterile hypopyon* and *sterile endophthalmitis* or *uveitis* are probably more appropriate for describing this syndrome than "toxic lens syndrome."

INTRAOCULAR LENS STERILIZATION. The method of sterilization of the intraocular lens itself is a potential source of postoperative anterior segment inflammation. In the early decades of intraocular lens use, intraocular lens sterilization was a problem. The history of the early sterilization of intraocular lenses and subsequent difficulties with sterile hypopyon was reviewed at length by Worst.[64] One of the earliest methods of sterilizing intraocular lenses used quaternary ammonium compounds such as cetrimide. These compounds were found to cause inflammatory reactions in the postoperative period, such as sterile hypopyon, intense anterior segment inflammation, and fibrosis. Mainly, because of these problems, different techniques using "wet-pack" sterilization of intraocular lenses with a caustic soda, such as sodium hydroxide, was developed.[65] Other methods of early intraocular lens sterilization included ultraviolet radiation, which was initially advocated by Binkhorst.[66] This method of sterilization was rapidly abandoned due to the question of possible damage to the polymethylmethacrylate (PMMA), which composed the intraocular lens. One unpublished attempt to use gamma irradiation sterilization resulted in a 100% incidence of sterile hypopyon and was quickly abandoned.

Wet-pack or sodium hydroxide sterilization of intraocular lenses was used extensively until the late 1970s. Before implantation of these intraocular lenses into the eye, they were rinsed in a sodium bicarbonate–neutralizing solution. Contamination of the sodium bicarbonate–neutralizing solution caused two major outbreaks of postoperative infections involving *Paecilomyces lilacinus* fungus[67] and *Pseudomonas aeruginosa*.[68] The Food and Drug Administration banned wet-pack sterilization after these outbreaks, and various techniques of dry sterilization of intraocular lenses using ethylene oxide gas were developed.

The use of ethylene oxide gas as sterilization or so-called dry pack sterilization was initially associated with increased anterior segment inflammation.[64,69] Stark and coauthors[70] found an increased incidence of postoperative anterior segment inflammation in a group of patients who received intraocular lenses using ethylene oxide sterilization compared with patients who received intraocular lenses using sodium hydroxide or wet-pack sterilization. Increasing experience using the ethylene oxide sterilization technique with proper aeration of the intraocular lenses led to a decrease in anterior segment inflammation because of intraocular lens sterilization. At this time, anterior segment inflammation resulting from sterilization of the intraocular lens itself is extremely rare.

RESIDUAL POLISHING COMPOUNDS. Residual polishing compounds on the intraocular lens surface were another source of potential anterior segment inflammation after cataract surgery. In 1980, Meltzer[71] reported several cases of sterile hypopyon after intraocular lens implantation. He further analyzed the intraocular lenses using energy-dispersive x-ray techniques and found residual polishing compound on the surface of the intraocular lenses that had not been removed. Similarly, Ratner[72] found surface films as well as small amounts of gross particular contaminants on the surface of several intraocular lenses by using energy-dispersive x-ray analysis. Improvements in manufacturing techniques and quality control of intraocular lenses have essentially eliminated this problem in the present day.

Intraocular Lens–Induced Postoperative Inflammation

Sterile postoperative anterior segment inflammation after cataract surgery may be directly related to the intraocular lens itself. Postoperative inflammation after cataract extraction with intraocular lens implantation may be related to mechanical factors such as intraocular lens design or type of lens implanted. Lens manufacturing as well as finish of the surface or edge of the intraocular lens is another important mechanical factor to be considered in inflammation secondary to the intraocular lens itself. Also, the biocompatibility of the polymers used to manufacture the different components of the intraocular lens must be considered. A final important factor when assessing anterior segment inflammation after implantation of an intraocular lens is the fixation of the intraocular lens itself within the anterior or posterior chamber of the globe. Contact between intraocular lens components and uveal structures may lead to breakdown of the blood–aqueous barrier with subsequent release of inflammatory mediators.

A study has suggested intraocular lens–induced low-grade chronic inflammation with capsulorhexis and "in-the-bag" fixation, especially when the opening is small. It is theorized that lens epithelial cell reaction to the PMMA optic is the causative factor.[73] All previous studies have suggested that capsule-fixated intraocular lenses have the best track record for maintaining the blood–aqueous barrier, so additional research in this area will be important in clarifying this issue.

INTRAOCULAR LENS FINISH AND DESIGN. Anterior segment inflammation after cataract surgery with intraocular lens implantation may be directly related to mechanical factors such as intraocular lens finish, manufacturing, and design. Ellingson[74] initially described a group of patients with a triad of postoperative findings consisting of uveitis, glaucoma, and hyphema (UGH) syndrome. This syndrome was initially noted in patients who had received poorly made copies of the Choyce Mark VIII style anterior chamber intraocular lens. Ellingson speculated that the UGH syndrome was due to warping of the intraocular lens footplates. However, Keates and Ehrlich[75] examined several similar lenses removed from patients with the UGH syndrome and found that the lenses were poorly finished with sharp, irregular edges. Subsequent evaluation of similar poorly manufactured copies of the choice anterior chamber lens using scanning electron microscopy demonstrated that sharp edges of the implant, rather than warped footplates, were the cause of the UGH syndrome in these patients.[76]

Problems with specific lens designs as well as manufacturing and finish may also contribute to postoperative anterior segment inflammation. Various closed-loop, poorly finished anterior chamber intraocular lenses were implanted in the early to mid 1980s. One of the first closed-loop anterior chamber intraocular lens that was found to be associated with the UGH syndrome postoperatively was the Azar 91Z lens.[77] Hagen[78] reported on a large group of patients who developed the UGH syndrome after implantation of the Azar 91Z intraocular lens. In addition to the UGH syndrome, patients had an associated vitreous hemorrhage which Hagen coined the "UGH+ syndrome." Cystoid macular edema and corneal decompensation are two other findings often associated with the UGH syndrome. Explanted Azar 91Z intraocular lenses examined using scanning electron microscopy at the University of Utah revealed that many of the lenses were poorly finished with sharp edges on the lens optic as well as large areas of gaping at the point where the haptic was staked to the optic.[79] Further analysis of globes that had received this implant also found problems, such as uveal erosion and synechiae formation, which were related to the closed-loop design with small, round polypropylene loops.

Other types of anterior chamber intraocular lenses with a closed loop design and small, round loops were found to have similar problems with anterior segment inflammation. It just took a little longer for the complications to appear than with the Azar lens. Reidy and coauthors[80] analyzed a large group of explanted Leiske-style, semiflexible closed-loop anterior chamber intraocular lenses. The patients who had received these lenses were also found to have extensive anterior segment inflammatory reactions such as the UGH syndrome. Finally, Isenberg and coauthors[81] found a similar association of the UGH syndrome and anterior segment inflammation with the Stableflex style anterior chamber intraocular lens. Findings from these and similar studies eventually led to the removal of this style of closed-loop, anterior chamber intraocular lenses from the market.[82]

Modern anterior chamber intraocular lenses with an open design with relatively broad haptics have led to a decrease in anterior segment inflammation associated with anterior chamber intraocular lenses. In addition, modern lens finishing techniques and quality control have resulted in a marked improvement in the finish of intraocular lenses.[76]

Anterior chamber intraocular lenses are responsible for most postoperative UGH syndromes. However, posterior chamber intraocular lenses have been associated with inflammation secondary to contact between the posterior iris and the intraocular lens. Johnson and coauthors[83] reported on a group of patients who were noted to have microhyphemas with associated iris transillumination defects, which were thought to be secondary to posterior iris chafing. Other authors have described similar findings of posterior iris chafing in patients with posterior chamber intraocular lenses that also had some associated pigmentary glaucoma, possibly caused by the intraocular lens/iris contact.[84,85] Iris chafing with a posterior chamber intraocular lens may also lead to intermittent episodes of decreased vision with either white blood cells or red blood cells leaking into the anterior chamber. This was called the intermittent visual white-out syndrome in patients with iris-plane intraocular lenses.[86] The incidence of these complications due to posterior iris chafing is fortunately low and generally only seen with nonangulated sulcus-fixated intraocular lenses. The incidence should decrease even more in the future with increasing placement of a posterior chamber intraocular lens within the capsular bag.

A final cause of anterior segment inflammation secondary to an intraocular lens that has been reported is anterior segment ischemia caused by erosion of a posterior chamber intraocular lens loop into the ciliary body. Apple and coauthors[87] describe a patient with anterior segment inflammation and an anterior segment ischemic syndrome that resulted from a posterior chamber intraocular lens loop, which eroded deeply into the ciliary sulcus occluding the major arterial circle of the iris. The subsequent anterior segment ischemia resulted in a severe anterior uveitis.

BIOCOMPATIBILITY OF LENS POLYMERS. The biocompatibility of various polymers used in the manufacture of intraocular lens components has been extensively covered in the literature.[3,88,89] At the present time, most of the commonly used polymers in intraocular lenses including PMMA, polypropylene, and various silicones appear to be relatively well tolerated within the eye. There is no direct evidence in the literature that various intraocular lens polymers directly cause postoperative inflammation.

The most common polymer in the manufacture of intraocular lens optics is PMMA. Various types of PMMA have been used as a lens material during the past 40 years, and PMMA has been shown to have excellent long-term biocompatibility within the eye after cataract surgery.[3,89] PMMA has not been shown to cause postoperative inflammation directly, and there is also no evidence of any surface degradation of PMMA within the eye.

Intraocular lens haptics have used several different materials throughout the period of evolution of intraocular lens designs. Nylon was initially used in the manufacture of various intraocular lens haptics. Drews and coauthors[90] initially described signs of surface degradation of nylon intraocular lens loops. This was especially prominent in areas of uveal contact. Studies at the University of Utah confirmed these findings of extensive intraocular surface degradation of nylon intraocular lens loops.[88] Although the nylon material itself was not shown to directly cause intraocular inflammation, this material was abandoned due to the surface degradation.

Polypropylene has been used extensively in the manufacture of intraocular lens haptics. Clayman[91] reviewed this material in 1981 and reported that polypropylene was relatively inert within the eye. An extensive review at the University of Utah[88] noted signs of superficial degradation of polypropylene loops. This was noted mainly in areas along the haptic that had been in direct contact with the uveal material for greater than 2 years' time. Once again, there has been no direct evidence that this small superficial degradation directly causes postoperative inflammation after cataract surgery. Furthermore, the present trend toward capsular bag fixation of posterior chamber intraocular lenses helps minimize any direct uveal contact with the intraocular lens haptic by sequestering them within the capsular bag. At the present time, most manufacturers have moved toward a one-piece posterior chamber intraocular lens design with haptics composed of PMMA.

The biocompatibility, manufacturing, and design of soft intraocular lens materials, such as silicone and hydrogel, have been reviewed at length.[3] There have been no clinical reports of major anterior segment toxicity that has been directly related to either modern silicone or hydrogel lenses. Christ and coauthors[92] have developed a detailed methodology for evaluating elastomeric silicone biomaterials used for intraocular lens implantation. They extensively reviewed the chemical, optical, and mechanical properties important in the characterization of elastomeric small-incision intraocular lens materials. These techniques are useful in evaluating the biocompatibility of soft intraocular lens materials. Chirila and coauthors[93] have reviewed the toxic effects of various hydrogel materials. They found that fully polymerized hydrogel materials were found to be safe with in vitro testing.

Irrigating Solutions and Intraocular Medications

Acute anterior segment inflammation in patients after cataract extraction with intraocular lens insertion may be noted in the immediate postoperative period. This acute anterior segment inflammation may be due to a toxic reaction as a result of one of the many intraocular solutions, medications, as well as additives and preservatives that are used during cataract surgery. Assessing the exact cause of this acute anterior segment inflammation is often difficult.

PRESERVATIVES. Preservatives used in various ophthalmic solutions are a potential source of anterior segment toxicity after cataract surgery.[94] Benzalkonium is used as a preservative in many topical drops. Although this material is not used in intraocular solutions, accidental injection or leakage of topical drops into the anterior segment may occur. Intraocular benzalkonium is highly toxic to the anterior segment.[95] Bisulfite is used as a stabilizer in certain formulations of epinephrine. This material is toxic to the corneal endothelium[96] and may cause diffuse anterior segment toxicity if this preserved epinephrine is accidentally irrigated into the anterior chamber. Dilute intracardiac or nonpreserved epinephrine, which is commonly mixed with balanced salt solution (BSS) in routine cataract surgery might be toxic to the corneal endothelium.[97] Finally, ethylenediaminetetraacetic acid (EDTA) is used as a stabilizer for various topical and intraocular medications. Fortunately, this material is not used in any intraocular solutions.

DISINFECTANTS. Various disinfectants used preoperatively to sterilize the skin around the eye may be toxic to the cornea and the anterior segment of the eye if they gain access to the eye during surgery. MacRae and coauthors[98] have reviewed the corneal toxicity of various presurgical skin antiseptics. The antiseptic chlorhexidine has been shown to have various toxic effects on both the corneal epithelium and endothelium.[99] Corneal edema with permanent endothelial damage has been reported secondary to accidental exposure of the eye to a chlorhexidine detergent preparation.[100] We are aware of three cases of permanent corneal damage in our own area resulting from chlorhexidine, so this is a much more common problem than reported. Thus, care must be taken when preparing the eye for surgery to insure that toxic disinfectants used around the eye do not gain access to the anterior segment of the globe.

BALANCED SALT SOLUTION. Intraocular irrigating solutions such as BSS are used extensively during both the phacoemulsification and irrigation/aspiration phase of cataract surgery. The effects of intraocular irrigating solutions on the corneal endothelium, as well as their toxicity, have been studied extensively in the past.[101–103] Changes or irregularities in various parameters such as pH, chemical composition, or osmolality of BSS solutions, could result in anterior segment inflammation as well as corneal endothelial cell, iris, and trabecular meshwork damage. Abnormalities in pH or ionic composition of irrigating solutions used during cataract surgery have been shown to cause significant adverse effects to the corneal endothelium.[104] Several cases of severe anterior segment inflammation after cataract surgery in the past were found to be due to an increase in the pH of the balanced salt solution used during cataract surgery.[105] Furthermore, episodes of unexplained postoperative inflammation and corneal edema were found to be secondary to a toxic substance within the seal around the port where the irrigating line was inserted into the BSS solution (Olson RJ, University of Utah, personal communication, July 1993).

Various different changes in the composition of BSS have been formulated to increase the tolerance of the corneal endothelium to the solutions. A study compared BSS to BSS+ and found a significant increase in corneal thickness one hour after BSS irrigation was instilled into the anterior chamber. However, only minimal changes were seen after BSS+ was used as an irrigating solution regardless of irrigation time.[103] No study to date has verified whether this difference is of clinical significance for routine anterior segment cases, however.

MIOTIC AGENTS. Miotic agents are often used at the conclusion of the cataract surgery to constrict the pupil. Miochol (1% acetylcholine chloride) may possibly cause injuries in both endothelial cell function and ultrastructure which could result in transient corneal edema. The effects of intraocular acetylcholine and carbachol on the anterior segment of the eye have also been compared.[107] The clinical significance of these effects of intraocular miotics on the corneal endothelium are unclear. Although controversial work has been presented that intraocular carbachol (Miostat) promotes a prolonged breakdown of the aqueous–iris barrier and increased inflammation compared to Miochol,[108] the clinical significance of this is not clear at present.

ANTIBIOTICS. Intraocular antibiotics are a potential source for postoperative anterior segment inflammation. Gentamicin has been shown to be a potential cause of retinal toxicity when it is inadvertently injected intraocularly in high doses.[109,110] Case reports of intraocular gentamicin toxicity after cataract surgery have been reported that were thought to be due to an inappropriate intraocular injection of gentamicin after the surgery.[111] Campochiaro and coauthors[112] have reported findings of aminoglycoside toxicity in a survey of retinal specialists. Of interest, there were twenty cases of macular infarction reported in association with prophylactic use of gentamicin after anterior segment surgery. In most cases, the presumed mechanism was an inadvertent intraocular injection. However, at least two of the cases were believed to have been associated with leakage of gentamicin into the eye through the cataract wound after subconjunctival injection without ocular penetration. Thus, leakage of subconjunctival antibiotics into the anterior chamber after their injection at the conclusion of cataract surgery is also a potential source of inflammation. To the best of our knowledge, this still has not been documented well in the literature.

VISCOELASTICS. Acute anterior segment inflammation after cataract surgery has also been attributed to reactions to viscoelastics. Kim[113] described several patients who developed acute anterior uveitis with subsequent pseudophakic bullous keratopathy after cataract surgery. He attributed this inflammation to residual denatured sodium hyaluronate viscoelastic, which was injected into the anterior chamber after sterilization of reusable cannulas. Furthermore, Sutphin and Papadimus[114] described seven patients who developed postoperative anterior segment toxicity and corneal edema. Once again, the cause of this postoperative inflammation was found to be due to denatured viscoelastic material after sterilization of a reusable cannula. In contrast to these findings, Ohguro and coauthors[115] found that neither heat-denatured, nor intact or untreated sodium hyaluronate alone had any adverse effect on the corneal endothelium in cats. They found that preservatives or chemical contaminants mixed with sodium hyaluronate caused substantial endothelial morphologic changes in these cat eyes which resulted in corneal edema. The use of disposable cannulas should help alleviate any problems due to residual or denatured viscoelastic material or any other residue or preservative found in reusable cannulas.

When a chondroitin sulfate–hyaluronic acid combination was first used, there were reported cases of rapid onset of band keratopathy. This problem was resolved by decreasing the phosphate buffer concentration.[116] Soon afterward, however, the same combination was pulled off the market for unexplained inflammation. Although the problem was resolved, the cause was never explained which underscores the sensitivity of the eye to any inflammatory substance.

Sterilization of Instruments and Tubing

Detergent or enzyme residues after sterilization of reusable instruments and tubing are potential sources of anterior segment inflammation after cataract surgery. Nuyts and coauthors[117] reported a series of patients who had acute corneal decompensation after routine cataract surgery. This was found likely to be secondary to a detergent residue within reusable intraocular irrigating cannulas. Breebaart and coauthors[118] have coined the term "toxic endothelial cell destruction" for this syndrome of patients who had corneal decompensation after cataract surgery. They attributed the findings in their patients to a 10-fold increase of detergent concentration in the ultrasonic cleaning solution used to clean their instruments. These patients were characterized by severe endothelial cell damage in the immediate postoperative period with endothelial cell loss leading to acute corneal decompensation. A further laboratory evaluation by this same group of authors[119] found that a combination of a 4% detergent solution in the ultrasound cleaning apparatus combined with insufficient flushing caused detergent remnants to remain in the narrow lumen of the cannulas used for ocular surgery.

Endotoxin contamination of sterilized instruments has also been shown to cause postoperative anterior segment inflammation. Richburg and coauthors[120] reported several patients who developed a sterile hypopyon in the immediate postoperative period after uncomplicated cataract surgery. Careful analysis of the rate of inflammation revealed that the instruments were being placed into an ultrasound cleaning solution which was contaminated by the end of each week. The instruments were found to have a heat-stable endotoxin that remained on them despite the autoclave process. Furthermore, Kreisler and coauthors[121] described a series of patients with increased anterior segment inflammation on the first postoperative day after cataract extraction. An analysis of the cause of this inflammation revealed that the ultrasound cleaning bath and the liquid detergent used to clean the instruments were contaminated by *Klebsiella pneumoniae* bacteria. This bacteria produced a heat-stable endotoxin that remained on the instruments after cleaning and sterilization, causing the postoperative inflammation. Daily changing of ultrasound bath solutions before sterilization as well as careful attention to the ultrasound bath itself should help alleviate this cause of anterior segment inflammation.

Particulate Contaminants

Particulate contaminants are sometimes suspected as a cause for postoperative inflammation. Talc has been mentioned as a potential source of postoperative inflammation after cataract surgery. Bene and Kranias[122] have reported a case of a patient with iritis postoperatively who was noted to have deposits on the surface of the intraocular lens that were thought to be secondary to contamination by surgical glove powder. On occasion, titanium flecks thought to be from the phacoemulsification tip have been found in the anterior chamber of an eye with an unexplained postoperative inflammation (Olson RJ, University of Utah, personal communication, July 1993). Also, fibers from either cotton or cloth used during cataract surgery have been noted in the anterior segment of eyes with unexplained inflammation. Whether or not these fibers are directly responsible for any of the anterior segment inflammation is unclear. An additional potential source of intraocular contamination is that of "coring." Ullman and coauthors[123] have noted several cases of a core of rubber stopper being pushed into the ocular irrigating solution when the plastic spike for the infusion line was inserted. Although this was not noted to cause any problems during the surgeries, this coring is a potential source for contamination.

Toxic Anterior Segment Syndrome

Finally, there is on occasion an acute anterior segment inflammation after uncomplicated cataract extraction with implantation of an intraocular lens in which no cause for the inflammation can be found. We have reported three unrelated cases of this inflammation from our center, which we have named the toxic anterior segment syndrome (TASS).[124,125] These patients were found to have signs of an acute anterior segment toxic reaction that was associated with diffuse corneal endothelial damage and edema as well as signs of iris damage with a fixed or dilated pupil. These patients also developed a secondary glaucoma. The inflammatory process was not the result of an endophthalmitis. An extensive work-up in these patients did not find any specific cause for the TASS syndrome.

One of the most important factors in evaluating postoperative patients who present with a presumed sterile postoperative inflammation or toxic reaction is to rule out a true infectious endophthalmitis. Although the constellation of symptoms and findings for these patients is usually distinct from that of an infectious endophthalmitis, there is extensive overlap in presentation. Aqueous and vitreous taps must be performed to rule out endophthalmitis if there is any question of an infectious cause. Patients with a true, noninfectious postoperative inflammation may be treated with a course of intense postoperative corticosteroids and followed closely. The sterile hypopyon and other anterior segment inflammation changes should begin to clear relatively rapidly after institution of this treatment. Sterile uveitis patients who show signs of recurrence of anterior segment inflammation after taper of corticosteroids should raise suspicion for another cause of their inflammation. Chronic or recurrent anterior segment inflammatory etiologies include chronic bacterial endophthalmitis, *Propionibacterium acnes* endophthalmitis, or possibly phacoanaphylactic endophthalmitis.

Cases of acute postoperative anterior segment inflammation after cataract surgery in which an infectious cause has been ruled out should be worked up for a possible toxic cause. Intraocular solutions, medications, or any other materials used during the cataract surgery should be saved, if at all possible. If the actual solutions used during the surgery have been discarded, samples from closely related batches or lot numbers should be taken and analyzed. A careful analysis of all of the operative procedures from sterilization of the instruments to mixing an injection of intraocular solution should then be undertaken. The actual surgical procedure, including all nursing and anesthesia notes should also be analyzed.

Careful analysis and reporting of all outbreaks of postoperative inflammation after cataract surgery will help to define possible etiologies and avoid complications from these problems in the future.

Inflammation Related to Residual Lens Cortex

Phacoanaphylactic Endophthalmitis

Chronic postoperative inflammation after cataract surgery may be due to inflammation related to residual lens cortex. This entity has been termed phacoanaphylactic endophthalmitis. The signs and symptoms, diagnosis, and treatment of this entity have been reviewed extensively in the existing literature.[126–131]

This entity was originally described in the literature by Verhoeff and Lemoine[130] who called it "endophthalmitis phaco-anaphylactica" and postulated that this reaction was a hypersensitivity to the patient's own lens protein after cataract rupture. In 1952, Irvine and Irvine[132] described the entity of phacoanaphylactic endophthalmitis as a sterile, granulomatous inflammatory reaction to retained lens cortex. Furthermore, Rahi and Garner[129] thought that the "phacoanaphylaxis" was not accurate because of the fact that there is no evidence of IgG involvement in this entity. Disruption of the normally intact lens capsule because of trauma or surgery can expose lens proteins, which are normally sequestered, to the immune system, which may lead to a chronic inflammation.

At the present time, the incidence of phacoanaphylactic endophthalmitis is not well known. Phacoanaphylaxis was not noted in the era of intracapsular cataract extraction. With the transition from intracapsular to extracapsular cataract extraction, there were several reports of phacoanaphylactic endophthalmitis.[126–128] There also has been an isolated case report of phacoanaphylactic endophthalmitis after phacoemulsification.[133]

The clinical course of phacoanaphylactic endophthalmitis is relatively indolent. The onset of the inflammation occurs most commonly between 1 and 14 days after surgical disruption of the lens capsule. The inflammation is characterized by a waxing and waning granulomatous-type of inflammation, which may initially respond to corticosteroid treatment.[126–128] Histologically, phacoanaphylactic endophthalmitis is characterized by a zonal granulomatous inflammatory reaction around the lens remnant. The central part of the reaction is characterized by polymorphonuclear cells that are surrounded by concentric layers of epithelioid and giant cells, and, finally, lymphocytes and plasma cells. The adjacent iris and ciliary body may also show an infiltrate of mononuclear inflammatory cells. Once an infectious cause is completely ruled out, and the diagnosis of phacoanaphylactic endophthalmitis is most likely, the treatment is surgical removal of the intraocular lens and any remaining lens cortex and capsule. Surgical removal of the lens and capsular remnants, along with aggressive corticosteroid treatment, should help quiet the inflammation.[128]

INFLAMMATION AFTER POSTERIOR SEGMENT SURGERY

Retina–Vitreous Surgery

Retinal detachments are the most common reason requiring retinal–vitreous surgery. Retinal detachments are the end result of a separation of the sensory retina from the underlying retinal pigment epithelium. There are many different causes of retinal detachments; however, there are three major types of retinal detachments: (1) rhegmatogenous retinal detachments that are caused by a tear or hole in the retina; (2) traction retinal detachments that are a result of traction to the retina from the vitreous or fibrous tissue proliferation which pulls on the surface of the retina, detaching it from the retinal pigment epithelium; (3) exudative retinal detachments that are caused by fluid exudation into the subretinal space from various retinal vascular or choroidal diseases, such as intraocular inflammation, vascular abnormalities, or tumors.[134] The repair of retinal detachments varies depending on the cause and the findings noted in the individual patient. Surgical repair of retinal detachment may include scleral buckling, vitrectomy with or without injection of gas or silicone, and adjunct cryotherapy or laser therapy.[135–139]

As with any anterior segment surgery, surgery within the posterior segment of the globe may elicit an inflammatory cell reaction that can lead to a compromise in the success of the surgery in various patients. There are several intraoperative complications that may also lead to increase in postoperative inflammation, such as vitreous hemorrhage, further retinal breaks or perforations, and a general breakdown of the blood–retinal barrier. Postoperative inflammation after retina–vitreous surgery with breakdown of the blood–retinal barrier contributes greatly to some of the most common postoperative complications seen after this surgery.

Proliferative Vitreoretinopathy

Proliferative vitreoretinopathy, an excessive wound-healing response to rhegmatogenous retinal detachment, is the most common cause of failed retinal detachment repair.[140,141] Vitreoretinal traction may prevent closure of the retinal break and reapposition of the retina to the retinal pigment epithelium, leading to a recurrence of the retinal detachment.[134] This proliferative retinopathy often requires secondary surgery with further vitrectomy therapy as well as further manipulation of the posterior segment of the globe which may lead to an ever-increasing inflammatory cell reaction. Ryan[142] in his Jackson Memorial lecture, has presented an outline of the final common pathway for the pathogenesis of tractional retinal detachments in trauma, proliferative vitreoretinopathy, and proliferative diabetic retinopathy. He found that the common feature in all of these conditions is the breakdown of the blood–retinal barrier that is associated with or leads to an inflammatory response including an infiltrate of leukocytes. He further states that "serum factors that leak from the vessels and cytokines released by the leukocytes, particularly macrophages and monocytes, cause proliferation and migration of retinal cells that form cellular membranes, the contraction of which exerts tractional forces on the retina." Ryan further delineates the final common pathway for tractional retinal detachments into five distinct steps[142]:

> Step One: An underlying disease process or inciting event leads to an inflammatory response that affects the posterior segment of the eye.
>
> Step Two: The resultant breakdown of the blood/retinal barrier, combined with abnormal vitreous, initiates the wound-healing response.
>
> Step Three: The migration and proliferation of cells within the posterior segment is a key element.
>
> Step Four: When these cells attain a critical mass, such that forces of contraction exceed the forces of attachment of the sensory retina, then tractional retinal detachment occurs.
>
> Step Five: When traction detachment begins, the detachment itself leads to further breakdown of the blood/retinal barrier and inflammation that leads to acceleration of the process with further retinal detachment in a vicious cycle.

One of the main underlying events that leads to this final common pathway for proliferative vitreoretinopathy is inflammation with breakdown of the blood–retinal barrier. This inflammation then leads to the release of extracellular factors that can lead to the migration and proliferation of cells that form contract membranes, which ultimately results in tractional forces that detach the retina.[143,144] Once this initial inflammatory process begins with breakdown of the blood–retinal barrier and release of inflammatory mediators, there is a migration and proliferation of various cells within the eye. This can include retinal pigment epithelial cells, glial cells, fibroblasts, myofibroblasts, and endothelial cells. All of these cells can migrate and proliferate, eventually leading to the laying down of extracellular matrix material including collagen.[142] The final result of this cellular proliferation and laying down of collagen is proliferative vitreoretinopathy with tractional forces on the retina from the many cellular membranes causing recurrent retinal detachments.

Proliferative vitreoretinopathy may occur both anterior and posterior to the insertion of the vitreous base. A complete review of the management of proliferative vitreoretinopathy is beyond the scope of this chapter. Aaberg[144] has extensively reviewed the management of anterior and posterior proliferative vitreoretinopathy in his Jackson Memorial lecture. In addition, Lopez and coauthors[145] have reviewed the pathogenetic mechanisms in proliferative vitreoretinopathy. Both visual and anatomic success rates have improved steadily over the past decade with advances in vitreoretinal surgical techniques and adjunct methods of obtaining intraocular tamponade, such as air, expansile gas, and silicone. Research is presently being done on ways to decrease the proliferative process after posterior segment surgery. Because inflammation with breakdown of the blood–retinal barrier is a major inciting factor in proliferative vitreoretinopathy, research into the reduction of this reactive inflammatory cell process that stimulates the cellular proliferation in the first place is important.

Preretinal Membrane Formation

Ocular inflammation after posterior segment surgery may also lead to a mild cellular proliferation on the surface of the macula forming a preretinal or epiretinal membrane on the surface of the macula. Epiretinal membranes have been previously reported to occur in approximately 8% of eyes after retinal detachment repair.[146] However, a histopathologic study of the effects of retinal detachment surgery on postmortem eyes by Wilson and Green[147] found that epiretinal membranes were present in approximately 75% of the eyes studied post mortem, and in 30.6% of these eyes these membranes caused some degree of macular pucker. Macular pucker from wrinkling of these epiretinal membranes may cause distortion of vision or metamorphopsia as well as decreased visual acuity in general. It is thought that epiretinal membranes occur as the result of cellular proliferation on the surface of the macula and may represent a mild form of proliferative retinopathy.[134] If the epiretinal membrane has caused a significant decrease in postoperative visual acuity, vitrectomy with pealing of the premacular membrane may successfully improve vision in this group of patients.[148]

Cystoid Macular Edema

Cystoid macular edema is a complication after posterior segment surgery caused by leakage of the parafoveal capillaries with subsequent accumulation of extracellular fluid around the macula, which may result in decreased visual acuity. Once again, inflammation after surgery is thought to be a major contributing factor in the development of cystoid macular edema with breakdown of the blood–retinal barrier in the area of the parafoveal capillaries. Cystoid macular edema is a relatively common complication after retinal detachment associated with retinal–vitreous surgery of any type. Several reports have assessed the incidence of cystoid macular edema after retinal detachment repair. The rate of cystoid macular edema postoperatively ranges from 9% to 25% phakic eyes and 29% to 64% aphakic eyes after retinal detachment repair.[149–151] A histopathologic study on the effects of retinal detachment in globes studied post mortem revealed that there was a 10.2% incidence of cystoid macular edema in these eyes.[147] The therapy for cystoid macular edema is similar to cystoid macular edema after cataract surgery. This includes surgical therapy as well as therapy with drug preparations, which can be used either topically or orally and include steroids, nonsteroidal antiinflammatories, or even carbonic anhydrase inhibitors.[152]

OCULAR SEQUELAE OF POSTOPERATIVE INFLAMMATION

Chronic postoperative inflammation or infection may ultimately lead to a large variety of ocular complications. The ocular sequelae of chronic uveitis and endophthalmitis have been thoroughly outlined in several ophthalmic textbooks.[153,154] It is once again beyond the scope of this chapter to discuss the various sequelae of ocular inflammation in depth. However, it is important to briefly review some of the more common ocular consequences of surgically-induced inflammation.

Cornea

The corneal endothelium is sensitive to inflammatory insults of any kind, including anterior segment surgery, especially cataract extraction with insertion of an iris-fixated, anterior chamber intraocular lens.[75–89] Chronic breakdown of the blood–aqueous barrier after anterior segment surgery may lead to chronic inflammatory complications such as the UGH syndrome. Anterior segment inflammation or glaucoma, as well as mechanical damage to the endothelium from an intraocular lens, may lead to endothelial damage, which may result in chronic stromal and epithelial edema. This leads to the condition of bullous keratopathy. Multiple studies have documented an increase in the incidence of pseudophakic bullous keratopathy since the late 1970s and throughout the 1980s.[155–159] A large study from our laboratory at the University of Utah[160] found that pseudophakic bullous keratopathy was the most common indication for penetrating keratoplasty in each year from 1984 through 1989 with a peak in 1987. Since that time, the incidence of pseudophakic bullous keratopathy cases has decreased. This decreasing incidence of bullous keratopathy may reflect the discontinued use of closed-loop, anterior chamber, and iris-plane intraocular lenses most commonly associated with this complication.

Among the many problems associated with chronic bullous keratopathy are decreased vision, pain, and possible infections. Ruptured bullae may become infected secondarily, which can lead to the formation of a corneal ulcer. In addition, chronic inflammation after ocular surgery of any kind can lead to possible vascularization of the cornea or band keratopathy with deposition of calcium beneath the corneal epithelium along Bowman layer in eyes that have been chronically inflamed. The causes of corneal decompensation after ocular surgery are related to either direct or indirect damage to the corneal endothelium. Anterior segment surgery may lead to direct intraoperative trauma to the corneal endothelium. Contact with surgical instruments or contact with implants, such as an intraocular lens or glaucoma seton, may directly injure endothelial cells. Direct contact between an intraocular lens and the surface of the endothelium may lead to a loss of endothelial cells.

The corneal endothelium may be further damaged by solutions or medications used during ocular surgery, as mentioned previously. Changes in the pH or the osmolality of irrigating fluids used in surgery may cause direct toxic effects to the corneal endothelium. In addition, various medications, additives, and disinfectants and preservatives may also cause direct damage to the corneal endothelium.

Mechanical factors related to intraocular lenses may also contribute to endothelial loss which can lead to corneal decompensation. These factors include improper sizing of an anterior chamber intraocular lens, poor lens position, and lens dislocation. Even properly sized and placed iris-fixated intraocular lenses have been found to lead to the so-called intermittent touch syndrome as described by Drews.[161] This syndrome of intermittent touch may lead to chronic inflammation, corneal changes that lead to edema, and cystoid macular edema. Anterior chamber lenses which were found to vault excessively, such as the closed-loop anterior chamber lenses,[162] were also found to cause intermittent touch and mechanical damage to the lens epithelium.

The most likely cause of pseudophakic bullous keratopathy occurring several years after the implantation of an iris-fixated or closed-loop, anterior chamber intraocular lens is due to chronic low-grade inflammation. Several of the closed-loop, anterior chamber intraocular lenses that were popular in the early 1980s were associated with a chronic low-grade UGH syndrome.[79–81] Chronic low-grade inflammation in this group of lenses was likely the cause of late-onset pseudophakic bullous keratopathy, as well as chronic cystoid macular edema, in these patients.[3,89] It was many of these complications that led to the withdrawal of the closed-loop style anterior chamber intraocular lenses from the market in 1987.[82]

Chronic inflammation leading to decompensation of the cornea may lead to other secondary complications. Corneas may show vascularization of the surface or scarring from chronic inflammation. In addition, ruptured bullae from chronic corneal edema may lead to corneal ulcer formation if they become secondarily infected. Severe corneal ulceration may lead to localized melting and frank perforation of the cornea with subsequent endophthalmitis or loss of vision. Finally, chronic inflammation of any kind in the anterior segment of the eye may lead to band keratopathy. This condition is characterized by a deposition of calcium beneath the corneal endothelium along Bowman layer.

Anterior Chamber

Chronic inflammation after ocular surgery may lead to a long-term breakdown of the blood–aqueous barrier. The chronic inflammatory cell reaction in the anterior chamber may lead to organization of the products of inflammation or chronic hemorrhage, leading to membrane formation in the anterior chamber. A retrocorneal fibrous membrane may form postoperatively, especially after penetrating keratoplasty. Retrocorneal or pupillary membranes may form as a result of organization of inflammatory cells and byproducts as well as through fibrous metaplasia or proliferation of cells within the eye secondary to chronic inflammation. Organized inflammatory fibrous membranes, as well as chronic hemorrhage, within the anterior chamber resulting from inflammation may close off or clog the anterior chamber angle, leading to chronic glaucoma.

Iris

The iris may undergo atrophic or necrotic changes as a result of chronic inflammation or mechanical changes. Iris chafing, erosion, and pigment dispersion have been noted secondary to the mechanical effects of intraocular lenses, especially poorly designed and finished iris-fixated and early anterior chamber intraocular lenses. Furthermore, chronic iris chafing leads to increased subsequent inflammation secondary to chronic breakdown of the blood–aqueous barrier with release of inflammatory cells and mediators into the anterior chamber. Recurrent microhyphemas within the anterior chamber, as well as pigment dispersion, may also add to these secondary inflammatory complications of the iris.

Synechia formation with adhesions of the iris to the peripheral cornea or to the intraocular lens or capsular remnants may occur as a result of chronic inflammation after ocular surgery. Peripheral anterior synechia may result from chronic irritation by lens loops or a footplate within the anterior chamber in the area of the angle. Synechia formation around many of the small diameter, round, closed-loop, anterior chamber intraocular lenses was noted commonly. Posterior synechia with adhesions between the iris and either lens capsular remnants, or posterior chamber intraocular lenses, or anterior lens capsule, may lead to seclusion of the pupil. A total posterior synechia or seclusion may cause pupillary block with subsequent forward bowing of the iris or iris bombé and subsequent pupillary block glaucoma. This may also result in secondary closed-angle glaucoma because of peripheral anterior synechia formation. Finally, chronic inflammatory changes after ocular surgery may lead to formation of fibrous membranes, either on the surface of the iris, or across the pupillary border or the pupillary space, forming a pupillary occlusion.

Ciliary Body

Chronic inflammation in the anterior or posterior segment of the globe may affect the ciliary body in several different ways. Chronic breakdown of the blood–aqueous barrier or chronic inflammatory cell insult made lead to membrane formation. A chronic inflammatory cell reaction in the posterior chamber may lead to organization and fibrosis behind the crystalline lens or intraocular lens and may extend posteriorly to the area of the vitreous base. A fibrous membrane in this area involving the pars plicata and extending posteriorly to the pars plana is termed a cyclitic membrane. Further organization and fibrosis of this cyclitic membrane may lead to contraction and shrinkage with detachment of the ciliary body as well as some of the peripheral retina. In addition, chronic intraocular inflammation may also lead to degeneration of the ciliary epithelium. Detachment of the ciliary body, as well as ciliary body degeneration, may lead to decreased production of aqueous humor and eventually to hypotony of the globe.

Retina/Vitreous

Cystoid Macular Edema

Cystoid macular edema is a retinal complication that can occur after all types of intraocular surgical procedures, both anterior and posterior. Cystoid macular edema is associated with disruption of the blood–aqueous barrier.[163,164] This disruption leads to increased vascular permeability in the parafoveal capillaries, which can lead to significant macular edema. Miyake[23] and Miyake and associates[164] have extensively reviewed the involvement of prostaglandins and other cyclooxygenase products in the pathogenesis of cystoid macular edema. Prostaglandins are produced mostly in the anterior segment of the eye (ie, the iris) in response to surgical trauma and are thought to accumulate within the eye because of damage to the tissues that normally affect the active transport of prostaglandins from ocular compartments. These prostaglandins may induce an increased vascular permeability with disruption of the blood–retinal barrier, which may lead to cystoid macular edema. A breakdown of the blood–aqueous barrier may lead to accumulation of inflammatory mediators, which then further disrupt the blood–retinal barrier posteriorly in the parafoveal and peridisc capillaries leading to leakage of fluid in these areas. Furthermore, there has been shown to be a mechanical component to cystoid macular edema after anterior segment surgery in which there is a direct effect of traction from the vitreous on the macula after removal of the crystalline lens. The end result of all of this is the accumulation of edema forming microcysts in the outer plexiform layer of Henle around the macula.

The incidence of macular edema after cataract surgery has been extensively reviewed in the literature. Stark and coauthors[165] initially presented an extensive review of cystoid macular edema in pseudophakia. In addition, Davidorf also presented an extensive review of pseudophakic cystoid macular edema in 1983.[24] There are several common findings in these earlier reviews of pseudophakic cystoid macular edema. It has been consistently shown that angiographically proven cases of cystoid macular edema are significantly higher in patients who had previously undergone intracapsular cataract extraction rather than extracapsular cataract extraction. In addition, complications occurring at the time of surgery, such as loss of vitreous or rupture of the posterior capsule, are important in the pathogenesis of cystoid macular edema. A third important factor in the development of cystoid macular edema postoperatively is the status of the patient's vascular and immune system. The presence of preexisting diseases that can affect the vascular system within the eye, such as uveitis and retinovascular disorders, are important.[152] Other factors, such as the type of intraocular lens used after cataract surgery and medications used both intraocularly and topically during the surgery, have also been implicated in postoperative cystoid macular edema.[12]

The treatment of cystoid macular edema includes various surgical and medical therapies. Wilkinson[152] provides a brief review of the surgical and medical options available for the treatment of cystoid macular edema. If there are obvious areas of incarcerated vitreous, surgical therapy to remove the vitreous, either using an anterior or posterior vitrectomy or an Nd:YAG laser vitreolysis, is helpful. Certain types of intraocular lenses, such as iris-fixated or closed-loop anterior chamber intraocular lenses, which are known to cause chronic inflammation may also require removal or exchange of the intraocular lens for treatment of cystoid macular edema.[3]

Medical therapy for cystoid macular edema has included the use of corticosteroids used topically, periocularly, and orally. More important, nonsteroidal antiinflammatory agents have been used to treat cystoid macular edema because of the suspected influence of prostaglandins on the breakdown of the blood–aqueous barrier, eventually leading to cystoid macular edema. Nonsteroidal inflammatory agents that inhibit the cyclooxygenase pathway leading to decreased production of prostaglandins have been shown to be helpful in the treatment of cystoid macular edema. Indomethacin was one of the first such pharmacologic methods used in the treatment of postoperative cystoid macular edema.[23,166] New nonsteroidal antiinflammatory agents, such as ketorolac, have shown effectiveness in the treatment of chronic aphakic and pseudophakic cystoid macular edema.[167,168] Ketorolac tromethamine has been shown to decrease the postoperative inflammation by decreasing the breakdown of the blood–aqueous barrier postoperatively.[18,19] In addition, another nonsteroidal antiinflammatory agent, diclofenac, has also been shown to decrease the breakdown of the blood–aqueous barrier after surgery using fluorophotometry.[20]

Other therapies that have been used in an attempt to treat cystoid macular edema include the use of acetazolamide.[169] Patients with cystoid macular edema resulting from inflammatory or inherited outer retinal disorders had a positive response to therapy with this carbonic anhydrase inhibitor. Finally, Pfoff and coauthors[170] have reported on the use of hyperbaric oxygen therapy on patients with chronic established cystoid macular edema. Although several patients showed improvement after this intense regimen of treatment, vision tended to regress with time after cessation of the treatment.

Retina

Intraocular inflammation anywhere within the eye and after all types of ocular surgery may result in inflammatory sequelae involving the retina. These retinal sequelae from uveitis or chronic intraocular inflammation have been well summarized by Yanoff and Fine.[153] Intraocular inflammation may cause a lymphocytic infiltrate surrounding blood vessels in the retina, leading to a retinal perivasculitis. This perivasculitis can result in vascular sheathing with thickening of the blood vessel walls and organization and cicatrization of the perivascular inflammatory infiltrate. Any ocular inflammation may also lead to scarring of the retina that may extend into the choroid. Similarly, the retinal pigment epithelium may be involved in chronic inflammation and may show either hypertrophy or atrophy. In addition, the retinal pigment epithelium is susceptible to undergoing hyperplasia after inflammation which is commonly seen in the end-stage inflammatory eye characterized by phthisis bulbi. Finally, the retina may become detached secondary to traction from organized vitreous or cyclitic membranes. In addition, retinal detachment itself may lead to further scarring as characterized by proliferative retinopathy discussed previously.

Vitreous

The vitreous cavity itself may become involved after ocular inflammation with inflammatory cells in the vitreous leading to the condition called vitritis. Although the vitreous itself is avascular and does not contribute directly to complications of postoperative inflammation, the vitreous may be involved secondarily due to blood vessels growing into the vitreous or secondary hemorrhage within the vitreous cavity. Also, more important, inflammatory cells and inflammatory byproducts within the vitreous may lead to organization of the vitreous with secondary fibrous membrane formation. This organization of the vitreous may lead to traction on various ocular structures, such as the ciliary body and the retina, leading to detachment of these structures.

End-Stage Inflammatory Complications

Chronic intraocular inflammation that is severe and of long duration may lead to end-stage reactions within the globe.[153,154] The condition of atrophia bulbi is characterized by ocular atrophy with shrinkage. Long-standing hypotony secondary to inflammation causes the globe to become soft and shrunken. The globe takes on a squared-off appearance at this point. There is also atrophy of many of the intraocular structures within the globe.

The final step in end-stage chronic intraocular inflammation is the condition called phthisis bulbi. This entity is also characterized by chronic hypotony with shrinkage of the globe and thickening of the sclera. In addition to atrophy of the intraocular structures, there is disorganization with widespread scarring. Finally, there can be metaplasia of the retinal pigment epithelium, leading to intraocular bony formation in addition to the disorganization.

References

1. Miyake K. blood/retinal barrier in eyes with long-standing aphakia with apparently normal fundi. Arch Ophthalmol 1982;100:1437–1441.
2. Obstbaum SA. The Binkhorst Medal Lecture: biologic relationship between poly (methylmethacrylate) intraocular lenses and uveal tissue. J Cataract Refract Surg 1992;18:219–231.
3. Apple DJ, Mamalis N, Olson RJ, Kincaid MC. Intraoc-

ular lenses: evolution, designs, complications, and pathology. Baltimore, Williams & Wilkins, 1989.

4. Cunha-Vaz JG. The blood/ocular barriers. Surv Ophthalmol 1979;23:269–296.
5. Klebanoff SJ, Clark RA. The neutrophil: function in clinical disorders. Amsterdam, North-Holland, 1978.
6. Ambache N. Properties of irin, a physiologic constituent of the rabbit iris. J Physiol (London) 1957; 135:114–132.
7. Ambache N, Brummer HC. A simple chemical procedure for distinguishing E from F prostaglandins, with application to tissue abstracts. Br J Pharmacol 1968;33:162–170.
8. Eakins KE. Prostaglandin and non-prostaglandin mediated breakdown of the blood/aqueous barrier. Exp Eye Res 1977;25:483–498.
9. Kass MA, Holmberg NJ. Prostaglandin and thromboxane synthesis in microsomes of rabbit ocular tissue. Inv Ophthalmol Vis Sci 1979;18:166–169.
10. Bhattacherjee P, Kulkarnia PS, Eakins KE. Metabolism of arachidonic acid in rabbit ocular tissues. Inv Ophthalmol Vis Sci 1979;18:172–178.
11. Flowlse RJ. Lipocortins. In: Samuelsson B, Paoletti R, Ramwell P, eds. Advances in prostaglandin, thromboxane, and leukotriene research. New York, Raven Press, 1978:577–580.
12. Jampol LE, Sanders DR, Kraff MC. Prophylaxis and therapy of aphakic cystoid macular edema. Surv Ophthalmol 1984;28:535–539.
13. Kraff MC, Sanders DR, Jampol LM, et al. Prophylaxis of pseudophakic cystoid macular edema with topical indomethacin. Ophthalmol 1982;89:885–890.
14. Sanders DR, Kraff MC. Steroidal and nonsteroidal antiinflammatory agents: effects on post-surgical inflammation and blood/aqueous humor barrier breakdown. Arch Ophthalmol 1984;102:1453–1456.
15. Yannuzzi LA, Landau AU, Turtz AI. Incidence of aphakic cystoid macular edema with the use of topical indomethacin. Ophthalmol 1981;88:947–954.
16. Miyake K. Prevention of cystoid macular edema after lens extraction by topical indomethacin: I. A preliminary report. Graefes Arch Clin Exp Ophthalmol 1977;203:81–88.
17. Yannuzzi LA. A prospective on the treatment of aphakic cystoid macular edema. Surv Ophthalmol 1984; 28:540–553.
18. Flach AJ, Lavelle CJ, Olander KW, et al. The effect of ketorolac tromethamine solution 0.5% in reducing postoperative inflammation after cataract extraction and intraocular lens implantation. Ophthalmology 88;95:1280–1284.
19. Flach AJ, Kraff MC, Sanders DR, et al. Quantitative effect of 0.5% ketorolac tromethamine solution and 0.1% dexamethasone sodium phosphate solution on postsurgical blood/aqueous barrier. Arch Ophthalmol 1988;406:480–483.
20. Kraff MC, Sanders DR, McGuigan L, et al. Inhibition of blood/aqueous humor barrier breakdown with diclofenac: a fluorophotometric study. Arch Ophthalmol 1990;108:380–383.
21. Miyake K, Mibu H, Hariguchi M, et al. Inflammatory mediators in postoperative aphakic and pseudophakic baboon eyes. Arch Ophthalmol 1990;108:1764–1767.
22. Obstbaum SA, Galin MA. Cystoid macular edema and ocular inflammation: the corneo-retinal inflammatory syndrome. Trans Ophthalmol Soc UK 1979;99:187–191.
23. Miyake K. Indomethacin and the treatment of postoperative cystoid macular edema. Surv Ophthalmol 1984;28:554–568.
24. Davidorf FH. Pseudophakic cystoid macular edema. Ophthalmic Forum 1983;1:83.
25. The Miami Study Group. Cystoid macular edema in aphakic and pseudophakic eyes. Am J Ophthalmol 1979;88:45–48.
26. Jaffe NS, Clayman HM, Jaffe NS. Cystoid macular edema after intracapsular and extracapsular cataract extraction with and without an intraocular lens. Ophthalmology 1982;89:25–29.
27. Taylor DM, Sachs SW, Stern AL. Aphakic cystoid macular edema: long-term clinical observations. Surv Ophthalmol 1984;28:437–441.
28. Smith RT, Campbell CJ, Koester CJ, et al. The barrier function in extracapsular cataract surgery. Ophthalmology 1990;97:90–95.
29. Ohrloff C, Schlnus R, Rothe R, et al. Role of the posterior capsule in the aqueous/vitreous barrier in aphakic and pseudophakic eyes. J Cataract Refract Surg 1990;16:198–201.
30. Samuelsson B. Leukotrienes and related compounds. In: Hayashi O, Yamamato S, eds. Advances in prostaglandin, thromboxane and leukotriene research, vol 15. New York, Raven Press, 1985:1–9.
31. Bhattacherjee P, Hammond B, Salmon JA, et al. Chemotactic response to some arachidonic acid lipoxygenase products in the rabbit eye. Eur J Pharmacol 1981;73:21–28.
32. Serhan CN, Smolen JE, Korchak HM, et al. Leukotriene B4 is a complete secretagogue in human neutrophils: Ca^{+2} translocations in liposomes and kinetics of neutrophil activation. In: Samuelsson B, Paoletti R, Ramwell P, eds. Advances in prostaglandins, thromboxane and leukotriene research. New York, Raven Press, 1983:53–62.
33. Galin MA, Tuberville AW, Obstbaum SA, et al. Mechanism of implant failure. Trans Ophthalmol Soc UK 1980;100:229–230.

34. Galin MA, Goldstein IM, Tuberville AW, et al. Intraocular lenses generate chemotactic activity in human serum. Arch Ophthalmol 1981;99:1434–1435.
35. Tuberville AW, Galin MA, Perez HD, et al. Complement activation by nylon and polypropylene-looped prosthetic intraocular lenses. Inv Ophthalmol Vis Sci 1982;22:727–733.
36. Mondino BJ, Nagata S, Glovsky MM. Activation of the alternative complement pathway by intraocular lenses. Inv Ophthalmol Vis Sci 1985;26:905–908.
37. Gobel RJ, Janatova J, Googe SM, et al. Activation of complement in human serum by some synthetic polymers used for intraocular lenses. Biomaterials 1987;8:285–288.
38. Janatova J, Teck BF, Prahl JW. Third component of human complement: Structural requirements for its function. Biochemistry 1980;19:4479–4485.
39. Goldstein IM, Perez HD. Biologically active peptides derived from the fifth component of complement. In: Spaeth TH, ed. Progress in hemostasis and thrombosis, vol 5. New York, Grune & Stratton, 1980:41–79.
40. Serhan CN, Hambert M, Samuelsson B. Lipoxins: novel series of biologically active compounds formed from arachidonic acid in human leukocytes. Proc Natl Acad Sci USA 1984;81:5335–5339.
41. Driebe WT Jr, Mandelbaum S, Forster RK, Schwartz LK, et al. Pseudophakic endophthalmitis: diagnosis and management. Ophthalmology 1986;93:442–448.
42. Forster RK, Abbott RL, Gelender H. Management of infectious endophthalmitis. Ophthalmology 1980;87: 313–319.
43. Olk RJ, Bohigian GM. The management of endophthalmitis: diagnosis and therapeutic guidelines including the use of vitrectomy. Ophthalmic Surg 1987;18:262–267.
44. Olson JC, Flynn HW Jr, Forster RK, Culbertson WW. Results in the treatment of postoperative endophthalmitis. Ophthalmology 1983;90:692–699.
45. Stern GA, Engel HM, Driebe WT Jr. The treatment of postoperative endophthalmitis: the results of differing approaches to treatment. Ophthalmology 1989;96:62–67.
46. Zaidman GW, Mondino BJ. Postoperative pseudophakic bacterial endophthalmitis. Am J Ophthalmol 1982;93:218–223.
47. Stark WJ, Worthen DM, Holladay JT, et al. The FDA report on intraocular lenses. Ophthalmol 1983; 90:311–317.
48. Mosier MA, Lusk B, Pettit TH, et al. Fungal endophthalmitis following intraocular lens implantation. Am J Ophthalmol 1977;83:1–8.
49. Stern WH, Tamura E, Jacob RA, et al. Epidemic postsurgical *Candida parapsilosis* endophthalmitis: clinical findings and management of fifteen consecutive cases. Ophthalmology 1985;92:1701–1709.
50. Davis JL, Koidou-Tsiligianni A, Pflugfelder SC, et al. Coagulase-negative staphylococcal endophthalmitis: increase in antimicrobial resistance. Ophthalmology 1988;95:1404–1410.
51. Ficker L, Meredith TA, Wilson LA, Kaplan HJ, et al. Chronic bacterial endophthalmitis. Am J Ophthalmol 1987;103:745–748.
52. Schanzlin DJ, Golberg DB, Brown SI. *Staphylococcus epidermidis* endophthalmitis following intraocular lens implantation. Br J Ophthalmol 1980;64:684–686.
53. Meisler DM, Mandelbaum S. *Propionibacterium*–associated endophthalmitis after extracapsular cataract extraction: review of reported cases. Ophthalmology 1989;96:54–61.
54. Meisler DM, Palestine AG, Vastine DW, et al. Chronic propionibacterium endophthalmitis after extracapsular cataract extraction and intraocular lens implantation. Am J Ophthalmol 1986;102:733–739.
55. Piest KL, Kincaid MC, Tetz MR, et al. Localized endophthalmitis: a newly documented cause of toxic lens syndrome. J Cataract Refract Surg 1987;13: 498–510.
56. Smith RE. Inflammation after cataract surgery. (Editorial) Am J Ophthalmol 1986;102:788–790.
57. Tetz MR, Apple DJ, Hansen SO, King MH, et al. "Localized endophthalmitis": a complication of extracapsular cataract extraction. Implants in Ophthalmology 1987;1:93–97.
58. Zambrano W, Flynn HW, Pflugfelder SC, Roussel TJ, et al. Management options for *Propionibacterium acnes* endophthalmitis. Ophthalmology 1989;96:1100–1105.
59. Ormerod LD, Paton BG, Haaf J, et al. Anaerobic bacterial endophthalmitis. Ophthalmol 1987;94: 799–808.
60. Alpar JJ. Toxic lens syndrome. J Ocul Ther Surg 1982;1:306–308.
61. Shepherd DD. The "toxic lens" syndrome. Contact Intraocul Lens Med J 1980;6:158–161.
62. Hunter JW. Early postoperative sterile hypopyons. Br J Ophthalmol 1978;62:470–473.
63. Parelman AG. Sterile uveitis and intraocular lens implantation. J Am Intraocul Implant Soc 1979;5: 301–306.
64. Worst JGF. A retrospective view on the sterilization of intraocular lenses and the incidence of sterile hypopyon. (Editorial) J Am Intraocul Implant Soc 1980;6:10–12.
65. Ridley F. Safety requirements for acrylic implants. Br J Ophthalmol 1957;41:359–367.
66. Binkhorst CD, Flu FP. Sterilization of intraocular acrylic lens prostheses with ultraviolet rays. Br J Ophthalmol 1956;40:665–668.
67. Pettit TH, Olson RJ, Foos RY, Martin WJ: Fungal en-

dophthalmitis following intraocular lens implantation: a surgical epidemic. Arch Ophthalmol 1980;98:1025–1039.

68. Gerding DN, Poley BJ, Hall WH, LeWin DP, et al. Treatment of *Pseudomonas* endophthalmitis associated with prosthetic intraocular lens implant. Am J Ophthalmol 1979;88:902–908.
69. Boyaner D, Soloman LD. Ocular reaction to the use of wet-pack versus dry-pack intraocular lenses. J Am Intraocul Implant Soc 1980;6:252–254.
70. Stark WJ, Rosenblum P, Maumenee AE, Cowan CL. Postoperative inflammatory reactions to intraocular lenses sterilized with ethylene-oxide. Ophthalmology 1980;87:385–389.
71. Meltzer DW. Sterile hypopyon following intraocular lens surgery. Arch Ophthalmol 1980;98:100–104.
72. Ratner BD. Analysis of surface contaminants on intraocular lenses. Arch Ophthalmol 1983;101:1434–1438.
73. Tsuboi S, Tsujioka M, Kusube T, Kojima S. Effect of continuous circular capsulorhexis and intraocular lens fixation on the blood/aqueous barrier. Arch Ophthalmol 1992;110:1124–1127.
74. Ellingson FT. Complications with the Choyce Mark VIII anterior chamber lens implant (Uveitis—Glaucoma—Hyphema). J Am Intraocul Implant Soc 1977;3:199–201.
75. Keates RH, Ehrlich DR. "Lenses of chance": complications of anterior chamber implants. Ophthalmology 1978;85:408–414.
76. Apple DJ, Brems RN, Park RB, Kavka-Van Norman D, et al. Anterior chamber lenses: I. Complications and pathology and a review of designs. J Cataract Refract Surg 1987;13:157–174.
77. Beehler CC. UGH syndrome with the 91Z lens. (Letter) J Am Intraocul Implant Soc 1983;9:459.
78. Hagen JC III. A comparative study of the 91Z and other anterior chamber intraocular lenses. J Am Intraocul Implant Soc 1984;10:324–328.
79. Mamalis N, Apple DJ, Brady SE, Notes RG, et al. Pathological and scanning electron microscopic evaluation of the 91Z intraocular lens. J Am Intraocul Implant Soc 1984;10:191–199.
80. Reidy JJ, Apple DJ, Googe JM, Richey MA, Mamalis N, et al. An analysis of semi-flexible, closed-loop anterior chamber intraocular lenses. J Am Intraocul Implant Soc 1985;11:344–352.
81. Isenberg RA, Apple DJ, Reidy JJ, Richards SC, et al. Histopathologic and scanning electron microscopic study of one type of intraocular lens. Arch Ophthalmol 1986;104:683–686.
82. Apple DJ, Olson RJ. Closed-loop anterior chamber intraocular lenses. (Letter) Arch Ophthalmol 1987;105:19–20.
83. Johnson SH, Kratz RP, Olson PF. Iris transillumination defects and microhyphema syndrome. Am Intraocul Implant Soc J 1984;10:425–428.
84. Masket S. Pseudophakic posterior iris chafing syndrome. J Cataract Refract Surg 1986;12:252–256.
85. Samples JR, Van Buskirk EM. Pigmentary glaucoma associated with posterior chamber intraocular lenses. Am J Ophthalmol 1985;100:385–388.
86. Lieppman ME: Intermittent visual "white-out": A new intraocular lens complication. Ophthalmology 1982; 89:109–112.
87. Apple DJ, Craythorn JM, Olson RJ, Little LE, et al. Anterior segment complications and neovascular glaucoma following implantation of a posterior chamber intraocular lens. Ophthalmology 1984; 91:403–419.
88. Apple DJ, Mamalis N, Brady SC, Loftfield K, et al. Biocompatibility of implant materials: a review and scanning electron microscopic study. J Am Intraocul Implant Soc 1984;10:53–66.
89. Apple DJ, Mamalis N, Loftfield K, Googe JM, et al. Complications of intraocular lenses: a historical and histopathological review. Surg Ophthalmol 1984;29: 1–54.
90. Drews RC, Smith ME, Okun N. Scanning electron microscopy of intraocular lenses. Ophthalmology 1978; 85:415–424.
91. Clayman HM: Polypropylene. Ophthalmology 1981; 88:959–964.
92. Christ FR, Fencil DA, Van Gent S, Knight PM. Evaluation of the chemical, optical, and mechanical properties of elastomeric intraocular lens materials and their clinical significance. J Cataract Refract Surg 1989;15:176–184.
93. Chirila TV, Walker LN, Constable IJ, Thompson DE, et al. Cytotoxic effects of residual chemicals from polymeric biomaterials for artificial soft intraocular lenses. J Cataract Refract Surg 1991;17:154–162.
94. Gasset AR, Ishii Y, Kaufman HE, Miller T. Cytotoxicity of ophthalmic preservatives. Am J Ophthalmol 1974;78:98–105.
95. Fraunfelder FT, ed. Drug-induced ocular side effects and drug interactions. Philadelphia, Lea & Febiger, 1989:477.
96. Hull DS, Chemotti MT, Edelhauser HF, Van Horn DF, et al. Effect of epinephrine on the corneal endothelium. Am J Ophthalmol 1975;79:245–250.
97. Olson RJ, Kolodner H, Riddle P, Escapini H Jr. Commonly used intraocular medications in the corneal endothelium. Arch Ophthalmol 1980;98:2224–2226.
98. MacRae SM, Brown B, Edelhauser HF. The corneal toxicity of presurgical skin antiseptics. Am J Ophthalmol 1984;97:221–232.
99. Green K, Livingston V, Bowman K, Hull DS. Chlorhexidine effects on corneal epithelium and endothelium. Arch Ophthalmol 1980;98:1273–1278.

100. Phinney RB, Mondino BJ, Hofbauer JD, et al. Corneal edema related to accidental Hibiclens exposure. Am J Ophthalmol 1988;106:210–215.
101. Edelhauser HF, Gonnering R, Van Horn DL. Intraocular irrigating solutions. Arch Ophthalmol 1978;96: 516–520.
102. Edelhauser HF, Van Horn DL, Schultz RO, Hyndiuk RA. Comparative toxicity of intraocular irrigating solutions on the corneal endothelium. Am J Ophthalmol 1976;81:473–481.
103. Glasser DB, Matsuda M, Ellis JG, Edelhauser HF. Effects of intraocular irrigating solutions on the corneal endothelium after in-vivo anterior chamber irrigation. Am J Ophthalmol 1985;99:321–328.
104. Gonnering R, Edelhauser HF, Van Horn DL, Durant W. The pH tolerance of rabbit and human corneal endothelium. Invest Ophthalmol Vis Sci 1979;18;373.
105. Googe JM, Mamalis N, Apple DJ, Olson RJ. BSS Warning. J Am Intraocul Implant Soc 1984;10:202.
107. Yee RW, Edelhouser HF. Comparison of intraocular acetylcholine and carbachol. J Cataract Refract Surg 1986;12:18–22.
108. Roberts C. Effect of intraocular miotics on postoperative inflammation. Boston, American Society of Cataract and Refraction Surgery, 1991.
109. McDonald AR, Schatz H, Allen AW, et al. Retinal toxicity secondary to intraocular gentamicin injection. Ophthalmology 1986;93:871–877.
110. Snider JD III, Cohen HB, Chenoweth RG. Acute ischemic retinopathy secondary to intraocular gentamicin. In: Ryan SJ, Division AK, Little HL, eds. Retinal diseases. New York, Grune & Stratton, 1985:227–232.
111. Waltz K, Margo CE. Intraocular gentamicin toxicity. (Letter) Arch Ophthalmol 1991;109:911.
112. Campochiaro PA, Conway BP: Aminoglycoside toxicity—a survey of retinal specialists: implications for ocular use. Arch Ophthalmol 1991;109:946–950.
113. Kim JH. Intraocular inflammation of denatured viscoelastic substance in cases of cataract extraction and lens implantation. J Cataract Refract Surg 1987;13:537–542.
114. Sutphin JE, Papadimus TJ. Post-cataract extraction corneal edema: Epidemiological intervention and control. Invest Ophthalmol Vis Sci 1989;30(Suppl): 165.
115. Ohguro N, Matsuda M, Kinoshita S. The effects of denatured sodium hyaluronate on the corneal endothelium in cats. Am J Ophthalmol 1991;112:424–430.
116. Nevyas AS, Raber IM, Eagle RC, Wallace IB, Nevyas HJ. Acute band keratopathy following intracameral Viscoat. Arch Ophthalmol 1987;105:958–964.
117. Nuyts RMMA, Breebaart AC, Pels E, Edelhauser HF. Acute corneal decompensation following routine cataract surgery. Invest Ophthalmol Vis Sci 1989; 30(Suppl):338.
118. Breebaart AC, Nuyts RMMA, Pels E, Edelhauser HF, et al. Toxic endothelial cell destruction of the cornea after routine extracapsular cataract surgery. Arch Ophthalmol 1990;108:1121–1125.
119. Nuyts RMMA, Edelhauser HF, Pels E, Breebaart AC. Toxic effects of detergents on the corneal endothelium. Arch Ophthalmol 1990;108:1158–1162.
120. Richburg FA, Reidy JJ, Apple DJ, Olson RJ. Sterile hypopyon secondary to ultrasonic cleaning solution. J Cataract Refract Surg 1986;12:248–251.
121. Kreisler KR, Martin SS, Young CW, Anderson CW, et al. Postoperative inflammation following cataract extraction caused by bacterial contamination of the cleaning bath detergent. J Cataract Refract Surg 1992;18:106–110.
122. Bene C, Kranias G. Possible intraocular lens contamination by surgical glove powder. Ophthalmic Surg 1986;17:290–291.
123. Ullman S, Clevenger CE, Parker GR. Coring—a potential source of intraocular contamination. (Letter) J Cataract Refract Surgery 1990;16:338.
124. Monson MC, Mamalis N, Olson RJ. Toxic anterior segment inflammation following cataract surgery. J Cataract Refract Surg 1992;18:184–189.
125. Olson RJ, Apple DJ. Unexplained intraocular toxicity after cataract/intraocular lens surgery. J Cataract Refract Surg 1987;13:688–689.
126. Apple DJ, Mamalis N, Steinmetz RL, et al. Phacoanaphylactic endophthalmitis associated with extracapsular cataract extraction and posterior chamber lens. Arch Ophthalmol 1984;102:1528–1532.
127. Apple DJ, Mamalis N, Steinmetz RL, et al. Phacoanaphylactic endophthalmitis following ECCE and IOL implantation. (Guest Editorial) J Am Intraocul Implant Soc 1984;10:423–424.
128. Marak GE. Phacoanaphylactic endophthalmitis. Surv Ophthalmol 1992;36:325–339.
129. Rahi AHS, Garner A. The lens. In: Rahi AHS, Garner A, eds. Immunopathology of the eye. Oxford, Blackwell Scientific Publications, 1976:204–220.
130. Verhoeff FH, Lemoine AN. Endophthalmitis phacoanaphylactica. Am J Ophthalmol 1922;5:737–745.
131. Wohl LG, Klein OR Jr, Lucier AC, Galman BD. Pseudophakic phacoanaphylactic endophthalmitis. Ophthalmic Surg 1986;17:234–237.
132. Irvine SR, Irvine AR. Lens-induced uveitis and glaucoma. Part I: Endophthalmitis phaco-anaphylactica. Am J Ophthalmol 1952;35:177–186.
133. Smith RE, Weiner P. Unusual presentation of phacoanaphylaxis following phacoemulsification. Ophthalmic Surg 1976;7:65–68.
134. American Academy of Ophthalmology. The repair of rhegmatogenous retinal detachments. Ophthalmology 1990;97:1562–1572.
135. Benson WE. Retinal detachment: diagnosis and management, Second ed. Philadelphia, JB Lippincott, 1988:113–155.

136. Hilton GF, McLean EB, Norton EWD. Retinal detachment, ed 4. San Francisco, American Academy of Ophthalmology, 1981:77–98.
137. Michels RG. Scleral buckling methods for rhegmatogenous retinal detachment. Retina 1986;6:1–49.
138. Williams GA, Aaberg TM. Technique of scleral buckling. In: Ryan SJ, Glazer BM, Michels RG, eds. Retina, vol 3. St. Louis, CV Mosby, 1989:114–149.
139. Packer AJ, ed. Manual of retinal detachment and repair. New York, Churchill Livingstone, 1989.
140. Rachal WF, Burton TC. Changing concepts of failures after retinal detachment surgery. Arch Ophthalmol 1979;1997:480–483.
141. Glaser BM, Lamor M. Pathobiology of proliferative vitreoretinopathy. In: Ryan SJ, ed. Retina, vol. 3. St. Louis, CV Mosby, 1989:369–383.
142. Ryan SJ. Traction retinal detachment: XLIX Edward Jackson Memorial Lecture. Am J Ophthalmol 1993;115:1–20.
143. Glaser BM, Cardin A, Biscoe B. Proliferative vitreoretinopathy: the mechanism of development of vitreoretinal traction. Ophthalmology 1987;94:327.
144. Aaberg TM. Management of anterior and posterior proliferative vitreoretinopathy: XLV Edward Jackson Memorial Lecture. Am J Ophthalmol 1988;106:519–532.
145. Lopez PF, Grossniklaus HE, Aaberg TM, et al. Pathologenetic mechanisms in anterior proliferative vitreoretinopathy. Am J Ophthalmol 1992;114:257–279.
146. Lobes LA, Burton TC. The incidence of macular pucker after retinal detachment surgery. Am J Ophthalmol 1978;85:72–77.
147. Wilson DJ, Green WR. Histopathologic study of the effect of retinal detachment surgery on 49 eyes obtained post-mortem. Am J Ophthalmol 1987;103: 167–179.
148. DeBustros S, Rice T, Michels R, et al. Vitrectomy for macular pucker: use after treatment of retinal tears or retinal detachment. Arch Ophthalmol 1988;106:758–760.
149. Meredith TA, Reeser FH, Topping TM, et al. Cystoid macular edema after retinal detachment surgery. Ophthalmology 1987;87:1090–1095.
150. Lobes LA, Grand MG. Incidence of cystoid macular edema following scleral buckling procedure. Arch Ophthalmol 1980;98:1230–1232.
151. Sabates NR, Sabates FN, Sabates R, et al. Macular changes following retinal detachment surgery. Am J Ophthalmol 1989;108:22–29.
152. Wilkinson CP. Retinal complications after cataract surgery: focal points. Am Acad Ophthalmol 1992;10:1–10.
153. Yanoff M, Fine BS. Ocular pathology: a text and atlas, ed 3. Philadelphia, JB Lippincott, 1989:60–65.
154. Apple DJ, Rabb MF. Ocular pathology: clinical applications and self-assessment. St. Louis: CV Mosby, 1985.
155. Arentsen JJ, Morgan B, Green WR. Changing indications for keratoplasty. Am J Ophthalmol 1976;81: 313–318.
156. Smith RE, McDonald HR, Nesburne AB, et al. Penetrating keratoplasty: changing indications, 1947–1978. Arch Ophthalmol 1980;98:1226–1229.
157. Robin JB, Gindi JJ, Koh K, et al. An update of the indications for penetrating keratoplasty: 1979 through 1983. Arch Ophthalmol 1986;104:87–89.
158. Mohamadi P, McDonnell JM, Irvine JA, et al. Changing indications for penetrating keratoplasty, 1984–1988. Am J Ophthalmol 1989;107:550–552.
159. Mamalis N, Craig MT, Coulter VL, et al. Penetrating keratoplasty 1981–1988: clinical indications and pathologic findings. J Cataract Refract Surg 1991;17:163–167.
160. Mamalis N, Anderson CW, Kreisler KR, et al. Changing trends in the indications for penetrating keratoplasty. Arch Ophthalmol 1992;110:1409–1411.
161. Drews RC. Intermittent touch syndrome. Arch Ophthalmol 100:1440–1441, 1982.
162. Duffin RM, Olson RJ. Vaulting characteristics of flexible loop anterior chamber intraocular lenses. Arch Ophthalmol 1983;101:1429–1433.
163. Cunha-Vaz JG, Travassos A. Breakdown of the blood/retinal barriers in cystoid macular edema. Surv Ophthalmol 1984;28:485–492.
164. Miyake K, Shirashawa E, Hikita M. Active transport system of prostaglandins: Clinical implications and considerations. J Cataract Refract Surg 1992;18:100–105.
165. Stark WJ, Maumenee AE, Fagadau W, et al. Cystoid macular edema in pseudophakia. Surv Ophthalmol 1984;28:442–451.
166. Jampol LM. Pharmacologic therapy of aphakic and pseudophakic cystoid macular edema: 1985 update. Ophthalmology 1985;92:807–810.
167. Flach AJ, Dolan BJ, Irvine AR. Effectiveness of ketorolac tromethamine 0.5% ophthalmic solution for chronic aphakic and pseudophakic cystoid macular edema. Am J Ophthalmol 1987;103:479–486.
168. Flach AJ, Jampol LM, Weinberg D, et al. Improvement in visual acuity in chronic and pseudophakic cystoid macular edema after treatment with topical 0.5% ketorolac tromethamine. Am J Ophthalmol 1991;112:514–519.
169. Cox SN, Hay E, Bird AC. Treatment of chronic macular edema with acetazolamide. Arch Ophthalmol 1988;106:1190–1195.
170. Pfoff DS, Thom SR. Preliminary report on the effect of hyperbaric oxygen on cystoid macular edema. J Cataract Refract Surg 1987;13:136–140.

Ophthalmic Surgery Complications: Prevention and Management,
edited by Judie F. Charlton and George W. Weinstein.

15

Richard F. Spaide

Postsurgical Cystoid Macular Edema

Cystoid macular edema (CME) may occur as a distal, secondary effect from almost any type of ocular surgery. CME occurs most commonly with cataract extraction,[1–15] but it may occur after neodymium: yttrium-aluminum-garnet (Nd:YAG) laser capsulotomy,[16–24] penetrating keratoplasty,[25] scleral buckling,[26] and, less commonly, after filtering procedures.[1–27] After uneventful cataract extraction, about 60% of patients with intracapsular[1] and 20% to 30% of patients with extracapsular surgery[2] develop CME. Although most of these cases spontaneously resolve, chronic CME with lasting degradation of visual acuity occurs in approximately 1% of patients undergoing extracapsular cataract extraction. CME is one of the most common causes of unexpected poor visual acuity after cataract surgery, a procedure performed more than 1 million times a year in the United States. Treatment of chronic CME offers the possibility of ameliorating the edema and improving the visual acuity in these patients.[28]

DIAGNOSIS

Clinical Examination

Many eyes with CME show some evidence of inflammation. Occasionally, patients have specific complaints of ocular irritation or nonspecific complaints that their "eye doesn't feel right." Perilimbal injection is not uncommon. Cell and flare in the anterior segment and cells in the vitreous may be observed. Many of these eyes have additional anatomic alterations, such as iris or vitreous incarcerated in the wound, intraocular lens pupillary capture, tilted or subluxated intraocular lenses (IOLs), retention of large amounts of lens cortex, or rupture of the hyaloid face.

CME is best seen with a fundus contact lens using careful biomicroscopic examination of the posterior pole (Fig. 15-1*A*). Examination with a direct or indirect ophthalmoscope is generally not effective. Use of the slit-lamp biomicroscope with a 78- or 90-diopter lens is more helpful; however, a contact lens, such as a Goldmann lens, is generally the best way to appreciate macular edema. The macula appears thicker and slightly more yellow than usual, and there is a loss of the foveal depression. With the illumination of the biomicroscope placed at an oblique angle, the cystoid spaces may be observed. These fusiform spaces are larger in the perifoveal region and become progressively smaller away from the center of the macula. The region of macular thickening is larger than the area involved by the cystoid spaces and may extend to the vascular arcades. Small splinter hemorrhages may be seen within the retina,[4] and blood may accumulate within the cystoid spaces. Some patients may have obscuration of the underlying choroidal details either from severe edema or a concomitant shallow serous detachment of the macula.

Epiretinal membranes, found in about 10% of patients,[3,5] may be diagnosed by observing a pellucid, grayish membrane on the surface of the retina. When the light beam is swept across the macula, glinting reflexes from the inner surface of the retina may be seen that do not follow a pattern expected from the cystoid spaces alone. With resolution of the CME, the potential for visual recovery may be limited by the epiretinal membrane.

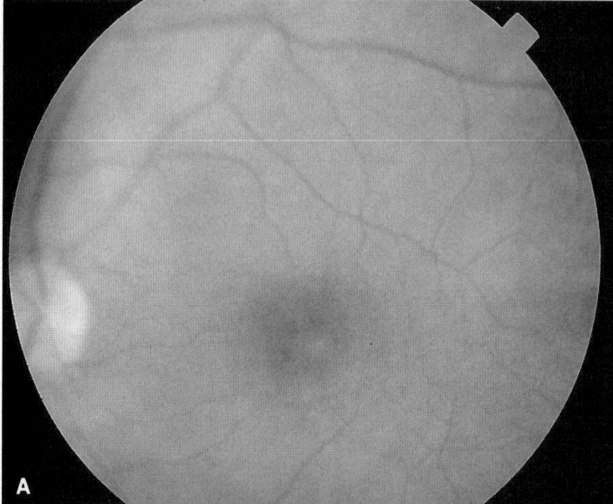

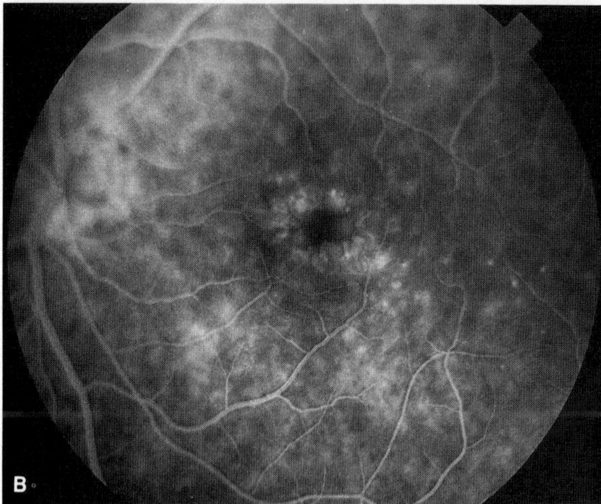

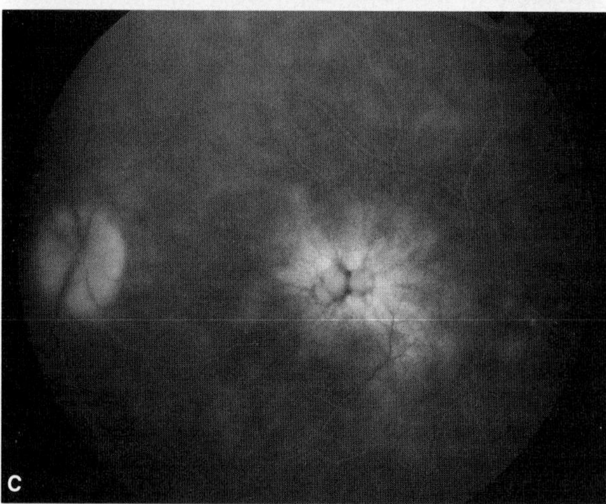

Figure 15-1. (A) Photograph of cystoid macular edema (CME) demonstrating foveal cysts. (See color plate after page xvi.) (B) Arteriovenous phase fluorescein angiogram of the same eye shows dye beginning to accumulate in the cystoid spaces of the macula. (C) Later in the fluorescein angiogram, the cystoid spaces, as well as the foveal cysts, are evident.

Patients with chronic edema may have a coalescence of the central cystoid spaces with the development of what is referred to as a foveal cyst but that is actually a foveal schisis cavity. Patients with foveal cysts generally have poorer vision and may be less likely to have satisfactory visual recovery. There may be an "unroofing" of the foveal cyst with the formation of an inner lamellar macular hole.[3,29] The resultant defect has the subtle, but characteristic appearance of a sharp step from the perifoveal cystoid spaces to a circular or ovular indented area in the foveal region with a different sheen from the surrounding retina.

Patients with chronic CME may develop punctiform mottling of the retinal pigment epithelium (RPE), possibly related to the presence of chronic subretinal serous fluid. With resolution of the CME, the granular clumping of the pigment does not change.

Swelling of the optic nerve head in some degree is found in almost every patient. Comparison with the optic nerve in the fellow eye may aid in the recognition of the nerve head edema. There generally is a slight thickening and elevation of the rim, a decrease in the cup size, and a slightly erythematous appearance of the entire optic nerve. The relative contribution of the nerve head swelling to decreased visual function, if any, is not known.

Fluorescein Angiography

The cystoid accumulation of edema fluid is particularly evident during fluorescein angiography (see Fig. 15-1*B* and *C*). Early in the fluorescein angiographic examination, capillary dilation and leakage are conspicuous. The fluorescein usually does not seem to leak diffusely from the perifoveal capillaries. Early in the angiographic study, fluorescein appears to leak from small points in the midsection of each capillary segment, implying that the leakage from the capillary segment is not uniform. The relative leakage from the RPE, if any, is not known.

The leakage continues during the course of the angiographic examination, and the fluorescein pools within cystic spaces in the outer plexiform layer of the retina. Because of the unique horizontal arrangement of the outer plexiform layer in the perifoveal macula (Henle fiber layer) cystoid accumulation of fluid creates fusiform spaces. Radial arrangement of the cystoid spaces in Henle layer gives rise to the familiar petalloid appearance of CME in the perifoveal region.

Patchy leakage of the macular capillaries occurs outside of the perifoveal region as well. This leakage is especially evident in the middle and late stages of the fluorescein angiogram as small ill-defined intraretinal areas of hyperfluorescence. In severe cases of CME, the cystoid spaces may form within the macula located outside of the immediate perifoveal region. In these areas, the outer plexiform layer is oriented vertically, and cystoid spaces that form have a honeycomb appearance.

There is late staining of the optic nerve in virtually every case of CME because of leakage of the capillaries in the optic nerve head. Improvement in the CME is accompanied by a parallel decrease in optic nerve staining. This finding suggests that factors causing macular capillary leakage also cause leakage from capillaries within the optic nerve head.

Fluorescein angiography may be technically difficult in certain patients, particularly those with pseudophakic bullous keratopathy, significant capsular opacities, or small pupils. The resultant fluorescein angiogram may be dark or indistinct. In these patients, details in the early and midphases of the angiogram may be barely visible, whereas an area of hyperfluorescence frequently can be seen in the later phases of the angiogram. The specific diagnosis of CME, as opposed to other conditions (such as choroidal neovascularization), may not be made with certainty in these patients based on the angiographic findings alone.

Fluorescein angiography is a sensitive tool in diagnosing CME, but the area of dye leakage seen during angiography correlates poorly with visual acuity.[5,30] Several possible explanations exist for this disparity. First, the actual amount of foveal thickening is one of the most important predictors of visual acuity.[30] The poor correlation between the angiographic findings and visual acuity suggests that the two-dimensional area of fluorescein leakage seen during angiography is not strictly related to the amount of macular, or foveal, thickening, which is in the third dimension. Second, the cystoid spaces seen during fluorescein angiography lie in the outer plexiform layer, and loss of visual acuity may depend on accumulation of fluid in other regions, such as within or under the photoreceptor layer. Third, there may be pathologic factors occurring in the retina besides the simple accumulation of fluid. These factors may contribute to the degradation of visual function without causing recognizable changes in the fluorescein angiogram.

HISTOPATHOLOGY

By histopathologic examination, maculae with CME exhibit cystoid spaces predominantly in Henle fiber layer.[31–38] Cystoid spaces may also be seen in the inner nuclear, ganglion, and nerve fiber layers. The fluid in the cystoid spaces appears to contain little protein or lipid. There is not universal agreement about the histopathologic mechanism of development of the cystoid spaces. Some authors[31] have stated that these spaces are extracellular accumulations of fluid, whereas others[36,38] have considered the possibility of Müller cell swelling and necrosis coupled with vascular decompensation, leading to the formation of the cystoid spaces. There may be shortening of the inner and outer segments of the photoreceptors and loss of Müller cells. Subretinal fluid may be present. Atrophy, vacuolization, and proliferation of the RPE may also occur.[37]

The perifoveal region appears to be much more susceptible to the formation of cystoid spaces than the macula outside of this area. This propensity has no accepted explanation, but may be related to the unique retinal anatomy and the peculiar capillary arrangement in the foveal and perifoveal area. It has been shown that active fluid transport from the retina occurs at the RPE and at the retinal vessels.[39] Inflammation may increase the fluid flux through the retina–fluid leaks from retinal capillaries (perhaps in a nonuniform manner). This same fluid is then resorbed by the retinal vessels and RPE. The macular region has an unusual vascular arrangement; an avascular area is bounded on all sides by a highly vascularized region. Fluid produced in the perifoveal region may spill into the avascular portions of the fovea where resorption may be limited.

In one study of CME, correlations between histopathologic findings and CME were made.[33] The presence of iritis did not show a statistically significant association with CME, whereas the presence of iridovitreal synechiae, cyclitis, vitritis, and retinal phlebitis did.[33] Every eye had a posterior vitreous detachment, and no eye had discernible, persistent, vitreomacular adhesions. A study of 31 eyes with vitreous incarceration in the wound found that only 6 had CME.[34] It is possible that other eyes in that study previously had CME that resolved. All eyes had a posterior vitreous detachment. Of the 6 eyes with CME, 6 had iridovitreal synechiae, 5 had periphlebitis, and in those that did not have diabetes as an additional risk factor for macular edema, all 4 had pars plicata distortion.[34]

Eyes with CME that do not have vitreous in the anterior chamber have profound fluorescein leakage from iris vessels during iris angiography and anterior chamber fluorophotometry.[40,41] Fluorophotometric studies have shown diffuse fluorescein leakage into the vitreous cavity.[42–43] Therefore, eyes with CME appear to have a global blood–ocular barrier breakdown.

To date, no animal model has been developed that fully emulates postsurgical CME seen in humans. After lens extraction, a group of rhesus monkeys did not develop fluorescein angiographic findings of either macular capillary abnormalities or CME.[44] Leakage from both the retinal vasculature and the RPE was found by horseradish peroxidase tracer studies. Histopathologic study, however, revealed Müller cell edema but no cystoid spaces. Lens extraction in young rhesus monkeys may not adequately emulate cataract extraction in an elderly human, who may be expected to have the vitreal, retinal vascular, and RPE changes associated with age. CME, nonetheless, has been reported in pediatric cataract extractions.[14]

Some aspects of postsurgical CME can be produced in rhesus monkeys given repeated intravascular talc injections.[45] With time, multifocal retinal infarctions caused by the talc results in cystoid degeneration in the outer plexiform layer throughout the posterior pole. Rhesus monkeys given repeated talc injections had fluorescein angiographic findings of retinal vascular leakage that are found in postsurgical CME; however, these monkeys also had precapillary arteriolar occlusion and capillary nonperfusion, which is not found in postsurgical CME.[45] The findings of this animal model suggest that some element of tissue ischemia may be involved in the formation of the cystoid spaces of postsurgical CME.

DIFFERENTIAL DIAGNOSIS

Branch Retinal Vein Occlusion

The typical age of patients with postcataract surgery CME is about 70 years[5]; patients this age frequently have ocular and systemic conditions that can mimic or exacerbate CME. Branch vein occlusions characteristically cause an acute sector-shaped area of intraretinal hemorrhage and edema. With time, the hemorrhage may clear leaving an area of retinal edema. Although occlusions of larger branches may result in dilation of the corresponding vessel, occlusions of smaller veins in the macular region may not. Some patients may develop small flecks of intraretinal lipid, which do not occur in postcataract surgery CME. Fluorescein angiography, particularly in the earlier phases, demonstrates asymmetric filling of the veins in the macula. There may be small patches of capillary nonperfusion as well. Later in the angiogram, intraretinal hyperfluorescence accumulates and is centered in the area of the branch retinal vein occlusion.

Diabetic Macular Edema

In one study of patients sent to a referral practice for CME, approximately 8% had diabetes.[5] Although patients with no preexisting diabetic macular edema may develop macular edema after surgery, patients with preexisting macular edema frequently have a severe exacerbation of their macular edema after cataract surgery.[46,47] In diabetic patients, the relative contribution of diabetic retinopathy and postsurgical CME may be difficult to estimate. As the treatment for each of these conditions differs, the determination is important. Diabetic patients frequently have microaneurysms and leakage from these microaneurysms; however, after ocular surgery many patients with diabetes regularly have diffuse capillary leakage. One important differentiating clue can be garnered from the fluorescein angiogram—optic nerve head staining does not come from background diabetic changes. In a diabetic patient with macular edema, the presence of optic nerve staining implies the macular edema is related, at least in part, to the surgical process.

Choroidal Neovascularization

Nonexudative age-related macular degeneration, common in patients of this age group, was found in almost 40% of patients in one study. In the Framingham Eye Study, 35.6% of the patients of a similar age had nonexudative age-related macular degeneration.[48] New vessel growth, the hallmark of exudative age-related macular degeneration, is heralded by a grayish-green discoloration in the area of choroidal neovascularization (CNV) associated with overlying neurosensory detachment, RPE detachments, flecks of subretinal lipid, and sub-RPE and subretinal hemorrhage. These findings are not seen in postsurgical CME. Occult neovascularization is a slower-growing variant of CNV and, as the name implies, may be more difficult to recognize. Not infrequently, occult CNV may cause CME and thus be confused with postsurgical CME. Patients with occult CNV have thickening at the level of the RPE, a shallow overlying neurosensory detachment, and possible flecks of subretinal lipid; however, they do not necessarily have sub-RPE or subretinal hemorrhage. The fluorescein angiographic findings of occult choroidal neovascularization include ill-defined hyperfluorescence at the level of the RPE, pinpoint leakage (ooze) from the RPE, and "thumbprints," which are small irregular folds of the RPE.[49–51] In occult CNV, the new vessels may not be visible during fluorescein angiography. There is no late staining of the optic nerve head in occult CNV.

Retinal Detachment

Shallow retinal detachments can extend into the macula and cause poor visual acuity, but not be readily apparent.[52] These detachments may cause folds in the macula that give the appearance of CME (Fig. 15-2). These patients may have angiographic evidence of CME, which may be related to either the previous cataract surgery or the retinal detachment. In one study of patients seen in a referral practice for CME, 9 of 150 (6%) were not eligible for the study because they actually had retinal detachments.[5] Patients with CME usually complain of blurry vision with some slight distortion. In addition to blurry vision, patients with shallow retinal detachment complain of wavy vision that changes with head position. These patients may notice that their visual acuity is better in the morning than in the evening. If the retinal detachment is particularly shallow, it may not be immediately visible by indirect ophthalmoscopic examination. With the illumination of the biomicroscope placed at an angle, shadows of the retinal blood vessels may be seen to be displaced from the vessels. There may be retinal folds in the macular region, something that does not occur in CME. These patients may have a more prominent accumulation of fluid under the inferior retina, which aids in the diagnosis. Contact B-scan ultrasonography can help confirm the diagnosis.

Endophthalmitis

Most cases of postoperative endophthalmitis start with an explosive onset of pain, loss of vision, and severe uveitis. Endophthalmitis from less virulent organisms, such as *Propionibacterium acnes or Candida parapsilosis*, may produce an indolent intraocular inflammation resulting in a less conspicuous

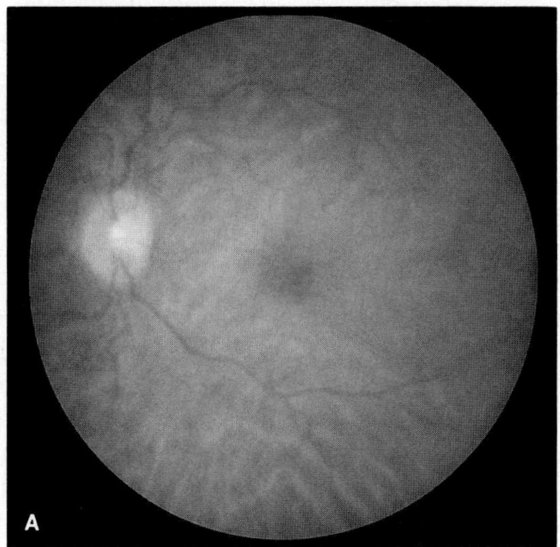

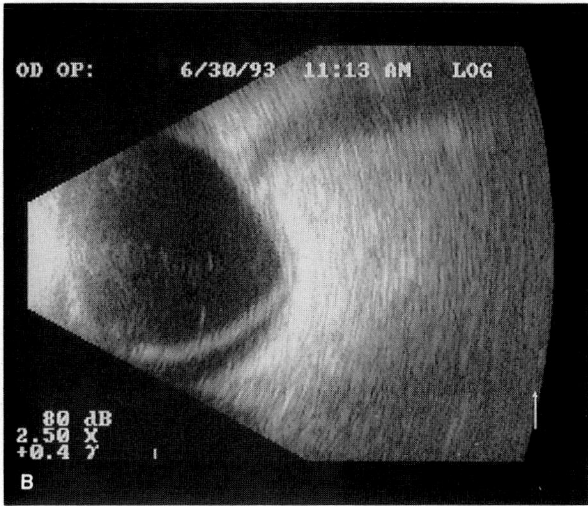

Figure 15-2. (A) Photograph of a patient with a shallow retinal detachment. The fine radiating retinal folds in the macula simulate CME (See color plate after page xvi.) (B) Contact B-scan ultrasonogram demonstrating the shallow detachment extending into the macula. The referring physician did not suspect the presence of a retinal detachment.

clinical presentation.[53] One case of *P. acnes* endophthalmitis has been reported following intracapsular cataract extraction (ICCE),[54] but *P. acnes* occurs after extracapsular cataract extraction (ECCE).[3,55] This anaerobic bacteria may become sequestered within the lens capsule, or between the lens capsule and the intraocular lens, causing a chronic intraocular inflammation with all of the sequelae of uveitis. This infection may be recognized by a chronic inflammatory response after cataract surgery that initially responds to topical corticosteroids but worsens over time in a patient with a white plaque on the posterior lens capsule. Vitrectomy, capsulectomy, culture, and intraocular antibiotic administration are indicated if this diagnosis is suspected.[53]

PREVALENCE

CME is rarely seen in the first week after surgery.[56] The peak prevalence as detected by fluorescein angiography occurs approximately 6 weeks postoperatively. Many of these cases are subtle and do not have pronounced biomicroscopic changes. At one time, many of these patients were considered to be asymptomatic; because the fluorescein angiogram was the principal sign indicating the presence of CME, the condition these patients demonstrated was referred to as *angiographic CME*. This term originated in the days of intracapsular surgery when final refractions were not performed until several months after surgery. With the widespread use of IOLs, it became apparent that many, but not all, of these patients were symptomatic. Most patients have spontaneous resolution of their CME in the ensuing months after surgery.

Six months after the onset of CME, a subset of patients remains with a chronic condition that is less likely to resolve spontaneously. Patients with chronic CME have a condition that has been termed *clinically significant CME*. The exact relationship that angiographic CME has to clinically significant CME is not known with certainty. It is possible that patients with clinically significant CME may have a chronic form of "angiographic" CME. Conversely, clinically significant CME may be a separate condition on a microscopic or pathophysiologic level that initially may not be differentiable from angiographic CME using conventional fluorescein angiographic examination techniques. After ICCE alone, about 1% to 2% of patients have decreased visual acuity from clinically significant CME. Iris-fixated IOLs implanted after ICCE were associated with a prevalence of clinically significant CME of 2% to more than 5% depending on the IOL geometry and how the IOL was manufactured.[57–59]

Cataract surgery continued to develop, and a shift in surgery technique to preserving the posterior capsule through ECCE and phacoemulsification occurred. Concurrently, posterior chamber IOLs became more popular. With these advances, the prevalence of clinically significant CME decreased to approximately 1%.[2] Some patients who develop clinically significant CME have had difficult surgery complicated by capsular rupture, vitreous loss, retention of lens cortex, and inadequate wound closure,[5,7] and thus do not neatly fit into either an ICCE or ECCE group. Part of the overall decrease in clinically significant CME is probably due to a general improvement in surgical technique as time has progressed.

After ECCE or phacoemulsification, many patients require Nd:YAG laser capsulotomy because they develop capsular opacities that limit visual acuity. This second surgical procedure is associated with the development of CME in a small proportion of patients. The prevalence of CME after Nd:YAG laser capsulotomy varies in reports by different groups,[16–24] with a weighted average of 1.5%. Many of these studies used power levels in excess of what is commonly used today, and so the actual prevalence using current technique may be somewhat lower.

Even though the prevalence of postcataract surgery CME has declined, it continues to be a significant disappointment for patients and ophthalmologists alike. Additional medical expenses are generated by postsurgical CME because of increased physician visits, fluorescein angiography, and added treatment requirements. In attacking the problem that CME poses, ophthalmologists have concentrated on two main areas. The first, and ultimately the most promising, is the prevention of CME through refinement of surgical technique. The prevalence of chronic CME after cataract surgery has been reduced by one half in a decade through improved surgical technique and IOLs. The second area of concentration is improved treatment of CME when it does occur. CME continues to be a problem requiring treatment because cataract extraction involves at least some degree of ocular trauma no matter how advanced the technique, operative complications continue to occur, and, finally, many patients develop CME for no obvious technique-related reason.

The goal of CME treatment is to improve visual acuity by decreasing macular edema once it forms. Elimination of the edema would also reduce the risk of subsequent pathologic events, such as foveal cysts and inner lamellar holes. The design and implementation of effective treatment hinges on a precise understanding of the pathophysiologic events in disease progression. Many different types of treatment have been attempted for CME, each based on some proposed aspect of the pathophysiology. Most treatment strategies for CME concentrated on either vitreous traction or inflammation as the primary etiology. Additional treatments have been suggested that try to ameliorate the edema without directly treating the cause for the edema formation.

THEORIES OF PATHOGENESIS

Vitreous Traction on the Macula

In 1953, Irvine[8] described a syndrome occurring after uncomplicated intracapsular cataract surgery in which he found delayed rupture of the anterior vitreous face, contact of the vitreous with the cataract wound with subsequent contraction of the vitreous, and resultant loss of vision associated with macular changes. Two years later Schepens[60] demonstrated attachments of the vitreous to the macula and suggested a role for the vitreous in the production of macular changes. Reese and associates[61] as well as Tolentino and Schepens[6] later enhanced the hypothesis and proposed that vitreous changes brought about by cataract surgery may lead to traction on the macula with the subsequent development of CME. Some authors[62,63] proposed the existence of "invisible" strands of vitreous inserting into the optic nerve and macula in CME as the explanation for the fluorescein angiographic pattern observed (ie, pooling of fluorescein in the cystoid spaces of the macula and late staining of the nerve head).

Gass and Norton[11] first discounted the theory of vitreous traction as the sole cause of CME because many of the patients in their series had no demonstrable vitreous attachment to the macula. This finding has been supported by other investigators. In a prospective vitrectomy study of 136 eyes with aphakic CME, only 5 (3.6%) had a demonstrable vitreous strand to the macula.[64] In a histopathologic study of eyes with CME,[35] and in eyes with CME and vitreous incarceration in the wound,[36] no attachment of the vitreous to the macula could be found.

Vitreous traction of the macula is undoubtedly *a* cause of CME, but it does not appear to be *the* predominant cause of CME in postcataract surgery patients. One condition caused by vitreous traction leading to macular edema is the vitreomacular traction syndrome.[65–67] This condition is caused by an incomplete posterior vitreous detachment where the vitreous remains attached to the macula and, usually, the optic nerve. Vitreomacular traction syndrome is relatively uncommon and may be seen in patients who never had ocular surgery. Because cataract extraction frequently precipitates posterior vitreous separation, it is possible that cataract extraction is associated with a higher prevalence of vitreomacular traction syndrome. During funduscopic examination, patients with vitreomacular traction syndrome are seen to have a cone of vitreous sweeping down toward the macula and optic nerve. The vitreous usually attaches to the posterior pole within the vascular arcades and causes a ridge-like distortion in the retina at the interface. There may be macular edema and distortion. These findings may also be appreciated in stereoscopic fluorescein angiograms.

Vitreous Incarceration in the Wound

Vitreous incarceration in the wound has been associated with CME. Follow-up study of eyes with CME has shown that eyes with vitreous incarceration were more likely to have macular edema than eyes without it.[11,12] The mean time for resolution of CME is much longer in eyes with than in eyes without vitreous incarceration.[11,12]

With changes in cataract surgery, including improved wound suturing, extracapsular surgery, posterior chamber IOLs, and improvements in handling operative complications, vitreous incarceration in the wound has become less common. In one study of patients with clinically significant CME, many of whom had complicated cataract surgery, 35% had vitreous incarceration in the wound.[5] In a histopathologic study, eyes with CME were not more likely to have vitreous incarceration than eyes without CME.

VITREOUS PROCEDURES IN THE TREATMENT OF CYSTOID MACULAR EDEMA

Vitrectomy for Vitreomacular Traction Syndrome

Vitreomacular traction syndrome is generally treated by vitrectomy. Occasionally, the vitreous spontaneously separates from the macula during the vitrectomy so that no actual "peeling" is necessary. If it does not, peeling the posterior vitreous face from the surface of the macula is relatively straightforward. After the surgery, the patient may have a decrease in the distortion as well as an improvement in visual acuity. Complete resolution of the macular edema may take months to occur.

Treatment of Vitreous Incarceration

Nd:YAG Laser Vitreolysis

If CME complicated with vitreous incarceration in the wound resolves more slowly than CME without vitreous incarceration, removing or cutting the offending vitreous might shorten the time for resolution of the associated CME. This strategy is the basis of several studies examining the role of both Nd:YAG laser vitreolysis and vitrectomy in the treatment of CME.

Nd:YAG laser vitreolysis has been reported to cause improvement of CME in some postcataract surgery patients.[68,69] The exact benefit of this treatment cannot be gauged with certainty at the present because of several reasons. First, the studies had no controls. Second, the patients were treated with corticosteroids after Nd:YAG laser vitreolysis, which may have a separate, beneficial, effect on CME. Third, many of the patients had CME for a short period[68,69] and may have spontaneously improved. Fourth, vitreous fibers chronically incarcerated in the wound become much more difficult to lyse. The corneal endothelium migrates over the vitreous strands and lays down basement membrane, making the strands more tenacious. The early treatment of the patients in these studies may have resulted in a higher anatomic success rate in terms of cutting the vitreous fibers than if the authors had waited longer to perform the procedure.

Nd:YAG laser vitreolysis is performed using a contact lens with an auxiliary button dioptric element (such as the Abraham lens). Patients who have corneal opacities or peripheral corneal edema require the use of a mirrored gonioscopy lens. Certain caveats in lysing vitreous strands merit special attention. First, the strands are always larger and broader than they first appear. Second, it is easy, especially using a gonioscopy lens, to strike the iris, which in an irritated eye may cause bleeding or increased inflammation. Third, iridovitreal synechiae posterior to the iris cannot be reliably lysed with a Nd:YAG laser. This problem may not be identified by slit-lamp examination, but can be recognized and treated during vitrectomy.

Vitrectomy

Using the same reasoning that CME with vitreous incarceration may resolve faster after the incarceration is relieved, several studies investigating vitrectomy have been performed. After publication of favorable results of nonrandomized vitrectomy studies in aphakic eyes,[70,71] a randomized clinical trial was conducted using vitrectomy to treat chronic aphakic CME with vitreous in the wound.[64,72] The proportion of patients who had an improvement in visual acuity after vitrectomy was greater than in the control group, but several patients in the vitrectomy group did not improve. The patients in the vitrectomy group were treated with topical atropine and corticosteroids; however, the patients in the control group were not, which might have favorably affected the vitrectomy group. After surgery, postvitrectomy patients may follow the same time course for resolution that patients with CME without vitreous incarceration would be expected to have.

Because of changes in cataract surgery as well as the improvement in anterior vitrectomy techniques, most patients with CME do not have vitreous incarceration. In addition, almost every patient undergoing cataract surgery has an intraocular lens implantation, and consequently is not aphakic. There are little data concerning vitrectomy for pseudophakic patients with CME who do not have vitreous incarceration. Preliminary study has suggested that vitrectomy may have a beneficial effect on CME for some patients with uveitis. Whether this may be beneficial in pseudophakic CME without vitreous incarceration remains to be proved.

Vitreous-Uveal Traction

Iridovitreal adhesions and vitreal distortion of the pars plicata have been correlated with the presence of CME. After a cataract extraction, iridovitreal adhesions may form after vitreous loss. It is possible for vitreous adhesions with the posterior iris, pars plicata, or both to form in eyes with or without vitreous loss. Pars plana vitrectomy can be used to relieve these adhesions. Removing the vitreous traction from the uveal structures may affect the prognosis of CME in several different ways. Vitreous traction may chronically stimulate the involved uveal tract to release inflammatory mediators. Vitreous traction on the pars plicata can alter aqueous humor dynamics and intraocular pressure, factors that may participate in the formation of CME.[74] Transport of prostaglandins from the eye occurs in the area of the ciliary body.[75] It is possible that chronic traction in this area may change the dynamics of inflammatory mediator transport within the eye leading to CME.

INFLAMMATION AS THE ORIGIN OF CYSTOID MACULAR EDEMA

Irvine considered inflammation as one of the causes of decreased vision in patients with spontaneous rupture of the vitreous face and macular changes. In 1954, Chandler described macular edema resulting in "cystic degeneration" after cataract surgery and considered prolonged postoperative inflammation as a predisposing cause.

Although eyes with CME do not necessarily have cell and flare, they commonly have other signs of intraocular inflammation. These eyes frequently are irritated and have perilimbal injection. Eyes with CME have evidence of blood–ocular barrier breakdown during fluorophotometry. Histopathologic study has shown inflammatory cells in the iris, ciliary body, and around the retinal blood vessels. The histopathologic finding of cyclitis, in particular, was strongly associated with chronic CME.

A study of 141 patients with visual loss from chronic CME revealed that iris incarceration in the wound was the most important predictor of poor vision.[5] In this study, the mean visual acuity of patients with hypertension, glaucoma, iritis, an IOL, or vitreous incarceration in the wound was not significantly different from the mean visual acuity of patients without these factors.[5] Almost 43% of patients with vitreous in the wound had iris in the wound. When analyzed by logistic regression, iris, but not vitreous, incarceration in the wound was predictive of visual acuity less than 20/200.

The iris is a metabolically active tissue capable of producing many different inflammatory mediators.[76] Incarceration of iris in the wound may cause the production and release of these mediators with CME formation as a possible distal effect. CME associated with iris clip lenses and rigid anterior chamber intraocular lenses appears to have chronic iris stimulation as the common element. The only factors found to be associated with a chronic breakdown of the blood–aqueous barrier in a study of patients after cataract surgery and posterior chamber lens implantation were abnormal pupil shape and posterior synechiae, both implying iris involvement.[77] Entrapment of the peripheral iris in the wound might cause chronic stimulation of the ciliary body leading to cyclitis, a histopathologic finding that has been strongly associated with chronic CME.[34]

CME has long been associated with certain forms of uveitis, such as pars planitis, bird-shot chorioretinitis, and idiopathic vitritis.[3] These syndromes share some similarities with postcataract surgery CME, such as evidence of inflammation in the region of the iris and ciliary body. Because uveitis can cause CME, and because eyes with CME seem to harbor some inflammation, it seems logical to presume that inflammation or mediators of inflammation play a role in the production or augmentation of postcataract surgery CME.

Possible Inflammatory Mediators in Cystoid Macular Edema

Several mediators of inflammation have been proposed to produce or enhance the formation of CME. Worst[78] suggested that potentially toxic substances, normally contained in the anterior segment, may diffuse back to the macula after cataract extraction. Worst[78] was the first author to suggest that prostaglandins may participate in the formation of CME by this mechanism.

The synthesis of prostaglandins starts with arachidonic acid, a 20-carbon acid derived from dietary linoleic acid. Arachidonic acid is released from cell membranes by the action of phospholipase A_2 in response to ischemia, trauma, and neuronal or hormonal stimuli. Cyclooxygenase converts arachidonic acid to cyclic endoperoxide intermediates that are then converted to prostaglandins.[79–81] Light exposure to the retina also has been suggested as a factor that may increase the production of prostaglandins mediated through the generation of free radicals.[82] Corticosteroids can indirectly block the action of phospholipase A_2, thus preventing the release of arachidonic acid. Nonsteroidal antiinflammatory drugs, such as aspirin, indomethacin, or ketorolac tromethamine, block the synthesis of prostaglandins from arachidonic acid by inhibiting cyclooxygenase.[79–81]

The causal link between prostaglandins and CME, though appealing, has been difficult to confirm. CME has not been induced in animal eyes through the injection of prostaglandins. Topical application of prostaglandins are being investigated as possible antiglaucoma medications in humans, and their use has not been associated with CME.[83,84] There are theoretic problems in looking at the actions of inflammatory mediators in isolation, however; the effect of one mediator is often modified by the milieu of other mediators that may be present.

Arachidonic acid may be metabolized by enzymes, such as the 5-lipoxygenase,[80] to produce leukotrienes and peptidoleukotrienes. Additional mediators, not produced from arachidonic acid, such as neuropeptides, cytokines, bradykinin, histamine, tumor necrosis factor, and platelet-activating factor, have been shown to have roles in inflammation. During an inflammatory response, a spectrum of these inflammatory mediators are produced. Inflammatory mediators implicated in ocular inflammation are listed in Table 15-1.[79–91]

Inflammatory mediators ordinarily interact in an orchestrated manner to effect the proper response. For example, neuropeptides can cause prostaglandin release in the eye. Prostaglandins require intact innervation in the eye, though, to produce inflammatory effects.[85] Denervation reduces the sensitivity of the eye to the inflammatory effects of prostaglandins.[85] Effects of platelet-activating factor are mediated through peptidoleukotrienes.[86] Platelet-activating factor may increase the release of arachidonic acid and the production of prostaglandins.[87] Prostaglandins and leukotrienes interact to increase vascular permeability. Tumor necrosis factor increases aqueous prostaglandin and leukotriene concentrations.[88] Tumor necrosis factor can also induce interleukin-1 (IL-1), which is a potent agent causing vascular leakage; IL-1 can, in turn, induce prostaglandins.[89]

Table 15-1
Mediators That May Promote Ocular Inflammation

Cytochrome p450 products
Histamine
Interferon-γ
Interleukins (especially 1, 2, 6, and 8)
Leukotrienes
Neuropeptides
Platelet-activating factor
Prostaglandins
Serotonin
Tumor necrosis factor

Table 15-2
Mediators That May Inhibit Intraocular Inflammation

α-Melanocyte-stimulating hormone
Endogenous glucocorticoids
Prostaglandins
Transforming growth factor–β
Vasoactive intestinal peptide

Many of these mediators promote inflammation, whereas others, such as transforming growth factor–beta (TGF-β), are immunosuppressive[92] (Table 15-2). These immunosuppressive mediators, which appear in the eye, participate in the maintenance of an altered immune response in the eye called anterior chamber–associated immune deviation (ACAID). TGF-β helps establish ACAID through a secondary mediator, prostaglandin E2.[92] (Thus, prostaglandins appear to both promote and suppress certain aspects of intraocular inflammation.) Ocular use of immunosuppressive cytokines, or analogues of these cytokines, may be one avenue to treat CME, and uveitis, in the future.

CME may be the distal result of a pathologic production or interaction of several different inflammatory mediators produced in the anterior segment. Reduction of any or all of the proinflammatory mediators may cause a decline in inflammatory activity, and prevent or ameliorate CME. Although corticosteroids inhibit the release of arachidonic acid as well as reducing the production or effect of several other autacoids, they are associated with many adverse effects. To sidestep the complications of corticosteroids, later studies have investigated the role of nonsteroidal antiinflammatory drugs (NSAIDs) in the treatment of CME. These studies have focused on prostaglandin synthesis inhibitors for two main reasons. First, because prostaglandins have proinflammatory effects and they also interact with other mediators of inflammation, reducing prostaglandin synthesis may modulate the entire inflammatory process. Second, prostaglandin synthesis inhibitors are commonly available, and there are relatively few known inhibitors of any of the other mediators of inflammation.[28]

ANTIINFLAMMATORY AGENTS IN THE TREATMENT OF POSTSURGICAL CYSTOID MACULAR EDEMA

Corticosteroids

Because corticosteroids improve CME related to uveitis syndromes, such as intermediate uveitis, it is understandable that corticosteroids were among the first medications used to treat postcataract surgery CME. Unfortunately, corticosteroids have never been the subject of a randomized double-blind study for the treatment of CME, making interpretation of the studies difficult.

Gehring[95] treated 17 patients with CME detected by contact lens examination. After treatment using 20 to 40 mg of systemically administered prednisone per day for varying periods, 13 patients (76%) improved to 20/30 and 15 patients (88%) improved by two or more lines of visual acuity. Several patients had recurrences of CME with discontinuance of prednisone, and they improved with resumption of prednisone. Though the results appear dramatic, many of the cases in this series were of relatively recent onset and may have spontaneously resolved without treatment.

Stern and colleagues[57] studied 50 patients who had chronic CME associated with iris-fixated lenses. Of the 50 patients, 49 were treated with varying combinations of oral, sub-Tenon, and topical corticosteroids. Eleven patients responded quickly with corticosteroids and had no recurrence of CME, although some of these patients were continued on a lower dose schedule. Thirty patients had recurrences after corticosteroids were tapered; with resumption of corticosteroids, 16 of these improved to 20/40 or better, and 14 had a final visual acuity between 20/40 and 20/80. Nine patients did not seem to respond to corticosteroids.

Despite the lack of randomized studies, corticosteroids are among the most commonly used drugs in the treatment of CME. Most patients seen in a referral practice have received at least one course of topical corticosteroids before referral. The efficacy of topical corticosteroids might be limited in this disorder because of poor penetration past the anterior segment of the eye. Similarly, uveitis syndromes associated with CME, such as intermediate uveitis, may not respond to topical corticosteroids but frequently respond to oral and sub-Tenon corticosteroids.

Corticosteroids have many adverse ocular and systemic side effects, particularly in older patients. The most common ocular complication in patients treated for CME with corticosteroids is elevated intraocular pressure. McEntyre[96] suggested that ocular hypertension induced by corticosteroid administration altered hydrostatic dynamics in the macula. He treated patients with enough corticosteroids to induce ocular hypertension and found these patients had a decrease in their CME. A complete account of the intraocular pressures for these patients was not reported. Most patients apparently had a pressure rise of 5 to 10 mmHg, but some had intraocular pressures as high as 38 mmHg. Melberg and Olk[97] compared the success rate of treatment for two groups of patients with postcataract surgery CME: one group that did have an elevation of intraocular pressure with treatment and a control group that did not. All 16 patients without vitreous attachment to anterior chamber structures who developed increased intraocular pressure had improvement of their CME. In contrast, only 4 of 14 control patients without an increase in intraocular pressure had improvement in their CME.[97]

Corticosteroid-induced ocular hypertension may affect the fluid flow from leaking macular capillaries by increasing the hydrostatic tissue fluid pressure. In the discussion of Melberg and Olk's article, Jampol[98] considered several possible explanations for the observed effect in addition to the rise in intraocular pressure affecting tissue hydrostatic pressure. Other possibilities considered were that the corticosteroid responders differed genetically, had different corticosteroid receptors, or had better drug penetration than the nonresponders. Another possibility suggested was that inflammation causes decreased intraocular pressure, and patients having the best response to antiinflammatory therapy would be expected to have a greater restoration of intraocular pressure than those who did not.[98]

Nonsteroidal antiinflammatory drugs, such as the cyclooxygenase inhibitors (COIs), decrease intraocular inflammation without causing elevated intraocular pressure.[99] As I discuss subsequently, studies have shown an improvement in CME in patients treated with COIs. With COIs, there appears to be a dissociation between increased intraocular pressure and improvement of CME. This finding may suggest that the increased intraocular pressure found in corticosteroid-treated patients may not be the sole mechanism causing improvement in CME.

Increased intraocular pressure induced by corticosteroids may be treated with additional medications, but lowering intraocular pressure may alter the therapeutic efficacy. Withdrawal of the corticosteroids may be the most prudent approach for patients with elevated intraocular pressure. Common systemic complications associated with corticosteroids in patients being treated for CME include hyperglycemia, hypertension, and neuropsychiatric problems. Sub-Tenon injection of corticosteroids reduces the potential for systemic complications, and possibly some of the ocular complications, such as glaucoma, as well. Many patients have at least a transient response to sub-Tenon injection of corticosteroids. There is no proof of any long-term improvement or alteration of the natural course of CME after dissipation of the corticosteroids. It is possible, though, that some severe sequelae, such as the formation of foveal cysts or inner lamellar holes, may be avoided with the reduction of edema.

Nonsteroidal Antiinflammatory Drugs

Prophylaxis of Postsurgical Cystoid Macular Edema

Corticosteroids have many adverse effects in older patients, whereas nonsteroidal antiinflammatory drugs generally have fewer and less severe detrimental effects. Numerous studies have been conducted to examine the efficacy of COIs both in the prophylaxis and treatment of CME.[100–116] Miyake and associates[101–103] used indomethacin, a prostaglandin synthesis inhibitor, to try to prevent CME after cataract surgery. A long-term follow-up study[103] found that patients treated with indomethacin had improvement in visual acuity early after surgery, but this effect did not persist. Other investigators found that patients treated prophylactically with topical indomethacin had a decreased incidence of angiographically demonstrable CME by approximately one half, but no improvement in visual acuity was found.[104,106] Systemic indomethacin used for prophylaxis was thought to reduce the incidence of CME 4 to 6 weeks after cataract surgery, but no improvement in visual acuity was found.[107] In one study, systemic aspirin did not appear to have an effect on visual acuity from postcataract-surgery CME.[108]

Many of the studies investigating indomethacin employed simultaneous corticosteroid treatment.[100] This use may obscure the true treatment benefit from indomethacin, but, conversely, corticosteroids are given to nearly all patients undergoing cataract extraction.

A well-controlled, paired comparison study by Flach and associates showed[105] that ketorolac tromethamine used without corticosteroids was effective in reducing the incidence of angiographic CME. Because no study has been done to evaluate the effectiveness of topical corticosteroids in reducing the incidence of angiographic CME, the practical benefit of this finding is difficult to quantify. The visual acuity of the patients was not mentioned in the results of this study.[105]

A major goal in prophylactic treatment would be to decrease the number of patients with clinically significant CME. No prophylaxis study has shown a statistically significant long-term reduction in the number of patients developing clinically significant CME. Because clinically significant CME is relatively uncommon, thousands of patients would have to be enrolled in a randomized study. As yet, no study of this size has been performed in the prevention of clinically significant CME.

Treatment of Clinically Significant Cystoid Macular Edema

A more pragmatic approach would be to treat patients with clinically significant CME.[110–115] Neither oral indomethacin[110] nor topical fenoprofen[111] caused a statistically significant improvement in visual acuity. Yannuzzi[112] treated 40 consecutive patients with CME using indomethacin and corticosteroids, and found 80% improved by two or more Snellen lines. There were no control patients. In several patients, the visual acuity declined with cessation of treatment and then improved with resumption of therapy. In another study by Peterson and associates,[113] use of topical indomethacin was associated with an improvement of three Snellen lines or more in 80% of patients treated. This particular study included only patients who could tolerate the medication for 8 weeks, and the study had no controls. Of the patients who initially responded, 53% displayed an "on-off" phenomenon when treatment was started and stopped.[113]

Two double-masked,[114,115] randomized trials showed that patients treated with topical ketorolac drops were more likely to have a visual acuity improvement of two or more lines of Snellen distance visual acuity than were patients given a placebo. A two-line improvement in Snellen acuity may be accomplished by as little as a 33% improvement in the visual acuity advancing from 20/80 to 20/60. At the present time, it is difficult to determine if there is a long-term effect or if the natural course of CME is changed by a limited course of ketorolac treatment. Although there was a statistically significant effect demonstrated under ketorolac treatment, this improvement may not be great enough to be of utility for all patients.

There are several possibilities why COIs have not caused a better improvement of visual acuity in CME. Chronic edema may produce profound architectural alterations in the fovea, causing lasting damage. The fovea may also suffer damage induced by inflammation. Eyes with CME may have Müller cell abnormalities as well as the possibility of ischemic damage contributing to the long-term visual loss. Finally, RPE changes caused by CME may also cause visual loss.

The limited success of prostaglandin synthesis inhibitors in these studies raises other questions concerning the role that prostaglandin synthesis inhibition has in the treatment of CME. It is also possible that the types and dosages of COIs were not used in an optimal dose. Oral COIs penetrate into the eye poorly.[109] Topical COIs penetrate to varying degrees, but the exact amount of prostaglandin synthesis inhibition needed, at different areas in the eye, is not known with certainty. Because of the many different classes of mediators released in inflammation, blocking prostaglandin synthesis alone may not be sufficient. A nonsteroidal drug that blocks production or dampens the effect of more than one type of inflammatory mediator might be more efficacious in treating CME. It may be possible to inhibit inflammation and its sequelae without experiencing the side effects of corticosteroids.

REDUCTION OF PHOTOTOXICITY

The dioptric mechanism of the eye focuses light on the retina where selected photochemical reactions ordinarily occur. The cataractous lens has chromophores that reduce the transmission of shorter-wavelength light. During removal of the cataractous lens, the retina is exposed to much light, and the relative proportion of shorter-wavelength light may be increased. In the postsurgical state, IOLs may allow a greater proportion of shorter-wavelength light to reach the retina than ordinarily would be possible. It has been theorized that this excess light causes or potentiates the tendency to form CME, possibly through increased formation of prostaglandins.[82]

Blocking ultraviolet (UV) light from the microscope has not been shown to have a statistically significant effect on the prevalence of CME.[116] Pupillary light occluders used during cataract surgery have not been found to have an effect on the prevalence of CME.[117] In one randomized study, UV-absorbing intraocular lenses have been shown to reduce the incidence of angiographically detected CME; however, no effect on the visual acuity was found.[118] In two other, much smaller, studies, no effect on the prevalence of CME was found in patients receiving UV-absorbing IOLs.[119–120]

Patients who were either scheduled for enucleation or who had a blind eye were exposed to the light of an operating microscope to investigate the phototoxic effects on the retina.[121–123] Extensive RPE necrosis and disruption of the outer lamellae of the photoreceptors was demonstrated.[123] Photic injury from the microscope could be produced with both infrared and UV filters in use.[122] Despite the intentional photic injury demonstrated in these studies, no patient developed CME.[121–123]

INTRAOCULAR LENS REMOVAL AND REPLACEMENT

Intraocular lenses have been associated with CME by several mechanisms. Certain earlier IOLs, through the method of packaging, poor quality of the finish, or impurities in the plastic, were associated with CME.[58] These problems have largely been eliminated with modern manufacturing techniques. Some IOLs, such as the iris clip and rigid closed-loop anterior chamber IOLs, appear to have chronically stimulated the iris and caused CME.[58,59,124,125] Monitoring by the Food and Drug Administration and ophthalmologists[59] led to recognition of this propensity; consequently, these lenses are either no longer available or not commonly used. CME may be more frequent in eyes that through implantation, migration,[126] or dislocation developed iris tuck by a haptic or capture of the iris by the lens.[126]

Many patients with intraocular lens-related CME also have concurrent problems, such as pseudophakic bullous keratopathy, glaucoma, hyphema, and chronic inflammation. These patients ultimately may require surgery with explantation or exchange of their IOLs as a part of a larger effort to salvage the eye.

In one study examining the effect of lens removal in IOL-related CME, 5 of 10 eyes attained a visual acuity of 20/50 or better.[127] In another study, 6 eyes had lens exchange, and 4 of the eyes had visual acuity improvement of two lines or more.[128] Many eyes with pseudophakic bullous keratopathy have concurrent CME, but the exact prevalence is difficult to determine because of the difficulty in performing fluorescein angiography. However, one study showed resolution of angiographic CME in 18 of 25 patients treated with penetrating keratoplasty, anterior chamber IOL removal, and replacement with a posterior chamber IOL.[129]

IMPROVEMENT OF RPE PUMP FUNCTION AND OTHER METHODS IN THE TREATMENT OF CYSTOID MACULAR EDEMA

Carbonic Anhydrase Inhibition

Carbonic anhydrase inhibitors, such as acetazolamide, have been shown in nonrandomized studies to decrease CME and improve visual acuity in patients who had cataract surgery[130–131] and scleral buckling.[132] These drugs have not been studied in a randomized trial, but patients displayed an on-off effect with initiation and cessation of treatment. Acetazolamide may work by improving the ability of the retinal pigment epithelium to pump fluid out of the retina.[133] The rationale is to remove the edema fluid within the retina rather than to treat the cause for the fluid accumulation. This drug has been effective in only a few patients, some of whom experience tachyphylaxis; the effect of the medication lasts only as long as the patients use the drug. Long-term carbonic anhydrase inhibitor use is associated with many adverse effects, particularly in older patients.

Grid Laser Photocoagulation

Grid laser was described as a method of treatment of postsurgical CME using ruby and argon laser photocoagulation. Using a ruby laser, Zweng and associates treated 17 patients.[134] Of the 5 patients who improved, 3 patients attained 20/30 or better visual acuity. Schepens[135] suggested using argon laser for grid photocoagulation to treat CME. He did not report the results of this treatment, however. Two pilot studies investigating argon laser for chronic CME unresponsive to medical therapy found that approximately one half of the treated patients showed improvement in their visual acuity.[136–137]

The results of treating a patient with postcataract-surgery CME are shown in Figure 15-3. This patient had CME for 6 months that was not responsive to corticosteroid treatment. Her visual acuity before laser treatment was 20/100. She was given a grid laser treatment with an argon laser using a 100-μm spot size and sufficient power to cause a light blanching of the RPE. Her visual acuity improved to 20/60− in 2 weeks and with time improved to 20/25−. A follow-up angiogram showed resolution of the CME but showed late staining of the optic nerve head. It is possible that the grid laser affected the pumping ability of the RPE. In this respect, grid laser photocoagulation may resemble carbonic anhydrase inhibitors in that the pumping ability of the RPE is modified without directly treating what is causing the CME to form originally.

Grid laser treatment has not been investigated in the context of a controlled clinical trial; therefore, no information is available concerning its efficacy or safety. It is possible that grid laser treatment, particularly in elderly patients, may induce or accelerate RPE atrophy in the macular region, which is an unacceptable trade-off causing detriment over time to the central vision.

Hyperoxic Therapy

Five patients with chronic CME after cataract extraction or secondary IOL implantation were treated with intermittent hyperbaric oxygen for 21 days and had an improvement in visual acuity.[138] The fluorescein angiography results did not improve after the conclusion of treatment in two patients and showed minimal change in a third patient. The visual acuity improvement did not seem to be correlated to the change in the fluorescein angiography result. The authors suggested that constriction of perifoveal capillaries by hyperbaric oxygen may facilitate the reformation of damaged junctional complexes in the capillary wall.[138] Although this explanation may be true, it does not adequately explain the rapid improvement in visual acuity without a parallel change in the amount of macular edema. The hyperbaric oxygen may also af-

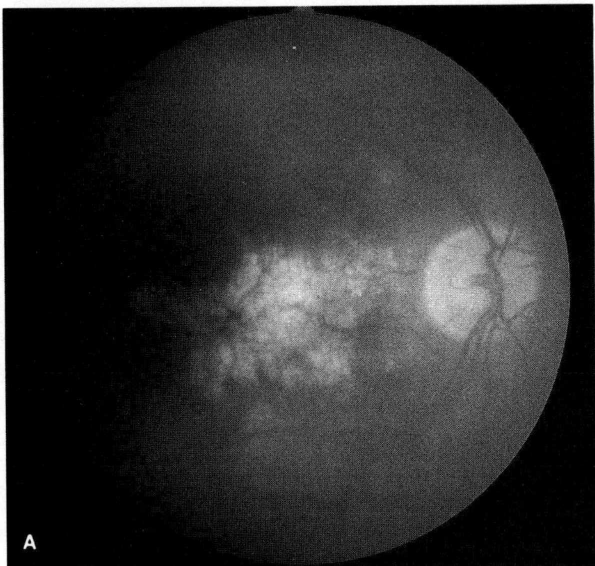

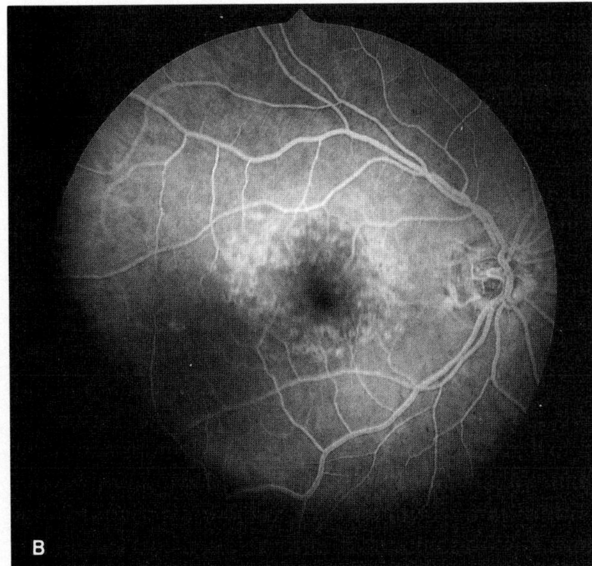

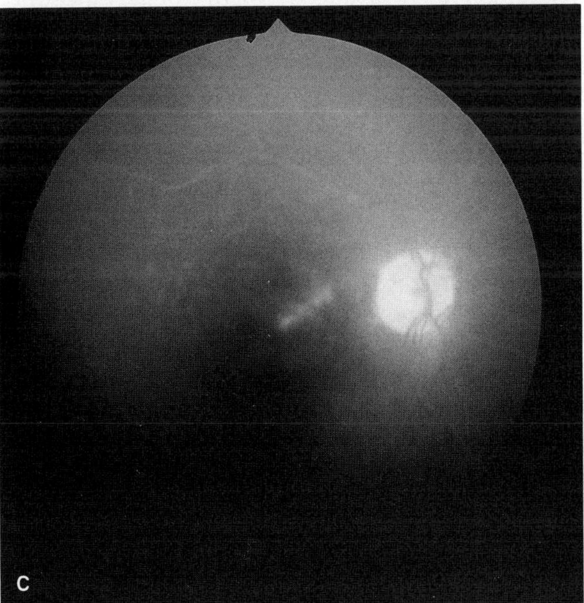

Figure 15-3. (**A**) Pretreatment fluorescein angiogram. (**B**) After laser treatment the patient had resolution of the CME. The grid laser pattern is evident in the arteriovenous phase of the angiogram. (**C**) In the later phases of the angiogram, no CME is evident, but there is persistent late staining of the optic nerve.

fect the anterior segment of the eye, or it may alter ischemia of the macula.

In a different study, high concentrations of oxygen were administered to three eyes with chronic aphakic CME through the use of modified swimmer's goggles.[139] All three patients had an improvement in visual acuity. Benner and Xiaoping[139] suggested that the locally administered oxygen increased the partial pressure of oxygen (Po_2) of the inner retina. Transcorneal delivery of oxygen has been shown to increase the Po_2 of the anterior segment,[140] but whether or not this approach also increases retinal oxygenation is a matter of speculation. It is also possible that the local increase of the Po_2 in the anterior segment altered the production or metabolism of inflammatory mediators produced.

CME TREATMENT ALGORITHM

This year more than 1 million patients will have cataract extractions in the United States. If 1% to 2% of these patients develop clinically significant CME, there will be 10,000 to 20,000 disappointed patients with potentially treatable visual loss. How should a patient with clinically significant CME be treated? The lack of randomized therapeutic trials limits the objective information available to base definitive recommendations for the treatment of CME. Given the imperfect nature of current knowledge, recommendations for treatment are formed from consolidating information from past therapeutic studies and considerations of the pathophysiology of CME.[141]

The best course of action for a patient with CME for only a few months after cataract surgery is to wait, as most of these patients will spontaneously resolve. Patients with chronic CME who have vitreous incarceration in the surgical wound usually merit a course of pharmacologic treatment before any attempts of surgical repair for the vitreous incarceration. Nd:YAG laser vitreolysis may be convenient for the physician and the patient, but has distinct technical limitations. In addition, there is little knowledge of the efficacy of Nd:YAG laser vitreolysis in more chronic cases of CME. Vitrectomy, either through an anterior or posterior approach, has the potential to effect a better repair of vitreous adhesions to the wound or iris, especially in more chronic cases. Iris incarceration may be repaired during the same procedure.

In cases in which pharmacologic therapy is indicated, what is the drug of choice, and how should it be delivered? This question cannot be definitively answered at the present time because of the lack of adequate studies examining and comparing various medications used in the treatment of CME. Corticosteroids are probably the most commonly used medications in the treatment for CME but have not been the subject of a randomized control trial. NSAIDs offer the possibility of less adverse systemic and ocular side effects. Oral NSAIDs do not appear to penetrate the eye well and have not been shown to be efficacious. Topical indomethacin is not available commercially, but the eye drops may be prepared by a pharmacist. Indomethacin eye drops commonly cause irritation, and less commonly cause punctate keratitis and corneal epithelial loss. The epithelial problems may be related to the high pH of 9 required to keep indomethacin in solution.

One topical NSAID, ketorolac tromethamine, has been shown to be effective in treating clinically significant CME; it is available as an eye drop but is not currently labeled for the treatment of CME. A few patients respond to ketorolac, but the amount of improvement experienced may not be satisfactory. Ketorolac has not been compared with corticosteroids in any reported clinical study for the treatment of clinically significant CME to date.

Studies using both corticosteroids and NSAIDs together suggest that some patients may respond to a short course of therapy without recurrence of CME. The withdrawal of corticosteroids and NSAIDs, though, has been associated with the recurrence of

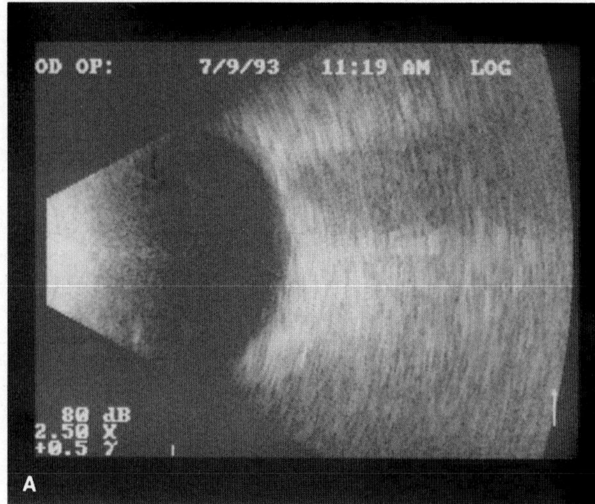

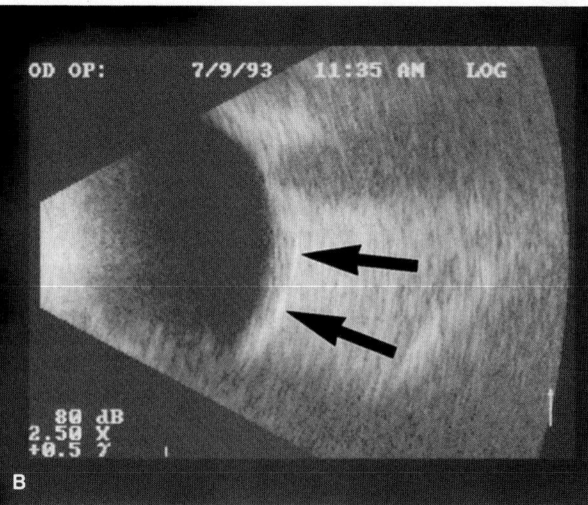

Figure 15-4. (**A**) Contact B-scan ultrasonogram before sub–Tenon injection of triamcinolone. (**B**) After injection of triamcinolone, a hyperechogenic collection is seen in Tenon space behind the macula, confirming the desired location of the injection.

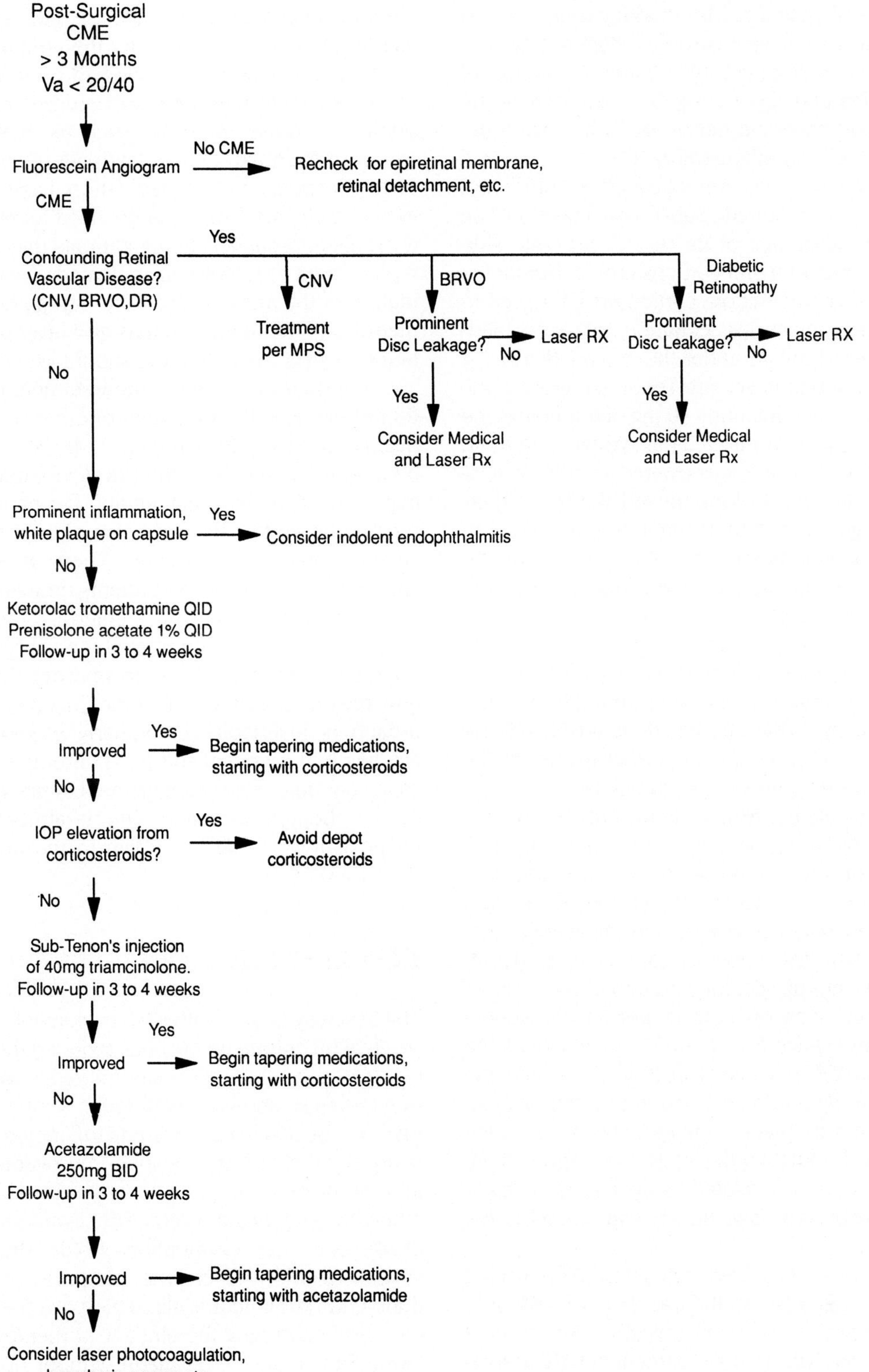

Figure 15-5. Cystoid macular edema (CME) treatment flow chart.

CME in several patients. This finding suggests that some patients may have a chronic inflammatory condition that may require chronic treatment. The use of corticosteroids and NSAIDs together may reduce the amount of corticosteroid necessary to achieve a desired amount of antiinflammatory effect.

If topical medications are not effective, sub-Tenon injection may be required. Sub-Tenon injection has the theoretic advantage of decreased systemic side effects compared with oral corticosteroids. Ocular hypertension after sub-Tenon corticosteroid injection appears to be relatively less common unless the medication dissects forward under the conjunctiva.

One technique to inject sub-Tenon corticosteroids is as follows: 1 mL containing 40 mg of triamcinolone acetonide is drawn up into a 3-mL syringe, and a ⅝-in. 25-gauge needle is then secured to the syringe. Patients are directed to look toward the tip of their nose, and the needle entry is made through the conjunctiva supertemporal to the globe, close to the equator. The needle is then slowly inserted, keeping the tip close to the globe. While the needle is being advanced, it is moved side to side in a sweeping motion that parallels the circumference of the globe. This maneuver makes inadvertent perforation of the sclera less likely. While the needle is advanced, the angle of the syringe is altered so that the tip of the needle follows the curvature of the globe.

After the needle is advanced to the hub, the syringe is aspirated to ensure that a vessel has not been cannulated. If not, the corticosteroid is slowly injected. The patient frequently feels nothing immediately but later has an increasing ache behind the eye after the injection. When the corticosteroid is properly injected, it does not dissect forward under the conjunctiva. It can be seen on contact B-scan ultrasonography in Tenon space[142] (Fig. 15-4). The effects of the injection on CME may take 1 or 2 weeks to become apparent. The patient notices an improvement in visual acuity and frequently remarks that colors seem brighter as well. Whether the subjective improvement in color perception is related to decreased macular edema or decreased optic nerve head edema is not known.

Although there has been no placebo-controlled study of corticosteroids in the treatment of CME after cataract surgery, sub-Tenon injection of corticosteroids is a mainstay in the treatment of CME associated with uveitis syndromes, such as intermediate uveitis. Glaucoma, even in steroid responders, is uncommon after sub-Tenon injection unless the corticosteroid dissects forward under the conjunctiva.

In patients who either have had no response to or could not receive sub-Tenon corticosteroids, a carbonic anhydrase inhibitor, such as acetazolamide, can be prescribed. Only a few patients have a satisfactory response to this medication. Lack of response to any medication suggests the need for evaluation of alternate approaches. Some patients may require IOL replacement or removal as indicated by careful examination of the anterior segment. Rarely, experimental methods of treatment, such as grid laser photocoagulation or hyperoxic therapy, should be considered.

Separate issues arise in the treatment of CME that do not occur in the treatment of other ocular inflammatory diseases. Postsurgical CME is a disappointment to the patient and the physician, both of whom expected improved visual acuity. The patient may express concern that the physician did not perform the cataract operation correctly. There is generally a strong pressure to treat patients immediately with postsurgical CME seen in a referral practice. Many times these patients are treated with several medications simultaneously to try to improve the vision by any means possible. In some instances, this approach is justifiable, particularly when the fellow eye has had a poor result from chronic CME. In any case, an organized management strategy is better than a shotgun approach. One treatment algorithm for postsurgical CME is shown in the flow diagram (Fig. 15-5).

CONCLUSION

The best way to deal with CME is to avoid it. Improved surgical technique already has reduced the incidence of CME, and refinements undoubtedly continue this trend. Newer surgical techniques should be examined prospectively to determine the incidence of clinically significant CME. Despite improvements, a certain proportion of patients will probably develop clinically significant CME. The evaluation of new drugs, as well as reevaluation of older drugs such as corticosteroid medications, requires randomized double-blind clinical trials, which are the gold standard in determining the efficacy of therapy. Such determinations cannot be made without ophthalmologists referring patients with clinically significant CME to randomized trials.

References

1. Hitchings RA, Chisholm IH, Bird AC. Aphakic macular edema: incidence and pathogenesis. Invest Ophthalmol 1975;14:68.
2. Wright PL, Wilkinson CP, Balyeat HD, et al. Angiographic cystoid macular edema after posterior chamber lens implantation. Arch Ophthalmol 1988;106: 740.
3. Gass JDM. Stereoscopic atlas of macular diseases. St. Louis, CV Mosby, 1987:368–380.
4. Bovino JA, Kelly TJ, Marcus DF. Intraretinal hemorrhages in cystoid macular edema. Arch Ophthalmol 1984;102:1151.
5. Spaide RF, Yannuzzi LA, Sisco LJ. Chronic cystoid macular edema and predictors of visual acuity. Ophthalmic Surg 1993;24:262.
6. Tolentino FI, Schepens CL. Edema of the posterior pole after cataract extraction: a biomicroscopic study. Arch Ophthalmol 1965;74:781.
7. Ruiz RS, Saatchi OA. Visual outcome in pseudophakic eyes with clinical cystoid macular edema. Ophthalmic Surg 1991;22:190.
8. Irvine SR. A newly defined vitreous syndrome following cataract surgery: interpreted according to recent concepts of the structure of the vitreous. Am J Ophthalmol 1953;36:599.
9. Reese AB, Jones IS, Cooper WC. Macular changes secondary to vitreous traction. Trans Am Ophthalmol Soc 1966;64:123.
10. Gass JDM, Norton EWD. Cystoid macular edema and papilledema following cataract extraction: a fluorescein funduscopic and angiographic study. Arch Ophthalmol 1966;76:646.
11. Gass JDM, Norton EWD. Follow-up study of cystoid macular edema following cataract extraction. Trans Am Acad Ophthalmol Otolaryngol 1969;73:665.
12. Wilkinson CP. A long-term follow-up study of cystoid macular edema in aphakic and pseudophakic eyes. Trans Am Ophthalmol Soc 1981;79:810.
13. Chandler PA. Complications after cataract surgery: clinical aspects. Tran Am Acad Ophthalmol Otolaryngol 1954;58:382.
14. Hoyt CS, Nickel D. Aphakic cystoid macular edema: occurrence in infants and children after transpupillary lensectomy and anterior vitrectomy. Arch Ophthalmol 1982;100:746.
15. Nicholls JVV. Macular edema in association with cataract extraction. Am J Ophthalmol 1954;37:665.
16. Keates RH, Steinert RF, Puliafito CA, Maxwell SK. Long-term follow-up of Nd:YAG laser posterior capsulotomy. Am J Intraocular Implant Soc 1984;10:164.
17. Johnson S, Kratz R, Olson P. Clinical experience with the Nd:YAG laser. Am J Intraocular Implant Soc 1984;10:452.
18. Chambless WS. Neodymium YAG laser posterior capsulotomy results and complications. Am J Intraocular Implant Soc 1985;11:31, 1985.
19. Winslow RL, Taylor BC. Retinal complications following YAG capsulotomy. Ophthalmology 1985;92: 785.
20. Stark WJ, Worthen D, Holladay JT, Murray G. Neodymium:YAG lasers: an FDA report. Ophthalmology 1985;92:209.
21. Liesegang TJ, Bourne WM, Ilstrup DM. Secondary surgical and neodymium-YAG laser discissions. Am J Ophthalmol 1985;100:510.
22. Shah GR, Gills JP, Durham DG, Asmus WH. Three thousand YAG lasers in posterior capsulotomies: an analysis of complications and comparison to polishing and surgical discission. Ophthalmology 1986;17: 473.
23. Bath PE, Frankhauser F. Long-term results of Nd:YAG laser posterior capsulotomy with the Swiss laser. J Cataract Refract Surg 1986;12:150.
24. Steinert RF, Puliafito CA, Kumar SR, Dudak SD, Patel S. Cystoid macular edema, retinal detachment and glaucoma after Nd:YAG laser posterior capsulotomy. Am J Ophthalmol 1991;112:373.
25. Kramer SG. Cystoid macular edema after aphakic penetrating keratoplasty. Ophthalmology 1981;88: 782.
26. Miyake K, Miyake Y, Maekubo K, Asakura M, Manabe R. Incidence of cystoid macular edema after retinal detachment surgery and the use of topical indomethacin. Am J Ophthalmol 1983;95:451.
27. Choplin NT, Bene CH. Cystoid macular edema following laser iridotomy. Ann Ophthalmol 1983;15: 172.
28. Spaide RF, Yannuzzi LA. Post-cataract surgery cystoid macular edema. In: Schwartz B, ed. Clinical signs in ophthalmology. St. Louis, Mosby–Year Book, 1992:2–16.
29. Gass JDM. Lamellar macular hole: a complication of cystoid macular edema after cataract extraction: a clinicopathologic case report. Trans Am Ophthalmol Soc 1975;73:231.
30. Nussenblatt RB, Kaufman SC, Palestine AG, Davis MD, Ferris FL. Macular thickening and visual acuity: measurement in patients with cystoid macular edema. Ophthalmology 1987;94:1134.
31. Gass JDM, Anderson DR, Davis EB. A clinical, fluorescein angiographic, and electron microscopic correlation of cystoid macular edema. Am J Ophthalmol 1985;100:82.
32. Yanoff M, Fine BS, Brucker AJ, Eagle RC Jr. Pathology of human cystoid macular edema. Surv Ophthalmol 1984;28:205.
33. Martin NF, Green WR, Martin LW. Retinal phlebitis in

the Irvine-Gass syndrome. Am J Ophthalmol 1977;83: 377.

34. McDonnell PJ, de la Cruz ZC, Green WR. Vitreous incarceration complicating cataract surgery: a light and electron microscopic study. Ophthalmology 1986;93:247.
35. Norton AL, Brown WJ, Carlson M, Pilger IS. Pathogenesis of aphakic macular edema. Am J Ophthalmol 1975;80:96.
36. Fine BS, Brucker AJ. Macular edema and cystoid macular edema. Am J Ophthalmol 1981;92:466.
37. Tso MOM. Pathology of cystoid macular edema. Ophthalmology 1982;89:902.
38. Streeten B. Discussion of Tso MOM: Pathology of cystoid macular edema. Ophthalmology 1982;89: 914.
39. Mutra JN, Cunha-Vaz JG, Sabo CA, Jones CW, Laski ME. Microperfusion studies on the permeability of retinal vessels. Invest Ophthalmol Vis Sci 1990; 31:471.
40. Kottow M, Hendrickson. P. Iris angiography in cystoid macular edema after cataract extraction. Arch Ophthalmol 1975;93:487.
41. Easty D, Dallas N, O'Malley R. Aphakic macular oedema following prosthetic lens implantation. Br J Ophthalmol 1977;61:321.
42. Cunha-Vaz JG, Travassos A. Breakdown of the blood retinal barriers and cystoid macular edema. Surv Ophthalmol 1984;28(Suppl):485.
43. Blair NP, Elman MJ, Rusin MM. Vitreous fluorophotometry in patients with cataract surgery. Graefes Arch Clin Exp Ophthalmol 1987;223:441.
44. Tso MOM, Shih CY. Experimental macular edema after lens extraction. Invest Ophthalmol Vis Sci 1977; 16:381.
45. Jampol LM, Setogawa T, Rednam KRV, Tso MOM. Talc retinopathy in primates: a model of ischemic retinopathy. I. Clinical studies. Arch Ophthalmol 1981;99:1273.
46. Jaffee GJ, Burton TC, Kuhn E, Prescott A, Hartz A. Progression of nonproliferative diabetic retinopathy and visual outcome after extracapsular cataract extraction and intraocular lens implantation. Am J Ophthalmol 1992;114:448.
47. Pollack A, Leiba H, Bukelman A, Oliver M. Cystoid macular edema following cataract extraction in patients with diabetes. Br J Ophthalmol 1992;76:221.
48. Liebowitz HM, Krueger DE, Maunder LR, et al. The Framingham Eye Study Monograph. Surv Ophthalmol 1980;24(Suppl):336.
49. Boldt HC, Folk JC. Slow leakage from the retinal pigment epithelium (ooze) in age-related macular degeneration. Retina 1990;10:244.
50. Frederick AR Jr, Morely MG, Topping TM, Peterson TJ, Wilson DJ. The appearance of stippled retinal pigment epithelial detachments: a sign of occult choroidal neovascularization in age-related macular degeneration. Retina 1993;13:3.
51. Schatz H, McDonald HR, Johnson RN. Retinal pigment epithelial folds associated with retinal pigment epithelial detachment in macular degeneration. Ophthalmology 1990;97:658.
52. Lakhanpal V, Schocket SS. Pseudophakic and aphakic retinal detachment mimicking cystoid macular edema. Ophthalmology 1987;94:785.
53. Fox GM, Joondeph BC, Flynn Jr HW, Pflugfelder SC, Roussel TJ. Delayed-onset pseudophakic endophthalmitis. Am J Ophthalmol 1991;111:163.
54. Chien AM, Raber IM, Fischer DH, Eagle RC, Naidoff MA. *Propionibacterium acnes* endophthalmitis after intracapsular cataract extraction. Ophthalmology 1992;99:487.
55. Meisler DM, Palestine AG, Vastine DW, et al. Chronic *Propionibacterium* endophthalmitis after extracapsular cataract extraction and intraocular lens implantation. Am J Ophthalmol 1986;102:733.
56. Klein RM, Yannuzzi L. Cystoid macular edema in the first week after cataract extraction. Am J Ophthalmol 1976;81:614.
57. Stern AL, Taylor DM, Dalburg LA, Cosentino RT. Pseudophakic cystoid maculopathy: a study of 50 cases. Ophthalmology 1981;88:942.
58. Apple DJ, Mamalis N, Loftfeld K. Complications of intraocular lenses: a historical and histopathological review. Surv Ophthalmol 1984;29:1.
59. Stark WJ, Worthen DM, Holladay JT, et al. The FDA Report on intraocular lenses. Ophthalmology 1983; 90:311.
60. Schepens CL. Fundus changes caused by alterations of the vitreous body. Am J Ophthalmol 1955;39:631.
61. Reese AB, Jones IS, Cooper WC. Macular changes secondary to vitreous traction. Am J Ophthalmol 1967;64:544.
62. Schubert HD. Cystoid macular edema: the apparent role of mechanical factors. In: Bito LZ, Stjernschantz J, eds. The ocular effects of prostaglandins and other eicosanoids. New York, Alan R. Liss, 1989: 277–291.
63. Jaffe NS. Vitreous traction at the posterior pole of the fundus due to alterations in the vitreous posterior. Trans Am Acad Ophthalmol Otolaryngol 1967;71: 642.
64. Fung WE, Vitrectomy-ACME Study Group. Vitrectomy for chronic aphakic cystoid macular edema: results of a national, collaborative, prospective, randomized investigation. Ophthalmology 1985;92:1102.
65. Smiddy WE, Michels RG, Green WR. Morphology, pathology and surgery of idiopathic vitreoretinal macular disorders. Retina 1990;10:288.
66. Smiddy WE, Green WR, Michels RG. Vitreomacular traction syndrome: ultrastructural characteristics. Am J Ophthalmol 1989;107:177.

67. Margherio RR, Trese MT, Margherio AR, Cartwright K. Surgical management of vitreomacular traction syndromes. Ophthalmology 1989;96:1437.
68. Katzen LE, Fleischman JA, Trokel S. YAG laser treatment of cystoid macular edema. Am J Ophthalmol 1983;95:589.
69. Steinert RF, Wasson PJ. Neodymium:YAG laser anterior vitreolysis for Irvine-Gass cystoid macular edema. J Cataract Refract Surg 1989;15:304.
70. Federman JL, Annesley WH Jr, Sarin LK, Remer P. Vitrectomy and cystoid macular edema. Ophthalmology 1980;87:622.
71. Fung WE. Anterior vitrectomy for aphakic cystoid macular edema. Ophthalmology 1980;87:189.
72. Fung WE. The national, prospective, randomized vitrectomy study for chronic aphakic cystoid macular edema: Progress report and comparison between control and nonrandomized groups. Surv Ophthalmol 1984;28(Suppl):569.
73. Dugel PU, Rao NA, Ozler S, Liggett PE, Smith RE. Pars plana vitrectomy for intraocular inflammation-related cystoid macular edema unresponsive to corticosteroids. Ophthalmology 1992;99:1535.
74. Zarbin MA, Michels RG, Green WR. Dissection of epiciliary tissue to treat chronic hypotony after surgery for retinal detachment with proliferative vitreoretinopathy. Retina 1991;11:208.
75. Bito LZ, Salvador EV. Intraocular fluid dynamics. III. The site and mechanism of prostaglandin transfer across the blood intraocular fluid barriers. Exp Eye Res 1972;14:233.
76. Bhattacherjee P, Kulkarni PS, Eakins KE. Metabolism of arachidonic acid in rabbit ocular tissues. Invest Ophthalmol Vis Sci 1979;18:172.
77. Ferguson VMG, Spalton DJ. Continued breakdown of the blood aqueous barrier following cataract surgery. Br J Ophthalmol 1992;76:453.
78. Worst JGF. Bioxizitat des Kammerwassers. Eine vereinheitlichende pathologische Theorie, begrundel auf hypothetische biotoxische Kammerwasserfaktoren. Klin Monatsbl Augenheilkd 1975;167:376.
79. Bazan NG, de Abreu MT, Bazan HE, Blfort R Jr. Arachidonic acid cascade and platelet-activating factor in the network of eye inflammatory mediators: therapeutic implications in uveitis. Int Ophthalmol 1990;14:335.
80. Williams KI, Higgs GA. Eicosanoids and inflammation. J Pathology 1988;156:101.
81. Smith WL. The eicosanoids and their biochemical mechanisms of action. Biochem J 1989;259:315.
82. Jampol LM. Aphakic cystoid macular edema: a hypothesis. Arch Ophthalmol 1985;103:1134.
83. Stjernschantz J, Bito LZ. The ocular effects of eicosanoids and other autocoids: historic background and the need for a broader perspective. In: Bito LZ, Stjernschantz J, eds. The ocular effects of prostaglandins and other eicosanoids. New York, Alan R. Liss, 1989:1-13.
84. Bito LZ, Camras CB, Gum GG, Resul B. The ocular hypotensive effects and side effects of prostaglandins on the eyes of experimental animals. In: Bito LZ, Stjernschantz J, eds. The ocular effects of prostaglandins and other eicosanoids. New York, Alan R. Liss, 1989:349–368.
85. Butler JM, Hammond BR. The effects of sensory denervation on the responses of the rabbit eye to prostaglandin E_2, bradykinin, and substance P. Br J Pharmacol 1980;69:495.
86. Muller A, Meynier F, and Bonne C. PAF-induced conjuctivitis in the rabbit is mediated by peptido-leukotrienes. J Ocul Pharmacol 1990;6:227.
87. Snyder F. Platelet-activating factor and related acetylated lipids as potent biologically active cellular mediators. Am J Physiol 259 (Cell Physiol) 1990;28: C697.
88. Fleisher LN, Ferrell JB, Smith MG, McGahan MC. Lipid mediators of tumor necrosis factor-alpha-induced uveitis. Invest Ophthalmol Vis Sci 1991;32: 2393.
89. De Vos AF, Hoekzema R, Kijlstra A. Cytokines and uveitis. Curr Eye Res 1992;11:581.
90. Franks WA, Limb GA, Stanford MR, et al. Cytokines in human intraocular inflammation. Curr Eye Res 1992; 11(Suppl):187.
91. Murray PI, Hoekzema R, van Haren MA, de Hon FD, Kijlstra A. Aqueous humor interleukin-6 levels in uveitis. Invest Ophthalmol Vis Sci 1990;31:917.
92. Streilein JW, Wilbanks GA, Taylor A, Cousins S. Eye-derived cytokines and the immunosuppressive intraocular microenvironment: a review. Curr Eye Res 1992;11(Suppl):41.
93. Lipton JM, Macaluso A, Hiltz ME, Catania A. Central administration of the peptide alpha-MSH inhibits inflammation in the skin. Peptides 1991;12:795.
94. Catania A, Arnold J, Macaluso A, Hiltz ME, Lipton JM. Inhibition of acute inflammation in the periphery by central action of salicylates. Proc Natl Acad Sci USA 1991;88:8544.
95. Gehring JR. Macular edema following cataract extraction. Arch Ophthalmol 1968;80:626.
96. McEntyre JM. A successful treatment for aphakic cystoid macular edema. Ann Ophthalmol 1978;10: 1219.
97. Melberg NS, Olk RJ. Corticosteroid-induced ocular hypertension in the treatment of aphakic or pseudophakic cystoid macular edema. Ophthalmology 1993;100:164.
98. Jampol LM. Discussion of Melberg NS, Olk RJ: Corticosteroid-induced ocular hypertension in the treatment of aphakic or pseudophakic cystoid macular edema. Ophthalmology 1993;100:167.
99. Gieser DK, Hodapp E, Goldberg I, Kass MA, Becker

B. Flurbiprofen and intraocular pressure. Ann Ophthalmol 1981;13:831.
100. Flach AJ. Cyclo-oxygenase inhibitors in ophthalmology. Surv Ophthalmol 1992;36:259.
101. Miyake K. Prevention of cystoid macular edema after lens extraction by topical indomethacin. I. A preliminary report. Albrecht von Graefes Arch Klin Exp Ophthalmol 1977;203:81.
102. Miyake K. Prevention of cystoid macular edema after lens extraction by topical indomethacin. II. A control study in bilateral extractions. Jpn J Ophthalmol 1978; 22:80.
103. Miyake K, Sakamura S, Miura H. Long-term follow-up study on the prevention of aphakic cystoid macular edema by topical indomethacin. Br J Ophthalmol 1980;64:324.
104. Yannuzzi LA, Landau AN, Turtz AL. Incidence of aphakic cystoid macular edema with the use of topical indomethacin. Ophthalmology 1981;88:947.
105. Flach AJ, Stegman RC, Graham J, Kruger LP. Prophylaxis of aphakic macular edema without corticosteroids. Ophthalmology 1990;97:1253.
106. Kraff MC, Sanders DR, Jampol LM, Peyman GA, Lieberman HL. Prophylaxis of pseudophakic cystoid macular edema with topical indomethacin. Ophthalmology 1982;89:885.
107. Klein RM, Katzin HM, Yannuzzi LA. The effect of indomethacin pretreatment on aphakic cystoid macular edema. Am J Ophthalmol 1979;87:487.
108. Shammas HJ, Milkie CF. Does aspirin prevent postoperative cystoid macular edema? J Am Intraocul Implant Soc 1979;5:337.
109. Abelson MB, Smith LM, Ormerod LD. Prospective, randomized trial of oral piroxicam in the prophylaxis of postoperative cystoid macular edema. J Ocular Pharmacology 1989;5:147.
110. Yannuzzi LA, Klein RM, Wallyn RH, Cohen N, Katz I. Ineffectiveness of indomethacin in the treatment of chronic cystoid macular edema. Am J Ophthalmol 1977;84:517.
111. Burnett J, Tessler H, Isenberg S, Tso MOM. Double masked trial of fenoprofen sodium treatment of chronic aphakic cystoid macular edema. Ophthalmic Surg 1983;14:150.
112. Yannuzzi LA. A perspective on the treatment of aphakic cystoid macular edema. Surv Ophthalmol 1984; 28(Suppl):540.
113. Peterson M, Yoshizumi MO, Hepler R, Mondino B, Kreiger A. Topical indomethacin in the treatment of chronic cystoid macular edema. Graefes Arch Clin Exp Ophthalmol 1992;230:401.
114. Flach AJ, Dolan BJ, Irvine AR. Effectiveness of ketorolac 0.5% solution for chronic aphakic and pseudophakic cystoid macular edema. Am J Ophthalmol 1987;103:479.
115. Flach AJ, Jampol LM, Weinberg D, et al. Improvement in visual acuity in chronic aphakic and pseudophakic cystoid macular edema after treatment with topical 0.5% ketorolac tromethamine. Am J Ophthalmol 1991;112:514.
116. Jampol LM, Kraff MC, Sanders DR, Alexander K, Lieberman H. Near-UV radiation from the operating microscope and pseudophakic cystoid macular edema. Arch Ophthalmol 1985;103:28.
117. Kraff MC, Lieberman HL, Jampol LM, Sanders DR. Effect of a pupillary light occluder on cystoid macular edema. J Cataract Refract Surg 1989;15:658.
118. Kraff MC, Sanders DR, Jampol LM, Lieberman HL. Effect of an ultraviolet-filtering intraocular lens on cystoid macular edema. Ophthalmology 1985;92: 366.
119. Komatsu M, Kanagami S, Shimizu K. Ultraviolet-absorbing intraocular lens versus non–UV-absorbing intraocular lens: comparison of angiographic cystoid macular edema. J Cataract Refract Surg 1989;15:654.
120. Clarke MP, Yap M, Weatherill JR. Do intraocular lenses with ultraviolet absorbing chromophores protect against macular edema? Acta Ophthalmol 1989; 67:593.
121. Robertson DM, Feldman RB. Photic retinopathy from the operating room microscope. Am J Ophthalmol 1986;101:561.
122. Robertson DM, McLaren JW. Photic retinopathy from the operating room microscope: study with filters. Arch Ophthalmol 1989;107:373.
123. Green WR, Robertson DM. Pathologic findings of photic retinopathy in the human eye. Am J Ophthalmol 1991;112:520.
124. Apple DJ, Olson RJ. Closed-loop anterior chamber lenses. Arch Ophthalmol 1987;105:52.
125. Smith PW, Wong SK, Stark WJ, Gottsch JD, Terry AC, Bonham RD. Complications of closed-loop intraocular lenses. Arch Ophthalmol 105:1987.
126. Lindstrom RL, Nelson JD, Neist RL. Anterior chamber lens subluxation through a basal peripheral iridectomy. J Am Intraocul Implant Soc 1983;9:53.
127. Smith SG. Intraocular lens removal for chronic cystoid macular edema. J Cataract Refract Surg 1989;15: 442.
128. Stark WJ, Gottsch JD, Goodman DF, Goodman GL, Pratzer K. Posterior chamber intraocular lens implantation in the absence of capsular support. Arch Ophthalmol 1989;107:1078.
129. Price FW, Whiston WE. Natural history of cystoid macular edema in pseudophakic bullous keratopathy. J Cataract Refract Surg 1990;16:163.
130. Cox SN, Hay E, Bird AC. Treatment of chronic macular edema with acetazolamide. Arch Ophthalmol 1988;106:1190.
131. Tripathi RC, Fekrat S, Tripathi BJ, Ernest JT. A direct correlation of the resolution of pseudophakic cystoid

macular edema with acetazolamide therapy. Ann Ophthalmol 1991;23:127.

132. Weene LE. Cystoid macular edema after scleral buckling responsive to acetazolamide. Ann Ophthalmol 1992;24:423.
133. Marmor MF, Maack T. Enhancement of retinal adhesion and subretinal fluid absorption by acetazolamide. Invest Ophthalmol Vis Sci 1982;23:121.
134. Zweng HC, Little HL, Peabody RR. Laser photocoagulation of macular lesions. Trans Am Acad Ophthalmol Otolaryngol 1968;72:377.
135. Schepens CL. Retinal detachment and allied diseases, vol 2. Philadelphia, WB Saunders, 1983:1018.
136. Perez R, Provenzano J, Muñoz D, Vazquez L. Argon laser for clinically significant pseudophakic foveal edema. Ophthalmology 1991;98(Suppl)250.
137. Haller JA. Grid photocoagulation for chronic cystoid macular edema. Invest Ophthalmol Vis Sci 1992; 33(Suppl):1316.
138. Pfoff DS, Thom SR. Preliminary report on the effect of hyperbaric oxygen on cystoid macular edema. J Cataract Refract Surg 1987;13:136.
139. Benner JD, Xiaoping M. Locally administered hyperoxic therapy for aphakic cystoid macular edema. Am J Ophthalmol 1992;113:104.
140. Jampol LM, Orlin C, Cohen SB, Zanetti C, Lehman E, Goldberg MF. Hyperbaric and transcorneal delivery of oxygen to the rabbit and monkey anterior segment. Arch Ophthalmol 1988;106:825.
141. Spaide RF, Yannuzzi LA. Cystoid macular edema after cataract surgery. Semin Ophthalmol 1993;8:121.
142. Freeman WR, Green RL, Smith RE. Echographic localization of corticosteroids after periocular injection. Am J Ophthalmol 103:281, 1987.

Ophthalmic Surgery Complications: Prevention and Management,
edited by Judie F. Charlton and George W. Weinstein.
J. B. Lippincott Company, Philadelphia

16

Ngoc Nguyen
Marc F. Lieberman

Postoperative Intraocular Pressure

Elevated intraocular pressure (IOP) after ophthalmic surgery is a ubiquitous complication, reported with nearly every type of ocular procedure. The severity and prevalence of this phenomenon reflect in part the vigilance of the surveillance. For example, if IOPs were monitored every few hours after vitrectomy surgery or corneal transplantation, the evidence for transient ocular hypertension would be even more compelling than the pressure results from a single reading 1 day after surgery. In fact, it can be safely assumed that most eyes experience elevated IOP in the immediate postoperative period, usually without sequelae.

The nature and consequences of postoperative IOP elevations depend as much on the previous ocular history as on the intraoperative events. Broadly speaking, elevated pressure sequelae have slightly different complexions in eyes with no history of previous glaucoma, eyes with an underlying predisposition to glaucoma (such as a history of angle recession or uveitis), or eyes with a history of treated glaucoma.

In simplistic terms, the "secondary glaucomas" are usually defined by pressure criteria alone (the detection of elevated intraocular tension) rather than on the development of disc and field changes (as is central to the definition of primary open-angle glaucoma). Accordingly, secondary glaucomas that occur after surgery are usually caused by embarrassment of the outflow system on either a transient or prolonged basis. This embarrassment may be due to either intercameral blockage, as from viscoelastics or blood, or compromised trabecular architecture, such as following corneal transplantation. The eye's rebound capacity determines whether the short-term impairment of outflow becomes a temporary or a permanent feature, requiring ongoing attention and medication.

Cataract surgery is the most common ophthalmic procedure performed, and thus has produced the largest literature regarding elevated IOP postoperatively. A review of this literature occupies most of this chapter. It will be followed by extensive discussions of IOP difficulties encountered after corneal surgery, retinal–vitreous surgery, and other miscellaneous procedures.

IOP ELEVATION AND CATARACT SURGERY

Anticipating Complications

Intimate knowledge of the ocular history, an examination before cataract extraction, and current knowledge of contemporary surgical trends (eg, risks of anterior chamber versus posterior chamber lens implantation) facilitate the surgeon's ability to deal with complications both intraoperatively and postoperatively. A rigorous preoperative evaluation of the patient elicits information such as the history of diabetes, known ocular trauma, and the use of systemic or topical steroid preparations, which could raise red flags as risk factors for glaucomatous vulnerability. The ocular examination requires gonioscopy (eg, for the detection of posterior synechiae or signs of iridodonesis from previous trauma), optic nerve evaluation (eg, for evidence of preexisting glaucoma), retinal evaluation (eg, for the detection of diabetes), and some form of visual field testing. The cataract surgeon who eschews these standards of ophthalmic practice invites unpleasant surprises.

Patients With No Prior Risk Factors

Even in the absence of a history of glaucoma or physical abnormalities on examination, the incidence of first-day postoperative elevated pressure after seemingly uncomplicated cataract surgery has been reported to be as high as 30% after a standard extracapsular cataract extraction (ECCE) and 8% after phacoemulsification with posterior chamber lens implant.[1] In studies that have measured IOPs several hours after surgery, pressure elevations of 25 mmHg or more have been seen in nearly 60% of patients, and spikes of 40 mmHg have been detected in about one in eight eyes.[2] This phenomenon of short-term ocular hypertension is complicated because it involves issues such as the use and evacuation of viscoelastic materials, the type of wound closure, and other confounding factors; many of these are discussed below.

Most cases of elevated tension spontaneously resolve in the first several days, although there are reports of secondary glaucoma persisting in about 3% to 4% of patients with no previously detected disease.[1,3] This small group of patients who go on to glaucoma after cataract extraction reinforces the fact that the long-term ophthalmic management of pseudophakic eyes is crucial, both because of the concurrence of glaucoma in the elderly population most likely to undergo cataract extraction, as well as the improved clarity of media, which allows the appreciation of subtle glaucomatous changes in the optic nerve and precise perimetric evaluation.

Patients Predisposed to Glaucoma

TRAUMA. Another group of patients who must be taken into account before cataract extraction are those who have had, either by history or examination, anterior segment trauma. Occasionally a patient relates a history of a convincing injury to the eye, but most frequently the slit-lamp examination alerts the physician. Tears in the pupillary margin, asymmetric pigment dusting of the corneal endothelium, or asymmetry in appearance of the irides are all valuable clues. Gonioscopy, however, is invaluable: here variations in the exposure of the scleral spur and ciliary body, evidence of "balling up" of iris processes, or signs of a phacodonesis or iridodonesis can be detected. Late contusion glaucoma may occur in as many as 2% to 10% of eyes.[4–6]

The rule of thumb is that about two thirds of the angle must be recessed before glaucoma will manifest itself; however, "false angles" can often be seen after trauma, and it is difficult to know precisely how much trabecular damage has actually occurred. Such information is valuable on three counts:

1. An eye with already embarrassed outflow will quite possibly experience ocular hypertension with retention of viscoelastic or lens debris, out of proportion to what would otherwise be expected in an open angle.
2. Evidence of anterior segment trauma may predispose to zonular disruption, leading to complications intraoperatively during maneuvering of the lens or implant.
3. A recessed angle may have little reserve if an anterior chamber lens implant is placed, and hence it may behave like an eye with chronic angle closure, possibly requiring a glaucoma procedure in combination with cataract extraction.

UVEITIS. Eyes with preexisting and treated uveitis embrace a wide spectrum of ocular conditions, many of which prove challenging to cataract extraction, and others that contraindicate such surgery. The incidence of cataracts is about 50% in patients with uveitis associated with juvenile rheumatoid arthritis,[7–9] pars planitis,[10] and Fuchs syndrome.[11–14] The cataracts (specifically posterior subcapsular changes) are often accelerated by the use of long-term steroid drops. Sometimes the eye may also manifest vitreous and macular changes, which will greatly affect the outcome of cataract surgery (eg, pars planitis).

It is often difficult to sort out the cause of the secondary glaucomas in the presence of uveitis: is the elevated tension due to particulate debris or humoral factors, or is it a response to steroid medications?[15] Another confounding feature is the presence or absence of peripheral anterior synechiae, which not only affect the capacity of outflow, but also make an anterior chamber lens implant considerably less desirable. Although lens implantation can safely be done in selected cases of uveitis, this requires great surgical discretion.[16–22]

DIABETES. A particularly common ocular condition that affects the surgeon's decisions during cataract extraction is the existence of diabetes. Iris neovascularization has been reported in 6% of patients with diabetes mellitus after ECCE and posterior chamber lens implant.[23] Both patient and surgeon should be prepared for a postoperative course with a higher incidence of unforeseen sequelae. In the presence of preproliferative and proliferative retinopathy, precataract panretinal photocoagulation (PRP) is recommended if it can be placed through the cataractous media before surgery.[24–27] If cataract prevents delivery of laser to the retina, the patient and surgeon should be prepared for laser treatment in the early period after cataract surgery.

Additionally, both the patient and surgeon should be aware of the greater risk of neovascular glaucoma with inadvertent capsular rupture during surgery. As expected, the presence of proliferative retinopathy leads to a much greater chance of complication than the presence of background retinopathy. For example, 40% of patients with proliferative disease who underwent intracapsular cataract extraction (ICCE) soon went on to develop neovascular glaucoma.[25,28,29] Poliner and colleagues[30] reported that 12% of eyes that had ECCE with opening of the posterior capsule developed rubeosis, compared with 0% in patients with intact capsules. Benson and associates,[23] however, found that an intact posterior capsule did not necessarily protect the eye from developing rubeosis. The ophthalmologist must carefully examine all pseudophakic eyes for signs of rubeosis, because prompt treatment with PRP can often effect regression of the new vessels.

The surgeon should also anticipate the long-term requirement for maximal pupillary dilation (for maximal fundus access) for the lifetime of the diabetic patient, and should conduct cataract surgery and postoperative care accordingly. Active proliferative diabetic retinopathy at the time of surgery is a poor prognostic indicator for final visual acuity and is associated with postoperative deterioration of retinopathy and fibrinous uveitis that can lead to posterior synechiae, preventing postoperative PRP.[31,32] The surgeon may elect to use long-term dilating drops and tolerate iris–intraocular lens (IOL) capture (if it will occur) to achieve maximal pupillary diameter. Again, because of the predilection for the posterior iris pigment epithelium to behave as though it were "sticky" in eyes with diabetes, there is a higher incidence of iris adherence to the lens implant, and a slightly greater risk for pupillary block glaucoma in these eyes. Although most contemporary phacoemulsification surgeons do not routinely use surgical iridectomy, this is a worthwhile maneuver in cataract operations on known diabetics.[33]

Previous History of Glaucoma

Both cataract and glaucoma often occur together (often without the patient's knowledge) simply because of the high age-related prevalence of each of these diseases. Similarly, the treatment for glaucoma may in itself contribute to cataract formation (eg, chronic miotic usage). More importantly, perhaps, the concurrent use of medications may greatly complicate cataract surgery, requiring additional iris manipulation, with a greater risk of capsular rupture and vitrectomy. Even the simple observation that the maximum extent of pupillary dilation in the office is only 5 mm may allow the surgeon to plan alternative approaches in the event the pupil is too small at the time of surgery.

The role of cataract extraction in patients with a known history of glaucoma raises many other interesting issues. The first question is: What is the behavior of glaucomatous eyes in response to the common transient elevation of pressure following a routine and uncomplicated cataract extraction? Such pressure spikes have been estimated to be five times more frequent in glaucomatous eyes.[34–36] Presumably, the agencies for trabecular embarrassment that occur in the normal eye, such as blockade of the trabecular outflow by viscoelastic or particulate debris, are potentiated in eyes with an already dysfunctional trabecular meshwork, manifested as glaucoma. In eyes with far advanced optic nerve and visual field loss, such sudden elevations of IOP could theoretically prove catastrophic. This apprehension derives from a retrospective study[37] of eyes with "split fixation" by Goldmann kinetic perimetry, some of which lost central vision through "central snuff-out," despite pressures that were only modestly elevated. However, this phenomenon may be rare.[38]

Fearful of such complications, the cataract surgeon has many medical options to reduce the IOP in the perioperative period, including intracameral miotics, topical beta blockers, miotic drops, powerful α_2-agonists (eg, apraclonidine hydrochloride), or oral carbonic anhydrase inhibitors.[39–41] A comprehensive prophylactic regimen, for example, would be the use of one drop of preoperative apraclonidine at the time of surgery, followed by acetazolamide (Diamox Sequels), 500 mg, twice a day for 36 to 48 hours postoperatively.

Another issue raised in the literature is whether there is a beneficial long-term effect on IOP control in glaucomatous eyes after cataract extraction alone.[42] Some authors mention that pressures may be reduced by cataract surgery alone in a significant fashion for many months to years[43–45] while others have commented that the need for topical medications may be reduced.[46,47] McGuigan and associates[35] reported that about half of glaucoma patients after cataract surgery retained the same normal medications, about a quarter required additional medications, and about a quarter required fewer medications at 18 months postoperatively.

CHRONIC OPEN-ANGLE GLAUCOMA. The consensus with respect to chronic open-angle glaucoma control with cataract extraction alone is that the placement of a lens implant is for all practical purposes a neutral process with respect to pressure control. For example, the beneficial effect of argon laser trabeculoplasty has been seen to persist after ECCE with or without lens implant.[48,49]

However, eyes with chronic open-angle glaucoma undergoing cataract surgery may have complicating features that make the surgery and postoperative course challenging. An uncommon association in eyes that had been on chronic miotics and have undergone lens implant surgery is the tendency for synechial adherence between the lens implant and the iris.[50–53] Much like the iris in diabetes,[33] such contact can lead to a focal iris neovascularization as well as significant capture of the lens implant. Neovascularization has been known to progress to total synechial closure, with a consequent glaucoma. Extensive pupillary capture has also been associated with forms of pupillary block.[54]

Another confounding feature of cataract surgery in glaucomatous eyes is that they may show a tendency toward greater inflammation, possibly due to the use of medications (especially miotics) preoperatively.[55] This sometimes requires an intensive postoperative regimen of topical steroids, which in itself can occasionally elicit a pressure rise in eyes with known glaucoma. In a similar fashion, inadvertent dispersion of iris pigment from lens implants[56] can sometimes overwhelm an already compromised trabecular meshwork. This is more common in lens implants that are slightly decentered or of inappropriate size, resulting in greater friction between the optic or haptic and the iris epithelium.

CHRONIC ANGLE-CLOSURE GLAUCOMA. The eye with chronic angle-closure glaucoma may predictably benefit from cataract extraction. Mechanistically speaking, the removal of a relatively large cataract can both relieve pupillary block due to iridolenticular touch and reduce shallowing or cramping of the anterior segment by a large lens. Nearly two thirds of patients with angle-closure glaucoma (in contrast with 14% of patients with chronic open-angle glaucoma) achieved a pressure reduction below 21 mmHg without medications after cataract extraction alone;[57] preexisting peripheral anterior synechiae posed few problems.

Eyes with chronic angle-closure glaucoma, however, raise two additional problems: first, the slightly increased association of ciliary block (malignant) glaucoma,[58] and second, the mechanical difficulty and possible contraindication of placing an anterior chamber lens implant in compromised angles if a posterior chamber lens implantation is impossible.

EYES WITH PREVIOUS FILTRATION SURGERY. In eyes that have established trabeculectomy blebs, there is a significant risk that the filtration will be impaired with the postoperative healing of cataract and lens implantation surgery; estimates range from 50% to 64% for reduced bleb function.[42] This has been ascribed to possible embarrassment of the filtration site by intracameral debris or inflammation, or stimulation to external episcleral scarring.[59] Moreover, such blebs cannot always be relied on to prevent postcataract IOP spikes. Anticipating such bleb failure, the surgeon may attempt to prolong preexisting filtration by the use of postoperative 5-FU injections; however, this has been reported primarily on an anecdotal basis.

Surgical Techniques

The selection of surgical approach for cataract in the glaucoma patient will lead the surgeon to anticipate certain kinds of complications. For example, in eyes with chronic miotic usage, strategies for dealing with small pupil, capsular rupture, suitability for anterior chamber lens implantation, and postoperative hyphema should be considered in advance. The selection of surgical approach is not a cavalier one, and each path has well-documented benefits and risks. The presence of an IOL implant itself does not significantly alter the long-term glaucoma outcome, but rather the perioperative and postoperative events involved in the surgery.[60–62]

The use of ICCE techniques has become increasingly uncommon, and special complications and forms of glaucoma once seen after ICCE are now mostly of historical interest. Specifically, the incidences of alpha-chymotrypsin secondary glaucoma and pupillary block glaucoma are considerably less common than in the past. However, the transition to ECCE and phacoemulsification surgery has led to the appearance of new forms of glaucoma, such as elevated pressures due to the use of viscoelastics (discussed later in this chapter).

The logic of combining cataract extraction with a glaucoma procedure becomes more compelling as technology allows for smaller and smaller wounds, and hence the congruence of the path of lens extraction and aqueous filtration. In fact, the possibility of total elimination of topical medications (at considerable cost and time investment by the patient) and the favorable outcome of combined procedures outweigh for many surgeons the minimal complication rate associated with combined cataract and filtration procedures.

Given the high incidence of postoperative pressure elevation, and the possible optic nerve vulnerability to such pressure spikes, combined procedures have been shown to prevent transient IOP elevations in several studies.[35,63] Much of this literature reflects the experience with classical (nonphacoemulsification) ECCE and lens implantation, and the results are impressive in the immediate postoperative period. Krupin and associates[64] reported that pressure elevations were significantly decreased in combined eyes (14% of cases), in contrast with the 69% of glaucomatous eyes that underwent cataract surgery alone. About 1 year after surgery, IOP control is often quite good, although an anatomic bleb is seen in fewer than 20% of cases.[65] At 2 years, IOP control has been reported to be similar to that of filtration surgery alone.[66]

Literature reflecting long-term phacoemulsification and filtration results is only now emerging, but it seems to show similar trends for excellent pressure control—even in the absence of significant anatomic blebs. Whether a combined procedure or ECCE alone is used, greater than 85% of eyes with glaucoma receiving IOLs achieve 20/40 vision or better, with retinal or optic nerve disease explaining the vast majority of eyes with vision less than this.[66] Indications for combined cataract and glaucoma surgery include eyes with:

1. Advanced glaucomatous damage that is medically controlled before lens extraction
2. Severe field loss near fixation, where a pressure spike could be detrimental to the preservation of vision, regardless of pressure control
3. A maximally tolerated medical therapy with no other therapeutic options in the event the pressure elevation becomes uncontrolled after cataract surgery
4. Uncontrolled IOP and cataract

Some surgeons advocate expanded criteria to include even eyes on minimal glaucoma topical therapy, with the expectation that surgically controlled IOP has advantages for the patient over the long-term use and expense of well-tolerated drops.

The ideal approach to eyes with a combination of cataract and chronic open-angle glaucoma has yet to be defined. The relatively large wound usually required for ECCE (6–11 mm), involving conjunctival healing over one or more superior quadrants, may make subsequent filtering surgery less successful. In contrast, a small-wound phacoemulsification and trabeculectomy, using an opening of less than 5 mm, can preserve an adjacent quadrant's "virgin conjunctiva" for later filtering surgery. Therefore, the combined phacoemulsification, IOL, and trabeculectomy operation, with adjunctive antimetabolites such as 5-FU or mitomycin C applications, is becoming popular. Nevertheless, the recommendation for any specific patient will depend on the visual needs and the surgeon's abilities.

Mechanisms of Postoperative Pressure Elevation

The advent of ECCE—and especially phacoemulsification—has resulted in technology that can subject the anterior chamber to a flow of fluids many times its natural volume during the course of surgery, with the atomization of natural cataractous materials (capsule and protein) and the introduction of synthetic viscoelastic substances. All of these can contribute, in the presence of a technically uncomplicated and perfect cataract extraction, to a transient elevated IOP postoperatively. This section deals with some circumstances implicated in these forms of secondary glaucoma occurring within the initial 4 to 7 days after glaucoma surgery. Some of these can be minimized with very discrete interventions; others cannot.

Secondary Open-Angle Glaucoma

ALPHA-CHYMOTRYPSIN GLAUCOMA. This interesting secondary glaucoma is of historical relevance, having appeared with the use of enzymatic digestion of the zonules during ICCE. The elevated pressure occurred 2 to 5 days after surgery.[67] The pressure rise, usually modest, was seen in over 70% of patients.[68,69] This was almost invariably a self-limited event, disappearing within 10 days. It was not confined to eyes with preexisting glaucoma, and it rarely led to long-term complications.

The mechanism of alpha-chymotrypsin glaucoma has remained controversial. Tonographic[70] and electron microscopic studies[71,72] have clearly demonstrated zonular fragments clogging the trabecular meshwork, thus impairing outflow facilities. There were also signs of microscopic inflammation, possibly due to the enzyme itself, but it was unclear whether there was any trabecular damage from possible contaminants in the enzyme preparation. What was unexpected, though, was that the pressure elevations reflected a dose-response curve, depending on the concentration of the enzyme used, the volume of enzyme injected into the anterior segment, and the duration of intracameral exposure. The severity and incidence of the pressure rise were greatly reduced by diluting the enzyme to the 1:10,000 range instead of the standard 1:5000 dilution and using an intraoperative volume of 0.5 cc instead of the standard 2 cc. Retention in the eye for less than 2 minutes with subsequent irrigation was also favorable in reducing IOP. Pretreatment with antiglaucoma medications was largely ineffective, as was the use of periocular steroids.

With the demise of intracapsular surgery techniques, this enzyme is now rarely used. In the uncommon instance when, for example, an IOL within the bag must be removed in toto, alpha-chymotrypsin might be useful. Using a high dilution, small volume, and vigorous irrigation is the most useful prophylactic measure.

RETAINED PARTICULATE MATERIAL. Microscopic amounts of blood, pigment, inflammatory debris, or retained cortical and nuclear lens fragments can also temporarily occlude the trabecular meshwork.[54] A transient rise in IOP has been reported in conjunction with heavy pigmentation of the trabecular meshwork, although the correlation between pigment and IOP is not always straightforward.[73] This pigment dispersion has been reported with iris-supported lens implants[56] as well as posterior chamber lenses.[74–77] The literature does not report whether there is any additive effect in eyes with already heavily pigmented angles, such as patients with pigment dispersion syndrome or pseudoexfoliation.

Elevated pressures do not always occur in the presence of retained lens material. The most common scenario is that retained fragments of lens cortex subsequently hydrate and appear as debris in the anterior chamber. These may or may not be associated with inflammation, depending largely on the intensity of the steroid regimen. However, there are reports of lens particles, protein, and possibly macrophages causing a phacolytic-like picture, which usually subsides with topical antiinflammatory therapy.[78] Accordingly, it is preferable to allow the eye to retain as little lens material as possible.

If nuclear fragments fall into the vitreous, significant and intractable intraocular inflammation can progress, occasionally leading to a genuine phacoanaphylactic complication.[79,80] Standard antiglaucoma medications and intensive steroid therapy are usually required, and often vitrectomy with removal of retained lens material is indicated. One rule of thumb is that any fragment of retained nuclear material thought to be larger than one fourth of a disc diameter in the vitreous cavity must be carefully watched, if not removed.[79,81]

Any disruption of the lens–capsular barrier from the vitreous not only allows lens material to fall posteriorly, but also allows vitreous material to come anteriorly. In eyes that have had extensive vitreous forward motion, in the absence of an anterior vitrectomy, postoperative glaucoma has been noted. Vitreous in the anterior chamber has also been associated with pupillary block and late peripheral anterior synechiae formation. If immediate removal of the vitreous is not done, vitrectomy may be performed at a later date, especially in the presence of cystoid macular edema or chronic inflammation.[80,81]

RETAINED VISCOELASTIC MATERIAL. In ways slightly reminiscent of alpha-chymotrypsin glaucoma, the details of how various viscoelastic substances elevate pressures remain obscure. The most commonly available material is sodium hyaluronate, with or without chondroitin sulfate or hydroxypropylmethylcellulose.[82] The clinical signs of retained viscoelastic are seen in the first 24 to 72 hours after surgery. There is an apparent suspension of particulate matter and cells in the anterior segment, as though they are immobile in a plastic-like medium. The IOP may or may not be elevated. The transient elevated pressure tends to peak at 12 to 16 hours but usually resolves within 24 to 72 hours.[83] Some reports have indicated that the response may be confined to only the first 8 hours postoperatively, and hence can go undiagnosed at the standard postoperative check 1 day after surgery.

There is little doubt that the glaucoma mechanism is from blockade of the trabecular outflow pathway, as measured by outflow facility studies.[84] Although in vitro studies show that removal of the sodium hyaluronate can improve outflow facility, this is not always the case clinically.[85] Two parameters that are difficult to assess clinically are the exact volume of retained viscoelastic in the eye and its exact location in the anterior segment. One study[86] suggested that with the use of less than 0.3 cc of sodium hyaluronate, pressure elevations postoperatively were rare. There are conflicting reports about the advantages and disadvantages of the various viscoelastic formulations.[85,87,88]

There are many suggestions on how best to prevent postoperative viscoelastic-induced pressure spikes. Maximal removal of the viscoelastic is advisable, even in the presence of a functioning filtering bleb. What is intriguing is the fact that IOP elevations can be seen even after the evacuation of the material from the anterior segment after cataract extraction.[85,89,90] The material's removal may simply reduce the incidence or the amplitude of the pressure elevation, rather than altogether eliminating the phenomenon.[85] Other studies[91] suggest that evacuation of the viscoelastic is irrelevant with respect to pressure spiking.

Various medical regimens have been formulated to prevent this pressure spike. Fry[92] found that the use of an intracameral miotic was particularly effective, as was the use of a beta blocker, carbonic anhydrase inhibitor, and postoperative miotic ointment. Apraclonidine was said not to be particularly useful. Other studies have advised pilocarpine ointment,[93] postoperative timolol,[94] and a combination of intracameral miotic and postoperative carbachol.[40,95–97]

As a historical footnote, a purified synthetic viscoelastic made of polyacrylamide polymer and marketed as Orcolon caused a severe, intractable secondary glaucoma in a few patients, requiring a high rate of secondary glaucoma surgery.[98] Despite attempts at experimentally recreating these regrettable cases of "Orcolon glaucoma," the perverse molecular circumstances that led to the secondary glaucomas have not been reproduced.

PUPILLARY BLOCK GLAUCOMA. The most common form of angle-closure glaucoma following cataract extraction, pupillary block glaucoma invariably results from some unintended impediment of flow between posterior and anterior chambers. It is rarely seen in the presence of a surgical iridectomy, and more than 75% of cases are reported in the first 2 weeks after surgery.[54]

In the days of ICCE, the incidence of aphakic pupillary block was 1% to 7%. A host of mechanisms have been associated with obstruction of flow from the posterior segment forward. These have been reported even in the presence of patent iridectomies that were insufficiently basal (>1 mm from the iris root). Reported circumstances include the presence of retained air in the anterior segment, occluding the pupil; iris–vitreous adhesions following the shallowing of the chamber from wound leak, with subsequent pupillary block; incomplete iridectomy (partial thickness); inflammatory seclusio pupillae (total posterior synechiae along the pupillary margin); obstruction of the pupil from iris apposition to an anterior chamber or iris-fixed lens implant; adherence of the posterior chamber lens implant to the pupillary margin; adherence of the capsule to the peripheral iridectomy; condensation of the hyaloid face or capsule to the iridectomy; and silicone oil occluding the superior iridectomy.[99–102]

There is often an overlap between these pseudophakic conditions and clinical entities that behave like ciliary block glaucoma.[58] In fact, only by sequentially addressing each potential blockade site can one reach an accurate diagnosis, adding additional iridotomies to eliminate pupillary block, perforating the posterior capsule centrally and peripherally to eliminate capsular adhesion, and perforating the hyaloid face centrally and peripherally to eliminate the possibility of aqueous misdirection.

Eyes with diabetes are thought to be at particular risk for the development of this whole spectrum of inflammatory forms of impaired aqueous flow. The best prophylaxis is a definitive, through-and-through basal peripheral iridectomy in all cataract and implantation surgeries in diabetic eyes. In the rare circumstance that silicone oil is injected into the vitreous cavity, the iridectomy should be performed inferiorly because the oil will float superiorly, leaving a layer of aqueous inferiorly.[103]

The postoperative treatment of these various forms of pupillary block usually requires vigorous attempts at maximum dilatation and cycloplegia, rather than the use of miotics, as is the case in phakic angle-closure glaucomas. Additional laser iridotomies, with either argon or neodymium:yttrium-aluminum-garnet (Nd:YAG), are appropriate. Various layers of the anterior segment must often be perforated before the issues are resolved.

In summary, the unusual occurrence of postcataract pupillary block secondary glaucoma can be avoided by the routine use of surgical iridectomy in eyes with diabetes or anterior chamber (or iris-fixed) lens implantations, and the use of antiinflammatory agents and vigorous surveillance in eyes prone to excessive inflammation postoperatively.

HEMORRHAGE-RELATED GLAUCOMAS. When surgery is performed in eyes treated with topical miotics or in the presence of anticoagulants (eg, warfarin [Coumadin]), postoperative hyphema can be encountered. A small amount of blood may be seen in the first 48 hours, although hemorrhage may occur up to 7 days postoperatively.[104–106] In such cases, the pressure elevation may be due to blockade of the trabecular meshwork by free red blood cells or by macrophage-laden red blood cells. In the case of combined cataract-filtering procedures, hemorrhagic and fibrinous debris may also occlude the filtering ostium. There is no large series on the treatment of postsurgical hyphemas comparable to the literature on traumatic hyphemas,[107] but eyes with pressures that cannot be controlled with topical and systemic medications after 48 hours should be considered for surgical irrigation of the hyphema. When there is hemorrhagic occlusion of the ostium of a combined procedure, this can usually be waited out for 3 to 5 days, especially if antimetabolites were applied at the time of surgery or postoperatively.

Another blood-related form of secondary glaucoma occurs about 4 to 6 weeks after surgery and is associated with the retention of red blood cells in the vitreous cavity, where they undergo erythroclastic degeneration into ghost cells.[108] This scenario requires capsular rupture and vitreous presentation into the anterior segment or erythrocytes accumulating posteriorly after vitrectomy, originating either from hyphema or vitreous hemorrhage. Over several weeks, these cell membranes can migrate into the anterior segment, often appearing on slit-lamp examination as a tan, layered hyphema. Sudden pressure elevations have been reported, and often surgical intervention is needed to irrigate the anterior segment.

Another scenario in which either hyphema or ghost cell glaucoma may occur is in eyes with proliferative retinopathy where there has been a violation of the vitreous during the cataract procedure, with subsequent neovascularization and bleeding.

STEROID-RESPONSE GLAUCOMA. Since the initial reports by Becker[109] that a few patients manifested an elevated IOP with prolonged and intensive use of topical steroid drops, this phenomenon has been observed and evaluated in many settings. The mechanism remains unclear,[110–114] but there is presumably some molecular impairment at the level of the trabecular meshwork where intracellular processing of aqueous is affected. It is a particular problem in eyes that have had long-term steroid usage, such as in cases of uveitis.[15]

In eyes that experience significant postoperative inflammation following cataract extraction, the IOP elevation from steroids may be seen 2 to 6 weeks after an intensive regimen. Often, concurrent antiglaucoma medications are required. Alternative strategies would be the substitution of weaker steroids (eg, fluorometholone or medrysone) or perhaps nonsteroidal antiinflammatory agents (eg, ketorolac).

It is unusual for steroid-response glaucoma by itself to go on to a longstanding disease process, unless there is unmasking of a tendency toward chronic open-angle glaucoma with subsequent disc and field changes. Such an unmasked glaucoma should be suspected on the basis of other risk factors, such as prior tension levels, family history, and so forth. The rule of thumb is that the duration of steroid usage mirrors the duration of time for the steroid effect to wear off.

SECONDARY INFLAMMATORY GLAUCOMAS. The most common scenario for inflammatory glaucoma is the activation or exacerbation of a preexisting uveitis. This can sometimes be confused after extracapsular surgery when there has been a significant amount of retained cortical debris, with subsequent inflammatory response. The issue of elevated pressures can be further complicated by trying to sort out the role of postoperative steroid drops.

There are specific syndromes where the surgeon can anticipate inflammatory glaucoma, depending on the choice of IOL implant. For example, anterior chamber lens implants have about twice the incidence of secondary glaucomas than posterior chamber lens implants.[115] A particularly important feature is whether the anterior chamber lens implants have flexible haptics with an open-loop design, or have a closed-loop design. The latter is associated with a particularly high incidence of synechial closure and inflammation.[116–118]

A specific syndrome has been described with the combination of inflammation, glaucoma, and microhemorrhage, referred to as the UGH syndrome (*u*veitis/*g*laucoma/*h*yphema).[119] This appeared more commonly with anterior chamber lenses with extensive iris–IOL friction, but has also been seen in instances of posterior IOL touching the posterior iris surface, or dislocation of the lens implant. Commonly, there are episodic rises in IOP, with impaired vision from symptomatic anterior iritis or even from symptomatic recurrent hemorrhage. Chafing of the iris surface apparently leads to both inflammation and rupture of iris vasculature, and subsequent cellular presentation into the anterior segment. The standard approach is to treat these episodes with antiglaucoma medications and steroids. With repeat episodes, one should consider removing or exchanging the lens implant. The goal is to minimize recurrence and chronic detrimental effects on the corneal endothelium, optic nerve, and macula. Like all inflammatory glaucomas, however, the potential for steroid-induced intraocular tension elevation must always be considered during management.

SUPRACHOROIDAL HEMORRHAGE. The presence of glaucoma is a significant risk factor for the development of suprachoroidal hemorrhage in eyes undergoing glaucoma surgery. The incidence of hemorrhage into the suprachoroidal space is about 0.25%.[120–123] The risk factors associated with suprachoroidal hemorrhage include old age, high myopia, history of vitreous loss during surgery, IOPs above 21 mmHg, generalized atherosclerosis, systemic hypertension, and diabetes.[123] Presumably, there is a rupture of one of the short posterior cellular arteries into the suprachoroidal space, the sequelae of which depend entirely on the severity of bleeding and its timing. If the eye is opened widely at the time of arterial rupture, the entire ocular contents can tragically be extruded. More commonly, there is pain in the eye 2 to 7 days after surgery, and a dark mound in the suprachoroidal space is appreciated by indirect ophthalmoscopy.

In the event of a postoperative suprachoroidal hemorrhage, there may be sufficient propulsion of the intraocular contents that there is shallowing of the anterior chamber. The hemorrhage can also be associated with a suprachoroidal effusion,[124] and hence the peripheral anterior chamber may be shallow from an annular choroidal swelling effect pushing forward. Elevated tension per se, however, is usually not an issue.

Sclerostomies, performed either at the time of the hemorrhage during surgery or afterward, can debulk the hemorrhage. Usually, it is best to wait about 4 to 5 days for lysis of the blood clot before sclerostomy. Some advise drainage within 2 weeks to achieve maximal visual potential.[125] In one small series, good vision was obtained in patients who underwent a secondary lens implantation after abortion of their primary cataract surgery.[126]

Malignant Glaucoma (Ciliary Block Glaucoma)

Although originally described as a complication of filtration surgery in eyes with angle-closure glaucoma, malignant glaucoma has been associated with many anterior segment procedures.[58] There are even reports of spontaneous occurrences associated with ciliary spasm, argon laser treatment to the trabecular meshwork, and so forth. Technically, it is a condition of abnormal permeability between the vitreous cavity and the anterior chamber; the hyaloid face and its annular ring adjacent to the ciliary processes are the presumed sites of malfunction. It has had many names, including aqueous misdirection syndrome, posterior aqueous secretion syndrome, ciliary block glaucoma, and hyaloid block glaucoma; the term *malignant glaucoma*, although not as anatomically correct, nevertheless remains useful for archival referencing.

Malignant glaucoma can occur with any form of cataract surgery, with or without a concomitant glaucoma procedure. Its presentation involves an inappropriately elevated pressure with both central and peripheral anterior chamber shallowing. The central, axial shallowing helps distinguish this disorder from other types of pupillary block. However, pupillary block glaucoma must be ruled out by verifying the presence of patent iridotomies or surgical iridectomies. If the pupillary block mechanism has been eliminated, the diagnosis of malignant glaucoma can be made.

According to some authorities, 50% of cases with malignant glaucoma can be medically corrected after 5 days of therapy.[127,128] This consists of intensive cycloplegics, IOP reduction with beta blockers and carbonic anhydrase inhibitors, topical steroids, and hyperosmotic solutions intravenously if necessary. In the absence of response, a more definitive intervention is required; the nature of this intervention depends on the status of the eye.

After a medical regimen, the nonsurgical responses to malignant glaucoma in the phakic eye are limited.[58] If there is an exceedingly large sector iridectomy—such as might have been performed at the time of a previous trabeculectomy or iridectomy—there are reports of argon laser treatments to the ciliary processes that have aborted the malignant glaucoma.[129] In the absence of such an exceptional circumstance, the intervention of choice is a vitreous aspiration or, preferably, a controlled anterior vitrectomy. Because this glaucoma is not caused by the lens, it need not be removed. However, sometimes these lenses become cataractous with multiple interventions, and a cataract extraction is performed at a later date.

In eyes that are either aphakic or pseudophakic, there is the possibility for definitive laser intervention.[130] The neodymium:yttrium-aluminum-garnet (Nd:YAG) laser has been successfully used to produce an anterior hyaloidectomy, which successfully allows fluid to pass from the vitreous cavity forward. This is a gratifying and immediate response, with deepening of the anterior chamber on the rupture of the hyaloid face.

However, it is sometimes useful to choose multiple laser sites and sequentially eliminate the possibility of pupillary block glaucoma, by adding additional iridotomies in areas of presumed aqueous loculation behind the iris; iridocapsular, by performing a posterior capsulotomy; and hyaloid block, by performing a hyaloidotomy centrally or peripherally (if visible through an iridectomy) to eliminate malignant glaucoma.

The occurrence of malignant glaucoma in one eye greatly increases the risk of its appearance in the fellow eye during intraocular surgery. Prophylactic iridectomy or the use of cycloplegics, or both, may be necessary. As with all cases of malignant glaucoma, miotics should be eschewed because of their tendency to precipitate an attack of ciliary block.

Membranous Obstruction of the Outflow Tracts

EPITHELIAL DOWNGROWTH. Although an increasingly rare occurrence, epithelial downgrowth after cataract extraction appeared in about 0.1% of cases when ICCE was the norm.[131,132] The resulting devastation from intractable glaucoma resulted in almost 20% of the eyes requiring enucleation. With the advent of smaller wounds from ECCE and phacoemulsification, the incidence of this phenomena after cataract surgery is close to 0%.[133] The condition is associated with complicated intraocular surgery, involving prolapse of the iris into the wound, or with vitreous wick formation, facilitating a postoperative wound gap through which the surface epithelium has access to the anterior segment.[134] In the initial phases, hypotony is encountered, but usually inflammation and epithelial proliferation lead to a profound glaucoma.

The basis of the epithelial downgrowth glaucoma can be from several factors.[135] The wound gape and its resultant hypotony and inflammation can lead to anterior chamber shallowing, with subsequent synechial closure of the angle. More troublesome is the proliferation of epithelium into the trabecular meshwork area, with later contraction of the iris forward. The associated inflammation and presumed trabeculitis also decrease outflow, which can be further exacerbated by the use of chronic steroids to prevent inflammation. There have even been reports of pupillary block glaucoma due to epithelial downgrowth over the pupil area itself, and hemorrhages from secondary neovascularization of the iris can lead to both a neovascular and particulate blockade of the trabecular outflow. Furthermore, if the chronic hypotony is self-limited or surgically corrected, the profoundly embarrassed trabecular meshwork may no longer be able to function, and a significant secondary glaucoma ensues.[136]

Glaucoma is said to occur in about 50% of eyes with epithelial ingrowth,[135] with onset usually manifested within the first several months after surgery. Early chronic hypotony, peaking of the pupil, visible fistula on gonioscopy, and aqueous leakage (positive Seidel test) can all be seen in the early stages of epithelial ingrowth. By the time there is actual proliferation into the anterior segment, it may be appreciated on the corneal endothelial surface by a scalloped and thickened leading edge. It may be suspected on the iris itself because of distortion of the focal architecture with flattening of the iris surface, or even a translucent gray membrane. Light argon laser coagulation can be reliably used to distinguish the border of epithelial cells on the iris, which responds to low-energy argon bursts (500 $\mu \times 100$ milliwatts $\times$ 0.1 second) with a characteristic white fluffy appearance, in contrast to the normal iris contraction in areas where epithelium is not present.[137] The corneal lesion can be verified by the use of specular microscopy.[138]

The differential diagnosis elaborated by Maumenee[139] remains comprehensive: fibrovascular ingrowth, associated with much slower onset and obvious appearance of vascular membrane; vitreous–corneal adhesion, with subsequent edema of the cornea; focal Descemet membrane detachment or shelved corneal incision, at the site of the cataract entry wound; and focal corneal edema from endothelial trauma at the time of surgery. Other than the fibrous ingrowth, the corneal lesions are almost all uniformly stable, and hence can be distinguished from epithelial downgrowth.

There is a very poor prognosis for this condition, despite many innovative surgical approaches. Extensive corneal scleral transplantation, often combined with iridectomy, vitrectomy, and cryotherapy, may be necessary.[134,137,140] The earlier the diagnosis, however, the better the odds are for confining damage to a focal area and salvaging the visual capacity of the eye.[137]

FIBROUS INGROWTH. As with epithelial downgrowth, the proliferation of a fibrovascular membrane into the anterior segment is historically associated with the large wounds of ICCE, with decreasing incidence with extracapsular procedures.[137,141,142] As with epithelial downgrowth, the risk factors of complicated surgery—with iris and vitreous prolapse, malposition of wound edges, and incarceration into the wound leading to gaping—set the stage for the advent of the fibrous ingrowth.

The histologic source of the fibroblast remains controversial; it is said to derive from subepithelial connective tissue, corneal or limbal stroma, or metaplasia of the epithelium. Nevertheless, the mechanisms of secondary glaucoma can be multiple: fibrovascular occlusion of the trabecular meshwork; chronic hypotony with secondary synechial closure from shallow anterior chamber peripherally, with later glaucoma; or recurrent hemorrhage from friable fibrovascular tissue.

Unlike epithelial downgrowth, which is frequently symptomatic with photophobia and inflammation, fibrovascular ingrowth often has a slow, quiet progression. When vessels are a prominent component of the membrane, the extent of the fibrous ingrowth over the iris and cornea is obvious. In other cases, only the corectopia, ectropion uvea, and pupillary membrane indicate extensive growth. Penetration into the vitreous cavity can lead to blinding retinal detachment. It is, however, considered less progressive and destructive than epithelial downgrowth. It also tends to be self-limited, which is fortunate because there is no documented treatment. Inflammation and glaucoma can be treated as they arise, but the fibrous ingrowth does not seem to respond to intensive steroid treatment.

Glaucoma Following Nd:YAG Laser Capsulotomy

A long-term consequence of cataract extraction is the need for opening the posterior capsule, in the presence of a posterior chamber lens implant. Although multiple complications of capsulotomy have been well documented (cystoid macular edema,[143] retinal detachment,[144–148] dislocation of the posterior chamber lens,[149] and *Propionibacterium acnes* endophthalmitis[150]), the tendency toward elevated IOP is of concern here.

After Nd:YAG laser capsulotomy, IOP elevations of at least 10 mmHg have been reported in as many as 30% of cases.[151,152] This incidence of pressure rise, however, has been reduced with the use of multiple glaucoma medications (timolol,[153] pilocarpine,[154] and apraclonidine[155,156]). The mechanism of the pressure rise after capsulotomy remains uncertain: perhaps there is trabecular blockade from both soluble and insoluble lens particles[130] or from a substance released from the vitreous gel at the time of laser application.[157]

Especially in eyes with preexisting glaucoma, it is advisable prophylactically to treat the eye to undergo capsulotomy with an α_2-agonist such as 1% apraclonidine.[158] Glaucoma control usually remains unaffected if there is no IOP spike after YAG laser capsulotomy. A malignant glaucoma has been seen after capsulotomy.[159]

Congenital Cataract Surgery

Glaucoma is often seen after congenital cataract surgery, but its diagnosis is often hampered by an ocular examination complicated by nystagmus, small pupillary openings, and limited cooperation. The incidence is between 5% and 16%.[160–162] However, a careful follow-up report by Simon and colleagues[163] reported a 41% incidence of glaucoma in 17 eyes followed for at least 5 years after surgery. A clinical rule of thumb is that glaucoma will appear about 5 years after surgery.

Since approximately 1980, the preferred technique for congenital cataract extraction has been a combination of lens removal and anterior vitrectomy. Although initially encouraging in terms of reducing the incidence of secondary glaucoma, such as pupillary block and cortical opacification through the visual axis,[160–164] pupillary block glaucoma has still been reported.[165] In fact, a 10% incidence of glaucoma following the lensectomy and vitrectomy technique was reported by Keech and colleagues[162] and a 24% incidence by Simon and coworkers.[163] There are several sources for glaucoma following congenital cataract surgery other than pupillary block. A trabecular or angle anomaly has been suspected with congenital lens opacity,[160] but this finding is not always obvious on gonioscopy.

As with most pediatric glaucomas, topical beta blockers are the main medical agent used; rarely, miotics and systemic carbonic anhydrase inhibitors are useful. More often, a trabeculectomy with or without antimetabolite, or glaucoma seton implantation (eg, Molteno) is required.

The visual prognosis from congenital cataract surgery—with or without glaucoma—is often grim. The only prophylactic measures thought to be useful include impeccable intraocular surgery and the intense treatment of intraocular inflammation, to reduce synechial formation and adhesions.

CORNEAL SURGERY

Glaucoma is a notorious risk factor for graft failure, and it is a common sequela after grafting, due to several causes, such as trabecular traction or synechial proliferation. The association of corneal surgery and glaucoma becomes further complicated when concomitant cataract surgery is performed, and when steroids are used in the long-term management for graft survival.

Glaucoma and Penetrating Keratoplasty

Preexisting Glaucoma

Although glaucoma is rarely a cause of corneal failure and subsequent need for penetrating keratoplasty, it is not uncommonly associated with the primary causes of corneal failure. This is particularly true in eyes with longstanding uveitis (herpetic or interstitial)[166] or anterior chamber inflammation.[167–169] Similarly, many corneal failures are precipitated by endothelial trauma associated with cataract extraction, which can also result in secondary glaucoma. A similar mechanism occurs in the unusual association of glaucoma following ocular trauma that sustains corneal failure and later requires transplantation. Although visualization through impaired cornea is not always possible, even a partial gonioscopic assessment is invaluable in anticipating glaucoma following transplantation.

The corneal surgeon's rule of thumb is that preexisting glaucoma *must* be controlled before undertaking a penetrating keratoplasty; the glaucomatologist's experience is that preexisting glaucoma is at significant risk of going out of control following penetrating keratoplasty.[170] Because of the importance of low IOP for corneal graft survival, antecedent glaucoma surgeries are often required. These would span the spectrum of interventions: trabeculectomies with antimetabolites such as mitomycin or 5-FU; glaucoma seton implants, such as Molteno or ACTSEB (*A*nterior *C*hamber *T*ube *S*hunt to *E*ncircling *B*and) devices;[171,172] or even transscleral YAG laser cyclophotocoagulation.[173]

Secondary Glaucoma From Corneal Disease

There is a high incidence of glaucoma following penetrating keratoplasty, with reports ranging from 13% to 38% in phakic eyes and 42% to 89% in aphakic eyes.[166,168,169,174] Noninflammatory sources of corneal failure, such as Fuchs dystrophy, keratoconus, and macular or granular corneal dystrophies, show the lowest risk of glaucoma.[175,176]

In the review by Kirkness and Ficker,[166] an interesting risk analysis was generated for the development of glaucoma, depending on the amount of anterior segment disorganization. For example, congenital anterior chamber dysgenesis syndromes allegedly have a risk of glaucoma 33 times greater than keratoconus after penetrating keratoplasty. In addition, traumatic corneal failure was said to lead to a risk 13 times higher for developing glaucoma, and iridocorneal endothelial syndrome carried a risk 10 times greater than keratoconus for developing glaucoma after an uncomplicated keratoplasty.

The incidence of postoperative pressure rise also depends on the type of surgical procedure. Penetrating keratoplasty alone had the lowest incidence (5%) compared with combined penetrating keratoplasty with ECCE (21%), or if vitrectomy was also done at the time of surgery (23%).[177,178] Intracapsular surgery combined with penetrating keratoplasty was said to have a 2.5 times greater risk for developing glaucoma than straightforward extracapsular surgery with penetrating keratoplasty; this risk increased to about 4.5 with the addition of anterior vitrectomy.[166]

Donor–Host Button Size

The cause of glaucoma following penetrating keratoplasty is multifactorial, but there is a significant implication of mechanical stress on the outflow system. Collapse of the trabecular meshwork is said to be associated with the loss of zonular and lenticular support in cases of aphakia,[179] or from the incision in the nearby Descemet membrane.[180] A frequent source of distortion in the past was a combination of tight suturing of the donor button, and the use of the same-size trephine for both the corneal button and the host bed. Since the observations by Zimmerman and coworkers[179] and Olson and Kaufman,[181] donor buttons are now routinely cut about 0.25 mm larger than the recipient bed, without affecting postoperative refractive error. Use of the oversize button is also said to decrease the incidence of wound leak and the formation of anterior peripheral synechiae. The size of the corneal graft also affects the trabecular stress: grafts of 7.5 to 8.0 mm are considered optimal, avoiding the compression that can be seen with smaller grafts and the crowding that can be seen with larger grafts.

The glaucoma that results from an incorrectly sized graft button can be formidable. There are reports of pressures of more than 50 mmHg in the first 7 days, with the associated risks of ischemic optic neuropathy, central retinal vein occlusion, and central retinal artery occlusion. Medications are often ineffective in treating this early postoperative rise. In one series, glaucoma surgery was required in almost 25% of cases.[169]

Miscellaneous Glaucomas

The three most common associations of glaucoma with corneal surgery have been discussed: preexisting primary open-angle glaucoma; secondary glaucoma, associated with corneal disease (Fuchs dystrophy, endothelial keratitis, iridocorneal endothelial syndrome, or herpetic disease); and difficulties with donor–host corneal button sizes. Other forms of glaucoma can also be seen in the perioperative period, and these are similar to those that occur at the time of cataract extraction. They include pupillary block with or without inflammation, peripheral angle shallowing from choroidal effusion or suprachoroidal hemorrhage, inflammatory glaucoma (particulate debris or prostaglandins), hemorrhagic or ghost cell glaucoma, lens-induced glaucoma, steroid-induced glaucoma, prostaglandin-related glaucoma, and viscoelastic-induced glaucoma.[182]

The long-term use of topical corticosteroids can often be a confounding issue in the development of IOP elevations following penetrating keratoplasty. It has been recommended that less potent steroids for stimulating IOP, such as fluorometholone, can maintain antiinflammatory activity[183] while reducing the incidence of steroid-induced glaucoma.

Perhaps because of the common phenomenon of microscopic wound dehiscence in nearly 5% of grafts,[184] retrocorneal fibrous proliferation and epithelial ingrowth appear in the corneal literature as late complications, sometimes with associated glaucoma. The symptoms and signs of these two conditions, as well as their dismal surgical responsiveness, have been mentioned previously.

Although the standard glaucoma medications must be used in the presence of any of the abovementioned situations of elevated IOP, early surgical intervention with trabeculectomy (with antimetabolite or glaucoma seton) may be required for the satisfactory control of glaucoma (as is commonly the case with the donor–host button glaucomas). Prolonged IOP can be toxic to the transplanted cornea endothelial surface.[185]

Surgical Management of Postkeratoplasty Glaucoma

Because of the extensive anterior segment surgery often associated with penetrating keratoplasty, several guidelines for glaucoma intervention should be kept in mind. Often, the conjunctiva in these eyes has been violated, with subsequent scarring, either during prior cataract surgery or at the time of transplantation and other anterior segment surgery. Accordingly, at the time of glaucoma surgery, it is useful to balloon up the conjunctiva with lidocaine or saline before initiating a limbus-based flap for dissection, to ensure that access to the limbus is possible. Antimetabolites may also be necessary at the time of trabeculectomy.

Although argon laser trabeculoplasty has been mentioned as an adjunct to antiglaucoma medications in this setting,[186,187] this is rarely a definitive intervention. A more aggressive laser technique, involving transpupillary argon laser photocoagulation of ciliary processes, has been described,[188] but this has failed to find widespread clinical utility. At least 25% of the total ciliary processes apparently need to be coagulated, and even this may be insufficient. Instrumentation for endoscopic cyclophotocoagulation has also been described.[189] A comparable approach was undertaken with endophotocoagulation during vitreous surgery, with extensive ciliary ablation of more than 75% of processes, but with only equivocal IOP control.[190,191]

The use of trabeculectomy to control postkeratoplasty glaucoma may not have as successful a long-term result as in other eyes; Gilvarry and coworkers[192] report a 50% success rate at 2 years. These trabeculectomy results may be improved by the use of antimetabolites, but possibly at the expense of the graft's endothelial viability. A normal endothelial cell loss of 4% per year is expected in grafts, but after the use of 5-FU, the decrease in cell count has been reported at 15% per year[193]; after the use of intraoperative mitomycin, the cell loss has been reported at 11% after only a few months' follow-up.[194]

Of considerable theoretic attractiveness is the use of the glaucoma implant setons for the management of postoperative glaucoma. They offer the advantage of having their plates far removed from the interpalpebral area, and with the placement of a silicone tube into the anterior segment, between the iris and host cornea, mechanical touching to the graft can be avoided. Nevertheless, the success rate is not necessarily predictable, and it may depend on the timing of the surgery: the greatest failure rate apparently occurs when seton surgery *follows* keratoplasty.[172] Results seemed to be similar with the use of either the Molteno or the ACTSEB seton.[171,172] Nevertheless, there seems to be a tendency for significant endothelial cell loss, as high as 24%.[171] Although frank graft failure does not necessarily ensue, careful monitoring of graft status and the frequent use of steroids may be necessary.

Cyclophotocoagulation was often the treatment of last resort for refractory glaucoma unresponsive to other medical or surgical interventions. However, the long-term complications of visual loss remain daunting. About 70% of either aphakic angle-closure glaucomas or open-angle glaucomas respond to 180° cyclocryotherapy.[195] Similar rates have been reported with the use of transscleral YAG laser cyclophotocoagulation. Because this laser modality causes less postoperative pain and inflammation, it may be more compatible with long-term graft survival.[196–198]

Refractive Corneal Surgery

With the evolving technology of incisional refractive corneal surgery, there seems to be no particular predilection toward glaucoma. Nevertheless, some caveats and situations should be mentioned. The first is the mechanical difficulty of accurate Goldmann tonometry in the presence of large radial incisions that leave too small a central optical zone. Accordingly, less standard measures, such as the Tonopen or other devices, are sometimes used—if at all. There is one anecdotal report of a patient who sustained profound bilateral visual loss from undiagnosed glaucoma because the symptoms of halos, glare, and discomfort were attributed to the radial keratotomies, and IOP measurements and disc evaluation were ignored.

A more common and predictable problem is the long-term use of topical corticosteroids in the management of some patients after refractive surgery, with the risk of elevated IOP in susceptible patients. Again, this phenomenon can only be known to exist if the IOP is consistently assessed. The use of less potent topical steroids (eg, fluorometholone or medrysone) or even nonsteroidal antiinflammatory agents (eg, ketorolac) may be more appropriate. Although no reported cases of glaucoma have yet been associated with laser refractive surgery, the same caveats apply: differentiate glaucoma symptoms from corneal symptoms, and periodically measure the IOP and evaluate the optic nerve.

IOP ELEVATIONS FOLLOWING RETINAL–VITREOUS SURGERY

Overview

Risk Factors for Open-Angle Glaucoma

As seen in patients with concomitant cataract and glaucoma, there are many retinal diseases that share risk factors with the development of open-angle glaucoma, and this may explain the association of some retinal conditions with presurgical glaucoma status. For example, the known association between myopia and glaucoma, and myopia and retinal detachment, may underlie the documented observation that open-angle glaucoma is more common in patients with rhegmatogenous retinal detachment.[199,200] Similarly, there is an association between type II diabetes and the development of glaucoma,[201] and hence with a possible relation between preexisting glaucoma in eyes that subsequently require vitrectomy. Another risk factor that must be considered is the higher incidence of advanced chronic open-angle glaucoma in African Americans. These points emphasize the need to thoroughly evaluate the IOP, gonioscopic status, and optic nerve health in the surgical and fellow eye with retinal disease.

Predisposition Toward Neovascular Glaucoma

DIABETES. Neovascular glaucoma is almost invariably related to some form of profound retinopathy. It is the feared sequela of uncontrolled proliferative diabetic retinopathy, and an estimated one third of cases of neovascular glaucoma are secondary to diabetes.[202,203] The prevalence of neovascular disease is related both to the duration of the diabetes and to concomitant vascular diseases such as systemic hypertension.

There is also an associated risk of neovascularization in eyes that have undergone vitrectomy, but it is difficult to sort out the causes and effects, such as differentiating early rubeosis from iris hyperemia, the unpredictable course of rubeosis iridis, and the association of rubeosis with other postoperative complications such as rhegmatogenous retinal detachment. In fact, vitrectomy in aphakic eyes is said to lead to irreversible neovascular glaucoma if there is an untreated rhegma.[204] A completely attached retina and aggressive PRP are of paramount importance in decreasing the risk of neovascular glaucoma following vitrectomy for complications of proliferative diabetic retinopathy. Some 83% of eyes with detached retina versus 4% of eyes with attached retina developed neovascular glaucoma.[205] Successfully reattached retina is associated with more regression of rubeosis iridis (76%) than if the retina was not reattached (27%).[206]

There is a similarly high association of neovascular glaucoma in eyes with diabetes when the intact lenticular–zonular barrier defining the interface of the anterior and posterior segments is violated at the time of cataract extraction, lensectomy, or vitrectomy. Changes in vitreous may result in the presentation of endogenous angiogenic factors.[207–209] Such a scenario would explain such clinical observations as the fact that rubeosis occurs twice as often in aphakic eyes as in phakic eyes[210] and the fact that the 5% to 8% incidence of rubeosis neovascular glaucoma following vitrectomy jumps to 12% to 36% if concomitant lensectomy was performed. The development of rubeosis after vitrectomy in patients with active proliferative diabetic retinopathy is a significant source of morbidity, with an estimated rate of blindness of about 10% after its detection.[204,211–213] Panretinal destruction, either by laser photocoagulation or laser destruction,[214,215] or peripheral cryoretinopexy[216] may be effective in causing the involution of the iris neovascularization. Glaucoma drainage procedures, such as trabeculectomy with antimetabolite, or glaucoma seton surgeries, can lead to stabilization or even involution of the neovascular glaucoma, possibly by providing filtration for angiogenic factors.

VASCULAR OCCLUSION. The other major source of neovascular glaucoma is from vascular occlusion, with resultant retinal ischemia. The most common form is central retinal vein occlusion, which itself has a high association of systemic risk factors such as systemic hypertension and the presence of diabetes. Although there is some controversy as to the fine points of epidemiology, it is a common clinical impression that there is an association of central vein occlusion with preexisting glaucoma or elevated ocular pressure.[217]

Although the nonischemic forms of central vein occlusion outnumber ischemic forms by about 4:1, the distinction between the two types of vein occlusion may require fine distinctions of fluorescein angiography, specific transit times of fluorescein passage through the retina, and specific B/A wave ratios on the electroretinogram—these may not be available in every clinical setting. Nevertheless, up to 85% of patients with ischemic central retinal vein occlusion go on to develop neovascular glaucoma, often within 3 to 5 months after the primary vascular occlusion.[218,219] Perhaps the most useful predictive factor for the development of neovascular glaucoma is decreasing B/A wave amplitude ratios on the electroretinogram.[220–223] Other findings include a decreased maximum saturated response (R_{max}) or decreased half-saturation intensities (log K). In the absence of electrophysiologic testing, however, careful clinical observation and angiography after the resolution of hemorrhage may show areas of capillary nonperfusion.

The delivery of PRP or pancryopexy can often cause neovascularization to involute before there is irreversible angle closure. In the event of progressive synechial fibrovascular proliferation, standard medical interventions are rarely sufficient, and surgical trabeculectomy or glaucoma setons are required. Special attention should be paid to the fellow eye, especially if it too has elevated IOP, because it may also be at risk for central retinal vein occlusion.

CAROTID ARTERIAL INSUFFICIENCY. The third common cause of neovascular glaucoma besides diabetes and vascular occlusion is carotid arterial insufficiency. This can be unilateral or bilateral, and can involve the common or internal carotid artery. The clinical picture may have a variable and complex presentation. With profound ischemia, IOP may be low despite the presence of a neovascular membrane in the angle, presumably due to hypoperfusion of the ciliary body. Aberrations in ciliary perfusion may also account for the wide swings of IOP sometimes seen. If the occluded carotid artery itself is surgically addressed, the IOP elevation can be rapid and high because of the increased aqueous production in the presence of a chronically embarrassed trabecular meshwork from neovascular growth. It is the anterior segment, of course, that is ischemic, and hence PRP is of limited value.

Treatment of Neovascular Glaucoma

Although overall this condition has a poor prognosis, the fundamental principle is to try to prevent the complications of hemorrhage from the fragile new vessels. Whenever possible, it is desirable to deliver PRP in the presence of proliferative diabetic retinopathy or ischemic retina following vein occlusion until involution of neovascularization is detected. Lensectomy should be avoided during vitrectomy in eyes with incipient neovascularization, and similarly capsular rupture should be avoided during cataract surgery.

When other surgeries, such as trabeculectomy or glaucoma seton implantation, must be done, PRP or peripheral retinal cryopexy should be delivered first, if possible.[224–229] In anticipating surgical manipulation of the iris, techniques have been described where presurgical photocoagulation of new vessels is done either on the iris surface or in the angle (goniophotocoagulation);[230,231] however, these recommendations have found limited clinical acceptance. Most clinicians think that these techniques do not truly forestall the possibility of bleeding in the event of an iridectomy, because deeper vessels remain unaffected, and clinically hemorrhage continues to be seen.

If absolute neovascular glaucoma ensues and remains unresponsive to maximum medical therapy, destruction of the ciliary body is the only recourse. Cyclocryotherapy in this setting has a high rate of complications, with intense iritis, hypotony, hemorrhage, cataract, and phthisis bulbi—all in association with a high risk for loss of vision. One technique in favor is to treat only 270° of the ciliary body, often in various sequences of two quadrants treated at a time, always leaving one fourth of the ciliary body untouched to reduce the possibility of phthisis.[232–235]

The current alternative to cyclocryotherapy is Nd:YAG laser cyclophotocoagulation therapy, which inflicts a considerably smaller amount of histologic damage because of the high degree of laser focus when delivered by a slit-lamp system or a fiberoptic system. The results of this technique are encouraging with respect to the reduction of IOP, and it seems to be less painful.[196,236–242] However, especially in eyes with a poor prognosis, such as those with neovascular glaucoma, the complications seen with cyclocryotherapy can also be seen with laser destruction of the ciliary body.

Ciliary body ablation has also been reported during vitrectomy by endolaser.[190] Because this treatment is mostly prophylactic in eyes with other forms of retinal disorder, it is difficult to extrapolate its utility to eyes suffering from neovascular glaucoma alone.

Complications of Panretinal Photocoagulation

The fundamental tenet of treating neovascular retinopathy is that thermocoagulation of the retinal and choroidal layers will, by some means, inhibit the elaboration of new blood vessels, and in fact will lead to the involution of existing neovascularization. Nevertheless, angle-closure glaucoma is a not uncommon complication of this often unavoidable laser intervention.

Shallowing of the anterior chamber and angle-closure glaucoma often occur because of effusions into the choroid anteriorly, in an annular distribution, with rolling forward of the ciliary body and hence narrowing of the outflow angle. This has been reported after extensive retinal photocoagulation, either by argon laser (1500 argon burns at 500 μ diameter) or xenon arc treatment (400 burns at 3° spot size, when delivered in a single session).[243–248] Blondeau and associates reported that angle closure can occur in as many as 30% of patients within 3 days of PRP, especially in eyes with preexisting shallow chambers or in eyes that receive extensive treatment in a solitary session.[243] Nevertheless, most of these pressure elevations are asymptomatic, manifesting as a mild corneal edema, pressures within the 20 to 50 mmHg range, and mild myopia from anterior displacement of the lens.

Three pathogenetic mechanisms are said to be activated at different time periods after PRP. The first is a transient, marked elevation of IOP at the time of either ruby laser or xenon arc photocoagulation, lasting only a fraction of a second.[249] This has not been observed with argon laser, and it is clinically of questionable significance. A more modest pressure elevation, but of longer duration, is seen after argon laser treatment, due to a confluence of factors: obstruction of the trabecular outflow system by protein-rich fluid, debris, or inflammation; increase in the total intraocular fluid content due to laser disruption of the blood–retinal barrier; congestion of the ciliary body, resulting in decreased uveal scleral outflow; possible laser damage to the ciliary nerves, with decreased muscle tone and reduced outflow facility; and the possible effects of prostaglandins.[243]

Similarly, the mechanism for angle-closure glaucoma that occurs in the first several days after extensive PRP is thought to be due primarily to the anterior rotation of the ciliary body from choroidal swelling, in response to the extensive laser treatment (Fig. 16-1).

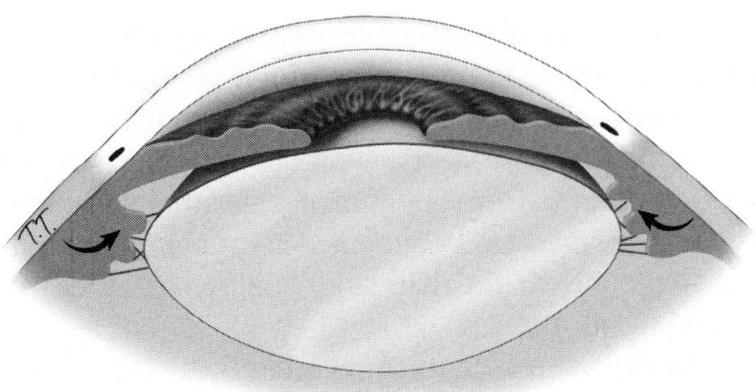

Figure 16-1. Shallowness of the anterior chamber and secondary angle-closure glaucoma can result from the anterior rotation of the ciliary body. This rotation is postulated to result from impaired venous drainage, which is thought to account for diffuse uveal edema following panretinal photocoagulation.

This has been documented by ultrasonography, showing ciliary body thickening after PRP.[248] The choroidal detachment is seen 6 to 18 hours after extensive laser treatment. However, it has also been suggested that the disruption of the blood–ocular barriers results in a fluid transudation into the vitreous from the choroid, which, in combination with an annular choroidal detachment, leads to anterior displacement of the lens-iris diaphragm and shallowing of the anterior chamber.[244] Pupillary block is rarely seen, but must be ruled out.

Because it is a temporary condition, medical treatment in combination with mydriatics and cycloplegics to lower the IOP is all that is usually needed. Unlike phakic pupillary block angle-closure glaucoma, miotics should be avoided: they can cause further anterior displacement of the lens-iris diaphragm. Most such annular effusions subside within 2 to 7 days. Rarely, if IOPs remain elevated and there is no resolution over days of the effusions, a surgical suprachoroidal drainage procedure can be done.

The complications of PRP can best be prevented by avoiding xenon and krypton red photocoagulation; by dividing large laser treatment sessions over time; by using less intense burn; and by using atropine prophylactically after PRP.[250–252]

IOP Elevations and Retinal Detachment Surgery

Schwartz Syndrome

Classically, the rhegmatogenous retinal detachment is said to reduce IOP in the affected eye by at least 2 mmHg compared with the fellow, normal eye.[253]

However, in 1973, Schwartz[254] reported patients with elevated IOPs in the presence of retinal detachment, with diminished outflow facility, open angles, and mild cell and flare in the aqueous humor. Some of these pressures were significantly elevated and unresponsive to medical treatment. After repair of the retinal detachment, the IOP and outflow facilities returned to normal.

The precise mechanism is unknown. Davidorf[255] suggested that these eyes may have sustained trabecular damage from previous trauma, which may have also contributed to the predilection for retinal detachment. It was thought that inflammation in association with the retinal detachment may have been responsible, causing a uveitis-like glaucoma from trabecular debris and cellular products.[254] In a similar fashion, pigment granules released by the retinal pigment epithelium, originally released into the subretinal space and now having access to the vitreous through the retinal hole, may have contributed to trabecular blockage.[255] A similar blockade from glycosaminoglycans—synthesized by photoreceptors and having access to the anterior segment through the rhegma—has been suggested as a possible source of obstruction as well.[256] Nevertheless, with repair of the retinal detachment, the temporary secondary glaucoma resolves.

Angle-Closure Glaucoma Following Retinal Detachment Repair

With the placement of a scleral indentation buckle for the successful resolution of a retinal detachment, transient angle-closure glaucoma (without pupillary block) has been reported in 1.4% to 4% of cases[200,257–259] (Fig. 16-2). The risk factors include a preoperative narrow angle, an anterior scleral buckle, postoperative ciliary choroidal attachment, large buckles, and encircling bands. As with the angle closure seen after PRP, many of the patients remain asymptomatic, or their symptoms are subsumed by the larger discomfort that follows major ophthalmic surgery.

A shallow anterior chamber is usually recognized within the first 96 hours after surgery and appears at the slit-lamp examination as both a central and peripheral shallowing, with pressures as high as 50 mmHg. Serous or hemorrhagic choroidal detachments are usually appreciated on funduscopy. Although most cases of anterior chamber shallowing and glaucoma subside spontaneously, sequelae of peripheral anterior synechiae with increased risk of secondary glaucoma are sometimes seen.

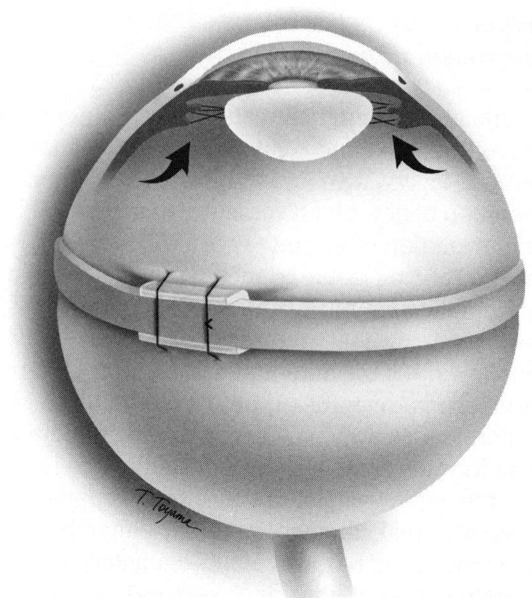

Figure 16-2. The axial elongation of the eye, and possibly embarrassed venous drainage, can result in anterior rotation of the ciliary body with subsequent secondary angle-closure glaucoma.

Because this angle-closure glaucoma can occur in the absence of pupillary block directly, one compelling explanation has been experimentally confirmed in primate eyes.[260] If the encircling band applied to the eye directly compresses one or more vortex veins, it can thus interfere with venous drainage from the uveal tract. This interference with uveoscleral outflow in turn leads to accumulation of supraciliary and suprachoroidal fluids, with subsequent swelling and anterior rotation of the ciliary body in an annular fashion, with anterior segment compromise. This mechanism is more likely than pupillary block, because this syndrome has been observed in aphakic eyes with patent iridectomies and with the hyaloid face well behind the iris surface. It is also thought that even a high scleral buckle with massive displacement of the intervitreous volume is unlikely to be the cause, because the angle-closure condition itself resolves while the buckle maintains its height.

Because this secondary angle-closure glaucoma spontaneously resolves in at most a few weeks, standard medical therapy of cycloplegics and antiglaucoma medications is likely to be sufficient. Miotics are avoided because they can cause the lens-iris diaphragm to move even more forward. If pupillary block or iris bombé occurs at the slit-lamp examination, laser iridotomies are advised. Similarly, argon laser peripheral iridoplasties may give a transient access to the trabecular meshwork and should be considered in cases that are not resolving and that have elevated pressures. Occasionally, drainage of the suprachoroidal fluid is necessary, as with reformation of the anterior segment. Although such events rarely lead to true glaucomatous optic nerve damage, the most common complication is the development of peripheral anterior synechiae, which may lead to a greater risk for secondary glaucoma in the future.

The incidence of anterior segment ischemia is about 3% of eyes with high buckles, especially if more than one rectus muscle needs to be disinserted during surgery. Clinically, corneal edema is appreciated, as well as anterior chamber shallowing centrally and peripherally, with a fibrinous anterior chamber reaction. If there is genuine and irreversible anterior segment ischemia, iris atrophy, extensive posterior and anterior synechiae, cataract formation, and corneal neovascularization have been detected.[259,260] Such a catastrophic event is particularly likely in patients with sickle cell hemoglobinopathy; 71% of patients with sickle cell disease are said to develop this complication after scleral buckling.[261] Although this may be ameliorated by exchange transfusions using hemoglobin A, this alarming finding makes it advisable to do a complete hemoglobin electrophoresis in retinal detachment patients at risk for sickle cell disease.

Glaucoma Following Vitrectomy Surgery

In the most common surgical context of vitrectomy and retinal surgery in eyes with diabetes, postoperative glaucoma is extremely common. Following pars plana vitrectomy, postoperative glaucoma has been reported to appear in 28% to 35% of cases, with a higher incidence in diabetic than nondiabetic eyes.[262,263] Similarly, about 25% of patients with diabetes experience an IOP elevation above 20 mmHg 1 year after uncomplicated vitrectomy.[263–265] The severity of the secondary glaucoma depends on whether there is background retinopathy or proliferative retinopathy. In the latter case, about 50% of patients have experienced intraocular hemorrhage, which tends to clear in 2 to 8 weeks after vitrectomy; there may be a 20% bleed rate several months after surgery. The site of the bleeding is presumably from residual or fragile neovascular tissues, either on the retinal surface or elsewhere in the eye. This in turn can lead to secondary glaucomas, such as ghost cell glaucoma,[108] or anterior segment blockade of the trabecular meshwork from intensive hyphema. Especially in patients with sickle cell hemoglobinopathy, postoperative glaucoma has been reported from mild hyphemas with sickling erythrocytes causing trabecular blockade.[266,267] However, there are special forms of elevated pressures when exogenous agents are introduced in the eye for internal tamponade.

Intraocular Gas

Because sterile room air cannot expand within the globe and is rapidly resorbed within 5 to 7 days, several forms of intraocular gas have been described, with desirable properties of expandability and long-term retention. Sulfur hexafluoride (SF_6) can double its volume within 48 hours and remain within the eye for up to 2 weeks. As might be expected, this can cause a pressure elevation of greater than 30 mmHg after injection in 26% to 45% of eyes, with the additional risk of central retinal artery occlusion.[268,269] Similar findings were seen with a comparable gas, perfluorocarbon: more than 60% of patients had pressure elevations higher than 22 mmHg, and a third had pressures of more than 40 mmHg in their first week postoperatively. Almost 25% of eyes required gas aspiration for IOP control alone.[270]

Risk factors for this form of glaucoma include the patient being in a supine or upright position, which allows the gas to push the lens-iris diaphragm anteriorly and precipitate pupillary block; hence, the patient should maintain a prone position. Similarly, a 40:60 measure of SF_6 gas is said to be less likely to cause the extremely high pressure elevations seen with the use of 100% SF_6. Lastly, eyes that demonstrate a fibrinous anterior chamber reaction are more likely to have pressure elevation, and this may be a useful warning sign. Because of the physics of IOP measurement, applanation tonometry is considered superior to pneumotonometry or Schiøtz indentation tonometry.

Mechanistically, it is simple to imagine that an expanding bubble within the vitreous cavity would elevate the IOP, but the extent depends on the rate of expansion. SF_6 gas rapidly expands in the first 6 hours postoperatively but does not reach its maximum size until 24 to 48 hours. However, in the absence of an expanding bubble, IOP elevation may also result from a combination of pupillary block, inflammatory debris, or pigmentary release into the trabecular meshwork.[271] This complication, expectedly transient, can often be managed with carbonic anhydrase inhibitors, hyperosmotic agents, or beta blockers. Techniques of removing the gas bubble, either through a knife incision in aphakic eyes or a tuberculin syringe–needle aspiration through the pars plana, have been described.

Intraocular Silicone Oil

In eyes with complicated retinal detachment and proliferative vitreal retinopathy, internal silicone tamponade has been increasingly used.[272–275] However, silicone oil can migrate throughout the eye and can have significant long-term complications, including corneal decompensation, cataract, and glaucoma.[276,277]

Secondary glaucoma is said to occur in 10% to 40% of cases after silicone injection.[278–280] Glaucoma has been reported to be the most serious long-term complication when silicone oil was used for repairing giant retinal tears, especially in aphakic eyes.[281] Occasionally, a tendency toward elevated IOPs can be masked by a concurrent ciliary body detachment. The glaucoma can be due either to a pupillary block mechanism (seen in about 3% of patients up to 3 weeks after surgery) or to globules of silicone oil in the anterior segment. Some authors have reported elevated pressures in more than 90% of eyes within 48 hours.[282,283] In Nguyen and coworkers' series,[283] more than 25% of eyes with uncontrolled postoperative IOPs required removal of silicone oil for this indication alone, and an additional 14% required glaucoma surgery.

The specifics of the glaucoma pathophysiology remain unresolved. Silicone oil can become emulsified and enter the trabecular meshwork. Although these fine globules may be seen in as many as 40% of cases, they may not be sufficient to elevate the pressure.[284] Other researchers have suggested that it is the phagocytosis of the globules by macrophages and trabecular cells that causes the decrease in aqueous facility.[274,285]

Because silicone oil is used only in eyes with extremely complicated retinal–vitreous disease, other mechanisms may also contribute to the glaucoma. Acute pupillary block has been reported in eyes without iridectomy; annular choroidal effusions following surgery, possibly worsened by scleral buckle, can also be contributory factors. Other possible mechanisms include concomitant neovascular disease, ghost cell glaucoma, persistent inflammatory debris, persistent retinal detachment and Schwartz syndrome, or retained lens particles.

The most important preventative measure for silicone oil glaucoma is to reduce the risk of pupillary block with an inferior iridectomy[103] and to limit the silicone oil's tendency to form a suspension. In the presence of large globules, the surgeon should insist on strict prone positioning for the first 24 hours after surgery. Prophylactic beta blockers, carbonic anhydrous inhibitors, or hyperosmotic agents may be useful. If medical therapy is unsuccessful, trabeculectomy is unlikely to succeed, due to the almost universal periocular and conjunctival scarring from prior surgery in such eyes. Glaucoma seton implants have been recommended, but these require the removal of silicone from the eye before placement of the tube either in the anterior segment or through the pars plana. If silicone must be retained in the eye, transscleral YAG laser cyclophotocoagulation (or possibly cyclocryotherapy) can be considered as well.

GLAUCOMAS FOLLOWING MISCELLANEOUS OPHTHALMIC PROCEDURES

Elevated IOPs following other ophthalmic surgeries have been reported, such as angle-closure glaucoma from local anesthesia for blepharoplasty,[286] but the reports are anecdotal and few conclusions can be drawn. Of course, the preoperative evaluation of the patient is critical, because eyes that are prone to glaucoma undergoing any procedure are likely to manifest the glaucoma postoperatively as well. In procedures such as strabismus surgery involving extraocular muscles, care must be taken to avoid damage to the vortex veins, which could then precipitate the form of angle-closure glaucoma and anterior ischemia seen after scleral buckling procedures. The most likely association of postoperative pressure elevations and other ophthalmic procedures is the use of topical steroids.

The ubiquitous use of retrobulbar injections can technically cause a mild pressure elevation of 4 to 6 mmHg, but this is transient and not particularly related to glaucomatous damage.[287] Similarly, the rare complication of a retrobulbar hemorrhage into the orbit can cause a sudden impairment of venous outflow and proptosis with sudden elevated IOP. This is a surgical emergency, and monitoring the central retinal artery pulsation is advised. The usual response is immediate and requires surgical fistulization to allow extravasation of the trapped orbital blood. This is often done through a lateral canthotomy. The use of hyperosmotic agents and carbonic anhydrase inhibitors may be useful, and resolution of elevated pressures can be followed over the next several days to weeks.[288]

References

1. Kooner KS, et al. IOP following ECCE, phacoemulsification, and PC-IOL implantation. Ophthalmic Surg 1988;19:643–646.
2. Gross JG, et al. Increased IOP in the immediate postoperative period after extracapsular cataract extraction. Am J Ophthalmol 1988;105:466–469.
3. Kooner K, Dulaney DD, Zimmerman TJ. IOP following ECCE and IOL implantation in patients with glaucoma. Ophthalmic Surg 1988;19:570–575.
4. Tonjum A. IOP and facility of outflow late after ocular contusion. Acta Ophthalmol 1968;46:886–908.
5. Kaufman J, Tolpin D. Glaucoma after traumatic angle recession—a 10-year prospective study. Am J Ophthalmol 1974;78:648–654.
6. Thiel H, Aden G, Pullhorn G. Changes in the chamber angle following ocular contusions. Klin Monatsbl Augenheilkd 1980;177:165–173.
7. Kaplan H, Diamond J, Brown S. Vitrectomy in experimental uveitis. I. Operative technique in rabbits. Arch Ophthalmol 1979;97:331–335.
8. Key SI, Kimura S. Iridocyclitis associated with juvenile rheumatoid arthritis. Am J Ophthalmol 1975;80: 425–429.
9. Wolf M, Lichter P, Ragsdale C. Prognostic factors in the uveitis of juvenile rheumatoid arthritis. Ophthalmology 1987;94:1242–1248.
10. Smith R, Godfrey W, Kimura S. Complications of chronic cyclitis. Am J Ophthalmol 1976;82:277–283.
11. Franceschetti A. Heterochromic cyclitis (Fuchs' syndrome). Am J Ophthalmol 1955;39:50–58.
12. Jain I, et al. Fuchs' heterochromic cyclitis: some observations on clinical picture and on cataract surgery. Ann Ophthalmol 1983;15:640–642.
13. Kimura S, Hogan M, Thygeson P. Fuchs' syndrome of heterochromic cyclitis. Arch Ophthalmol 1955;54: 179–186.
14. Liesgang T. Clinical features and prognosis in Fuchs' uveitis syndrome. Arch Ophthalmol 1982;100:1622–1626.
15. Yaldo MK, Lieberman MF. The management of secondary glaucoma in the uveitis patient. Ophthalmol Clin North Am 1993;6:147–157.
16. Seamone C, Deschenes J, Jackson W. Cataract extraction in uveitis: comparison of aphakia and posterior chamber lens implantation. Can J Ophthalmol 1992;27:120–124.
17. Forster D, Rao N, Smith R. Cataract extraction in intermediate uveitis. Dev Ophthalmol 1992;23:212–218.
18. Hooper P, Rao N, Smith R. Cataract extraction in uveitis patients. Surv Ophthalmol 1990;35:120–144.
19. Pleyer U, et al. Clinical aspects, follow-up and results of cataract extraction in uveitis. Ophthalmology 1992;89:295–300.
20. Daus W, et al. Results of extracapsular cataract extraction with IOL implantation in eyes with uveitis and Fuchs' heterochromic iridocyclitis. Ger J Ophthalmol 1992;1:399–402.
21. Sherwood D, Rosenthal A. Cataract surgery in Fuchs' heterochromic iridocyclitis. Br J Ophthalmol 1992; 76:238–240.
22. Foster R, et al. Extracapsular cataract extraction and posterior chamber IOL implantation in uveitis patients. Ophthalmology 1992;99(8):1234–1241.
23. Benson W, et al. Extracapsular cataract extraction with placement of a posterior chamber lens in patients with diabetic retinopathy. Ophthalmology 1993;100:730–738.
24. Diabetic Retinopathy Study Research Group. Preliminary report on effects of photocoagulation therapy. Am J Ophthalmol 1976;81:383–396.
25. Aiello LM, Wand M, Liang G. Neovascular glaucoma and vitreous hemorrhage following cataract surgery in patients with diabetes mellitus. Ophthalmology 1983;90:814–820.
26. Cunliffe I, et al. Extracapsular cataract surgery with lens implantation in diabetics with and without proliferative retinopathy. Br J Ophthalmol 1991;75(1):9–12.
27. Wand M, et al. Effects of panretinal photocoagulation on rubeosis iridis, angle neovascularization, and neovascular glaucoma. Am J Ophthalmol 1978;86: 332–339.
28. Vignanelli M. Progression of diabetic retinopathy following cataract extraction. Klin Monatsbl Augenheilkd 1990;196:334–337.
29. Beasley H. Rubeosis iridis in aphakic diabetics. JAMA 1970;213:128.
30. Poliner L, et al. Neovascular glaucoma after intracapsular and extracapsular cataract extraction in diabetic patients. Am J Ophthalmol 1985;100:637–643.
31. Hykin P, Gregson R, Hamilton A. Extracapsular cataract extraction in diabetes with rubeosis iridis. Eye 1992;6(pt 3):296–299.
32. Hykin P, et al. Extracapsular cataract extraction in

proliferative diabetic retinopathy. Ophthalmology 1993;100:394–399.
33. Weinreb RN, et al. Pseudophakic pupillary block with angle-closure glaucoma in diabetic patients. Am J Ophthalmol 1986;102:325–328.
34. Kooner K, Dulaney D, Zimmerman T. IOP following extracapsular cataract extraction and posterior chamber IOL implantation. Ophthalmic Surg 1988; 19:471–474.
35. McGuigan L, et al. Extracapsular cataract extraction and posterior chamber lens implantation in eyes with preexisting glaucoma. Arch Ophthalmol 1986; 104:1301–1308.
36. Tuberville A, et al. Postsurgical IOP elevation. Am Intraocular Implant Soc J 1983;9:309–312.
37. Kolker A. Visual prognosis in advanced glaucoma: a comparison of medical and surgical therapy for retention of vision in 101 eyes with advanced glaucoma. Trans Am Ophthalmol Soc 1977;75:539–555.
38. Martinez JA, et al. Risk of postoperative visual loss in advanced glaucoma. Am J Ophthalmol 1993;115: 332–337.
39. Wiles SB, MacKenzie D, Ide CH. Control of IOP with apraclonidine hydrochloride after cataract extraction. Am J Ophthalmol 1991;111:184–188.
40. Wood TO. Effect of carbachol on postoperative IOP. J Cataract Refract Surg 1988;14:654–656.
41. Lewen R, Insler MS. The effect of prophylactic acetazolamide on the IOP rise associated with Healon-aided IOL surgery. Ann Ophthalmol 1985;17:315–318.
42. Greve EL, ed. Surgical management of coexisting glaucoma and cataract. Amsterdam/Berkeley, Kugler Publications, 1987.
43. Steuhl KP, et al. IOP and anterior chamber depth before and after extracapsular cataract extraction with posterior chamber lens implantation. Ophthalmic Surg 1992;23:233–237.
44. Miller J, Morin J. IOP after cataract extraction. Am J Ophthalmol 1968;66:523–528.
45. Gormaz A. Ocular tension after cataract surgery. Am J Ophthalmol 1962;53:832.
46. Obstbaum SA. Glaucoma and IOL implantation. J Cataract Refract Surg 1986;12:257–261.
47. Handa J, et al. Extracapsular cataract extraction with posterior chamber lens implantation in patients with glaucoma. Arch Ophthalmol 1987;105:765–769.
48. Brown S, et al. Effect of cataract surgery on IOP reduction obtained with laser trabeculoplasty. Am J Ophthalmol 1985;100:373–376.
49. Thomas J, Simmons R, Belcher C. ALT in the presurgical glaucoma patient. Ophthalmology 1982;89: 187–197.
50. Apple D, et al. Anterior segment complications and neovascular glaucoma following implantation of a posterior chamber IOL. Ophthalmology 1984;91: 403–419.
51. Johnson S, Kratz R, Olson P. Iris transillumination defect and microhyphema syndrome. J Am Intraocul Implant Soc 1984;10:425–428.
52. Masket S. Pseudophakic posterior iris chafing syndrome. J Cataract Refract Surg 1986;12:252–256.
53. Smith J. Pigmentary open-angle glaucoma secondary to posterior chamber IOL implantation and erosion of the iris pigment epithelium. J Am Intraocul Implant Soc 1985;11:174–176.
54. Tomey K, Traverso C. The glaucomas in aphakia and pseudophakia. Surv Ophthalmol 1991;36:79–112.
55. Sherwood MB, et al. Long-term morphologic effects of antiglaucoma drugs on the conjunctiva and Tenon's capsule in glaucomatous patients. Ophthalmology 1989;96:327–335.
56. Ballin N, Weiss D. Pigmentary dispersion and IOP elevation in pseudophakia. Ann Ophthalmol 1982; 14:627–630.
57. Wishart PK, Atkinson PL. Extracapsular cataract extraction and posterior chamber lens implantation in patients with primary chronic angle-closure glaucoma: effect on IOP control. Eye 1989;3:706–712.
58. Lieberman MF. Management of malignant glaucoma. In: Lee D, Higginbotham E, eds. Clinician's guide to difficult glaucomas. Oxford, Blackwell Scientific, 1993.
59. Regan E, Day R. Cataract extraction after filtering procedures. Trans Am Ophthalmol Soc 1970;68:96–104.
60. McMahan L, Monica M, Zimmerman T. Posterior chamber pseudophakes in glaucoma patients. Ophthalmic Surg 1986;17:146–150.
61. Monica M, Zimmerman T, McMahan L. Implantation of posterior chamber lenses in glaucoma patients. Ann Ophthalmol 1985;17:9–10.
62. Shepard D. IOL implantation—analysis of 500 consecutive cases. Ophthalmic Surg 1977;8(3):57–63.
63. Hunsaker J, Kass M. Combined procedures for cataract and glaucoma. Intl Ophthalmol Clin 1984;24(3): 33–42.
64. Krupin T, Feitl ME, Bishop KL. Postoperative IOP rise in open-angle glaucoma patients after cataract or combined cataract-filtration surgery. Ophthalmology 1989;96:579–584.
65. Simmons R, et al. The glaucomas and extracapsular cataract surgery with posterior chamber lens implantation. Trans New Orleans Acad Ophthalmol 1985;33:27–54.
66. Longstaff S, et al. Glaucoma triple procedures: efficacy of IOP control and visual outcome. Ophthalmic Surg 1990;21:786–792.
67. Kirsch R. Glaucoma following cataract extraction associated with use of alpha-chymotrypsin. Arch Ophthalmol 1964;71:612.

68. Lantz J, Quigley J. IOP after cataract extraction: effects of alpha-chymotrypsin. Can J Ophthalmol 1973; 8:339–343.
69. Menezo J, Marco M, Mascarell E. Enzymatic ocular hypertension: a statistic study. J Fr Ophthalmol 1978; 1:289–294.
70. Kirsch R. Further studies on glaucoma following cataract extraction associated with the use of alpha-chymotrypsin. Trans Am Acad Ophthalmol Otolaryngol 1965;69:1011–1023.
71. Anderson D. Experimental alpha-chymotrypsin glaucoma studied by scanning electron microscopy. Am J Ophthalmol 1971;71:470–476.
72. Kalvin N, Hamasaki D, Gass J. Experimental glaucoma in monkeys. I. Relationship between IOP and cupping of the optic disc and cavernous atrophy of the optic nerve. Arch Ophthalmol 1966;76:82–93.
73. Sugiyama K, Kitazawa Y. Trabecular pigmentation following extracapsular cataract extraction and posterior chamber IOL implantation. Ophthalmic Surg 1990;21:700–703.
74. Caplar M, Brown R, Love L. Pseudophakic pigmentary glaucoma. Am J Ophthalmol 1988;105: 320–321.
75. Samples J, Van Buskirk F. Pigmentary glaucoma associated with posterior chamber IOLs. Am J Ophthalmol 1985;100:385–388.
76. Watt R. Pigmentary dispersion syndrome associated with silicone posterior chamber IOLs. Cataract Refract Surg 1988;14:431–433.
77. Woodham J, Lester J. Pigmentary dispersion glaucoma secondary to posterior chamber IOLs. Ann Ophthalmol 1984;16:852–855.
78. Murphy G. Acute phacolytic glaucoma with primary IOL implantation after intracapsular cataract extraction. Am Intraocular Implant Soc 1981;7:266–267.
79. Gitter K, Cohen G. Complications of vitrectomy. In: Gitter K, ed. Current concepts of the vitreous including vitrectomy. St. Louis, CV Mosby, 1976.
80. Emery I, Little J. Phacoemulsification and aspiration of cataracts: surgical techniques, complications, and results. St. Louis, CV Mosby, 1979.
81. Gilliland GD, Hutton WL, Fuller DG. Retained intravitreal lens fragments after cataract surgery. Ophthalmology 1992;99:1263–1267.
82. Lane SS, Lindstrom RL. Viscoelastic agents: formulations, clinical applications and complication. In: Ostbaum SA, ed. Cataract and intraocular lens surgery. Philadelphia, WB Saunders, 1991:313–330.
83. Becker B, Shaffer RN. Glaucoma from viscoelastic substances. In: Hoskins HD, Kass MA, eds. Diagnosis and therapy of the glaucomas, 6th ed. St. Louis, CV Mosby, 1989:321.
84. Berson F, Patterson M, Epstein D. Obstruction of aqueous outflow by sodium hyaluronate in enucleated human eyes. Am J Ophthalmol 1983;95:668–672.
85. Lane S, et al. Prospective comparison of the effects of Occucoat, Viscoat, and Healon on IOP and endothelial cell loss. J Cataract Refract Surg 1991;17:21–26.
86. Polack F. Penetrating keratoplasty using MK stored corneas and Na-hyaluronate Healon. Trans Am Ophthalmol Soc 1982;80:248.
87. Embriano PJ. Postoperative pressures after phacoemulsification: sodium hyaluronate vs. sodium chondroitin sulfate-sodium hyaluronate. Ann Ophthalmol 1989;21(3):85–90.
88. Fry LL. Postoperative IOP rises: a comparison of Healon, Amvist, and Viscoat. J Cataract Refract Surg 1989;15:415–420.
89. Ruusuvaara P, Pajari S, Setälä K. Effect of sodium hyaluronate on immediate postoperative IOP after extracapsular cataract extraction and IOL implantation. Acta Ophthalmologica 1990;68:721–727.
90. Passo MS, Ernest JT, Goldstick TK. Hyaluronate increases IOP when used in cataract extraction. Br J Ophthalmol 1985;69:572–575.
91. Stamper R, DiLoreto D, Schacknow P. Effect of intraocular aspiration of sodium hyaluronate on postoperative IOP. Ophthalmic Surg 1990;21:486–491.
92. Fry LL. Comparison of the postoperative IOP with Betagan, Betoptic, Timoptic, Iopidine, Diamox, Pilopine Gel, and Miostat. J Cataract Refract Surg 1992; 18:14–19.
93. Ruiz R, et al. Management of increased IOP after cataract extraction. Am J Ophthalmol 1987;103:487–491.
94. Anmarkrud N, Bergaust B, Bulie T. The effect of Healon and timolol on early postoperative IOP after extracapsular cataract extraction with implantation of a posterior chamber lens. Acta Ophthalmologica 1992;70:96–100.
95. Hollands R, Drance S, Schulzer M. The effect of acetylcholine on early postoperative IOP. Am J Ophthalmol 1987;103:749–753.
96. Hollands R, Drance S, Schulzer M. The effect of intracameral carbachol on IOP after cataract extraction. Am J Ophthalmol 1987;104:225–228.
97. Gupta A, Bansal RK, Grewal SPS. Natural course of IOP after cataract extraction and the effect of intracameral carbachol. J Cataract Refract Surg 1992;18: 166–169.
98. Siegel MJ, et al. Secondary glaucoma and uveitis associated with Orcolon [letter]. Arch Ophthalmol 1991;109:1496–1498.
99. Miller S. Total pupillary capture. J Am Intraocul Implant Soc 1983;9:192–193.
100. Van Buskirk E. Pupillary block after IOL implantation. Am J Ophthalmol 1983;95:55–59.

101. Kielar R, Stambaugh J. Pupillary block glaucoma following IOL implantation. Ophthalmic Surg 1982; 13(8):329–333.
102. Shrader C, et al. Pupillary and iridovitreal block in pseudophakic eyes. Ophthalmology 1984;91:831–837.
103. Laganowski HC, Leaver PK. Silicone oil in the aphakic eye: the influence of a 6 o'clock peripheral iridectomy. Eye 1989;3(Pt 3):338–348.
104. Petrelli E, Wiznia R. Argon laser photocoagulation of inner wound vascularization after cataract extraction. Am J Ophthalmol 1977;84:58–61.
105. Speakman J. Recurrent hyphema after surgery. Can J Ophthalmol 1975;10:299–304.
106. Swan K. Hyphema due to wound vascularization after cataract extraction. Arch Ophthalmol 1973;89:87.
107. Read J. Traumatic hyphema: surgical vs. medical management. Ann Ophthalmol 1975;7:659–670.
108. Campbell D, Simmons R, Grant W. Ghost cells as a cause of glaucoma. Am J Ophthalmol 1976;81:441–450.
109. Becker B. IOP response to topical corticosteroids. Invest Ophthalmol 1965;4:198.
110. Armaly M. Effects of corticosteroids on IOP and fluid dynamics. I. The effect of dexamethasone in the normal eye. Arch Ophthalmol 1963;70:482.
111. Francois J. The importance of the mucopolysaccharides in IOP regulation. Invest Ophthalmol 1975; 14:173–176.
112. Miller D, Peczon J, Whitworth C. Corticosteroids and functions in the anterior segment of the eye. Am J Ophthalmol 1965;59:31.
113. Southren A, et al. Altered cortisol metabolism in cells cultured from trabecular meshwork specimens obtained from patients with primary open-angle glaucoma. Invest Ophthalmol Vis Sci 1983;24:1413–1417.
114. Weinreb R, Mitchell M, Polansky J. Prostaglandin production by human trabecular cells: in vitro inhibition by dexamethasone. Invest Ophthalmol Vis Sci 1983;24:1541–1545.
115. Stark W, et al. The FDA report on IOLs. Ophthalmology 1983;90:311–317.
116. Apple D, et al. Complications of IOLs—a historical and histopathological review. Surv Ophthalmol 1984;29(1):1–54.
117. Bergman M, Laatikainen L. IOP level in glaucomatous and nonglaucomatous eyes after complicated cataract surgery and implantation of an AC-IOL. Ophthalmic Surg 1992;23:378–382.
118. Hansen TE, Naeser K, Rask KL. A prospective study of IOP 4 months after extracapsular cataract extraction with implantation of posterior chamber lenses. J Cataract Refract Surg 1987;13:35–38.
119. Ellingson F. The uveitis-glaucoma-hyphema syndrome associated with the Mark VIII anterior chamber lens implant. Am Intraocul Implant Soc J 1978; 4(2):50–53.
120. Holland G. Zur Klinik der expulsiven Blutung nach Kataraktoperation. Klin Monatsbl Augenheilkd 1966; 149:859–864.
121. Taylor D. Expulsive hemorrhage: some observations and comments. Trans Am Ophthalmol Soc 1974;82: 157–169.
122. Payne J, et al. Expulsive hemorrhage: its incidence in cataract surgery and a report of four bilateral cases. Trans Am Ophthalmol Soc 1985;83:181–204.
123. Davison J. Acute intraoperative suprachoroidal hemorrhage in extracapsular cataract surgery. J Cataract Refract Surg 1986;12:606–622.
124. Maumenne AE, Schwartz MF. Acute intraoperative choroidal effusion. Am J Ophthalmol 1985;100(1): 147–154.
125. Gressel MG, Parrish R, Heuer DK. Delayed nonexpulsive suprachoroidal hemorrhage. Arch Ophthalmol 1984;102:1757–1760.
126. Bryant WR. Secondary IOL implantation in eyes that experienced suprachoroidal hemorrhage during primary cataract surgery. J Cataract Refract Surg 1989; 15:629–634.
127. Simmons R. Malignant glaucoma. Br J Ophthalmol 1972;56:263–272.
128. Simmons R. Malignant glaucoma. In: Ritch R, Shields M, eds. The secondary glaucomas. St. Louis, CV Mosby, 1982;1251–1263.
129. Herschler J. Laser shrinkage of the ciliary processes. Ophthalmology 1980;87:1155–1158.
130. Epstein D, Jedziniak J, Grant W. Obstruction of aqueous outflow by lens particles and by heavy-molecular-weight soluble lens proteins. Invest Ophthalmol Vis Sci 1978;17:272–277.
131. Bernardino V, Kim J, Smith T. Epithelialization of the anterior chamber after cataract extraction. Arch Ophthalmol 1969;82:742–750.
132. Theobald G, Hass J. Epithelial invasion of the anterior chamber following cataract extraction. Trans Am Acad Ophthalmol Otolaryngol 1948;52:470.
133. Merenmies L, Tarkkanen A. Causes of enucleation following cataract surgery. Acta Ophthalmol 1977;55: 347–352.
134. Maumenee A, et al. Review of 40 histologically proven cases of epithelial downgrowth following cataract extraction and suggested surgical management. Am J Ophthalmol 1970;69:589–603.
135. Weiner M, et al. Epithelial downgrowth: a 30-year clinicopathological review. Br J Ophthalmol 1989;73: 6–11.
136. Anseth A, Dohlman C, Albert D. Epithelial downgrowth—fistula repair and keratoplasty. Refract Corneal Surg 1991;7(1):23–27.

137. Stark W, et al. Surgical management of epithelial ingrowth. Am J Ophthalmol 1978;85:772–780.
138. Laing R, et al. Epithelialization of the anterior chamber: clinical investigation with the specular microscope. Arch Ophthalmol 1979;97:1870–1874.
139. Maumenee A. Treatment of epithelial downgrowth and intraocular fistula following cataract extraction. Trans Am Ophthalmol Soc 1964;62:153.
140. Brown S. Treatment of advanced epithelial downgrowth. Trans Am Acad Ophthalmol Otolaryngol 1973;77:618–622.
141. Blodi F. Cause and frequency of enucleation after cataract extraction. Intl Ophthalmol Clin 1965;5:257–269.
142. Allen J. Epithelial and stromal ingrowths. Am J Ophthalmol 1968;65:179–182.
143. Albert D, et al. A prospective study of angiographic cystoid macular edema 1 year after Nd:YAG posterior capsulotomy. Ann Ophthalmol 1990;22:139–143.
144. Ambler J, Constable I. Retinal detachment following Nd:YAG capsulotomy. Aust N Z J Ophthalmol 1988; 16:337–341.
145. Fastenberg D, Schwartz P, Lin H. Retinal detachment following neodymium:YAG laser capsulotomy. Am J Ophthalmol 1984;97:288–291.
146. Koch D, et al. Axial myopia increases the risk of retinal complications after neodymium:YAG laser posterior capsulotomy. Arch Ophthalmol 1989;107: 986–990.
147. Rickman-Barger L, et al. Retinal detachment after neodymium:YAG laser posterior capsulotomy. Am J Ophthalmol 1989;107:531–536.
148. Terry A, et al. Neodymium:YAG laser for posterior capsulotomy. Am J Ophthalmol 1983;96:716–720.
149. Clayman H, Jaffe N. Spontaneous enlargement of neodymium:YAG posterior capsulotomy in aphakic and pseudophakic patients. J Cataract Refract Surg 1988;14:667–669.
150. Meisler D, Mandelbaum S. *Propionibacterium*-associated endophthalmitis after extracapsular cataract extraction—review of reported cases. Ophthalmology 1989;96:54–61.
151. Flohr M, Robin A, Kelley J. Early complications following Q-switched neodymium:YAG laser posterior capsulotomy. Ophthalmology 1985;92:360–363.
152. Kraff K, Sanders D, Lieberman H. IOP and the corneal endothelium after neodymium:YAG posterior capsulotomy—relative effects of aphakia and pseudophakia. Arch Ophthalmol 1985;103:511–514.
153. Migliori M, Beckman H, Channel M. IOP changes after neodymium:YAG laser capsulotomy in eyes pretreated with timolol. Arch Ophthalmol 1987;105:473–475.
154. Brown S, et al. Effect of pilocarpine in treatment of IOP elevation following neodymium:YAG laser posterior capsulotomy. Ophthalmology 1985;92:354–359.
155. Brown R, et al. ALO 2145 reduces the IOP elevation after anterior segment laser surgery. Ophthalmology 1988;95:378–384.
156. Pollack I, et al. Effectiveness of apraclonidine preventing the rise in IOP after neodymium:YAG posterior capsulotomy. Trans Am Ophthalmol Soc 1988; 86:461–469.
157. Schubert H, et al. The role of the vitreous in the IOP rise after neodymium:YAG laser capsulotomy. Arch Ophthalmol 1985;103:1538–1542.
158. Silverstone DE, et al. Prophylactic use of apraclonidine for IOP increase after Nd:YAG capsulotomies. Am J Ophthalmol 1992;113:401–405.
159. Halkias A, Magauran DM, Joyce M. Ciliary block (malignant) glaucoma after cataract extraction with lens implant treated with YAG laser capsulotomy and anterior hyaloidotomy. Br J Ophthalmol 1992;76:569–570.
160. Chrousos G, Parks M, O'Neill J. Incidence of chronic glaucoma, retinal detachment and secondary membrane surgery in pediatric aphakic patients. Ophthalmology 1984;91:1238–1241.
161. Francois J. Late results of congenital cataract surgery. Ophthalmology 1979;86:1586–1598.
162. Keech R, Pongue A, Scott W. Complications after surgery for congenital and infantile cataracts. Am J Ophthalmol 1989;108:136–141.
163. Simon JW, et al. Glaucoma after pediatric lensectomy/vitrectomy. Ophthalmology 1991;98:670–674.
164. Parks M. Visual results in aphakic children. Am J Ophthalmol 1982;94:441–449.
165. Eustis HS Jr, Walton RC, Ball SF. Pupillary block glaucoma following pediatric cataract extraction. Ophthalmol Surg 1990;21:413–415.
166. Kirkness CM, Ficker LA. Risk factors for the development of postkeratoplasty glaucoma. Cornea 1992;11: 427–432.
167. Irvine A, Kaufman H. IOP following penetrating keratoplasty. Am J Ophthalmol 1969;68:835–844.
168. Karesh J, Nirankari V. Factors associated with glaucoma after penetrating keratoplasty. Am J Ophthalmol 1983;96:160–164.
169. Foulks G. Glaucoma associated with penetrating keratoplasty. Ophthalmology 1987;94:871–874.
170. Karesh J, Nirankari V. Factors associated with glaucoma after penetrating keratoplasty. Am J Ophthalmol 1983;96:160–164.
171. McDonnell P, et al. Molteno implant for the control of glaucoma in eyes after penetrating keratoplasty. Ophthalmology 1988;95:364–369.
172. Beebe W, et al. The use of Molteno implant and anterior chamber tube shunt to encircling band for the treatment of glaucoma in keratoplasty patients. Ophthalmology 1990;97:1414–1422.

173. Beckman H, Waeltermann J. Transscleral ruby laser cyclocoagulation. Am J Ophthalmol 1984;98:788–795.
174. Kirkness C, et al. The success and survival of repeat corneal grafts. Eye 1990;4(pt 1):58–64.
175. Kirkness C, Moshegov C. Postkeratoplasty glaucoma. Eye 1988;2(suppl):S19–S26.
176. Simmons R, et al. Elevated IOP following penetrating keratoplasty. Trans Am Ophthalmol Soc 1990;87:79–91.
177. Chien A, et al. Glaucoma in the immediate postoperative period after penetrating keratoplasty. Am J Ophthalmol 1993;115:711–714.
178. Meyer R, Musch D. Assessment of success and complications of triple procedure surgery. Am J Ophthalmol 1987;104:233–240.
179. Zimmerman T, et al. Transplant size and elevated IOP postkeratoplasty. Arch Ophthalmol 1978;96: 2231–2233.
180. Olson R, Kaufman H. A mathematical description of causative factors and prevention of elevated IOP after penetrating keratoplasty. Invest Ophthalmol Vis Sci 1977;16:1085–1092.
181. Olson R, et al. Refractive variation and donor tissue size in aphakic keratoplasty—a prospective randomized study. Arch Ophthalmol 1979;97:1480–1481.
182. Barron B, et al. Comparison of the effects of Viscoat and Healon on postoperative IOP. Am J Ophthalmol 1985;100:377–384.
183. Litoff D, Krachmer J. Complications of corneal surgery. Intl Ophthalmol Clin 1992;32(4):79–96.
184. Binder P, et al. Keratoplasty wound separations. Am J Ophthalmol 1975;80:109–115.
185. Charlin R, Polack F. The effect of elevated IOP elevation on the endothelium of corneal grafts. Cornea 1982;1:241–249.
186. Van Meier W, et al. Laser trabeculoplasty for glaucoma in aphakic and pseudophakic eyes after penetrating keratoplasty. Arch Ophthalmol 1988;106:185–188.
187. Shields S, Stewart WC, Shields MB. Transpupillary argon laser cyclophotocoagulation in the treatment of glaucoma. Ophthalmic Surg 1988;19:171–175.
188. Lee P. Argon laser photocoagulation of the ciliary processes in cases of aphakic glaucoma. Arch Ophthalmol 1979;97:2135–2138.
189. Shields MB. Intraocular cyclophotocoagulation. In: Krupin T, Wax MB, eds. New techniques in glaucoma surgery. Philadelphia, WB Saunders, 1988:167–173.
190. Zarbin M, et al. Endolaser treatment of the ciliary body for severe glaucoma. Ophthalmology 1988;95: 1639–1648.
191. Patel A, et al. Endolaser treatment of the ciliary body for uncontrolled glaucoma. Ophthalmology 1986;93: 825–830.
192. Gilvarry A, et al. The management of postkeratoplasty glaucoma by trabeculectomy. Eye 1989;3:713–718.
193. Fluorouracil Filtering Surgery Study Group. Fluorouracil filtering study 1-year follow-up. Am J Ophthalmol 1989;108:625–635.
194. Pastor S, et al. Corneal endothelial cell loss following trabeculectomy with mitomycin C. J Glaucoma 1993;2:112–113.
195. Caprioli J, et al. Cyclocryotherapy in the treatment of advanced glaucoma. Ophthalmology 1985;92:947–954.
196. Schuman J, Puliafito C. Laser cyclophotocoagulation. Intl Ophthalmol Clin 1990;30(2):111–119.
197. Schuman J, et al. Contact transscleral Nd:YAG laser cyclophotocoagulation—midterm results. Ophthalmology 1992;99:1089–1095.
198. Royal G, et al. One-year follow-up of Nd:YAG contact transscleral laser cyclophotocoagulation. Invest Ophthalmol Vis Res. 1992;33:1268.
199. Becker B. Discussion of Smith JL. Retinal detachment and glaucoma. Trans Am Acad Ophthalmol Otolaryngol 1963;67:731.
200. Phelps C, Burton T. Glaucoma and retinal detachment. Arch Ophthalmol 1977;95:418–422.
201. Klein F, Klein R, Moss S. IOP in diabetic persons. Ophthalmology 1984;91:1356–1360.
202. Grant W. Management of neovascular glaucoma. In: Leopold I, ed. Symposium on ocular therapy. St. Louis, CV Mosby, 1974.
203. Madsen P. Rubeosis of the iris and haemorrhagic glaucoma in patients with proliferative diabetic retinopathy. Br J Ophthalmol 1971;55:368–371.
204. Michels R. Vitrectomy for complications of diabetic retinopathy. Arch Ophthalmol 1978;96:237–246.
205. Wand M, et al. Neovascular glaucoma following pars plana vitrectomy for complications of diabetic retinopathy. Ophthalmic Surg 1990;21(2):113–118.
206. Scuderi J, Blumenkranz M, Blankenship G. Regression of diabetic rubeosis iridis following successful surgical reattachment of the retina by vitrectomy. Retina 1982;2(4):193–196.
207. Glaser B, et al. Retinal pigment epithelial cells release inhibitors of neovascularization. Ophthalmology 1987;94:780–784.
208. Glaser B, et al. The demonstration of angiogenic activity from ocular tissues (preliminary report). Ophthalmology 1980;87:440–446.
209. Patz A. Clinical and experimental studies on retinal neovascularization. XXXIX Edward Jackson Memorial Lecture. Am J Ophthalmol 1982;94:715–743.
210. Blankenship G, Cortez R, Machemer R. The lens and pars plana vitrectomy for diabetic retinopathy complications. Arch Ophthalmol 1979;97:1263–1267.
211. Charles S. Endophotocoagulation. Retina 1981;1: 117–120.

212. Michels R, Ryan S. Results and complications of 100 consecutive cases of pars plana vitrectomy. Am J Ophthalmol 1975;80(1):24–29.
213. Aaberg T, Van Horn D. Late complications of pars plana vitreous surgery. Ophthalmology 1978;85(2): 126–140.
214. Michels R. Vitreous surgery in proliferative diabetic retinopathy. In Acta XXIII Concilium Ophthalmologicum: Proceedings of the XXIII International Congress of Ophthalmology, Kyoto, Japan, 1978. Kyoto, Amsterdam-Oxford, Excerpta Medica.
215. Little H, et al. The effects of panretinal photocoagulation on rubeosis iridis. Am J Ophthalmol 1976;81: 804–809.
216. Ramsay R, Cantrill H, Knobloch W. Cryoretinopexy for proliferative diabetic retinopathy. Can J Ophthalmol 1982;17(1):17–20.
217. Cole M, Dodson P, Hendeles S. Medical conditions underlying retinal vein occlusion in patients with glaucoma or ocular hypertension. Br J Ophthalmol 1989;73:693–698.
218. Gutman F. Evaluation of a patient with central retinal vein occlusion. Ophthalmology 1983;90:481–483.
219. Hayreh S. Clarification of central retinal vein occlusion. Ophthalmology 1983;90:458–474.
220. Breton M, et al. Electroretinogram parameters at presentation as predictors of rubeosis in central retinal vein occlusion patients. Ophthalmology 1989;96: 1343–1352.
221. Johnson M, et al. Neovascularization in central retinal vein occlusion—electrographic findings. Arch Ophthalmol 1988;106:348–352.
222. Kaye S, Harding S. Early electroretinography in unilateral central retinal vein occlusion as a predictor of rubeosis iridis. Arch Ophthalmol 1988;106:353–356.
223. Sabates R, Hirose T, McMeel W. Electroretinography in the prognosis and classification of central retinal vein occlusion. Arch Ophthalmol 1983;101:232–235.
224. Callahan M. Photocoagulation and rubeosis iridis [letter]. Am J Ophthalmol 1974;78:873–874.
225. Hovener G. Photocoagulation for central vein occlusion. Klin Monatsbl Augenheilkd 1978;173:392–401.
226. Jacobson D, Murphy R, Rosenthal A. The treatment of angle neovascularization with panretinal photocoagulation. Ophthalmology 1979;86:1270.
227. Laatikainen L, et al. Panretinal photocoagulation in central retinal vein occlusion: a randomised controlled clinical study. Br J Ophthalmol 1977;61:741–753.
228. Laatikainen L. Preliminary report on effect of retinal panphotocoagulation on rubeosis iridis and neovascular glaucoma. Br J Ophthalmol 1977;61:278–284.
229. May D, et al. Xenon arc panretinal photocoagulation for central retinal vein occlusion: a randomised prospective study. Br J Ophthalmol 1979;63:725–734.
230. Simmons R, et al. Goniophotocoagulation for neovascular glaucoma. Trans Am Acad Ophthalmol Otolaryngol 1977;83(1):80–89.
231. Simmons R, Depperman S, Dueker D. The role of goniophotocoagulation in neovascularization of the anterior chamber angle. Ophthalmology 1980;87:79–82.
232. Boniuk M. Cryotherapy in neovascular glaucoma. Trans Am Acad Ophthalmol Otolaryngol 1974;78: 337–343.
233. Feibel R, Bigger J. Rubeosis iridis and neovascular glaucoma—evaluation of cyclocryotherapy. Am J Ophthalmol 1972;74:862–867.
234. Goldstein A, Ide C. Cyclocryotherapy for secondary glaucoma due to rubeosis iridis—case reports. Mo Med 1972;69:736–739.
235. Krupin T, Mitchell K, Becker B. Cyclocryotherapy in neovascular glaucoma. Am J Ophthalmol 1978; 86(4):24–26.
236. Balazsi G. Noncontact thermal mode Nd:YAG laser transscleral cyclocoagulation in the treatment of glaucoma—intermediate follow-up. Ophthalmology 1991;98:1858–1863.
237. Brancato R, et al. Contact transscleral cyclophotocoagulation with Nd:YAG laser in uncontrolled glaucoma. Ophthalmic Surg 1989;20:547–551.
238. Hampton C, et al. Evaluation of a protocol for transscleral neodymium:YAG cyclophotocoagulation in 100 patients. Ophthalmology 1990;97:910–917.
239. Kermani O, et al. Contact cw-Nd:YAG laser cyclophotocoagulation for treatment of refractory glaucoma. Ger J Ophthalmol 1992;1(2):74–78.
240. McAllister J, O'Brien C. Neodymium:YAG transscleral cyclocoagulation: a clinical study. Eye 1990;4(pt 5): 651–656.
241. Schuman JS, et al. Contact transscleral continuous wave neodymium:YAG laser cyclophotocoagulation. Ophthalmology 1990;97:571–580.
242. Trope GE, Ma S. Midterm effects of neodymium:YAG transscleral cyclocoagulation in glaucoma. Ophthalmology 1990;97:73–75.
243. Blondeau P, Pavan P, Phelps C. Acute pressure elevation following panretinal photocoagulation. Arch Ophthalmol 1981;99:1239–1241.
244. Boulton P. A study of the mechanism of transient myopia following extensive xenon arc photocoagulation. Trans Ophthalmol Soc UK 1973;93:287–300.
245. Mensher J. Anterior chamber depth alteration after retinal photocoagulation. Arch Ophthalmol 1977;95: 113–116.
246. Schiodte S. Changes in eye tension after panretinal xenon arc and argon laser photocoagulation in normotensive diabetic eyes. Acta Ophthalmol 1982;60: 692–700.
247. Huamonte F, et al. Immediate fundus complications after retinal scattered photocoagulation. I. Clinical

picture and pathogenesis. Ophthalmic Surg 1976; 7(1):88–99.

248. Phelps C. Angle-closure glaucoma secondary to ciliary body swelling. Arch Ophthalmol 1974;92:287–290.
249. Fraunfelder F, Viernstein L. IOP variation during xenon and ruby laser photocoagulation. Am J Ophthalmol 1971;71:1261–1266.
250. Bloom S, Brucker A. Complications of photocoagulation. In: Bloom SM, Brucker AJ, eds. Laser surgery of the posterior segment. Philadelphia, JB Lippincott, 1991:311.
251. Doft B, Blankenship G. Single versus multiple treatment sessions of argon laser panretinal photocoagulation for proliferative diabetic retinopathy. Ophthalmology 1982;89:772–779.
252. Weiter I, Brockhurst R, Tolentino F. Uveal effusion following panretinal photocoagulation. Ann Ophthalmol 1979;11:1723–1727.
253. Burton T, Arafat N, Phelps C. IOP in retinal detachment. Intl Ophthalmol 1979;1(3):147–152.
254. Schwartz A. Chronic open-angle glaucoma secondary to rhegmatogenous retinal detachment. Am J Ophthalmol 1973;75:205–211.
255. Davidorf F. Retinal pigment epithelial glaucoma. Ophthalmol Digest 1976;38:11.
256. Baruch E, et al. Glaucoma due to rhegmatogenous retinal detachment: Schwartz syndrome. Glaucoma 1981;3:229.
257. Perez R, Phelps C, Burton T. Angle-closure glaucoma following scleral buckling operations. Trans Am Acad Ophthalmol Otolaryngol 1976;81:247–252.
258. Smith T. Acute glaucoma after scleral buckling procedures. Am J Ophthalmol 1967;63:1807.
259. Ansem R, Bastiaensen L. Glaucoma following retinal detachment operations. Doc Ophthalmol 1987;67: 19–24.
260. Hayreh S, Baines J. Occlusion of the vortex veins: an experimental study. Br J Ophthalmol 1973;57:217–238.
261. Ryan S, Goldberg M. Anterior segment ischemia following scleral buckling in sickle cell hemoglobinopathy. Am J Ophthalmol 1971;72:35–50.
262. Campbell D, et al. Glaucoma occurring after closed vitrectomy. Am J Ophthalmol 1977;83:63–69.
263. Weinberg R, Peyman G, Huamonte F. Elevation of IOP after pars plana vitrectomy. Graefes Arch fur Klin und Exp Ophthalmol 1976;200(2):157–161.
264. Faulborn J, Conway B, Machemer R. Surgical complications of pars plana vitreous surgery. Ophthalmology 1978;85:116–125.
265. Ghartey K, et al. Closed vitreous surgery. XVII. Results and complications of pars plana vitrectomy. Arch Ophthalmol 1980;98:1248–1252.
266. Jampol L, et al. An update on vitrectomy surgery and retinal detachment repair in sickle cell disease. Arch Ophthalmol 1982;100:591–593.
267. Goldberg M. Sickled erythrocytes, hyphemas and secondary glaucoma. I. The diagnosis and treatment of sickled erythrocytes in human hyphemas. Ophthalmic Surg 1979;10(4):17–31.
268. Sabates W, et al. The use of intraocular gases—the results of sulfur hexafluoride gas in retinal detachment surgery. Ophthalmology 1981;88:447–454.
269. Abrams G, Swanson D, Sabates W. The results of sulfur hexafluoride gas in vitreous surgery. Am J Ophthalmol 1982;94:165–171.
270. Chang S, et al. Perfluorocarbon gases in vitreous surgery. Ophthalmology 1985;92:651–656.
271. Abrams G, et al. Dynamics of intravitreal sulfur hexafluoride gas. Invest Ophthalmol 1974;13:863–868.
272. Scott J. Treatment of the detached immobile retina. Trans Ophthalmol Soc UK 1972;92:351–357.
273. Scott J. The treatment of massive vitreous retraction. Trans Ophthalmol Soc UK 1973;93:417–423.
274. Grey R, Leaver P. Silicone oil injection in massive preretinal retraction. Trans Ophthalmol Soc UK 1977; 97:238–241.
275. Wilson-Holt N, Leaver P. Extended criteria for vitrectomy and fluid/silicone oil exchange. Eye 1990;4(pt 6):850–854.
276. Franks W, Leaver P. Removal of silicone oil—rewards and penalties. Eye 1991;5(pt 3):333–337.
277. Riedl K, et al. Intravitreal silicone oil injection: complications and treatment of 415 consecutive patients. Graefes Arch Klin Exp Ophthalmol 1990;228:19–23.
278. Federman J, Schubert H. Complications associated with the use of silicone oil in 150 eyes after retinal-vitreous surgery. Ophthalmology 1988;95:870–876.
279. Pang M, Peyman G, Kao G. Early anterior segment complication after silicone oil injection. Can J Ophthalmol 1986;21:271–275.
280. Leaver P, Grey R, Garmer A. Silicone oil injection in the treatment of massive preretinal retraction. II. Late complications in 93 eyes. Br J Ophthalmol 1979;63: 361–367.
281. Leaver P, Billington B. Vitrectomy and fluid/silicone oil exchange for giant retinal tears: 5 years follow-up. Graefes Arch Klin Exp Ophthalmol 1989;227:323–327.
282. deCorral L, Cohen S, Peyman G. Effect of intravitreal silicone oil on IOP. Ophthalmol Surg 1987;18:446–449.
283. Nguyen QH, et al. Incidence and management of glaucoma after intravitreal silicone oil injection for complicated retinal detachments. Ophthalmology 1992;99:1520–1526.
284. Laroche L, et al. Ocular findings following intravitreal silicone injection. Arch Ophthalmol 1983;101: 1422–1425.

285. Ni C, et al. Intravitreous silicone injection—histopathologic findings in a human eye after 12 years. Arch Ophthalmol 1983;101:1399–1401.
286. Gayton JL, Ledford JK. Angle-closure glaucoma following a combined blepharoplasty and ectropion repair. Ophthalmol Plast Reconstr Surg 1992;8:176–177.
287. Meyer D, et al. Effect of combined peribulbar and retrobulbar injection of large volumes of anesthetic agents on the IOP. Can J Ophthalmol 1992;27:230–232.
288. Feitle ME, Krupin T. Retrobulbar anesthesia. In: Zahl K, Meltzer M, eds. Regional anesthesia for intraocular surgery. Philadelphia, WB Saunders, 1990:83–91.

Ophthalmic Surgery Complications: Prevention and Management, edited by Judie F. Charlton and George W. Weinstein.

17

Thomas G. Chu

Expulsive and Delayed Suprachoroidal Hemorrhage

Suprachoroidal hemorrhage (SCH), either during and or after intraocular surgery, can be a devastating complication of ophthalmic surgery. The first reported case of choroidal hemorrhage in the setting of ophthalmic surgery was in 1760, by Baron de Wetzel.[1] The term "expulsive hemorrhage" was coined by Terson in 1894 to denote an acute hemorrhage of the choroid resulting in poor visual outcome and partial or total loss of vision.[2] The first reported successfully managed case of expulsive choroidal hemorrhage was in 1915 by Verhoeff.[3] Since then, much has been written about the cause, risk factors, and management of this condition. A better understanding of this condition can enable the ophthalmic surgeon to correctly manage patients at risk and to help in the treatment of patients suffering from SCH.

ANATOMIC CONSIDERATIONS

The physiology of the suprachoroidal space has been well described elsewhere.[4] The suprachoroidal space is a potential space between the choroid and the sclera. When filled with blood or fluid, it becomes a true space, of which the boundaries are the scleral spur anteriorly and the optic disc posteriorly. The choroid is firmly attached to the sclera at the ampullae of the vortex veins. These attachments are responsible for the typical lobular appearance of a large choroidal detachment. The outer surface of the ciliary body and the choroid are closely attached to the sclera by a series of fine collagen fibrils arranged in tangential sheets.[4] The suprachoroidal space normally contains about 10 μL of fluid.[5]

DEFINITIONS

Choroidal detachment and SCH are two distinct entities. A choroidal detachment is a separation of the uvea from the sclera. Choroidal detachment is secondary to effusion of serous fluid within the suprachoroidal space. Hypotony and inflammation appear to be responsible for the accumulation of fluid in the suprachoroidal space.[4,6] SCH is defined as blood, as opposed to serous fluid, within the suprachoroidal space. SCH can be classified in several ways: by the size and extent of hemorrhage, by their relation to intraocular surgery, or by precipitating events.

When categorized with respect to size, SCH can vary from a small area of involvement to a massive degree of involvement. Suprachoroidal hematomas are small loculated collections of blood within the suprachoroidal space. These lesions are benign, resolve spontaneously, and are distinct from SCH associated with intraocular surgery.[7] Hoffman and coworkers defined small areas of suprachoroidal blood in postintracapsular cataract extraction patients as "limited" choroidal hemorrhage.[8] These hemorrhages are most likely the postoperative equivalent of spontaneous suprachoroidal hematomas. Massive SCH represents the other end of the size spectrum. A massive hemorrhage into the suprachoroidal space can be large enough to force the inner retinal surfaces into direct apposition, usually within the center of the posterior chamber. This extensive type of hemorrhage is commonly termed a kissing SCH; an analogous term is a massive SCH with central retinal apposition.

The timing of development of SCH with relation to intraocular surgery is another method of classification. SCH may develop at the time of intraocular surgery (intraoperative SCH). Typically, the development of an intraoperative SCH is associated with a massive degree of hemorrhage, resulting in the expulsion of intraocular contents through the surgical wound. Such a forceful SCH is called an expulsive SCH. If, however, SCH develops in the postoperative period, it is termed either postoperative or delayed SCH. Delayed SCH occurs in a closed system and therefore is not associated with expulsion of intraocular contents. Nevertheless, it may be extensive enough to result in a kissing-type configuration.

Finally, SCH can be categorized by precipitating events. In particular, SCH can occur in the setting of either penetrating or blunt trauma. Traumatic SCH behaves differently from SCH associated with intraoperative surgery and should be considered a separate entity. Traumatic SCH will not be discussed in this chapter.

PATHOPHYSIOLOGY

There are several theories about how SCH develops in nontraumatized eyes.[9–12] Hypotony appears to be the major precipitating factor, resulting in a rupture of a necrotic long or short posterior ciliary artery.[10] Another theory is that hypotony causes a choroidal effusion that stretches and ruptures a long or short posterior ciliary artery.[9] Obstruction of venous outflow from the vortex veins may also be a precipitating factor that initiates the cascade of events leading to SCH.[11]

Histopathologic studies using experimental animal models or human autopsy eyes have been performed to try to elucidate the precise cause of expulsive SCH. Using histologic evidence from a rabbit model, Beyer and coworkers[12] suggested four stages in the development of expulsive SCH:

1. Engorgement of the choriocapillaris
2. Serous effusion into the suprachoroidal space, mainly in the posterior pole
3. Stretching and tearing of the vessels and attachments at the base of the ciliary body as the effusion enlarges, resulting in
4. Massive extravasation of blood from torn ciliary body vessels, leading to SCH and expulsion of intraocular contents through the surgical wound.

Human histopathologic studies appear to confirm the postulate that hypotony, followed by ciliochoroidal effusion, can lead to rupture of the long posterior ciliary arteries and therefore can be responsible for SCH.[9,13,14] One histopathologic study appears to illustrate that stage in the development of ciliochoroidal effusion in a perforated human eye at which the change from effusion to expulsive SCH is beginning.[14] The long posterior ciliary arteries appear especially vulnerable to rupture during separation of the choroid from the sclera—from ciliochoroidal effusion—because their connections between the scleral exit and the outer choroid are short.[14]

INCIDENCE

During intraocular surgery and in the postoperative period, SCH is relatively rare. It has been reported in all types of intraocular procedures: cataract extraction,[15–18] penetrating keratoplasty,[19,20] glaucoma-filtering surgery,[15,21–24] and vitreoretinal surgery.[15,25,26] Its incidence is difficult to estimate reliably because it is so infrequent. Numerous authors have retrospectively studied the incidence of expulsive SCH during intraocular surgery for various surgical procedures. The results of these studies, as well as studies of the incidence of delayed SCH, are summarized in Table 17-1. With cataract surgery, the overall incidence of expulsive SCH has been widely regarded to be about 0.2%.[16] This figure appears to be independent of the type of cataract extraction method (intracapsular or extracapsular cataract extraction or phacoemulsification).[15] Secondary intraocular lens implantation surgery appears to carry a similar risk of expulsive SCH.[15]

Studies examining the risk of SCH in relation to glaucoma-filtering surgery must be separated based on the type of SCH. The incidence of expulsive SCH during glaucoma-filtering surgery has been reported to be about 0.15%.[15] Several studies have reported the incidence of delayed SCH following glaucoma-filtering surgery. Givens and Shields[22] examined 305 consecutive cases of glaucoma-filtering procedures and found an incidence of 1.6% following this type of surgery. Ruderman and colleagues[24] reported a similar incidence of delayed SCH of 2.0% following 500 consecutive cases of glaucoma surgical procedures.

It is not surprising that the incidence of delayed SCH is about 10-fold greater than that of expulsive SCH. The opportunity to develop delayed SCH following glaucoma surgery appears to be particularly great.

Table 17-1
Incidence of Expulsive and Delayed Suprachoroidal Hemorrhage

STUDY	SURGERY TYPE	NUMBER OF PROCEDURES	NUMBER OF SCH	INCIDENCE (%)	SCH TYPE
Cataract Surgery					
Taylor[16]	ICCE	58,735	115	0.2	Expulsive
Straatsma et al[27]	CE	8,285	4	0.05	Expulsive
Speaker et al[15]	ECCE/Phaco	22,262	34	0.15	Expulsive
	ICCE	6,440	12	0.19	Expulsive
	2° IOL	1,782	3	0.17	Expulsive
Corneal Surgery					
Holland et al[49]	PK	115	1	0.087	Expulsive
Ingraham et al[20]	PK	830	9	1.08	Expulsive
Speaker et al[15]	PK	1,436	8	0.56	Expulsive
Glaucoma Surgery					
Givens and Shields[22]	Glaucoma	305	5	1.60	Delayed
Ruderman et al[24]	Glaucoma	500	10	2.00	Delayed
Speaker et al[15]	Glaucoma	1,329	2	0.15	Expulsive
Vitreoretinal Surgery					
Speaker et al[15]	Vitreoretinal	2,210	9	0.41	Expulsive
Hawkins and Schepens[5]	Retinal	1,500	15	1.0	Expulsive
Intraocular Surgery					
Cantor et al[21]	Intraocular	1,638	12	0.73	Expulsive

CE, cataract extraction; ECCE, extracapsular cataract extraction; ICCE, intracapsular cataract extraction; Phaco, phacoemulsification; PK, penetrating keratoplasty; SCH, suprachoroidal hemorrhage; 2° IOL, secondary intraocular lens.

Indeed, delayed SCH is precipitated by prolonged postoperative hypotony and inflammation, which are not uncommon after glaucoma procedures. Also, delayed SCH varies from small limited suprachoroidal hematomas to massive hemorrhages, but expulsive SCH usually is a severe, massive hemorrhage.

Expulsive SCH has also been rarely reported after penetrating keratoplasty and vitreoretinal surgery. The incidence of expulsive SCH during penetrating keratoplasty has been reported to vary between 0.56% and 1.08%.[15] The cumulative incidence, incorporating the data from all reported studies, is about 0.75%. Penetrating keratoplasty surgery typically involves a greater period of intraocular hypotony than in cataract surgery. Furthermore, this type of surgical procedure affords a greater opportunity for scleral collapse and displacement of intraocular structures. This may account for the higher incidence of expulsive SCH following this type of surgery. Two studies have systematically examined the relation between expulsive SCH and vitreoretinal surgery; the reported incidence during this type of surgery varies from 0.41%[15] to 1.0%.[5] Typically, prolonged intraocular hypotony does not occur during vitreoretinal surgery. Expulsive SCH, however, may be related to direct trauma to the choroid during drainage of subretinal fluid or creation of pars plana sclerotomies, or due to compression and trauma to vortex veins during placement of scleral buckling elements.

PATIENT CHARACTERISTICS

Retrospective studies and anecdotal case reports indicate that certain patient risk factors are associated with the development of SCH, both during and after intraocular surgery. These systemic, ocular, intraoperative, and postoperative risk factors are summarized in Table 17-2.

Table 17-2
Risk Factors for Suprachoroidal Hemorrhage

Systemic
Advanced age
Arteriosclerosis
Hypertension
Blood dyscrasia or coagulation defect
Diabetes mellitus
Ocular
Choroidal arteriolar sclerosis
Glaucoma
Myopia
Aphakia or pseudophakia
Choroiditis
Recent intraocular surgery
Suprachoroidal hemorrhage in fellow eye
Perioperative
Retrobulbar anesthesia without epinephrine
Precipitous drop in intraocular pressure
Valsalva maneuvers
Vitreous loss
Intraoperative systemic hypertension
Postoperative trauma

Numerous systemic findings have been implicated with the development of SCH. In particular, sclerosis and fragility of choroidal vessels associated with advanced age, systemic hypertension, and arteriosclerosis have been frequently described as predisposing factors.[6,8,19,27] In an extensive case control study of risk factors for expulsive SCH, Speaker and associates[15] reported that generalized atherosclerosis is a significant systemic risk factor. This study also reported an association between the development of SCH in the perioperative period with a history of liver disease and preoperative use of digoxin.

Various ocular conditions have been associated with SCH, including glaucoma, elevated intraocular pressure (IOP), aphakia, axial myopia, and inflammation.[15,21–24,28,29] Again, in the most extensive case control study for expulsive SCH, glaucoma, elevated IOP, and increased axial length were reported to be highly significant.[15] The mechanism by which these ocular risk factors are believed to affect the development of SCH is similar. They are presumed to weaken the integrity of the long posterior ciliary arteries by promoting vascular necrosis. This, in turn, would make these vessels more susceptible to rupture. In surgical aphakia, the absence of the lens and zonular support is believed to allow more stretching and separation of the uvea from the sclera during ciliochoroidal effusions. Loss of scleral rigidity or choroidal vascular fragility is also believed to be responsible for the association between SCH and axial myopia.

In anecdotal case reports, certain intraoperative maneuvers have been implicated in the development of SCH. Numerous authors have cautioned that general anesthesia may be a risk factor for SCH.[30–32] Speaker and colleagues[15] found an association between expulsive SCH and an intraoperative pulse rate above 90 beats per minute. They also reported a protective effect when epinephrine was in the anesthetic mixture used for a lid block, and also when the eye was softened before surgery. Complete lid and globe akinesia appears to be a prudent precaution to avoid SCH regardless of the anesthetic agent.

Coughing, straining, nausea, vomiting, and Valsalva-type maneuvers have all been implicated in precipitating SCH, either from bucking during general anesthesia or in the postoperative period.[20,21,24,30,33,34] These maneuvers are believed to increase episcleral venous pressure, resulting in an increased pressure gradient across the wall of necrotic ciliary vessels, thereby promoting their rupture.

Hypotony in the postoperative period has been reported to contribute to the development of delayed SCH.[23,24] As mentioned, hypotony is believed to initiate the development of ciliochoroidal effusion, thereby starting the cascade of events ending in SCH. In addition, the hypotonous eye may be more susceptible to episcleral venous pressure fluctuations induced by Valsalva maneuvers, and therefore may be more vulnerable to rupture of ciliary arteries.[24] The Fluorouracil Filtering Surgery Study Group,[29] when examining risk factors for SCH following filtering surgery, did not find postoperative hypotony to be statistically significant when comparing eyes with SCH versus eyes without hemorrhage. The incidence of SCH in this study was low (6%), however, so this study may not have had the statistical power to detect a difference between these two populations of patients.

CLINICAL CONSIDERATIONS

Prophylactic Measures

Certain preoperative preventive measures should be used in patients at high risk for the development of SCH. As outlined in Table 17-3, these measures should be undertaken before, during, and after sur-

Table 17-3
Prophylactic Measures

Preoperative
- Complete ophthalmic evaluation
- Complete medical evaluation
- Avoid aspirin and other anticoagulants

Operative
- Use minimal preoperative phenylephrine to avoid systemic hypertension
- Use epinephrine in lid blocks
- Lower intraocular pressure before incision
- Avoid rapid decompression of globe
- Avoid Valsalva maneuvers
- Early recognition of suprachoroidal hemorrhage if it occurs

Postoperative
- Avoid eye trauma or eye pressure
- Avoid hypotony
- Avoid Valsalva maneuvers

gery. Attention to these details may help avoid the occurrence of SCH.

A thorough preoperative examination should be performed, paying particular attention to systemic and ocular risk factors for SCH (see Table 17-2). A complete medical evaluation should be undertaken, looking for evidence of cardiovascular disease such as hypertension and arteriosclerosis. Patients should be screened for evidence of liver disease or the use of digoxin. Any underlying blood dyscrasia or coagulation defect should be addressed. Patients should be encouraged to avoid the use of aspirin or other nonsteroidal antiinflammatory agents. Diabetic patients should be under satisfactory blood glucose control.

Preoperatively, the physician should be alerted to the high-risk patient by the presence of certain findings in the ophthalmic history. Patients at highest risk for the development of SCH usually have a history of chronic glaucoma and are aphakic or pseudophakic. Other risk factors to be wary of include high myopia, choroidal arteriolar disease, recent intraocular surgery, and the the presence of SCH in the fellow eye.

Prophylactic measures should be used in the perioperative period. Increased preoperative IOP and a sudden decompression of the globe during intraocular surgery have been implicated as risk factors for the development of SCH.[15] It would seem prudent, therefore, to undertake aggressive medical management of IOP before the onset of surgery. The eye should be softened at the beginning of the operative procedure, using intravenous hyperosmotic agents or carbonic anhydrase inhibitors. Compressive maneuvers, however, should be avoided, because they may contribute to choroidal hyperemia or may facilitate the rupture of a weakened artery.

Hypertension and increased intraoperative heart rate have also been implicated as risk factors for SCH. In patients with hypertension and tachycardia, efforts should be made at the time of surgery to lower the heart rate and blood pressure. Labetalol, a rapidly acting intravenous agent with alpha- and beta-adrenergic antagonist activity, has been suggested for use in such high-risk patients.[15] The use of preoperative phenylephrine should also be restricted to help avoid systemic hypertension.

General anesthesia may also be a risk factor for SCH. Consideration should be given to performing surgery under monitored local anesthesia rather than under general anesthesia. A protective effect of epinephrine added to the lid block was reported in one study[15] and therefore should be considered when using this form of anesthesia.

During and after surgery, Valsalva maneuvers should be avoided. Laxatives and antiemetics are therefore recommended in high-risk patients. Postoperatively, the patient must be instructed to avoid any eye trauma or eye pressure, because this may precipitate the rupture of ciliary arteries. Postoperative inflammation must be vigorously controlled because inflammation may contribute to serous fluid accumulation in the suprachoroidal space, thereby starting the cascade of events leading to SCH.

In glaucoma-filtrating surgery, every effort should be made to avoid postoperative hypotony. In this regard, the use of a scleral flap rather than a full-thickness procedure may theoretically result in less marked hypotony. Also, tight wound closure with restoration of IOP to normal levels at the end of surgery is recommended regardless of the type of surgical procedure.

Intraoperative Diagnosis and Management

Expulsive (intraoperative) and delayed (postoperative) SCH requires prompt recognition and careful management. If expulsive SCH occurs during intraocular surgery, the surgeon must be prepared to react quickly and decisively. Clinically, early signs of intraoperative SCH include a sudden increase in IOP with firming of the globe, loss of a red reflex, shallowness of the anterior chamber with forward displacement of the iris and lens or lens implant, and vitreous prolapse. The magnitude of the problem and prognosis is directly correlated with the size of the ruptured vessel, time of recognition, and type of surgery being performed.

If intraoperative SCH is suspected, immediate tamponading of the open globe is required. This can be accomplished by direct digital pressure or by rapid suturing of all wounds. Closure of the eye allows the IOP to rise to a sufficient level to tamponade the bleeding vessel. If intraocular contents are noted to be expelling, they should be reposited as quickly as possible. If the intraocular contents cannot be replaced in the globe, the eye can be softened by performing posterior sclerotomies. The long-term benefit of performing posterior sclerotomies acutely at the time of initial presentation of SCH is debatable. Verhoeff originally advocated the use of emergency posterior sclerotomies to salvage such eyes.[3] Blood in the suprachoroidal space clots extremely rapidly, and quite often the SCH has already clotted by the time the emergency sclerotomies are made. If the hemorrhage has not clotted, the eye usually softens enough to allow for the repositing of intraocular tissue. With the acute drainage of SCH, however, the tamponading effect of increased IOP in a closed eye is lost, and frequently the SCH recommences hemorrhaging. Therefore, the surgeon must be wary of worsening an already bad situation.

Several other maneuvers may be performed acutely. Reformation of the anterior chamber by saline or air injection is recommended. Decreasing systolic blood pressure, intravenous hyperosmotic agents, and sedation for agitated patients may be helpful. Removal of the lid speculum and bridle sutures may also decrease direct pressure on the globe, preventing further extrusion of intraocular contents.

Postoperative Diagnosis and Management

Delayed or postoperative SCH behaves differently from expulsive SCH. This type of SCH usually presents after uncomplicated glaucoma-filtering surgery. Typically, the patient experiences a sudden onset of severe ocular pain with loss of vision. Headache, nausea, and vomiting may accompany the ocular pain. These symptoms may occur after a Valsalva-type maneuver or may be severe enough to arouse the patient from sleep. Clinically, patients with delayed SCH can have markedly decreased vision. On slit-lamp examination, there may be shallowness of the anterior chamber, vitreous prolapse into the anterior chamber in aphakic and pseudophakic eyes, and loss of a red reflex (Fig. 17-1). On funduscopic examination, dark elevated dome-shaped lesions may be seen to arise from the peripheral retina, but they may also be seen to extend posteriorly (Fig. 17-2). These lesions do not transilluminate well. IOP may be low, normal, or elevated.

Regardless of the cause of SCH, whether expulsive or delayed, the immediate postoperative management is similar. If the IOP is elevated, aggressive medical therapy is advocated with a topical β-blocker and

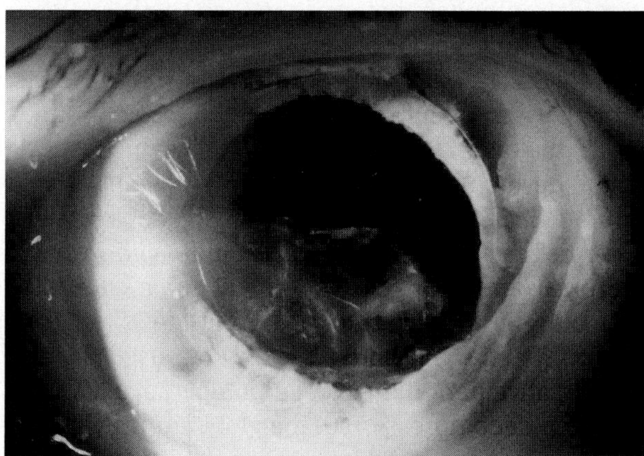

Figure 17-1. An 89-year-old woman with an ocular history of chronic glaucoma. She underwent uncomplicated cataract extraction, anterior chamber intraocular lens placement, and trabeculectomy. On the second postoperative day, she was awakened from sleep by severe eye pain. Notice the shallowed anterior chamber and forward displacement of the vitreous and anterior chamber lens. (See color plate after page xvi.)

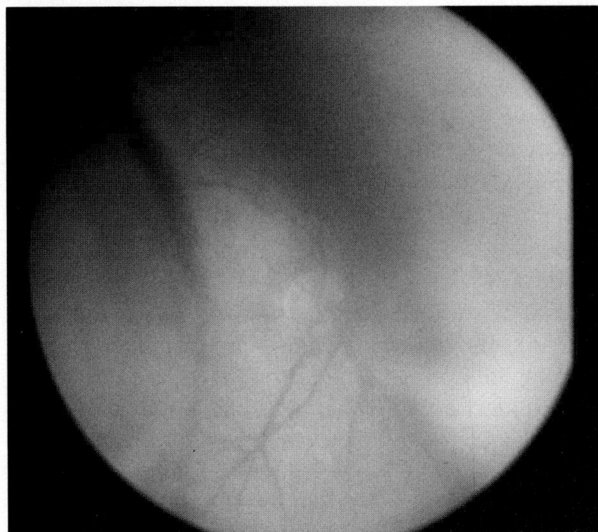

Figure 17-2. Same patient as in Figure 17-1. Notice the large, darkly colored dome-shaped elevations arising from the peripheral retina and extending toward the optic nerve. (See color plate after page xvi.)

an oral carbonic anhydrase inhibitor. Inflammation should be controlled by liberal use of a topical steroid. Oral prednisone may be necessary with severe intraocular inflammation. Pain, which can be considerable due to stretching of ciliary nerves, can be managed with adequate cycloplegia and analgesics; aspirin and nonsteroidal agents, however, are contraindicated because they may contribute to further hemorrhaging.

Echography

Suprachoroidal hemorrhage may be difficult to diagnose in the presence of opaque media. Patients with SCH may have corneal changes, breakthrough vitreous hemorrhage, or a kissing configuration that makes adequate visualization of the posterior chamber impossible. Echography is extremely useful in the diagnosis and management of these cases. Standardized echography can help establish an accurate diagnosis.[35] Echography can determine the location and extent of SCH, as well as the status of the retina and vitreous. Hemorrhagic choroidal detachment and serous choroidal effusion can be differentiated using A-scans and B-scans.[36]

The echographic evaluation should be performed as early in the postoperative period as possible in cases with opaque media. This examination can be done directly through the lids, with minimal direct pressure on the globe. Echographically, on B-scan, patients with SCH exhibit highly elevated choroidal detachments with a typical dome-shaped appearance (Fig. 17-3). In severe cases, broad central retinal apposition can be seen, illustrating a kissing-type configuration. The suprachoroidal space is typically filled

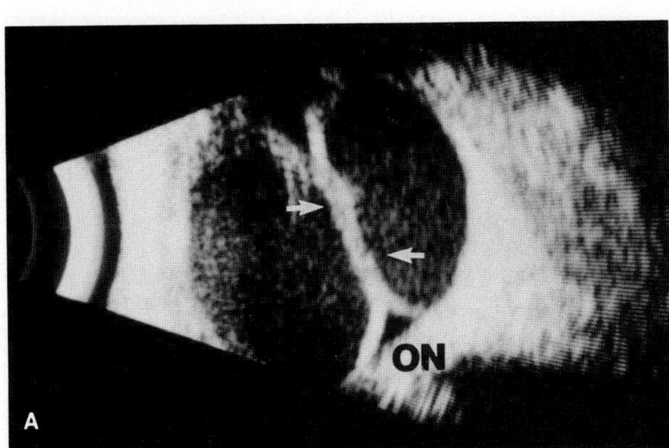

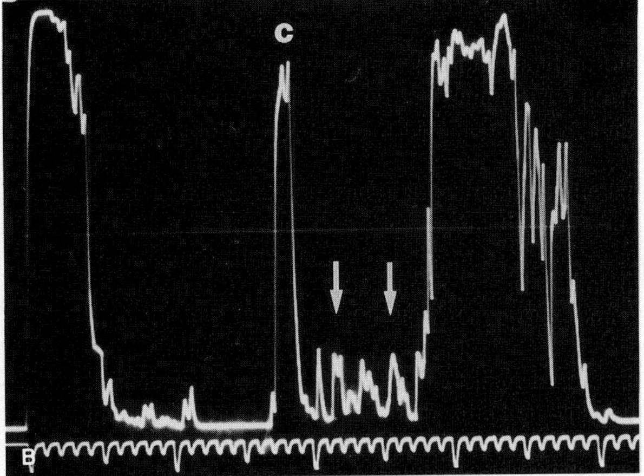

Figure 17-3. (**A**) B-scan echogram (longitudinal view) demonstrating a massive suprachoroidal hemorrhage with central retinal apposition. Note the typical dome-shaped appearance and broad central apposition of the detached choroid (*arrows*). The suprachoroidal space is filled with opacities denoting the presence of blood. ON, optic nerve. (**B**) A-scan echogram demonstrating a steeply rising, double-peaked, wide spike (**C**) characteristic of a choroidal detachment; the spikes of lower reflectivity (*arrows*) in the suprachoroidal space represent hemorrhage. (Chu TG, Cano MR, Green RL, Liggett PE, Lean JS. Massive suprachoroidal hemorrhage with central retinal apposition: a clinical and echographic study. Arch Ophthalmol 1991;109:1575–1581. Copyright 1991, American Medical Association.)

with opacities denoting the presence of clotted blood. On A-scan evaluation, a steeply rising, double-peaked wide spike is seen, characteristic of a choroidal detachment, with lower reflective spikes in the suprachoroidal space indicating the presence of clotted hemorrhage.

The density of choroidal hemorrhage varies with time. Echography is an excellent way to follow patients, with or without opaque media, for the lysis of the hemorrhage. On initial evaluation, all patients with SCH have dense clotted hemorrhage seen on ultrasonography. Fresh clots are seen echographically as a high-reflective, solid-appearing mass with irregular internal structure and irregular shape (Figs. 17-4 and 17-5). On follow-up, these blood clots decrease in size. A lower and more regular internal reflectivity, due to increased homogeneity of the internal structure of these clots, can be noted on ultrasonography (see Fig. 17-5). During dynamic echographic examination, fluid blood can be seen moving freely within the suprachoroidal space. Eventually, complete liquefaction of these hemorrhages can be seen, with the suprachoroidal space being filled with diffuse, low-reflective mobile opacities (see Fig. 17-5). The time to liquefaction of such hemorrhages was reported to vary from 7 to 14 days.[28,37] Once liquefaction has occurred, the height of the choroidal detachment slowly diminishes with time (Fig. 17-6). Patients should be followed clinically for this reduction in height.

Several reports have questioned the ability of ultrasonography to help in the diagnosis and management of SCH.[23,24] In contrast, my colleagues and I find echography to be useful in the management of such cases. Blood clots can be readily identified in the suprachoroidal space (see Figs. 17-4 and 17-5), as can the progression of clot lysis. In our patients, complete liquefaction of the clot occurred between 6 and 25 days.

If early surgical drainage of a massive SCH is warranted, echography may be a helpful adjunct in determining the optimal time for drainage. In our patients who underwent early surgical intervention, drainage was delayed until echographic evidence was obtained indicating liquefaction of the hemorrhage. By allowing for complete liquefaction of the hemorrhage, one can avoid probing the suprachoroidal space for residual clots, a maneuver that may cause further bleeding or retinal damage, yet facilitate the evacuation of the hemorrhage and restoration of normal ocular anatomy. Surgical intervention appears to be most effective when clot lysis is complete; however, whether complete liquefaction of the hemorrhage is necessary for successful hemorrhage drainage remains unknown. In our series, the mean time for clot lysis was 14 days, as determined by echography. Welch, Lambrou, Lakhanpal, and their colleagues,[18,38,39] advocated delaying drainage for 7 to 14 days.

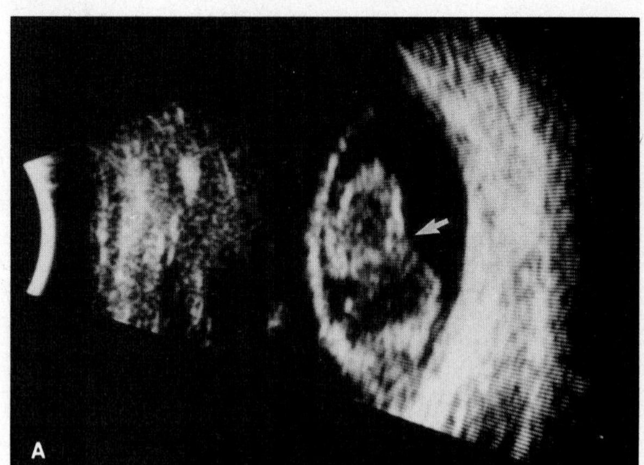

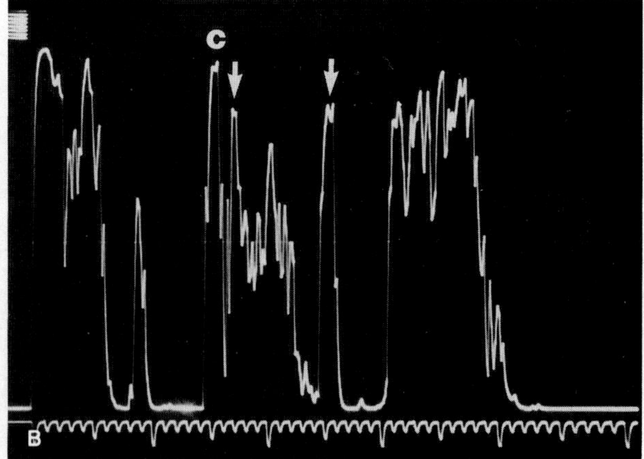

Figure 17-4. (**A**) B-scan echogram of a patient with a suprachoroidal hemorrhage performed 2 days after the hemorrhage occured. The blood clot (*arrow*) in the suprachoroidal space is easily identified. (**B**) Corresponding A-scan shows the choroidal detachment (**C**) and the edges of the clot (*arrows*) with a low-to-medium, irregular internal reflectivity. (Chu TG, Cano MR, Green RL, Liggett PE, Lean JS. Massive suprachoroidal hemorrhage with central retinal apposition: a clinical and echographic study. Arch Ophthalmol 1991;109:1575–1581. Copyright 1991, American Medical Association.)

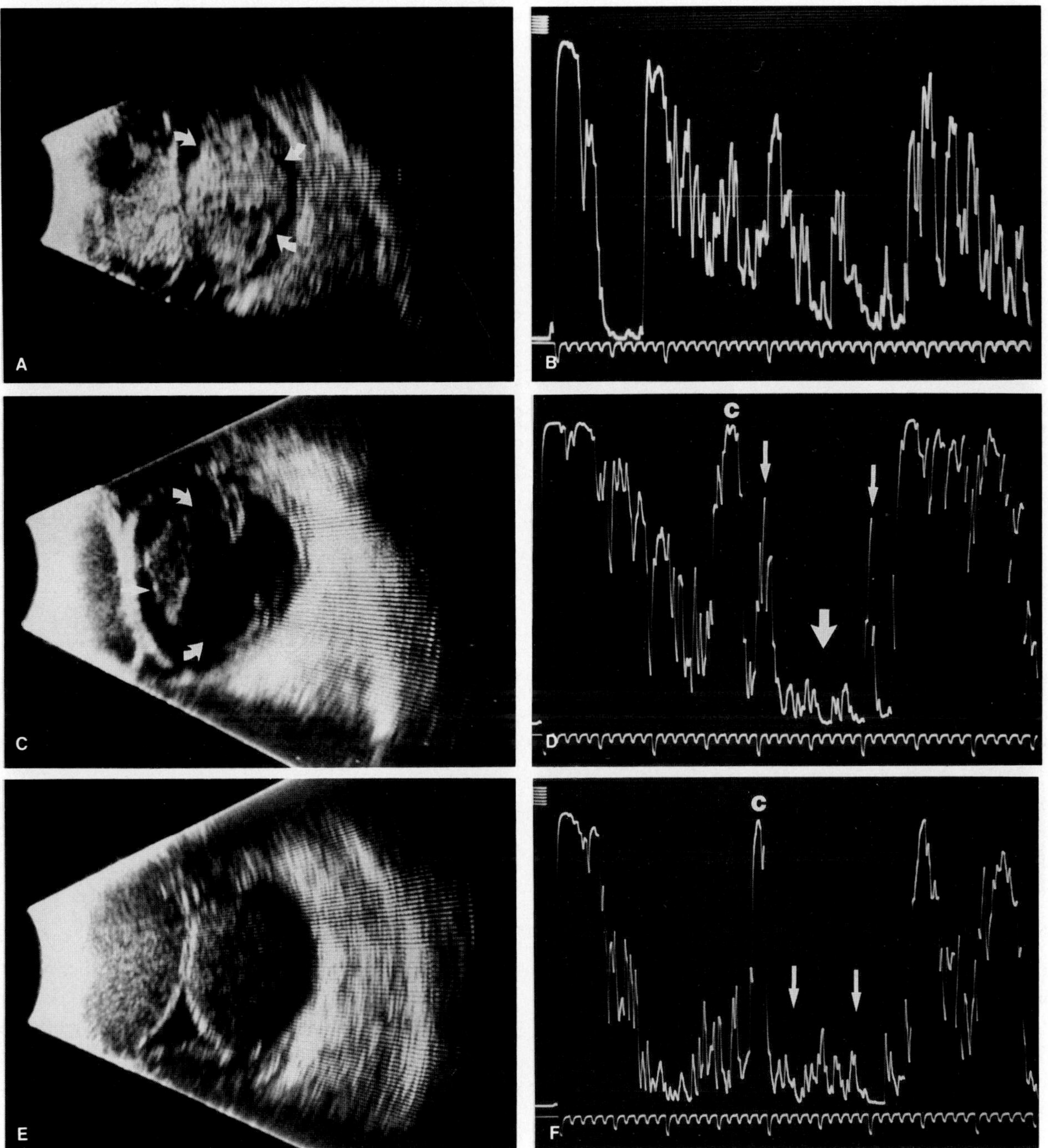

Figure 17-5. (**A**) B-scan echogram performed 24 hours after repair of a cataract wound dehiscence. Note the massive suprachoroidal hemorrhage with central retinal apposition; the solid-appearing mass in the suprachoroidal space (*arrows*) represents a large blood clot. (**B**) A-scan echogram showing the high and irregular reflectivity of the fresh clot. (**C**) B-scan echogram performed 5 days later. The large clot is still present (*arrows*); however, it now appears more homogeneous (echolucent). (**D**) A-scan spikes from the edges of the clot (*small arrows*). The internal reflectivity of the clot itself is lower and more homogeneous (*large arrow*). (**E**) B-scan echogram performed 2 weeks after occurrence of massive suprachoroidal hemorrhage. The suprachoroidal space is filled with fine diffuse opacities which are mobile during dynamic examination and indicate clot lysis. (**F**) Corresponding A-scan echogram performed 2 weeks after hemorrhage, exhibiting choroidal detachment (**C**) and low regular internal reflectivity of the liquefied blood (*arrows*). (Chu TG, Cano MR, Green RL, Liggett PE, Lean JS. Massive suprachoroidal hemorrhage with central retinal apposition: a clinical and echographic study. Arch Ophthalmol 1991;109:1575–1581. Copyright 1991, American Medical Association.)

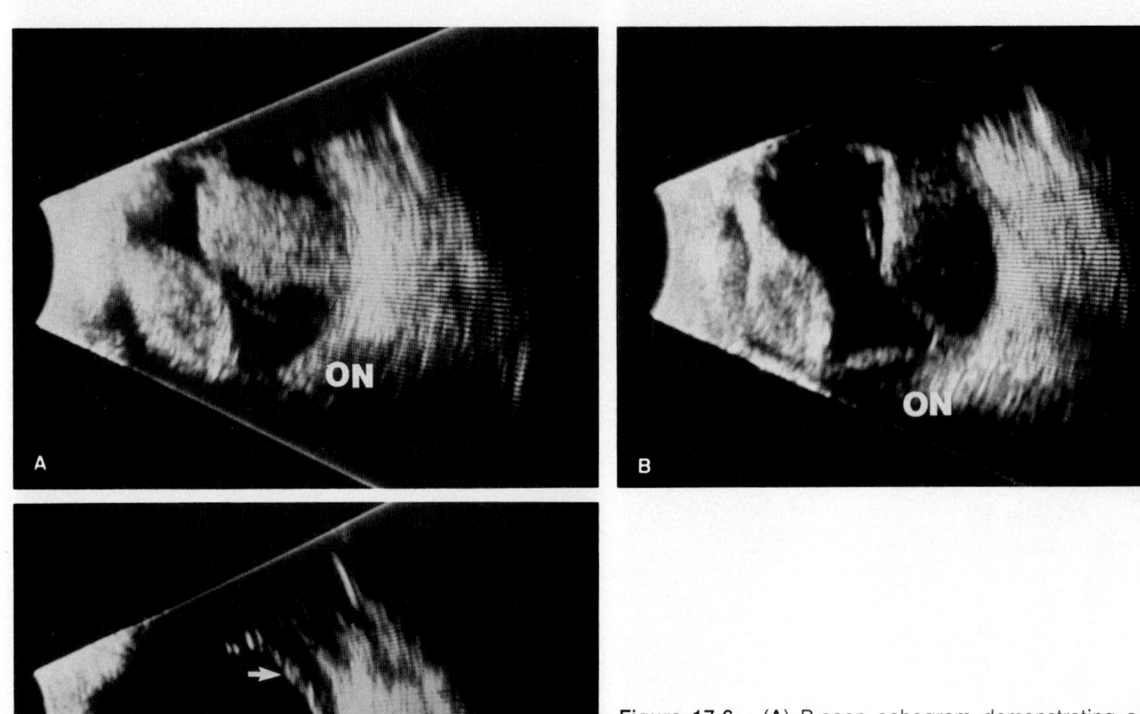

Figure 17-6. (A) B-scan echogram demonstrating a massive suprachoroidal hemorrhage with retinal apposition occurring 24 hours after the hemorrhage. (B) Echographic examination 2 weeks later shows a decrease in the elevation of the choroidal hemorrhage. (C) Resorption of the suprachoroidal hemorrhage is seen 5 weeks after hemorrhage. A shallow suprachoroidal hemorrhage is seen peripherally (*arrows*). ON, optic nerve. (Chu TG, Cano MR, Green RL, Liggett PE, Lean JS. Massive suprachoroidal hemorrhage with central retinal apposition: a clinical and echographic study. Arch Ophthalmol 1991;109:1575–1581. Copyright 1991, American Medical Association.)

Indications For Secondary Surgical Management

The decision to reoperate on patients with postoperative SCH is controversial. Many reports have advocated early surgical intervention in the management of SCH.[23,33,34,38–40] However, these reports encompass different subgroups of SCH. In analyzing these reports, we must distinguish expulsive from delayed SCH, because their long-term prognosis may differ. Regardless of the cause of SCH, however, several indications for early surgical drainage have been proposed.[39,40] Particular concerns include retinal detachment, central retinal apposition, vitreous incarceration into a surgical wound, breakthrough vitreous hemorrhage, increased IOP, retained lens material during cataract surgery, and intractable eye pain.

Frequently, a retinal detachment can be seen in the postoperative period, identified either on funduscopic examination or by echography. A distinction must be made, however, between retinal detachments of a serous cause and retinal detachments of a tractional or rhegmatogenous cause. Typically, serous retinal detachments are dome-shaped, low-lying, and situated over areas of choroidal hemorrhage. In contrast, tractional retinal detachments are taut areas of retinal separation, with apparent areas of vitreoretinal traction. Rhegmatogenous retinal detachments are usually more elevated and bullous in nature, and may not be overlying an area of choroidal hemorrhage. The presence of a rhegmatogenous retinal detachment in the postoperative period remains an absolute indication for surgical intervention.

With regard to serous retinal detachments, my colleagues and I reported on a series of 18 patients with massive SCH and central retinal apposition, with SCH in 12 patients either expulsive or delayed.[28] Six of these 12 patients exhibited a shallow posterior serous elevation of the retina once the choroidal detachments began to decrease in elevation (Fig. 17-7). The detachment in only one of these patients progressed to a more extensive retinal detachment; the other five detachments resolved spontaneously. Therefore, serous retinal detachments should be observed closely for regression or progression.

Central retinal apposition has traditionally been considered an absolute indication for surgical intervention. Berrocal[41] reported that retinal surfaces in apposition can become fixed. In our study,[28] my associates and I reported on the natural history of central retinal apposition without surgical intervention. Echographically, all patients, including those who underwent intraoperative drainage, exhibited highly elevated hemorrhagic choroidal detachments with a kissing configuration. Follow-up examination revealed that the duration of central retinal apposition in SCH ranged from 10 to 25 days. A rapid decrease in elevation was noted after the third week, although slight choroidal elevation persisted peripherally for longer than 6 weeks in all these patients (see Fig. 17-6). Despite this prolonged period of apposition of retinal surfaces, no evidence of persistent retinal adherence was noted either clinically or echographically. Therefore, central retinal apposition may be a relative rather than an absolute indication for early surgical intervention.

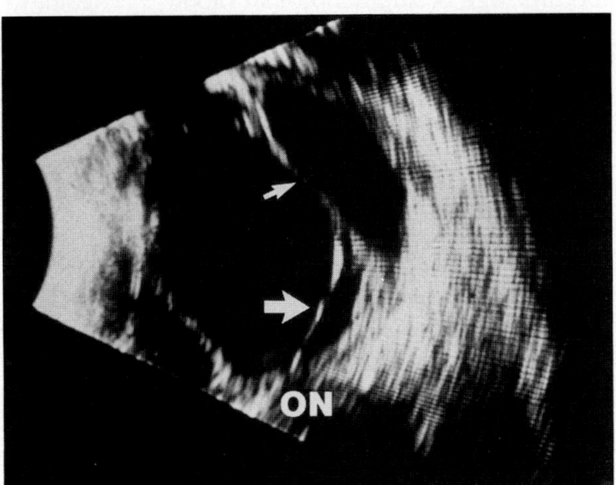

Figure 17-7. B-scan echogram demonstrates a shallowly elevated, high-reflective membrane (*large arrow*) inserting into the optic nerve (ON), representing a shallow posterior retinal detachment. Note the moderate elevation of the choroidal detachment (*small arrow*). (Chu TG, Cano MR, Green RL, Liggett PE, Lean JS. Massive suprachoroidal hemorrhage with central retinal apposition: a clinical and echographic study. Arch Ophthalmol 1991;109:1575–1581. Copyright 1991, American Medical Association.)

In direct contrast to our study, Reynolds and colleagues[37] advocated early surgical intervention in patients with central retinal apposition. In their study, 13 of 20 eyes with SCH and central retinal apposition underwent a secondary surgical procedure. Of these 13 eyes, 6 had a visual acuity of 20/200 or better compared with none of the 7 eyes observed. Several factors may be responsible for the discrepancy between this study and ours. Reynolds and associates did not specify the etiology of SCH in their patients with central retinal apposition. If the unoperated eyes suffered SCH after trauma, the prognosis would be poor regardless of surgical intervention. Also, the Reynolds study did not specify whether any of the patients with central retinal apposition had concomitant rhegmatogenous retinal detachments. Certainly, if the eyes that were simply observed had a concomitant retinal detachment, the final visual outcome would be expected to be poor. Lastly, the Reynolds study had follow-up of only 3 months; our study followed patients from 6 months to 2 years.

SURGICAL TECHNIQUES

When reoperation is considered in patients with SCH, the surgical approach can be one of two choices: drainage procedures, to remove the SCH and reestablish normal IOP; or vitreoretinal surgery in combination with a drainage procedure, to remove vitreous hemorrhage or retained lens material, relieve vitreoretinal traction, and reestablish the normal anatomic configuration of the posterior segment. Even when contemplating only a surgical drainage procedure, the surgeon should consult a vitreoretinal surgeon. Commonly, posterior segment complications such as retinal dialysis and retinal detachment can arise during anterior segment approaches to drainage of SCH.

Drainage Procedures

Anterior segment approaches are usually restricted to drainage procedures with or without anterior vitrectomy. When considering a drainage procedure, the time of intervention can be critical for success. As previously mentioned, mean clot lysis time has been reported to be between 7 and 14 days. Attempts to drain this type of hemorrhage before clot lysis are typically unsuccessful. Furthermore, vigorous attempts to remove clotted blood from the suprachoroidal space can result in additional injury to the globe. Therefore, drainage procedures in patients with SCH should be deferred for 1 to 2 weeks, preferably with clot lysis confirmed by echography.

Originally, Verhoeff[3] recommended the use of drainage sclerotomies at the time of expulsive SCH to enable closure of the surgical wound and to reduce IOP. He advocated the use of scleral punctures with a Graefe knife, and he suggested that scleral punctures be made as quickly as possible at the time of expulsive SCH and that the scleral opening be V-shaped, with excision of the apex of the V to facilitate the continued escape of blood postoperatively.

The technique of postoperative drainage of SCH initially suggested was not unlike the method recommended by Verhoeff for intraoperative management of SCH.[42,43] Shaffer advocated the use of a T-shaped posterior sclerotomy, with diathermy to the lips of the wound to cause scleral shrinkage.[43a] He also recommended that the anterior chamber be reformed with an air bubble or saline injection. More recently, several authors have suggested the use of drainage-type procedures in the postoperative management of SCH. The surgical principles of all these methods are essentially the same. Drainage sclerotomies are created in the quadrant or quadrants of the involved SCH. The IOP is then maintained by continuously injecting a vitreous substitute into the globe. Usually, an anterior chamber approach is recommended, as most of these eyes are aphakic or pseudophakic. The reestablishment of IOP by these methods facilitates the egress of lysed blood through the drainage sclerotomies in a controlled fashion. These methods are ideally suited for management of SCH where there is little remaining vitreous in the eye, when vitreoretinal traction is absent, and when a retinal detachment is also not present.

In most cases of expulsive SCH, the vitreous at the time of initial surgery is expelled by the force of the SCH. There may be some remaining vitreous in these eyes, with vitreoretinal traction extending from the surgical wound to the posterior pole. In these cases, care must be taken when reestablishing IOP by instilling a vitreous substitute that undue retinal traction is not created. In contrast, the vitreous is usually still present in cases of delayed SCH. Vitreoretinal traction, however, is usually absent if the surgical wound is not violated.

Several vitreous substitutes have been recommended for reestablishing IOP, all with advantages and disadvantages. Balanced salt solution and viscoelastic solutions have been advocated as vitreous substitutes.[44,45] Balanced salt solution can be instilled using a limbal approach by means of a gravity infusion system. Drainage sclerotomies are created posteriorly in a radial fashion before engagement of the infusion system. The anterior and posterior chambers are maintained with balanced salt solution as the choroidal blood is drained from the sclerotomies. The sclerotomies are then held open with forceps, allowing drainage of the suprachoroidal space as the eye is reformed with solution. A cyclodialysis spatula can also be gently introduced into the suprachoroidal space to facilitate removal of persistent blood clots. If a viscoelastic solution is used, it can be injected into the globe from a limbal approach with a syringe. Both of these methods afford excellent visualization of the posterior chamber during drainage of suprachoroidal blood. Their disadvantage, however, is the potential of uncontrolled IOP. Syringe injection of viscoelastic agents is not ideal because maintenance of IOP is imprecise. A gravity infusion system for balanced salt infusion is preferable, but care must be taken not to allow the globe to become hypotonous (which may lead to recurrent SCH) or the IOP to become too great (which may result in retinal incarceration).

Instead of balanced salt solution or viscoelastic agents, sterile air can be used to hydraulically aid in the drainage of suprachoroidal blood.[22,40] Again, radial incisions are made in the sclera into the suprachoroidal space. The eye is then insufflated with sterile air by using a continuous-infusion air pump through a 25-, 27-, or 30-gauge needle inserted through the limbus. The air pump insufflation pressure is preset to 20 to 30 mmHg. The sclerotomies are then held open with forceps, allowing drainage of the suprachoroidal space as the eye is reformed with air. Again, a cyclodialysis spatula can also be gently introduced into the suprachoroidal space to facilitate the removal of persistent blood clots. When drainage is complete, the insufflation needle is withdrawn and the sclerotomies can be closed with sutures. A major advantage of this technique is the use of a continuous-infusion air pump rather than a syringe. The IOP can be maintained at a predetermined level, preventing hypotony and excessive pressure. A potential disadvantage is the loss of detailed visualization of the retina due to air/fluid interface reflections. This method may therefore make it difficult to identify peripheral retinal tears and persistent vitreoretinal traction at the time of surgery.

Vitreoretinal Surgical Approaches

As mentioned above, when retinal detachment, vitreoretinal traction, vitreous hemorrhage, or dislocated lens fragments are present in the setting of SCH, vitreoretinal surgery at the time of the SCH drainage procedure is usually advisable. This surgical approach may be preferable to drainage-only procedures, because vitreoretinal surgery addresses the underlying pathologic changes in this condition. Indeed, vitreoretinal surgery reestablishes the normal anatomic configuration of the globe by the removal of vitreous and vitreous debris (ie, blood, lens remnants), the relief of vitreoretinal traction, and reattachment of the detached retina.

The sequence of surgical maneuvers, when vitreoretinal surgery is planned in combination with a drainage procedure, is important. Typically, in the presence of SCH, the normal anatomic location of the pars plana, anterior retina, and vitreous base is distorted. Therefore, entry into the posterior segment of the globe by means of a pars plana approach is dangerous and can result in iatrogenic damage to the anterior retina. Drainage of hemorrhage from the suprachoroidal space is therefore initially required before the creation of any pars plana incisions. The choice of the vitreous substitute used to reestablish IOP during this drainage procedure is usually limited to clear liquid solutions, to enable good visualization during vitrectomy. Balanced salt solution and viscoelastic agents can be used to accomplish drainage of suprachoroidal blood, as outlined in the previous section.

Perfluorocarbon liquids (PFLs) have been recommended as a surgical adjunct in cases of complex vitreoretinal pathology (Fig. 17-8). These agents are clear liquids with a specific gravity higher than water. When instilled into the vitreous cavity, these liquids sink to the posterior pole of the eye, forcing all other ocular fluids, both within the vitreous cavity (ie, aqueous, vitreous, and saline) and within the suprachoroidal space (ie, hemorrhage), anteriorly. These physiochemical properties make them ideally suited for use in drainage of SCH. Indeed, perfluoroperhydrophenanthrene, a PFL, has been used successfully in the drainage of SCH.[46] Unlike the above methods, when using a PFL, the drainage sclerotomies should be placed anteriorly, about 4 mm off the limbus. A 30-gauge needle attached to a syringe containing PFL is then introduced through the limbus. PFL is then slowly injected, and it immediately moves posteriorly. As it fills the posterior chamber, the PFL flattens the posterior pole while forcing suprachoroidal blood anteriorly, thereby allowing complete removal of this blood through anteriorly placed sclerotomies. An added benefit of PFL in these circumstances is that this liquid tamponades the retina against the inner wall of the eye, while forcing vitreous and vitreous debris anteriorly. This allows for easier removal of vitreous or lens components during vitrectomy, while protecting the retina from iatrogenic damage.

After the SCH is drained using PFL, the normal anatomic relations at the pars plana should be reestablished. A conventional three-port pars plana vitrectomy configuration can then be created. The settled PFL is left undisturbed and residual vitreous is re-

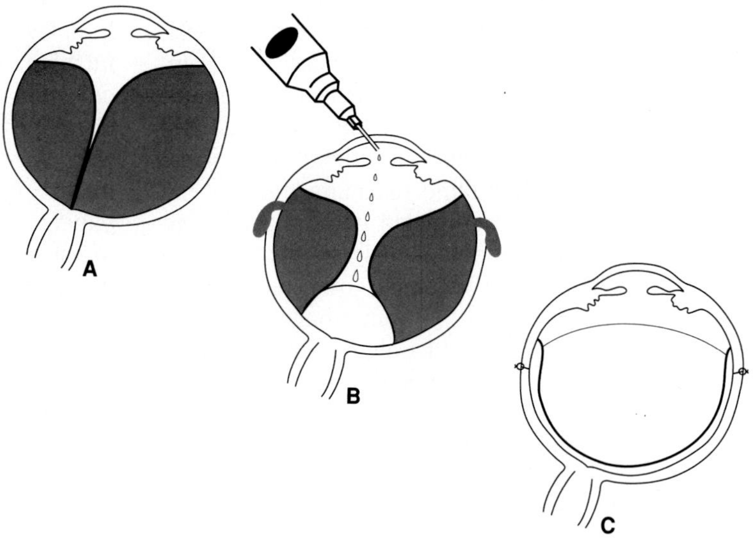

Figure 17-8. (**A**) A large suprachoroidal hemorrhage is present, with central retinal apposition. The hemorrhage is in a liquefied state. (**B**) Drainage sclerotomies are placed anterior to the equator. A 30-gauge needle attached to a syringe containing perfluorocarbon liquid (PFL) is then introduced through the limbus. PFL is slowly injected, reattaching the retina while forcing suprachoroidal blood anteriorly through the drainage sclerotomies. (**C**) The vitreous cavity is completely filled with PFL. The drainage sclerotomies are sutured closed. A standard three-port pars plana vitrectomy configuration can now be employed.

moved using vitrectomy. Vitreous strands causing vitreoretinal traction can be severed. If a rhegmatogenous retinal detachment is present, the retinal break can then be treated with retinopexy (photocoagulation or cryopexy). Finally, the PFL can be removed using either a fluid/fluid exchange with infusion fluid or a PFL/air exchange. A scleral buckling procedure can then be performed if residual vitreoretinal traction persists or if support to areas of retinal breaks is required. Internal tamponade with a long-acting intraocular gas or silicone oil may also be required.

PROGNOSIS

Expulsive Subchoroidal Hemorrhage

In expulsive SCH, in the absence of a rhegmatogenous retinal detachment, both early surgical intervention and observation and medical management have been advocated. Taylor[16] reported severe visual loss in four of five patients with expulsive SCH. Despite early surgical drainage of the hemorrhage in a study by Lakhanpal and colleagues,[39] only one of five patients with expulsive SCH regained visual acuity greater than 20/200. Lambrou and associates[38] also reported early surgical drainage in six patients with SCH; only one patient recovered visual acuity to the 20/200 level. Welch and colleagues[18] were more encouraged by early surgical drainage in expulsive SCH in their group of patients with vitreous but not retinal incarceration. Five of seven patients who underwent early surgical drainage recovered visual acuity of 20/200 or better, although some patients required subsequent vitreoretinal surgery for retinal detachments. Four of our 18 patients developed massive SCH intraoperatively.[28] All four underwent intraoperative placement of sclerotomies to facilitate drainage and wound closure, as previously described. All of these patients, however, had rapid reaccumulation of the hemorrhage. The reaccumulated hemorrhages were allowed to resolve spontaneously in all of these cases. All four patients obtained good initial visual acuity after resolution of the hemorrhage; however, all four had a poor visual outcome because of subsequent retinal detachment without repair, or progression of their underlying ocular disease.

Therefore, it does not appear that all patients with an expulsive SCH should undergo a secondary surgical procedure. Secondary surgery, however, should be contemplated on an individual level, based on clearly defined indications for intervention.

Delayed Subchoroidal Hemorrhage

Abrams, Lakhanpal, and Gressel, and their associates,[23,39,40] and Frenkel and Shin[34] believed that early surgical drainage may be beneficial in patients with delayed SCH. Gressel and colleagues[23] reported five cases of delayed SCH, with only one patient undergoing early surgical drainage. This patient was the only one in their study who maintained a visual acuity better than hand motions. Ruderman and associates[24] described nine patients who underwent surgical drainage within 72 hours of SCH after filtration surgery. Of these nine, only two regained prehemorrhage visual acuity. Ariano and Ball[33] presented five cases of delayed SCH, with three patients undergoing surgical drainage. Two of these three recovered their prehemorrhage visual acuity. Of the two remaining patients in that study, one maintained prehemorrhage visual acuity without the need for surgical drainage. Abrams and colleagues[40] reported the greatest success with early surgical drainage in patients with delayed SCH. In their study, three of seven patients maintained prehemorrhage visual acuity, and two of seven patients had a final visual acuity better than their prehemorrhage visual acuity. Frenkel and Shin[34] described two patients who recovered baseline visual acuity after prompt surgical drainage.

In direct contrast with the above studies, my colleagues and I observed that good initial visuai outcome can be attained without early surgical drainage in delayed SCH, and that echography may be a helpful adjunct in the treatment of patients in whom surgical drainage is warranted.[28] Eight of our 18 patients developed delayed SCH. In this group, all five patients who were followed up without surgical drainage maintained their prehemorrhage visual acuity. Two patients underwent early surgical drainage, and both maintained preoperative vision. Despite surgical drainage and sophisticated vitreoretinal surgery at 1 month, the eye of another patient developed phthisis bulbi. Our findings suggest that not all patients with delayed SCH need to undergo early surgical decompression of the choroidal hemorrhage. Gressel, Abrams, and their coworkers,[23,40] mentioned that delayed SCH may be more serous in nature than expulsive SCH and therefore easier to drain. We did not find this to be the case either clinically or echographically.

NEW FRONTIERS

Despite our increased knowledge of the cause of SCH, expulsive and delayed SCH continues to be a devastating condition. Several new treatment prospects hold promise. As mentioned above, the use of PFLs to help drain suprachoroidal blood is a tremendous tool for the vitreoretinal surgeon.[46] Another new treatment is the use of intravenous tissue plasminogen activator to accelerate clot lysis.[47] This form of treatment is experimental and clinical benefit remains to be proven. Lastly, the use of silicone oil tamponade following vitreoretinal surgery for SCH has been recommended,[48] but it should be reserved for the most desperate cases.

SUMMARY

Suprachoroidal hemorrhage, both expulsive and delayed, remains a rare but severely debilitating complication of intraocular surgery. A thorough understanding of the pathophysiology, risk factors, and clinical outcome of patients who develop SCH can help the ophthalmic surgeon avoid this complication in patients at risk, as well as help in the postoperative management of patients who develop SCH during or after intraocular surgery.

References

1. Pfingst AO. Expulsive choroidal hemorrhage complicating cataract surgery. South Med J 1936;29:323.
2. Terson A. Hemorragies sous-choroidiennes traumatiques et expulsives. Arch Ophthal Paris 1907;27:446.
3. Verhoeff FH. Scleral puncture for expulsive subchoroidal hemorrhage following sclerotomy: scleral puncture for postoperative separation of the choroid. Ophthalmic Rec 1915;24:55–59.
4. Brubaker RF, Pederson JE. Ciliochoroidal detachment. Surv Ophthalmol 1983;27:281–289.
5. Hawkins WR, Schepens CL. Choroidal detachment and retinal surgery. Am J Ophthalmol 1966;62:813–819.
6. Davison JA. Acute intraoperative suprachoroidal hemorrhage in extracapsular cataract surgery. J Cataract Refract Surg 1986;12:606–622.
7. Augsburger JJ, Coats TD, Lauritzen K. Localized suprachoroidal hematomas: ophthalmoscopic features, fluorescein angiography, and clinical course. Arch Ophthalmol 1990;108:968–972.
8. Hoffman P, Pollack A, Oliver M. Limited choroidal hemorrhage associated with intracapsular cataract extraction. Arch Ophthalmol 1984;102:1761–1765.
9. Maumenee AE, Schwartz MF. Acute intraoperative choroidal effusion. Am J Ophthalmol 1985;100:147–154.
10. Manschot WA. The pathology of expulsive hemorrhage. Am J Ophthalmol 1955;40:15–24.
11. Zauberman H. Expulsive choroidal haemorrhage: an experimental study. Br J Ophthalmol 1982;66:43–45.
12. Beyer CF, Peyman GA, Hill JM. Expulsive choroidal hemorrhage in rabbits—a histopathologic study. Arch Ophthalmol 1989;107:1648–1653.
13. Wolter JR. Expulsive hemorrhage: a study of histopathological details. Graefes Arch Clin Exp Ophthalmol 1982;219:155–158.
14. Wolter JR, Garfinkel RA. Ciliochoroidal effusion as precursor of suprachoroidal hemorrhage: a pathologic study. Ophthalmic Surg 1988;19:344–349.
15. Speaker MG, Guerriero PN, Met JA, et al. A case-control study of risk factors for intraoperative suprachoroidal expulsive hemorrhage. Ophthalmology 1991; 98:202–209.
16. Taylor DM. Expulsive hemorrhage. Am J Ophthalmol 1978;78:961–966.
17. Payne JW, Kameen AJ, Jensen AD, Christy NE. Expulsive hemorrhage: its incidence in cataract surgery and a report of four bilateral cases. Trans Am Ophthalmol Soc 1985;83:181–204.
18. Welch JC, Spaeth GL, Benson WE. Massive suprachoroidal hemorrhage—follow-up and outcome of 30 cases. Ophthalmology 1988;95:1202–1206.
19. Purcell J Jr, Krachmer JH, Doughman DJ, Bourne WM. Expulsive hemorrhage in penetrating keratoplasty. Ophthalmology 1982;89:41–43.
20. Ingraham HJ, Donnenfeld ED, Perry HD. Massive suprachoroidal hemorrhage in penetrating keratoplasty. Am J Ophthalmol 1989;108:670–675.
21. Cantor LB, Katz LJ, Spaeth GL. Complications of surgery in glaucoma: suprachoroidal expulsive hemorrhage in glaucoma patients undergoing intraocular surgery. Ophthalmology 1985;92:1266–1270.
22. Givens K, Shields MB. Suprachoroidal hemorrhage after glaucoma filtering surgery. Am J Ophthalmol 1987;103:689–694.
23. Gressel MG, Parrish R, Heuer DK. Delayed nonexpulsive suprachoroidal hemorrhage. Arch Ophthalmol 1984;102:1757–1760.
24. Ruderman JM, Harbin T Jr, Campbell DG. Postoperative suprachoroidal hemorrhage following filtration procedures. Arch Ophthalmol 1986;104:201–205.

25. Fastenberg DM, Perry HD, Donnenfeld ED, Schwartz PL, Shakin JL. Expulsive suprachoroidal hemorrhage with scleral buckling surgery (letter). Arch Ophthalmol 1991;109:323.
26. Lakhanpal V, Schocket SS, Elman MJ, Dogra MR. Intraoperative massive suprachoroidal hemorrhage during pars plana vitrectomy. Ophthalmology 1990;97: 1114–1119.
27. Straatsma BR, Khwarg SG, Rajacich GM, Meyer KT, Pettit TH. Cataract surgery after expulsive choroidal hemorrhage in the fellow eye. Ophthalmic Surg 1986;17:400–403.
28. Chu TG, Cano MR, Green RL, Liggett PE, Lean JS. Massive suprachoroidal hemorrhage with central retinal apposition—a clinical and echographic study. Arch Ophthalmol 1991;109:1575–1581.
29. Fluorouracil Filtering Surgery Study Group. Risk factors for suprachoroidal hemorrhage after filtering surgery. Am J Ophthalmol 1992;113:501–507.
30. Campbell JK. Expulsive choroidal hemorrhage and effusion—a reappraisal. Ann Ophthalmol 1980;12:332–342.
31. Taylor DM. Expulsive hemorrhage: some observations and comments. Trans Am Ophthalmol Soc 1974; 82:157–169.
32. Wheeler TM, Zimmerman TJ. Expulsive choroidal hemorrhage in the glaucoma patient. Ann Ophthalmol 1987;19:165–166.
33. Ariano ML, Ball SF. Delayed nonexpulsive suprachoroidal hemorrhage after trabeculectomy. Ophthalmic Surg 1987;18:661–666.
34. Frenkel RE, Shin DH. Prevention and management of delayed suprachoroidal hemorrhage after filtration surgery. Arch Ophthalmol 1986;104:1459–1463.
35. Ossoinig KC. Standardized echography: basic principles, clinical applications, and results. Int Ophthalmol Clin 1979;19:127–210.
36. Nasr A, Weingeist TA. The importance of standardized echography in the assessment of postsurgical choroidal detachments. In: Ossoinig KC, eds. Ophthalmic echography. Dordrecht, The Netherlands, Martinus Nijhoff, 1987:345–346.
37. Reynolds MG, Haimovici R, Flynn H Jr, et al. Suprachoroidal hemorrhage—clinical features and results of secondary surgical management. Ophthalmology 1993;100:460–465.
38. Lambrou F Jr, Meredith TA, Kaplan HJ. Secondary surgical management of expulsive choroidal hemorrhage. Arch Ophthalmol 1987;105:1195–1198.
39. Lakhanpal V, Schocket SS, Elman MJ, Nirankari VS. A new modified vitreoretinal surgical approach in the management of massive suprachoroidal hemorrhage. Ophthalmology 1989;96:793–800.
40. Abrams GW, Thomas MA, Williams GA, Burton TC. Management of postoperative suprachoroidal hemorrhage with continuous infusion air pump. Arch Ophthalmol 1986;104:1455–1458.
41. Berrocal JA. Adhesion of the retina secondary to large choroidal detachment as a cause of failure in retinal detachment surgery. Mod Probl Ophthalmol 1979;20: 51–52.
42. Vail D. Posterior sclerotomy as a form of treatment in subchoroidal expulsive hemorrhage. Am J Ophthalmol 1938;21:256–260.
43. Duehr PA, Hogenson CD. Treatment of subchoroidal hemorrhage by posterior sclerotomy. Arch Ophthalmol 1947;38:365–367.
43a. Shaffer RN. Posterior sclerotomy with scleral cautery in the treatment of expensive hemorrhage. Am J Ophthalmol 1966;61:1307.
44. Davison JA. Vitrectomy and fluid infusion in the treatment of delayed suprachoroidal hemorrhage after combined cataract and glaucoma filtration surgery. Ophthalmic Surg 1987;18:334–336.
45. Baldwin LB, Smith TJ, Hollins JL, Pearson PA. The use of viscoelastic substances in the drainage of postoperative suprachoroidal hemorrhage. Ophthalmic Surg 1989;20:504–507.
46. Desai UR, Peyman GA, Chen CJ, et al. Use of perfluoroperhydrophenanthrene in the management of suprachoroidal hemorrhages. Ophthalmology 1992;99:1542–1547.
47. Liu JC, Peyman GA, Oncel M. Treatment of experimental suprachoroidal hemorrhage with intravenous tissue plasminogen activator. Int Ophthalmol 1990;14: 267–270.
48. Alexandridis E. Silicone oil tamponade in the management of severe hemorrhagic detachment of the choroid and ciliary body after surgical trauma. Ophthalmologica 1990;200:189–193.
49. Holland EJ, Daya SM, Evangelista A, et al. Penetrating keratoplasty and transscleral fixation of posterior chamber lens. Am J Ophthalmol 1992;114: 182–187.

Ophthalmic Surgery Complications: Prevention and Management,
edited by Judie F. Charlton and George W. Weinstein.
J. B. Lippincott Company, Philadelphia © 1995.

18

Ranjit S. Dhaliwal
Travis A. Meredith

Endophthalmitis

Infectious endophthalmitis is a condition in which there is microbial invasion and inflammation of one or more coats of eye and the interior cavities. Clinically, most clinicians consider the presence of a vitritis necessary for the clinical suspicion of the presence of an infectious endophthalmitis. Although the most common causative agents of infectious endophthalmitis are bacteria, important pathogens may include fungi, parasites, and viruses.

From a diagnostic and therapeutic viewpoint, it is convenient to classify endophthalmitis according to the manner of spread of organism to the eye as well as on the time course of the disease. Exogenous endophthalmitis occurs when microorganisms invade the eye, usually through a break in the outer wall secondary to surgical intervention or to trauma. Endogenous endophthalmitis occurs when the microorganisms spread to the eye from a distant body site by means of the bloodstream. Most cases of infectious endophthalmitis occur after intraocular surgery, and more than 90% of these cases are caused by bacteria. Classifying the time course of the disease as acute, subacute, or delayed onset is helpful in selecting therapy for specific bacterial pathogens. The visual prognosis in many cases of infectious endophthalmitis is related to prompt diagnosis and initiation of therapy. Therefore, the clinician must maintain a high index of suspicion for the development of postoperative infectious endophthalmitis and consider intervention in those clinical settings where the pain and intraocular inflammation are in excess of typical expectations.

In this chapter, we explore the current concepts related to prophylaxis of infectious endophthalmitis, methods for obtaining cultures, initial choices for administration of antibiotics, and controversies in medical and surgical management. This discussion is limited to cases of exogenous endophthalmitis occurring after ocular surgery and repair of penetrating eye trauma.

ORIGIN AND PATHOGENESIS OF POSTOPERATIVE INFECTION

Postoperative infectious endophthalmitis remains a feared complication of intraocular surgery, although there has been an improvement in recent years in the visual prognosis of affected eyes. This improvement in prognosis has been related to prompt surgical intervention, improved culture techniques, and the development of new antibiotic regimens. A survey of 23,625 cases of extracapsular cataract extraction at a major teaching hospital demonstrated a rate of clinical diagnosis of infectious endophthalmitis of 0.089%.[1] A similar rate for extracapsular extractions was found in a national survey of the Medicare data base by Javitt and colleagues[2]; they also noted that the rate for intracapsular extractions was significantly higher (0.11%). These percentages are remarkably similar to the results from a study performed nearly 20 years earlier, during the intracapsular era when the incidence was 0.0865% in 30,000 cases.[3] At the current surgical rate of approximately 1.2 million cataract extractions per year in the United States, there are probably at least 1000 cases per year of endophthalmitis after cataract. Rates of infection after some anterior segment procedures are somewhat higher than after extracapsular cataract extraction (penetrating keratoplasty 0.11%; secondary intraocular lens implant, 0.30%).[1]

The human conjunctival sac is frequently populated by a wide variety of bacteria, many capable of causing endophthalmitis. Approximately 75% of preoperative cultures demonstrate viable organisms, although the exact species vary widely from one study to another.[4–6] Gram-positive organisms, particularly coagulase-negative *Staphylococcus* organisms, predominate, but gram-negative organisms are also isolated. Molecular epidemiologic studies show that the infecting organisms in postoperative endophthalmitis after cataract extraction are largely those of the patient's own periocular flora introduced into the eye during surgery.[6] Aqueous fluid samples taken during cataract surgery are observed to be positive in as many as 43% of eyes.[7,8] Cohen and associates[9] have reported that 6% of 33 consecutive eyes undergoing primary pars plana vitrectomy had culture-positive vitreous cavity aspirates.

Organisms may also be introduced into the eye from other sources during surgery. Contaminated irrigating solutions have been reported as the source of fungal endophthalmitis epidemics,[10–12] and colonization of the donor corneal rim may lead to endophthalmitis after corneal grafting.[13]

Microbes may gain access to the eye after surgery as well. Driebe and colleagues[14] documented wound abnormalities in 22% of 83 cases. Vitreous wicks may provide a route for inward microbial migration[15] as can inadequately buried sutures.[16] Postoperative manipulation of sutures may initiate an infection,[17] and transscleral fixation sutures have been associated with infection.[18]

Because bacteria enter the eye frequently during surgery, but relatively few eyes become infected, the pathogenesis of infection must be complex. The size of the inoculum, virulence of the organism, surgical status of the eye, type of implanted material, and host factors probably all play a role. *S epidermidis* introduced into the rabbit eye in large numbers, for example, produces a short-term infection, but the vitreous cavity rapidly becomes sterile without any treatment.[19] A case control study of endophthalmitis demonstrated that when communication between the anterior and posterior chambers occurred during surgery (such as a posterior capsular tear or the development of a complication requiring vitrectomy), the risk of endophthalmitis increased by a factor of 14.[20] The anterior chamber has been demonstrated to clear bacteria efficiently,[21] but the posterior chamber may have a more difficult time accomplishing this goal because of physical or chemical factors.

Host factors, such as immunosuppression medically or the acquired immunodeficiency syndrome, may increase the risk for postoperative infection. Patients with diabetes have a higher rate of endophthalmitis than the nondiabetic population.[1,22]

An epidemiologic study has demonstrated that bacteria adhere to intraocular lenses (IOLs) with Prolene haptics preferentially when compared with all-polymethylmethacrylate (PMMA) lenses.[23] These lenses are associated with endophthalmitis 4½ times more frequently than all-PMMA lenses.[20]

PREVENTION OF ENDOPHTHALMITIS

Reducing the number of periocular bacteria before surgery as prophylaxis is of clear importance. Routine preoperative examination for chronic blepharitis, conjunctivitis, canaliculitis, or dacryocystitis should be performed and these problems addressed before undertaking surgery. Preoperatively, facial scrubs and the use of topical antibiotics may be less frequently employed with the current trends toward outpatient surgery across North America. Meticulous preoperative povidone-iodine (which exerts its action by release of free iodine) has been demonstrated to be effective in reducing periocular bacterial flora.[4,24] Speaker and colleagues[25] reviewed their experience with preoperative antimicrobial prophylaxis with povidone-iodine compared with a silver protein solution involving 88063 patients. They noted a statistically significant reduction in culture-positive endophthalmitis in the group prepared with povidone-iodine with no attendant adverse effects. They also suggest routine applications of povidone-iodine solution preoperatively in all surgical cases in which the globe is closed and the patient does not have an allergy to iodine.

In general, surgical evidence now exists that prophylactic systemic antibiotics given within 2 hours of the incision significantly reduce the incidence of postoperative infection.[26,27] In ophthalmology, as well, the preponderance of evidence favors prophylactic use of perioperative antibiotics to reduce the incidence of postoperative endophthalmitis.[28] However, controversy persists as to the antibiotic choice, dosing frequency, and routes of administration. Topical gentamicin has been consistently demonstrated to be an effective drug, but the literature remains inconclusive as to the best antimicrobial choice for antibiotic prophylaxis.[28] More recently, the use of ciprofloxacin or a third-generation cephalosporin presents attractive alternatives to the use of aminoglycoside antibiotics. When choosing a particular antibiotic and its route of administration, it is important to consider the risk–benefit ratio of one versus another. Campochiaro and Conway[29] and Campochiaro and associates[30] have described more than 20 cases of macular infarction after routine subconjunctival injection of an aminoglycoside postoperatively. Inadvertent penetration of the eye during injection was thought to be responsible for achieving toxic levels of drugs in the eye in some cases; however, entry through the surgical wound was believed to be a possible cause in others. Although similar consequences may result from the use of alternative antibiotics, this has prompted concern about periocular injections of aminoglycosides.

No definitive studies exist demonstrating the best antibiotic dosing frequency or route of administration for postoperative prophylaxis. There is conflicting information from several studies concerning the role of topical versus subconjunctival perioperative antibiotic use. In a large study of perioperative antibiotic regimens,[31] 54,000 cases at a cataract camp in Pakistan were reviewed. No significant decrease in the rates of endophthalmitis in 10,000 patients administered postoperative subconjunctival antibiotics compared with 44,000 patients who were not administered subconjunctival antibiotics was noted. A later, smaller series from the same hospital demonstrated that the combination of preoperative topical antibiotics with subconjunctival antibiotics administered at the end of the procedure was more effective in reducing infections than the use of preoperative topical antibiotics alone.[32] In contradistinction, another smaller study demonstrated no significant reduction in the incidence of postoperative infection.[33] Animal studies have demonstrated the benefits of postoperative subconjunctival antibiotic injections postoperatively in prophylaxis of endophthalmitis. Clinical infection was reduced in treatment groups that receive subconjunctival injections of ceftazidime,[34] gentamicin,[35] or ciprofloxacin[36] compared with control groups who did not receive subconjunctival injections, although studies of antibiotic penetration into the vitreous cavity after subconjunctival injection typically demonstrate negligible levels of intraocular penetration.[37]

If postoperative subconjunctival antibiotic prophylaxis is performed, it is important to consider the cost, toxicity, allergenicity, and spectrum of coverage in selecting the appropriate drug. Prophylaxis against infection should combine careful preoperative evaluation, meticulous perioperative preparation, and administration of perioperative antibiotics. The role or prophylactic subconjunctival antibiotics at the end of surgery remains unclear.[38] Recommendations modified from Speaker and Menikoff are summarized in Table 18-1.

Table 18-1
Recommendations for Prophylaxis of Postoperative Endophthalmitis

Recognition and treatment of preoperative external disease
Topical antibiotics preoperatively
  Ciprofloxacin 0.3% or an aminoglycoside q3–5h the day before surgery and every 15 min q4h before surgery
Topical antiseptic preparation of the eye for surgery
  Providone-iodine 5% solution, 2 drops in the conjunctival sac
  Providone-iodine 5% solution to the eyelid margins and lashes
  Providone-iodine 10% solution to prepare the skin
Adhesive-backed plastic drapes to cover the eyelid margins and lashes
Subconjunctival antibiotic injection or collagen shield delivery of antibiotic postoperatively
  Vancomycin, 25 mg
    and
  Ceftazidime, 100 mg

(Adapted from Speaker ML, Menikoff JA. Int Ophthalmol Clin 1993;33:63)

CLINICAL PRESENTATIONS OF EXOGENOUS ENDOPHTHALMITIS

In the evaluation of postoperative infectious endophthalmitis, it is of particular importance to note the length of time from the surgical insult or trauma to the onset of symptoms as well as to the time that has passed since the onset of symptoms. The use of antibiotics or steroids postoperatively should be noted, and a thorough ocular examination performed to search for any possible route of entry of the infecting organism. Bacterial replication, toxin release, and attendant inflammation may lead to rapid tissue destruction and significant visual loss even with successful eradication of invading organisms. It is imperative in acute situations to choose a treatment strategy and antibiotic regimen, and to begin therapy on an empiric basis as quickly as possible. In general, we can suspect specific pathogens based on clinical presentation. Recognition of specific clinical syndromes may thus influence our therapeutic decisions.

Acute Postoperative Endophthalmitis

Acute postoperative endophthalmitis presents within the 1st week after surgery. The typical symptomatic onset is heralded by an increase in postoperative discomfort (usually beginning after the examination performed the day after surgery) followed by progressive loss of vision. Findings in the early stage include increased perilimbal conjunctival hyperemia and chemosis, increased anterior chamber reaction, and vitritis; differentiation from sterile inflammation may be difficult at this stage.[39] The presence of hypopyon strongly suggests infection. In more advanced presentations, hypopyon is severe, the cornea is thickened and perhaps infiltrated, and the fundus view is lost because of significant vitreous inflammation. Gram-positive organisms are responsible for 60% to 80% of acute infections in all large series, and staphylococcal species account for more than two thirds of all cases (Table 18-2). Of these, coagulase-negative staphylococci, which are the prevalent species colonizing skin and mucous membranes, are recognized as the most common causative agents in postoperative endophthalmitis.[14,40–42] The rise in incidence of pathogenic behavior of *S epidermidis* in human infections has paralleled the use of indwelling catheters in the newborn nursery and the implantation of IOLs in ophthalmic surgery. Coagulase-negative staphylococci have been commonly reported as *S epidermidis*, although there are at least 10 species included in this group. *S epidermidis, S warneri, S hominis, S haemolyticus, S capitis,* and *S simulans* have all been demonstrated as pathogens in postoperative endophthalmitis.[43] Coagulase-negative staphylococcal endophthalmitis tends to have a slow onset with a crescendo of symptoms during a 5- to 7-day period postoperatively; diagnosis may be delayed for more than 1 week in many cases.

S aureus is the second most commonly isolated organism in clinical cases of postoperative bacterial endophthalmitis (one third of gram-positive cases). *S aureus* usually produces a virulent, rapidly progressive intraocular infection. *S aureus* produces many enzymes, including catalase, which correlates with its pathogenicity. In addition, *S aureus* is capable of producing several different exotoxins that incite inflammation in the surrounding tissue. Less commonly encountered are streptococcal species. Finally, gram-negative organisms account for approximately 10% to 20% of cases. Among gram-

Table 18-2
Distribution of Isolates in Culture-Positive Postoperative Cases (%)

	DIAMOND[105] (1981)	OLSON AND COLLEAGUES[109] (1983)	DRIEBE AND ASSOCIATES[14] (1986)	BOHIGIAN AND OLK[114a] (1986)	WEBER AND associates[42] (1986)
Gram positive	79	90	76	82	90
Coagulase negative Staphylococci	41	34	38	34	58
Gram negative	11	15	16	18	10
Fungal	8	8	8	0	0

negative organisms, *Pseudomonas* is the most frequent cause of endophthalmitis. *P aeruginosa* accounted for 23% of all gram-negative cases; *Haemophilus influenzae* caused 19% of cases in one series.[44] Culture-negative cases can account for 25% to 45% of cases of pseudophakic endophthalmitis[14]; some may be the result of infection with organisms that die quickly after producing an inflammatory response, whereas others may reflect problems in obtaining the specimen or the organisms with culturing.[19]

Subacute Postoperative Infectious Endophthalmitis

Subacute onset infectious endophthalmitis occurs after 1 to 3 weeks. This course usually reflects the less virulent forms of coagulase-negative staphylococci; one third of these cases present more than 1 week after the inoculating event.[45] Other organisms may uncommonly produce a similar course.[46] A subacute presentation may also reflect the slow growth of fungal species (particularly *Candida parapsilosis*).[10,12,47] The clinical course of subacute-onset infectious endophthalmitis is usually days to weeks after surgery, and the clinical manifestations are those of inflammation that often respond to suppression by topical steroid therapy initially.[46] Breakthrough of the inflammation occurs; increasing steroid dosage frequency may suppress it again until the appearance of hypopyon or uncontrollable inflammation leads to a diagnostic and therapeutic intervention.

Delayed-Onset Postoperative Endophthalmitis

The onset of intraocular inflammation weeks to several months postoperatively is characteristic for endophthalmitis caused by *Propionibacterium acnes*, fungi, and, occasionally, coagulase-negative staphylococci. *P acnes* is a gram-positive anaerobic bacillus inhabitant of the conjunctiva causing an endophthalmitis that characteristically produces a granulomatous inflammation 1 to 2 months after surgery. A typical finding is the presence of white plaque on the lens capsule after the eye has been fully dilated. Fungal cases are much less specific regarding their findings, and their diagnosis is usually made by Gram stain, Giemsa stain, and culture on Sabouraud medium.[47] Fungal cases have been commonly identified in epidemic form, traced to contaminated irrigating solutions.[11,12] Close cooperation with the microbiology department in the diagnosis of these chronic forms of postoperative endophthalmitis is essential and requires communication by the ophthalmologist so that appropriate measures for proper identification of these organisms can be undertaken. Anaerobic and fungal cultures are critical, and cultures should be kept for a minimum of 2 weeks, particularly when *P acnes* is suspected, because these organisms may grow slowly.

Postoperative Bleb-Associated Infectious Endophthalmitis

Bleb-associated endophthalmitis can be seen after cataract extractions or after filtering procedures.[48] It typically presents in a delayed fashion weeks to months after the initial surgery, and is preceded by a period of irritation and redness of the eye. The classic initial finding is "white on red" as the white bleb fills with inflammatory material and is highlighted against the redness of the surrounding conjunctiva. Streptococcal species are the infecting organisms in approximately 60% of these cases. Streptococci are facultative anaerobic organisms or obligate anaerobes that are spherical or ovoid, and found in pairs or chains. They are gram positive, nonspore forming, catalase negative, and nonmotile. In the laboratory, they exhibit fastidious growth, replicating best on complex media and often requiring carbon dioxide.

Postoperative bleb-associated infectious endophthalmitis may also be caused by *H influenzae*. *H influenzae* is a small, non–spore- forming bacterium that is a strict parasite of humans. It is a common upper respiratory tract organism that spreads continuously to areas adjacent to the nasopharynx. Most infections are caused by nonencapsulated forms.

Posttraumatic Infectious Endophthalmitis

Posttraumatic endophthalmitis accounts for approximately 25% of all cases of intraocular infection. These cases present difficult therapeutic problems because of the direct effects of the injury as well as the more virulent spectrum of bacteria that are involved in traumatic infections.[49–55]

Many cases of posttraumatic endophthalmitis present at the same time the patient is being evaluated for trauma. Particularly with occult penetrations or unsuspected intraocular foreign bodies, it is the symptoms and signs of infection that lead the patient to seek care. In other instances, endophthalmitis presents as a complication after the trauma repair. When endophthalmitis presents after surgery for severe ocular trauma, its signs and symptoms may be difficult to separate from the effects of the trauma. Increasing pain and inflammatory signs in the early postoperative period lead to the suspicion of infection. The appearance of hypopyon makes endophthalmitis the likely diagnosis. Fungal cases and those caused by *Nocardia* make a late appearance weeks after the surgical repair. Infiltration of opaque material in the anterior chamber, focal fluffy infiltrates in the vitreous cavity, or increasing chronic inflammation should raise the suspicion of fungal disease. Rates of infection after trauma vary from 2% to 3% after penetrating injuries to 11% to 17% after industrial intraocular foreign bodies.[51] A series of rural injuries produced endophthalmitis in 30% of the eyes.[50] A wide variety of organisms are implicated in traumatic endophthalmitis, and both the patient's flora and organisms from the environment of the injury may be the responsible pathogens. Although staphylococci are still commonly identified, other organisms rarely seen in postsurgical endophthalmitis, such as *Bacillus* spp, are common. Mixed infections involving more than one organism are much more frequent than in postoperative cases. Incidence data for causative organisms in posttraumatic endophthalmitis are listed in Table 18-3.

Bacillus spp are commonly identified after injuries involving farm materials and are implicated as the causative organisms in approximately 25% to 30% of posttraumatic cases.[50,52–54] The most common intraocular pathogen is *B cereus* with *B subtilis* identified occasionally. *Bacillus* is an aerobic spore-forming rod that is gram positive or gram variable in staining. These organisms may grow singly, in chains, or in diplobacillary forms. In nature, they are found in decaying organic matter, dust, soil, vegetables, water, and as human flora. An infection by *B cereus* is particularly virulent and may destroy the eye in 12 to 24 hours. *Bacillus* along with clostridial infections are the only causes of endophthalmitis to induce fever and leukocytosis. Clinically, *Bacillus* infections present with severe ocular pain developing within 24 hours after injury and with signs of chemosis, periorbital swelling, and proptosis. Ring corneal infiltrates may occur within 48 hours.[54] The outcome in *Bacillus* endophthalmitis is almost universally poor, and many involved eyes require enucleation.

MANAGEMENT

Goals and Objectives

The goal of endophthalmitis therapy is to salvage the eye with the best possible recovery of vision. This result is accomplished by pursuing the twin objec-

Table 18-3
Distribution of Isolates in Traumatic Endophthalmitis (%)

	BRINTON AND COWORKERS[51] (1984)	AFFELDT AND ASSOCIATES[49] (1987)	BOLDT AND COLLEAGUES[50]* (1989)
Gram positive	89	60	71
Coagulase-negative staphylococci	37	29	25
Staphylococcus aureus	15	4	21
Streptococci	10	13	
Bacillus	26	20	46
Gram negative	5	20	29
Fungal	0	17	
Mixed	5	10	42

*Adds to more than 100% because of multiple organisms.

tives of killing the invading microorganisms and controlling the intraocular inflammatory process. Killing the pathogens is primarily accomplished by antimicrobial therapy, although pars plana vitrectomy also increases the efficiency and speed of microbial eradication.[56,57] Controlling inflammation is accomplished by administration of antiinflammatory agents, particularly corticosteroids, and by vitrectomy. Inflammation may increase despite the death of microorganisms,[19] and rapid lysis of bacteria may actually worsen inflammation.

Antibiotic Selection and Delivery

The goal of antimicrobial therapy for endophthalmitis is to provide adequate intravitreal concentrations of appropriate antibiotics for a sufficiently long time to eradicate microorganisms while avoiding concentrations of the drugs that can induce iatrogenic tissue damage. The initial choice of antibiotics must be made before the infecting organism has been identified by culture; choices are, therefore, largely empiric and based on the clinical setting and individual patient characteristics.

Historically, antibiotics delivered intravenously alone or in combination with topical medication resulted in few cures because the target area for antimicrobial therapy in infectious endophthalmitis is the vitreous cavity. Indeed, a survey of 103 published cases between 1944 and 1966 revealed that 73% had final visual acuities of hand motion or worse.[58] These poor results were in large part due to poor penetration of antibiotics through the blood–retinal barrier with little improvement by the use of frequent subconjunctival injections.[37,59–61] The concentrations of antimicrobial agents in the vitreous cavity after subconjunctival injection are insignificant in comparison with those achieved after intravitreal injection; therapeutic levels are rarely achieved when antimicrobial is administered by the subconjunctival route alone.[61] The use of intravitreal injection of antibiotics (sulfa compounds and penicillin) was introduced by Leopold and coworkers.[63–65] After a period of skepticism followed by lengthy controversy, intravitreal antibiotic injections are now well accepted as the mainstay of therapy in the management of postoperative infectious endophthalmitis.[66]

Antibiotics are generally injected directly into the vitreous cavity as primary therapy, or at the completion of a vitrectomy procedure. The antimicrobial is mixed so that the appropriate dose is contained in 0.1 mL of diluent (usually saline or balanced salt solution). For broad-spectrum coverage, two antibiotics are usually required; they are commonly diluted and administered separately to avoid problems of incompatibility of the solutions.

Antibiotic administration as part of the infusion fluid has been advocated by some as part of the vitrectomy procedure. This has the advantage of exposing the organisms to antibiotics earlier in the surgical case and has been recommended at concentrations of 8 μg/mL gentamicin in the infusion bottle.[66] However, this would amount to only one third of the concentration achieved by injecting 100 μg into a 4-cm^3 eye (25 μg/mL); therefore, the peak dosage and effective duration of action would be significantly reduced. Because of the potential problems associated with inaccurate antibiotic mixing when delivered by this method and because of the beneficial experience of intraocular injection of antibiotics, we generally do not employ antibiotic administration in the infusion fluid. Exceptions, perhaps, would be in cases with suspected virulent organisms (eg, *Bacillus* in posttraumatic cases) or when the use of a postoperative gas bubble limits postoperative intravitreal administration.

Whether or not intravenous antibiotic administration is necessary for cure of endophthalmitis remains an unanswered question.[67] Successful outcomes have been reported without intravenous antibiotics, even when the infection was caused by virulent organisms.[68] The major problem with intravenous administration of antimicrobials for endophthalmitis therapy is poor penetration into the vitreous cavity.[70]

Topical antibiotics are commonly employed in treating infectious endophthalmitis, although they add little to intraocular concentrations of drug. Administration three or four times daily is probably sufficient in most cases. When the endophthalmitis is associated with a corneal ulcer, stitch abscess, or infected bleb, frequent applications are important.

A recent review summarizes dilution procedures for preparation of intraocular injections and fortified eye drops.[70] Characteristics for antibiotics to be used in the management of infectious endophthalmitis include the following attributes:

1. *Bactericidal properties.* Like the central nervous system, the eye is relatively immune privileged. Because treatment with bacteriostatic antibiotics relies on host immune defenses to fight the

infection, they are probably less appropriate choices than bactericidal drugs.

2. *Broad spectrum of antimicrobial coverage.* Initial therapy must cover gram-positive organisms (including methicillin-resistant staphylococci and in trauma cases *Bacillus* spp) and gram-negative organisms.
3. *Excellent therapeutic ratios (activity/toxicity) after intravitreal injection.* After intravitreal injections, antibiotic concentrations in the vitreous cavity are frequently higher than those reached by the antimicrobial in other tissues. Retinal toxicity usually defines the upper limits of allowable intravitreal concentrations. The rabbit is most often the subject of toxicity studies because of availability and expense. Toxicity, commonly defined by histologic and electron microscopic studies in addition to electroretinographic testing, is often inadequately documented because of the limitations of testing in the avascular rabbit retina model. The paucity of vascularized primate retina studies, for example, may have delayed the recognition of vascular occlusive complications related to intravitreal aminoglycoside administration.[71,72]
4. *Good therapeutic ratios after intravenous injection.* Because of the blood–retinal barrier, the use of oral or intravenous microbials have infrequently been demonstrated consistently to reach vitreous levels above the minimal inhibitory concentration (MIC) for the important pathogens in endophthalmitis.[73–77] Generally, lipid-soluble antibiotics have better potential for intraocular penetration after systemic administration than do hydrophilic antibiotics that include aminoglycosides and β-lactam antibiotics. The pH of the system influences the lipid-solubility of the antibiotics chosen (ionized molecules being less able to travel across the blood–retinal barrier). The problem of poor penetration must be weighed against the significant systemic toxicities associated with some antimicrobials, especially the nephrotoxicity associated with aminoglycosides and amphotericin. Additionally, cumulative toxicities with combination systemic therapy must be considered (eg, ototoxicity associated with the concurrent use of vancomycin and aminoglycosides).
5. *Favorable pharmacokinetic properties.* The effects of inflammation and surgery itself enhance the intraocular penetration of certain antibiotics after intravenous administration.[37,69,75] Repeat dosing with intravenous antibiotics may enhance the intraocular penetration into inflamed eyes, as with ceftazidime.[75] After injection into the vitreous cavity, antimicrobials may be eliminated either by an anterior or a posterior route.[78–80] β-Lactam antimicrobials are generally eliminated by a posterior route, predominately across the retinal surface. Because of this wider area for elimination, their half-lives are generally short, ranging from 6 to 10 hours. Antimicrobials eliminated anteriorly (including aminoglycosides and vancomycin) have longer half-lives, presumably because they must traverse around the lens to reach the anterior chamber. Half-lives of these antimicrobials may be between 20 and 30 hours. Vitreous removal shortens the half-life of all antimicrobial agents studied in animal models.[69,81,82] Lens removal and inflammation each may shorten the half-life of anteriorly eliminated antibiotics, such as aminoglycosides.[74,82] However, inflammation may prolong the half-life of those antimicrobials eliminated posteriorly, such as β-lactam antibiotics, particularly if an active pump mechanism is involved.[75]

Antimicrobial Agents Used in Infectious Endophthalmitis

Multiple factors are involved in the ability of antimicrobial agents to kill bacteria. These include drug concentrations, duration of exposure, sites of infection, and the particular interaction between a given pathogen and the specific antimicrobial used. There are five commonly used groups of antimicrobial agents in the management of infectious endophthalmitis.

Cephalosporins

The cephalosporins are synthetic β-lactam antibiotics that are active against the bacterial cell wall. This class of antibiotic is well tolerated systemically. Cefazolin has been shown to be a relatively safe drug when 2.25 mg is injected intravitreally into the aphakic eye, and levels remain above MICs of common pathogens for about 48 hours.[75] Ceftazidime has similar properties.[69] Cephalosporins have good broad-spectrum coverage for gram-positive and for some gram-negative organisms, but the first-generation drugs are weak against enterococcus and methicillin-resistant staphylococcal organisms. Cefazolin concentrations in inflamed vitrectomized eyes well above the MICs for sensitive organisms can be achieved after repeated intravenous dosages.[75] Ceftazidime is a third-generation semisynthetic cephalosporin with excellent coverage for gram-negative organisms. It has an excellent therapeutic ratio after intraocular injection.[70,79,83] Ceftazidime also penetrates into the vitreous cavity after intravenous administration. Its concentration in the vitreous cavity of the inflamed aphakic-vitrectomized eye is nine times the MIC for *Pseudomonas* 2 hours after infusion.[69] Studies of gram-negative endophthalmitis demonstrate that almost all organisms involved were susceptible to ceftazidime and that there was no advantage in spectrum of coverage for the aminoglycosides over ceftazidime.[44,84]

Vancomycin

Vancomycin is a complex glycopeptide that inhibits cell wall assembly in addition to damaging protoplasts and inhibiting ribonucleic acid synthesis. The intraocular therapeutic ratio for vancomycin is good, although the half-life has not been well studied.[85] Systemic toxicity is seen after high intravenous dosages and is additive with the concurrent use of aminoglycosides. Vancomycin is well established as the drug of choice for gram-positive endophthalmitis because it covers essentially all staphylococcal organisms, *Streptococcus, P acnes,* and *Bacillus*.[86,87] Unfortunately, vancomycin has essentially no gram-negative coverage, and an additional agent for initial intravitreal injection is required to cover these organisms (eg, an aminoglycoside or ceftazidime).

Aminoglycosides

Aminoglycosides act by binding ribosomal subunits and thereby inhibiting protein synthesis. Aminoglycosides have a spectrum including both gram-positive and gram-negative organisms, but retinal toxicity after intraocular injection is a case for concern.[29,30,71,88,89] Retinal vascular infarction has been reported after the use of gentamicin in particular but also after intravitreal amikacin administration.[30,71] This complication limits the amount given for initial intravitreal doses, and the concentrations of these antibiotics stay above the pertinent MICs for only 24 to 36 hours. The penetration of aminoglycoside antibiotics in the human eye after intravenous administration does not reach therapeutic levels after single doses.[90] Systemic toxicities associated with the use of intravenous aminoglycosides include nephrotoxicity, ototoxicity (frequently irreversible), and neuromuscular paralysis.[86,91]

Quinolones

The quinolones are structurally related to nalidixic acid and interrupt the supercoiled state of bacterial DNA by inhibiting DNA gyrases. Their spectrum of coverage is broad and includes good coverage against gram-negative aerobes (including *Pseudomonas*), but they are weak against streptococci and anaerobes. Initial reports of the toxicity of intraocular ciprofloxacin suggest a low therapeutic ratio.[92] However, the intravenous therapeutic ratio is acceptable for ciprofloxacin, although in uninflamed eyes it reaches concentrations in the vitreous cavity above the MICs for target organisms inconsistently after intravenous administration.[76,77] Resistance of gram-positive organisms has developed rapidly to ciprofloxacin.

Antifungal Agents

Antifungal agents act by disrupting fungal cell membranes by combining with ergosterols (natamycin, amphotericin, or ketoconazole) or by blocking fungal thymidine synthesis (flucytosine). Amphotericin is still considered the gold standard in antifungal therapy and is recommended in a dose of 5 μg intravitreally.[81] The half-life of 9.1 days after intraocular injection is decreased by inflammation and vitreous removal. Systemic amphotericin administration is associated with significant renal toxicity, and the penetration into the eye is relatively poor.[73] Flucytosine or ketoconazole may have a role in treatment because they may penetrate the eye better than amphotericin and may be given orally.

Current Recommendations for Antibiotic Combinations

Based on the information obtained from clinical and experimental models of antibiotic pharmacokinetics and therapeutic ratios, we employ a combination of intravitreal, topical, and systemic antimicrobial

Table 18-4
Treatment of Endophthalmitis Antimicrobial and Antiinflammatory Agents

	INTRAOCULAR	PERIOCULAR	TOPICAL	SYSTEMIC
Acute postoperative traumatic and bleb-associated endophthalmitis	Vancomyin, 1 mg Ceftazidime, 2 mg	Vancomycin, 25 mg Ceftazidime, 100 mg Dexamethasone, 12–24 mg	Vancomycin, 50 mg/mL Ceftazidime, 50 mg/mL Corticosteroids Cycloplegics	Vancomycin, 1 gm IV q12h Ceftazidime, 1–2 g IV q8h Methylprednisolone sodium succinate (Solu-Medrol), 40–80 mg/d or Prednisone, 1 mg/kg/d
Delayed-onset postoperative endophthalmitis (depends on Gram and Giemsa stains or culture)	Vancomycin, 1 mg or Amphotericin, 5 μg	Vancomycin, 25 mg Dexamethasone, 12–24 mg	Vancomycin, 50 mg/mL Corticosteroids Cycloplegics	Vancomycin, 1 g IV q12h or Amphotericin B or Fluconazole

IV, intravenously.

agents. Our preferred antibiotic selections and dosages are presented in Table 18-4.

Role of Corticosteroid Administration

The adverse effects of endophthalmitis on the eye and the visual prognosis are related not only to the presence of specific pathogens but are also mediated by the attendant inflammatory process. Indeed, inflammation can increase even when microbes are no longer viable because of the antibiotic-related death of the bacteria itself. Corticosteroid administration has long been recognized as useful in the goal of controlling intraocular inflammation. In therapy for meningitis (an infection similar to endophthalmitis in many respects), better functional outcomes have been demonstrated when antimicrobial therapy is combined with systemic corticosteroid administration.[93,94] The therapeutic effects of corticosteroids are mediated by their ability to inhibit production of soluble mediators of inflammation, induce macrocortin (a protein that inhibits the production of prostaglandins and leukotrienes), decrease vascular permeability, and alter leukocyte migration. Topical administration of corticosteroids are given in frequent dosages after vitreous tap or surgery and antibiotic injection. Systemically administered corticosteroids have been shown to reduce intraocular inflammation independent of the effects of surgery in animal models of *S epidermidis* endophthalmitis.[95–97] We employ the use of oral corticosteroids, 1 mg/kg, with frequent topical corticosteroids in the postoperative management of acute endophthalmitis. Another alternative is intravenous methylprednisolone sodium succinate (Solu-Medrol), 40 to 80 mg/d, when systemic corticosteroids are not contraindicated.[98] The role of intraocular corticosteroid administration is less certain at this time, although this route of administration is recommended by several authorities.[98,99] Intraocular injection of corticosteroids was first advocated by Graham and Peyman,[96] Coats and Peyman,[100] and Peyman and Herbst[101] in the treatment of animal models of endophthalmitis and is reported to be beneficial in several treatment series of clinical endophthalmitis. Graham and Peyman[96] demonstrated in the rabbit model of *Pseudomonas* endophthalmitis that there was a beneficial effect of concurrent intraocular administration of gentamicin and corticosteroids if given within a few hours of a large bacterial inoculum; no benefit, however, was demonstrable once the infection became established.[96] Meredith and colleagues[97] demonstrated a beneficial effect of intraocular corticosteroid administration in a rabbit model of *S epidermidis* endophthalmitis, equivalent to but not superior to systemic administration. A beneficial effect of intraocular corticosteroids was also shown histopathologically in a similar model by Maxwell and coworkers.[102] In a model of *S aureus* endophthalmitis treated with vitrectomy, intraocular antibiotic injection, and intraocular corticosteroid injection, there was an increase in inflammatory scores, corneal opacity, and incidence of retinal necrosis compared with omission of intraocular corticosteroids.[103] Hence, intraocular corticosteroid administration may not result in a beneficial effect in all cases of postoperative endophthalmitis. The dosage advocated by most investigators for intraocular administration is 400 μg of dexamethasone, which is much lower than the 800-μg dose known experimentally to cause retinal toxicity.[104] Subconjunctival corticosteroid administration at the end of surgery can achieve intraocular levels of drug within the first hours after surgery, but the efficacy of this route of administration has not been rigorously tested in clinical or animal trials.

MANAGEMENT STRATEGIES

Management of Acute Postoperative Endophthalmitis

Initial Strategy: Pars Plana Vitrectomy Versus Culture and Injection of Intraocular Antibiotics

Controversy exists about the best initial approach to the management of postoperative endophthalmitis. In current clinical management, the surgeon must determine the initial management strategy and proceed immediately because time is of the essence to begin to sterilize the vitreous cavity and control the inflammatory process. One school of thought contends that the best initial management is to obtain a vitreous culture and inject antibiotics into the vitreous cavity, reserving vitreous removal for initially nonresponsive cases. An alternative approach is to perform vitrectomy immediately, obtaining a specimen for culture and injecting antibiotics into the eye either during or at the close of the surgical procedure.

Pars plana vitrectomy provides for faster eradication of organisms and control of inflammation in experimental animals, and is widely used in the management of endophthalmitis, analogous to drainage of an abscess. Recommendations for the immediate implementation of pars plana vitrectomy have included the following: (1) severer presentation (defined by loss of red reflex, loss of light projection, afferent pupillary defect, associated corneal ring infiltrate, and clinical worsening 24 to 48 hours after intraocular antibiotic administration); (2) infectious endophthalmitis with gram-negative organisms seen after initial vitreous tap[105]; (3) more fulminant course with inability to examine the retina[106]; (4) cases not responding to initial medical treatment;[107] and (5) vitreous abscess.[105,107] Vitrectomy has been clinically used by some investigators in all acute cases of endophthalmitis, by others for more severe cases only, and by some only when other treatments have failed.

The surgical results for endophthalmitis treated with vitrectomy have been reported to be less favorable compared with outcomes of management obtained by vitreous tap and injection of intraocular antibiotics alone. This result may reflect a bias toward the use of pars plana vitrectomy techniques in those cases with more severe presentations.[14,105,108,109] Animal data, conversely, have generally demonstrated advantages for vitrectomy and intraocular antibiotic administration compared with intraocular antibiotic treatment alone. Models of *S epidermidis* endophthalmitis show that vitrectomy without intraocular antibiotics is not efficacious in curing experimental intraocular infections. A combination of surgery and intraocular antibiotics, however, resulted in more negative cultures 1 week after treatment compared with the use of intraocular antibiotics alone.[56] Meredith and colleagues[97] demonstrated the beneficial effects of vitrectomy on reducing inflammation and opacities of the media in experimental *S epidermidis* models. Talley and colleagues[110] as well as Aguilar and coworkers[57] studied experimental *S aureus* endophthalmitis. Compared with antibiotic therapy alone, vitrectomy and intraocular antibiotic administration more often sterilized the vitreous cavity, reduced posttreatment inflammation,[57] and produced more eyes with clear media.[110]

The Endophthalmitis Vitrectomy Study (EVS) is a randomized controlled clinical trial designed to determine the best management for patients with acute postoperative infectious endophthalmitis.[67] In the EVS, patients are randomized to initial management by vitreous tap and injection of antibiotics, or to vitrectomy and injection of intraocular antibiotics. A second randomization allocates patients in each of these two groups to the use of intravenous antibiotics or not, creating a total of four subgroups for comparison. Patients with a progressive downhill course after tap and injection are allowed to undergo a vitrectomy procedure. The results of this important study should help define the initial management of acute postoperative endophthalmitis as well as address the efficacy of intravenous antibiotic therapy. This study is not designed to address the management of chronic, bleb-related, or posttraumatic endophthalmitis specifically.

CULTURE TECHNIQUES. Management of suspected infectious endophthalmitis begins with obtaining appropriate cultures and initiating appropriate antibiotic therapy. Although an anterior chamber culture is, on rare occasions, positive without a positive vitreous culture, the importance of obtaining a vitreous specimen for culture cannot be overemphasized because the vitreous is often positive when the anterior chamber is negative.[14,40,108,111,112] Although the value of an anterior chamber tap performed at the time of vitreous sampling remains controversial, it may be expedient to obtain the sample under controlled conditions for separate culturing.[14,108,111,113,114] A vitreous tap obtaining a small amount of material has a lower rate of successfully identifying organisms than culturing the entire specimen collected in the vitrectomy cassette during a vitrectomy procedure.[115]

When it is elected to begin therapy with antibiotics alone and not do initial vitrectomy, specimens may be obtained either in the office or in the operating room. If the wound is not intact, the patient should be taken to the operating room and the wound reinforced before further manipulating the eye. In a tap procedure, the goal should be to remove no more than a total of 0.3 to 0.4 mL to avoid significant hypotony; typically, 0.2 mL of fluid is injected as part of the antibiotic therapy and helps reestablish intraocular pressure. The anterior chamber is entered with a 25- to 27-gauge needle on a tuberculin syringe on the corneal edge of the corneoscleral limbus, and 0.1 mL is withdrawn and sent for culture. In the office, this procedure is completed at the slit lamp; however, an assistant is required to stabilize the patient's head and pull out the plunger while the surgeon monitors the needle position.

A vitreous aspiration can be obtained at the slit lamp or in the operating room after employing retrobulbar anesthesia. If the eye is aphakic, the vitreous may be reached through the pupil or a peripheral iridectomy; the needle may be initially passed through the limbus and into a position behind the iris. While the needle point is monitored to make sure vitreous does not become entrapped, gentle suction is used to aspirate 0.1 to 0.3 mL into a tuberculin syringe. If significant resistance to suction is encountered, especially if vitreous is incarcerated in the tip, the procedure should be aborted and another approach adopted. When a posterior chamber intraocular lens prevents access to the vitreous by means of a limbal approach, then entry may be made between 3 and 4 mm posterior to the limbus transconjunctivally and transsclerally. The aspiration technique is unchanged. Particular care is taken not to incarcerate vitreous and exert traction on the peripheral retina. If this approach fails either in the operating room or the clinic, an operating procedure with a vitreous cutting instrument is indicated. The previous incisions may be enlarged or a new 20-gauge incision created. The suction tubing from the vitreous cutter is divided 2 inches from the probe and the free end attached to a tuberculin syringe. The vitreous specimen should be obtained before turning on the infusion during vitrectomy to obtain an undiluted specimen. After entering the sclerotomy made 3 mm posterior to the limbus and directing the vitrectomy instrument tip into the midvitreous, automated cutting is engaged with gentle aspiration on the 3-mL syringe by the assistant. A total of 0.3 mL of vitreous specimen is adequate for vitreous culture and provision of space for the injection of intravitreal antibiotics with a 30-gauge needle, using the same sclerotomy site.

After obtaining this undiluted vitreous sample, the assistant should directly inoculate the specimen onto blood agar, chocolate agar, brain-heart infusion, and Sabouraud media or broth, and inject into thioglycolate broth. Material is also placed onto two glass slides which are sent immediately to the microbiology lab for Gram and Giemsa staining.

PARS PLANA VITRECTOMY. Vitreous taps may be performed with local anesthesia but if an extensive procedure is contemplated by the surgeon, then general anesthesia may be preferred because of the difficulty of obtaining adequate local anesthesia in the inflamed and painful eye. Local anesthesia is preferred in those situations when the patient's medical condition precludes the use of general anesthetic.

In most cases the vitrectomy will be carried out in a standard three port fashion. The conjunctiva is first incised to allow sclerotomy sites to be placed in the clock hours above and below the lateral rectus and above the medial rectus. The conjunctiva covering the wound should not be disturbed if possible. A wound leak or wound instability is repaired with interrupted 9-0 or 10-0 monofilament suture. A technical problem that initially confronts the surgeon is placement of the infusion cannula. Because the incision and placement of the infusion port is easier in a firm globe, it may be worthwhile to secure an inferotemporal port with a suture initially. It is important to visualize the port inside the eye either by shining the illumination probe through the cornea or by examination with the indirect ophthalmoscope. If the infusion port cannot be visualized, this infusion should not be turned on until clearance of opacity of the media allows verification of its position. Some surgeons prefer to add epinephrine to the infusate to help control intraoperative bleeding.

The clarity of the cornea and anterior chamber as well as the presence of the crystalline lens or a pseudophakos determines the first incision into the eye. The iris and central anterior vitreous are often impossible to visualize adequately because of corneal epithelial edema and folds, and the presence of significant amounts of anterior chamber fibrin and hypopyon. To clear the anterior chamber, initial incisions may be made in the limbus at approximately the 9:30- and 2:30-o'clock positions, modifying the location as necessary, depending on the presence of a previous surgical wound and presence of a filtering bleb. Through these incisions, an angled 20- through 27- gauge needle may be used to irrigate the anterior chamber while using the vitrectomy probe through the other incision to clear the anterior chamber of debris. This approach allows the intraocular pressure to be maintained at a constant level and reduces the chance for hemorrhage while making passage of the instruments into the limbal incisions easier.

An inflammatory membrane often extends over the lens or intraocular lens onto the surface of the iris. This membrane should be removed from the surface of the lens for better visualization of the posterior segment. It may be initially incised with a myringotomy blade or other sharp instrument, and then elevated for removal with a cutting instrument. Alternatively, it may be engaged with a hooked needle and rolled onto the needle to clear the visual axis.[116] Removal of the inflammatory membrane from the surface of the crystalline lens should begin over the iris, close to the pupillary border, if it is thought that the lens can be spared. Often, however, the lens in phakic eyes may be removed because of poor visualization of the internal structures and poor dilation of the pupil.

The anterior chamber may also be cleared by means of a posterior approach by making a peripheral iridectomy from the posterior side with the cutting instrument and entering the anterior chamber with the instrument. Suction of debris is easily accomplished with this method, but there is not great flexibility to manipulate fibrin membranes. In severe cases, the cornea and anterior chamber may become totally opaque. The initial approach in these eyes may be to remove a central corneal button and then proceed with an open sky vitrectomy followed by suturing in a donor corneal button.

Removal of an intraocular lens is not necessary to attain a bacteriologic cure of endophthalmitis, and the lens should be left in position if at all possible. Occasionally, interruption of capsular support during the procedure causes a partial dislocation, which may be managed with fixation sutures.

The pupil is usually midposition or smaller in infected eyes, adding to the problem of creating a adequate posterior view. During the anterior chamber lavage, synechiae between the pupil and lens may be opened by inserting a spatula between iris and lens to break the adherence. If the pupil remains unacceptably small, a sector iridectomy may be created with the cutting port, although bleeding often occurs. Other alternatives are to use pupil sutures to enlarge the pupil or to insert iris tacks through the limbus in positions where it is not compromised by previous surgery.

Once the anterior vitreous is easily seen, a pars plana incision 3.5 mm from the limbus is created. Material for culture and stain should be obtained from the eye early in the case as described in the previous section. If indicated, and providing the visualization is adequate, the surgeon may elect to perform a complete core vitrectomy. The objective of surgery is to remove as much vitreous as possible with safety. The central vitreous cavity is first cleared of vitreous debris followed by removal of pockets of more heavily infiltrated peripheral vitreous. Aggressive removal of infiltrated vitreous in the basal area should be discouraged because this can result in retinal tears owing to traction on inflamed peripheral retina. Because of difficulty with visibility, however, more than a core vitrectomy is frequently impossible. Surgery is easiest when there is a complete posterior vitreous detachment. If the vitreous remains attached posteriorly, attempts to remove it may create retinal breaks. In those eyes with a posterior vitreous detachment, one often finds a white mound of inflammatory debris lying over the posterior pole region. If this mound proves to be solid and adherent, it is unwise to attempt to remove large portions. However, if the material is flocculent and unorganized, attempts at removal with gentle suction using a passive vacuum technique can sometimes be successful but should be attempted with caution only. Retinal breaks in inflamed or necrotic peripheral retina are difficult to seal and may ultimately lead to failure of the procedure. If, after clearing the anterior chamber, visibility of the posterior vitreous cavity is poor, then it is more prudent to discontinue the surgical procedure than to risk retinal damage because of poor visualization.

After a water-tight closure of the sclerostomy sites, a 30-gauge needle is inserted though one of the sites and, if possible, visualized behind the IOL. With the bevel pointed anteriorly, the intraocular antimicrobial is slowly injected; sequential injections are made when two antimicrobials are administered. Closure of the conjunctival incisions and injection of subconjunctival antibiotics conclude the surgery.

The most commonly encountered intraoperative complications include hemorrhage and retinal detachment. Anterior hemorrhages from the surgical wound site and iris root may be controlled by increasing the intraocular pressure by raising the height of the infusion level. If a point source of hemorrhage is visualized, it usually can be controlled with intraocular bipolar, unimanual diathermy. Retinal breaks are a major surgical problem. If the vitreous traction is released from the breaks, these regions can be treated with intraocular argon laser or external cryotherapy. After relieving vitreous traction, posterior breaks can be managed with gas tamponade. However, the use of gas tamponade itself makes the administration of intraocular antibiotic problematic. If the vitreous remains attached to the breaks, then one should consider a scleral buckle in addition to external cryotherapy or internal argon laser. Choroidal hemorrhaging may also occur with hypotony during the procedure, and every effort should be made to keep the intraocular pressure constant during the entire procedure. Should choroidal hemorrhage ensue, the intraocular pressure should be immediately elevated in an attempt to close the bleeding vessels.

Management of Delayed-Onset Endophthalmitis

The onset of endophthalmitis 1 week or later after surgery without a predisposing cause, such as a filtering bleb, may be due to coagulase-negative staphylococci, *P acnes*, or a host of relatively uncommon pathogens. Usually, onset during the 2nd week is a result of less virulent forms of staphylococci. *P acnes* should be suspected in cases of chronic recurrent granulomatous inflammation several months after cataract surgery with implantation of a posterior chamber intraocular lens.[117] Especially suggestive is the presence of an equatorial white capsular plaque seen with the pupil fully dilated. Findings in fungal endophthalmitis are less specific and include chronic inflammation for months after cataract surgery; vitreous inflammation may be diffuse, or the classic focal infiltrates ("fluff-balls") may be appreciated. White infiltrates may appear in the vitreous as a "string of pearls" or on the lens capsule.[10,47,85]

When the onset is late and the course of inflammation is indolent, there is often time to obtain information before initiating therapy. Antimicrobial choice varies, depending on the pathogen identified; a close working relationship with the laboratory technicians is important so that they may take special measures for identification of the suspected organisms. An outpatient tap of the eye as described earlier may be helpful in establishing the diagnosis by culture, although obtaining the vitreous sample by vitrectomy may be preferable.[47] Proper management of the specimens for stain and culture is critically important because therapy is significantly different for some of the possible pathogens. Specimens obtained should be directly inoculated onto solid anaerobic media as well as in thioglycolate broth to identify *P acnes*, Sabouraud media for fungi, and blood and chocolate agar plates for staphylococcal and other species. The microbiology lab should be notified to hold these anaerobic cultures for a minimum of 2 weeks because the growth of *P acnes* is fastidious, and fungal growth may be slow. Giemsa and calcofluor stains for fungi may be particularly helpful in diagnosis of fungal disease. Gram stains may be useful to identify many gram-positive organisms but are rarely helpful in *P acnes* infections.[47] A surgical intervention may not be necessary until a differentiation between fungal and bacterial pathogenesis has been established.

In both fungal disease and *P acnes* infection, a pars plana vitrectomy is almost always necessary for successful management.[47,118] If a distinction has not been made between bacterial and fungal origin of the endophthalmitis, the laboratory technicians should be alerted to prepare stains immediately from material obtained during the first phase of the operation; this strategy may allow proper choice of antimicrobial agent for injection at the close of the procedure.

When the causative agent is *P acnes*, a partial capsulectomy (to include a portion of white plaque material identified) is an important goal of the surgery. The white plaque apparently sequesters viable organisms in most if not all cases. Only enough capsule is removed so that cultures can be made, and the zonular and capsular support for the intraocular lens remain.[47,118,119] If infection persists, removal of the posterior chamber intraocular lens and capsular remnants should be undertaken (using α-chymotrypsin enzyme to aid in complete removal) before insertion of a suture-fixated posterior chamber intraocular lens or an anterior chamber intraocular lens.

Intravitreal vancomycin is the antibiotic of choice for treatment of endophthalmitis caused by *P acnes*.[47,118,119] Anaerobic organisms like *P acnes* are relatively resistant to aminoglycoside antibiotics, and their use is unnecessary.

Vitrectomy is performed for therapeutic as well as diagnostic reasons for suspected fungal endophthalmitis.[47,120] At the time of vitrectomy for fungal endophthalmitis, we perform an intraocular injection of amphotericin B, 5 μg in 0.1 mL solution, without concurrent intraocular corticosteroids. Systemic therapy with intravenous amphotericin B, 0.25 to 1.0 mg/kg body weight, or oral ketoconazole, 200 to 600 mg daily, is often used based on the clinical setting,[47] but fungal endophthalmitis can be successfully managed with intravitreal therapy alone.[120] It is important to have an internist working in tandem to monitor the nephrotoxic effects of amphotericin B as well as to manage any concurrent systemic problems.

Because inflammation is chronic and indolent in these patients, postoperative management with topical corticosteroids is usually sufficient. Patients with delayed-onset endophthalmitis caused by fungi or *P acnes* have a high rate of recurrence after apparent initial successful therapy, and this will usually be manifested as a recrudescence of inflammation. Repeat cultures and antimicrobial injections are frequently necessary. A second operative procedure to remove vitreous or lens capsule harboring microbes may be necessary.

Management of Bleb-Related Endophthalmitis

In general, bleb-related endophthalmitis has a poor visual outcome, and initial vitrectomy is recommended for these cases.[48] Because of a high occurrence of cataract in the filtering bleb patients, a lensectomy is often performed at the time of vitrectomy. In some cases (particularly in phakic eyes), however, the initial infection may be confined to the anterior segment without vitreous involvement; therefore, systemic and intensive topical antibiotics may achieve good therapeutic levels in the anterior chamber and aqueous, thus curing the condition without vitrectomy surgery. The culture techniques are the same as those outlined earlier in the discussion of acute postoperative bacterial endophthalmitis.

Because of the relative resistance of the most commonly cultured organisms in bleb-related endophthalmitis to cefazolin and gentamicin, vancomycin has become the recommended antibiotic to be used intraocularly and systemically.[48]

Management of Posttraumatic Endophthalmitis

Vitrectomy is usually indicated in posttraumatic endophthalmitis because of the severity of the injuries, severity of infection, and the more adverse outcome reported in these cases.[49] Vitrectomy allows treatment of the residual intraocular effects of the trauma, such as retained lens cortex, vitreous hemorrhage, and retinal breaks as well as removal of infected vitreous, bacteria, and toxins. Culture techniques are the same as those outlined in the discussion of acute postoperative endophthalmitis and the most commonly encountered organisms include *Bacillus* sp, *Staphylococcus* sp, and rare fungal cases from retained plant or vegetable matter.

Because of the risk of *Bacillus* sp infection, vancomycin is the antibiotic of choice in acute infections for broad-spectrum coverage of gram-positive organisms; ceftazidime is added to cover gram-negative organisms. When the symptomatic onset is late and the course is indolent, a fungal etiology is likely; culturing and antimicrobial choice should reflect the most probable diagnosis.

Controversy arises regarding the management of intraocular foreign bodies vis-à-vis their risk for the development of endophthalmitis. Reported incidence data for endophthalmitis in this setting is reported in the 13% to 30% range.[50,121] Mieler and associates[122] reported that the culture was positive from aqueous, vitreous, or foreign-body specimens in 37% of eyes without clinically visible inflammation. A high index of suspicion for the development of endophthalmitis in this clinical setting is certainly justified with a relatively low threshold to consider systemic and possibly intraocular antibiotics.

Another clinical dilemma arises in the setting of posttraumatic endophthalmitis with the delivery of intraocular antibiotics in an eye requiring the use of intraocular gas for treatment of an associated retinal detachment. Traumatic endophthalmitis with retinal breaks or detachment has a poor visual prognosis; Brinton and colleagues[51] reported an anatomic failure rate of 100% in eyes with a retina break or retinal detachment. The eye is commonly filled with gas as part of the procedure to seal a retinal break or reattach the retina. Little fluid may remain in the eye, creating potential toxicity to the retina from high concentrations of antibiotic if the normal dose is injected in the gas-filled cavity. Two approaches that have been proposed are (1) use of 50% gas fill after vitrectomy and then injecting 50% of recommended doses of antibiotics,[123] (2) injecting them in their usual doses and performing a gas–fluid exchange after waiting several minutes for equilibration to occur.[124] Another option is to use antibiotics in the infusion line during the vitrectomy, although no toxicity studies have been performed exposing the detached retina, particularly the photoreceptors, to otherwise safe concentrations of antimicrobials.

POSTOPERATIVE MANAGEMENT AND COMPLICATIONS OF SURGERY

General Considerations

Patients usually have a dramatic improvement in ocular pain by the 1st postoperative day after the management outlined earlier. Narcotics are often used in the postoperative period but should be used judiciously because progressive reduction in pain can be used to monitor resolution of the infectious process.

Preliminary culture results are sometimes available 24 hours after surgery with a complete report 48 hours after the specimen is obtained. Once this information is available, the antibiotic therapy may be appropriately modified. If only staphylococci are identified, for example, coverage for gram-negative organisms may be discontinued. Systemic antibiotics are usually given for 2 to 7 days postoperatively depending on the response of the eye clinically and the bacteria identified. Drops are also used in fortified concentrations pending the culture and sensitivity results from the microbiology laboratory. Frequent topical application is particularly indicated with infected blebs and suture abscesses. Clinical and laboratory studies show that failure to sterilize the vitreous cavity after a single injection is not an uncommon problem. In 22 of 42 consecutive culture-positive eyes that were retapped, 12 (54%) were, indeed, culture positive.[125] Driebe and coworkers[14] cultured 18 eyes after intraocular antibiotic injection and found six positive cultures. Stern and colleagues[126] reported five patients with persistent infection after a single antibiotic injection.[126] Irvine and colleagues[44] found 14 culture- positive results in 19 retaps performed on 53 eyes with gram-negative endophthalmitis. Aguilar and associates[57] demonstrated 25% culture positivity 48 hours after intraocular injection of vancomycin or cefazolin in experimental *S aureus* endophthalmitis. The failure of a single injection of antibiotic to sterilize the intraocular space may be attributable to (1) lack of sensitivity of the organism to the initial choice of antibiotic, (2) slow growth rate of the organism (eg, *P acnes* and fungi), (3) delay in delivery of intraocular antibiotics (heavy inoculum), and (4) rapid clearance of the antibiotics injected in eyes that have undergone vitrectomy.

Reinjection of antibiotics can be considered after the first 48 hours if (1) the initial culture sensitivities show that the organism is resistant to the antibiotic originally injected; (2) the eye appears to respond poorly to the initial treatment; or (3) in eyes infected with *Streptococci*, gram-negative organisms, *P acnes*, or fungi.[108,109,125]

Control of inflammation is essential to success particularly in severer cases. Frequent topical steroids are almost always employed. Beginning systemic corticosteroids either simultaneously with initiation of antimicrobial therapy or within the first several days afterward is often indicated.

Complications of Surgery

The cornea is often edematous in the early postoperative period and the epithelial edema clears before the stromal edema during the ensuing weeks. The frequent administration of fortified topical medications also may cause corneal epithelial toxicity, requiring some modification in the antibiotic selection and dosing regimen. Pigmented cells may be seen on the posterior surface of the cornea for months after surgery for endophthalmitis.

More common than an elevated intraocular pressure is persistent hypotony postoperatively, even in the face of a sterile vitreous cavity. The hypotonous eye may demonstrate the presence of choroidal detachments on ultrasonography. The persistence of hypotony should prompt a search for a persistent wound leak and aggressive control of the inflammatory process.

Anterior segment inflammation may persist for weeks after successful surgery, and often flare is more prominent than cells. The persistence of bacterial endotoxins (in gram-negative infections) and exotoxins (in gram-positive infections) can result in the recurrence of anterior segment fibrin and cells within 24 hours of complete vitrectomy. We have found that injection of 0.05 to 0.10 mL of 10 μg/mL tissue plasminogen activator intracamerally at the slit lamp in the postoperative period has been useful in particularly severe cases to clear the fibrin clots. If there is evidence of persistence or worsening of the anterior segment inflammation despite aggressive medical management, then one should consider retapping the vitreous cavity with intraocular antibiotic injection or repeat vitrectomy surgery. Postoperatively, there may be the development of a cataract or persistence of opacities of the vitreous that interfere with vision. If the cataract and opacities interfere with an ophthalmoscopic evaluation of the retina, then ultrasound should be employed to follow the status of the posterior segment. Pars plana vitrectomy may be considered later for rehabilitation of vision in eyes with persistent opacity of the vitreous. Cataract extraction in phakic eyes may also be considered once inflammation has resolved.

Retinal detachment occurring soon after surgery is the most feared complication of surgery in endophthalmitis and is associated with a poor visual prognosis in most clinical series.[41,127] These eyes are at increased risk for the development of proliferative vitreoretinopathy and sympathetic ophthalmia has also been reported.[50,127,128]

As discussed earlier, a small percentage of eyes injected with aminoglycosides at surgery have been noted to develop vascular occlusion in the posterior pole. Macular infarction and poor vision result.[29,30,71]

VISUAL RESULTS

Although reported clinical series are difficult to compare, there has been a trend toward improvement in the clinical outcomes of treatment for postoperative endophthalmitis during the past decade. Factors important in this trend include (1) higher incidence of endophthalmitis produced by less virulent organisms,[1] (2) earlier diagnosis and treatment, (3) widespread acceptance of the use of intravitreal antibiotic therapy, (4) improved techniques and instrumentation in vitrectomy surgery, and (5) administration of corticosteroids to control inflammation.

The difficulties in comparing the reported series arise from the numerous variables involved. Most series mix endophthalmitis cases of differing causes (postoperative, traumatic, and endogenous) and include multiple organisms of differing virulence. The indications and timing for vitrectomy surgery differ from one series to another, and there is no uniformity in antibiotic selection or routes of administration.[29] Finally, the definition of success varies in the different series reported. However, the achievement of 20/400 posttreatment vision is a commonly used outcome measure.

Of the prognostic factors evaluated in outcome studies, the most important factor appears to be the virulence of the infecting organism. In culture-negative cases, 53% to 94% of eyes obtain at least 20/400 vision[14,109,129]; for *S epidermidis*, 65% to 91%[40–43,130]; for *P acnes* or fungal (*Candida*) endophthalmitis, 75% to 89%[47,119,120]; and for gram-negative and streptococcal endophthalmitis, 25% to 50%.[44,48,131,132] Salvage of useful vision is almost never reported for those cases involving *P aeruginosa* or *Bacillus* sp (Table 18-5).[52,54,114,133]

Another prognostic factor of importance is the time to onset of treatment after symptoms begin. Delays of more than 24 to 36 hours are associated with a worse visual outcome.[134,135] Animal models of Pseudomonas endophthalmitis demonstrated a reduced ability of antimicrobial agents to sterilize the vitreous cavity when injected more than 24 hours after onset of infection.[136]

The visual acuity at initial presentation also correlates with visual prognosis after treatment. Of those cases with initial visual acuities of 20/400 or better, 87% had maintained this level of vision after treatment; of those with light-perception initial vision, 21% improved to visual acuities of 20/400 or better.

Table 18-5
Endophthalmitis Treatment Results Percentage 20/400 or Better

CULTURE RESULTS	ROWSEY AND COWORKERS[106] (1982)	DRIEBE AND ASSOCIATES[14] (1986)	OLSON AND COLLEAGUES[109] (1983)	ORMEROD AND COWORKERS[45] (1983)	IRVINE AND COLLEAGUES[44] (1993)	MAO AND ASSOCIATES[132] (1992)
Negative	53	94	91			
Staphylococcus epidermidis	65	78	64	69		
S. aureus	25	64	43			
Streptococci		40	25			31
Gram negative		40	50		49	

Posttraumatic endophthalmitis and cases with proliferative vitreoretinopathy have worse visual prognoses.[49,114]

FUTURE DIRECTIONS

Prompt clinical recognition in conjunction with improved rapid laboratory diagnostic techniques should help in the initial management and antibiotic selection in cases of postoperative endophthalmitis. The proper role and timing of vitrectomy should be further defined; results of the EVS will play an important role.

In the future, improvements in our understanding of antibiotic pharmacokinetics and improved antibiotic spectra will likely result in more optimal treatment of postoperative endophthalmitis and improvement in visual results. Studies of ocular toxicity with new antibiotics will allow selection of drugs with better therapeutic ratios for intraocular injection. Prolonging intravitreal antimicrobial activity by developing delivery systems involving liposomes or synthetic polymers may simplify and improve drug therapy. Studies of newer antibiotics with better intraocular penetration after intravenous administration should improve the management of these difficult cases. The necessity for reinjection, potential toxicity of reinjection of various antibiotics, and the proper timing of reinjections require additional study as well. We will need further information concerning the role of corticosteroids in the management of endophthalmitis, and defining the optimal route and timing for its administration. Other agents and methods to control intraocular inflammation may also find a place in the treatment armamentarium.

Acknowledgment

Preparation of this chapter was supported in part by National Eye Institute grant RO 1 EY 05794-04A1.

References

1. Kattan HM, Flynn HW, Pflugfelder SC, et al. Nosocomial endophthalmitis survey: current incidence of infection following intraocular surgery. Ophthalmology 1991;98:227.
2. Javitt JC, Vitale S, Canner JK, et al. National outcomes of cataract extraction: endophthalmitis following inpatient surgery. Arch Ophthalmol 1991;109:1085.
3. Allen HF, Mangiaracine AB. Bacterial endophthalmitis after cataract extraction. II. Incidence in 36,000 consecutive operations with special reference to preoperative topical antibiotics. Tran Am Acad Ophthalmol Otolaryngol 1973;77:581.
4. Boes DA, Lindquist TD, Fritsche TR, et al. Effects of povidone-iodine chemical preparation and saline irrigation on the perilimbal flora. Ophthalmology 1992;99:1569.
5. Walker CB, Claoue CMP. Incidence of conjunctival colonization by bacteria capable of causing postoperative endophthalmitis. J R Soc Med 1986;79:520.
6. Speaker MG, Menikoff JA. Prophylaxis of endophthalmitis with topical povidone-iodine. Ophthalmology 1991;98:1769.
7. Sherwood DR, Rich WJ, Jacob SJ, et al. Bacterial contamination of intraocular and extraocular fluids during cataract extraction. Eye 1989;3:308.
8. Dickey JB, Thompson KD, Jay WM. Anterior chamber aspirate cultures after uncomplicated cataract surgery. Am J Ophthalmol 1991;112:278.

9. Cohen SM, Benner JC, Landers MB, et al. Intraocular fluid cultures after primary pars plana vitrectomy. Am J Ophthalmol 1992;114:697.
10. Stern WH, Tamura E, Jacobs RA, et al. Epidemic postsurgical *Candida parapsilosis* endophthalmitis: clinical findings and management of 15 consecutive cases. Ophthalmology 1985;92:1701.
11. O'Day DM. Value of a centralized surveillance system during a national epidemic of endophthalmitis. Ophthalmology 1985;92:309.
12. Pettit TH, Olson RJ, Foos RY, et al. Fungal endophthalmitis following intraocular lens implantation: a surgical epidemic. Arch Ophthalmol 1980;98:1025.
13. Cameron JA, Antonios SR, Cotter JB, et al. Endophthalmitis from contaminated donor corneas following penetrating keratoplasty. Arch Ophthalmol 1991;109:54.
14. Driebe WT Jr, Mandelbaum S, Forster RK, et al. Pseudophakic endophthalmitis: diagnosis and management. Ophthalmology 1986;93:442.
15. Lindstrom RL, Doughman DJ. Bacterial endophthalmitis associated with vitreous wick. Ann Ophthalmol 1979;11:1775.
16. Confino J, Brown SI. Bacterial endophthalmitis associated with exposed monofilament sutures following corneal transplantation. Am J Ophthalmol 1985;99:111.
17. Gelender H. Infectious endophthalmitis following cutting of sutures after cataract surgery. Am J Ophthalmol 1982;94:528.
18. Heilskov T, Joondeph BC, Olsen KR. Late endophthalmitis after transscleral fixation of a posterior chamber intraocular lens. Arch Ophthalmol 1989;107:1427.
19. Meredith TA, Trabelsi A, Miller MJ, et al. Spontaneous sterilization of experimental *Staphylococcus epidermidis* endophthalmitis. Invest Ophthalmol Vis Sci. 1990;31:181.
20. Menikoff JA, Speaker MG, Marmor M, et al. A case-control study of risk factors for post-operative endophthalmitis. Ophthalmology 1991;98:1761.
21. Maylath FR, Leopold IH. Study of experimental intraocular infection. I. The recoverability of organisms, inoculated into ocular tissues and fluids. II. The influence of antibiotics and cortisone, alone and combined, on intraocular growth of these organisms. Am J Ophthalmology 1955;40:86.
22. Verbraeken H, Rysslerlaere M. Bacteriological study of 92 cases of proven infectious endophthalmitis treated with pars plana vitrectomy. Ophthalmologica 1991;203:17.
23. Raskin E, Speaker M, Pelton-Herior K, et al. Polypropylene haptics increase bacterial adherence to intraocular lenses. (Abstract) Invest Ophthalmol Vis Sci 1992;33:1420.
24. Apt L, Isenberg SJ, Yoshimori R. Outpatient topical use of povidone-iodine in preparing the eye for surgery. Ophthalmology 1989;96:289.
25. Speaker MG, Milch FA, Shah MK. Role of external bacterial flora in the pathogenesis of acute postoperative endophthalmitis. Ophthalmology 1991;98: 639.
26. Wenzel RP. Preoperative antibiotic prophylaxis. N Engl J Med 1992;326:337.
27. Classen DC, Evans RS, Pestotnik SL, et al. The timing of prophylactic administration of antibiotics and the risk of surgical wound infection. N Engl J Med 1992;326:281.
28. Starr MB. Prophylactic antibiotics for ophthalmic surgery. Surv Ophthalmol 1983;27:353.
29. Campochiaro PA, Conway BP. Aminoglycoside toxicity: a survey of retinal specialists. Arch Ophthalmol 1991;109:946.
30. Campochiaro PA, Lin JI, Aminoglycoside Study Group. Aminoglycoside toxicity in the treatment of endophthalmitis. Arch Ophthalmol 1994;112:48.
31. Christy NE, Lall P. Postoperative endophthalmitis following cataract surgery: effects of subconjunctival antibiotics and other factors. Arch Ophthalmol 1973;90:361.
32. Christy NE, Sommer A. Antibiotic prophylaxis of postoperative endophthalmitis. Ann Ophthalmol 1979;11:1261.
33. Chalkley THF, Shoch D. An evaluation of prophylactic subconjunctival antibiotic injection in cataract surgery. Am J Ophthalmol 1967;64:1084.
34. Shockley RK, Fishman P, Aziz M, et al. Subconjunctival administration of ceftazidime in pigmented rabbit eyes. Arch Ophthalmol 1986;104:266.
35. Elliott RD, Katz HR. Inhibition of pseudophakic endophthalmitis in a rabbit model. Ophthalmic Surg 1987;1987:538.
36. Parks DJ, Cyryin AS, Sarfarazi FA, et al. Subconjunctival ciprofloxacin inhibits pseudophakic endophthalmitis in a rabbit model. Invest Ophthalmol Vis Sci 1991;34(Suppl 4):706.
37. Barza M. Factors affecting the intraocular penetration of antibiotics. The influence of route, inflammation, animal species and tissue pigmentation. Scan J Infect Dis 1978;14(Suppl):151.
38. Meredith TA. Prevention of postoperative infection. (Editorial) Arch Ophthalmol 1991;109:944.
39. Irvine WE, Flynn HW, Murray TG, et al. Retained lens fragments after phacoemulsification manifesting as marked intraocular inflammation with hypopyon. Am J Ophthalmol 1992;114:610.
40. Bode DD Jr, Gelender H, Forster RK. A retrospective review of endophthalmitis due to coagulase-negative staphylococci. Br J Ophthalmol 1985;69:915.
41. Ficker LA, Meredith TA, Wilson LA, et al. The role of

vitrectomy in *Staphylococcus epidermitis* endophthalmitis. Br J Ophthalmol 1987;72:386.
42. Weber DJ, Hoffman KL, Thoft RA, et al. Endophthalmitis following intraocular lens implantation: report of 30 cases and review of the literature. Rev Infect Dis 1986;8:12.
43. Ormerod LD, Ho DD, Becker LE, et al. Endophthalmitis caused by the coagulase-negative staphylococci. I. Disease spectrum and outcome. Ophthalmology 1993;100:715.
44. Irvine WD, Flynn HW Jr, Miller D, et al. Endophthalmitis caused by gram negative organisms. Arch Ophthalmol 1993;110:1450.
45. Ormerod LD, Becker LE, Cruise RJ. Endophthalmitis caused by the coagulase-negative staphylococci. II. Factors influencing presentation after cataract surgery. Ophthalmology 1993;100:724.
46. Ficker L, Meredith TA, Wilson LA, et al. Chronic bacterial endophthalmitis. Am J Ophthalmol 1987;103:745.
47. Fox GM, Joondeph BC, Flynn HW. Delayed-onset pseudophakic endophthalmitis. Am J Ophthalmol 1991;111:163.
48. Mandelbaum S, Forster RK, Gelender H, et al. Late onset endophthalmitis associated with filtering blebs. Ophthalmology 1985;92:964.
49. Affeldt JC, Flynn HW Jr, Forster RK, et al. Microbial endophthalmitis resulting from ocular trauma. Ophthalmology 1987;94:407.
50. Boldt HC, Pulido JS, Blodi CS, et al. Rural endophthalmitis. Ophthalmology 1989;96:1722.
51. Brinton GS, Topping TM, Hyndiuk RA, et al. Posttraumatic endophthalmitis. Arch Ophthalmol 1984;102:547.
52. Davey RT Jr, Tauber WB. Posttraumatic endophthalmitis: the emerging role of *Bacillus cereus* infection. Rev Infect Dis 1987;9:110.
53. Hamady R, Zaltas M, Paton B. Bacillus-induced endophthalmitis: new series of 10 cases and review of the literature. Br J Ophthalmol 1990;74:26.
54. O'Day DM, Smith RS, Gregg CR, et al. The problem of *Bacillus* species infection with special emphasis on the virulence of *Bacillus cereus.* Ophthalmology 1981;88:833.
55. Stern GA, Engel HM, Driebe WT Jr. The treatment of postoperative endophthalmitis: results of differing approaches to treatment. Ophthalmology 1988;96:62.
56. Cottingham AJ Jr, Forster RK. Vitrectomy in endophthalmitis: results of study using vitrectomy, intraocular antibiotics, or a combination of both. Arch Ophthalmol 1976;94:2078.
57. Aguilar HE, Meredith TA, Drews CD, et al. Treatment of experimental *S. aureus* endophthalmitis with vancomycin, cetazolin, and corticosteroids. Invest Ophthalmol Vis Sci. 1990;31(Suppl):308.
58. Leopold IH. Management of intraocular infection. Trans Ophthalmol Soc UK 1971;91:575.
59. Barza M, Kane A, Baum J. Oxacillin for bacterial endophthalmitis: subconjunctival, intravenous, both, or neither? Invest Ophthalmol Vis Sci 1980;19:1348.
60. Barza M, Kane A, Baum J. Ocular penetration of subconjunctival oxacillin, methicillin, and cefazolin in rabbits with *Staphylococcal* endophthalmitis. J Infect Dis 1982;145:899.
61. Barza M, Lynch E, Baum JL. Pharmacokinetics of newer cephalosporins after subconjunctival and intravitreal injection in rabbits. Arch Ophthalmol 1993;111:121.
62. Von Sallmann L, Meyer K, DiGrandi J. Experimental study on penicillin treatment of ectogenous infection of vitreous. Arch Ophthalmol 1944;32:179.
63. Leopold IH, Scheie HG. Studies with microcrystalline sulfathiazole. Arch Ophthalmol 1943;29:811.
64. Leopold IH. Intravitreal penetration of penicillin and penicillin therapy of infections of the vitreous. Arch Ophthalmol 1945;33:211.
65. Baum J, Peyman GA, Barza M. Intravitreal administration of antibiotic in the treatment of bacterial endophthalmitis. III. Consensus. Surv Ophthalmol 1982;26:204.
66. Peyman GA. Aminoglycoside toxicity. Arch Ophthalmol 1992;110:446.
67. Doft BH. The endophthalmitis vitrectomy study. Arch Ophthalmol 1991;198:487.
68. Pavan PR, Brinser JH. Exogenous bacterial endophthalmitis treated without systemic antibiotics. Am J Ophthalmol 1987;104:121.
69. Meredith TA. Antimicrobial pharmacokinetics in endophthalmitis treatment: studies of ceftazidime. Trans Am Ophthalmol Soc 1994.
70. Gardner S. Treatment of bacterial endophthalmitis. III. Ocular Ther Manag 1991;2:14.
71. Conway BP, Campochiaro PA. Macular infarction after endophthalmitis treated with vitrectomy and intravitreal gentamicin. Arch Ophthalmol 1986; 104:367.
72. Conway BP, Tabatabay CA, Campochiaro PA, et al. Gentamicin toxicity in the primate retina. Arch Ophthalmol 1989;107:107.
73. O'Day DM, Head WS, Robinson RD, et al. Intraocular penetration of systemically administered antifungal agents. Curr Eye Res 1985;4:131.
74. Kane A, Barza M, Baum J. Penetration of ocular tissues and fluids by moxalactam in rabbits with staphylococcal endophthalmitis. Antimicrob Agents Chemother 1981;20:595.
75. Martin DF, Ficker LA, Aguilar HA, et al. Vitreous cefazolin levels after intravenous injection: effects of inflammation, repeated antibiotic doses, and surgery. Arch Ophthalmol 1990;108:411.
76. Keren G, Alhalel A, Bartov E. The intravitreal penetra-

tion of orally administered ciprofloxacin in humans. Invest Ophthalmol Vis Sci 1991;32:2388.

77. El Baba FZ, Trousdale MD, Gauderman WJ, et al. Intravitreal penetration of oral ciprofloxacin in humans. Ophthalmology 1992;99:483.
78. Barza M. Antibacterial agents in the treatment of ocular infections. Infectious Dis Clin North Am 1989;3:533.
79. Maurice DM. Injection of drugs into the vitreous body. In: Leopold IJ, Burns RP, eds. Symposium on ocular therapy, vol 9. New York, Wiley, 1976:59.
80. Maurice DM, Mishima S. Ocular pharmacokinetics. In: Sears ML, ed. Pharmacology of the eye. New York, Springer-Verlag, 1984:19.
81. Doft BH, Weiskopf J, Nillson-Ehle I, et al. Amphotericin clearance in vitrectomized versus non-vitrectomized eyes. Ophthalmology 1985;92:1601.
82. Mandell BA, Meredith TA, Aguilar E, et al. Amikacin levels after intravitreal injection. Am J Ophthalmol 1993;115:770.
83. Campochiaro PA, Green WR. Toxicity of intravitreal ceftazidime in primate retina. Arch Ophthalmol 1992;110:1625.
84. DeVaro JM, Donahue SP, Jewart BH, et al. Are aminoglycosides necessary in the empiric therapy of bacterial endophthalmitis? Invest Ophthalmol Vis Sci 1992;33(Suppl):746.
85. Pflugfelder SC, Hernandez E, Fleisler SJ, et al. Intravitreal vancomycin. Arch Ophthalmol 1987;105:831.
86. Flynn HW, Pulido JS, Pflugfelder SC. Endophthalmitis therapy: changing antibiotic sensitivity patterns and current therapeutic recommendations. Arch Ophthalmol 1991;109:175.
87. Smith MA, Sorenson JA, Lowy FD. Treatment of experimental methicillin-resistant *Staphylococcus epidermidis* endophthalmitis with intravitreal vancomycin. Ophthalmology 1986;93:1328.
88. D'Amico DJ, Libert J, Kenyon KR. Comparative toxicity of intravitreal aminoglycoside antibiotics. Am J Ophthalmol 1985;100:264.
89. Talamo JH, D'Amico DJ, Hanninen LA. The influence of aphakia and vitrectomy on experimental retinal toxicity of aminoglycoside antibiotic. Am J Ophthalmol. 1985;100:840.
90. Rubinstein E, Goldfarb J, Keren G, et al. The penetration of gentamicin into the vitreous humor in man. Invest Ophthalmol Vis Sci 1983;24:637.
91. Lietman PS. Aminoglycosides and spectinomycin: aminocyclitols. In: Mandell GL, Douglas GR, Bennett JE, eds. Principles and practice of infectious disease, ed 3. New York, Churchill Livingstone, 1990:269.
92. Slana VS, Marchese AL, Jay WM. Ocular toxicity of intravitreal ciprofloxacin injection in pigmented rabbit eyes. Invest Ophthalmol Vis Sci 1992;33:727.
93. Lebel MH, Freij BJ, Syrogiannopoulous GA, et al. Dexamethasone therapy for bacterial meningitis: results of two double-blind, placebo-controlled trials. N Engl J Med 1988;319:964.
94. McCracken GH Jr, Lebel MH. Dexamethasone therapy for bacterial meningitis in infants and children. Am J Dis Child 1989;143:287.
95. Baum JL, Barza M, Lugar J, et al. The effect of corticosteroids in the treatment of experimental bacterial endophthalmitis. Am J Ophthalmol 1975;80:513.
96. Graham RO, Peyman GA. Intravitreal injection of dexamethasone: treatment of experimentally induced endophthalmitis. Arch Ophthalmol 1974;92:149.
97. Meredith TA, Aguilar HE, Trabelsi A, et al. Comparative treatment of experimental staphylococcus epidermidis endophthalmitis. Arch Ophthalmol 1990; 108:857.
98. Speaker MG, Menikoff JA. Postoperative endophthalmitis: pathogenesis, prophylaxis, and management. Int Ophthalmol Clin 1993;33:51.
99. Flynn HW, Pflugfelder SC, Culbertson WW. Recognition, treatment, and prevention of endophthalmitis. Semin Ophthalmol 1989;4:69.
100. Coats ML, Peyman GA. Intravitreal corticosteroids in the treatment of exogenous fungal endophthalmitis. Retina 1992;12:46.
101. Peyman GA, Herbst R. Bacterial endophthalmitis: treatment with intraocular injection of gentamicin and dexamethasone. Arch Ophthalmol 1974;91:416.
102. Maxwell DP, Brent BD, Diamond JG, et al. Effect of intravitreal dexamethasone on ocular histopathology in a rabbit model of endophthalmitis. Ophthalmology 1991;98:1370.
103. Meredith TA, Aguilar HE, Drews CD, et al. Intraocular dexamethasone produces a harmful effect in the treatment of experimental *S. aureus* endophthalmitis. Invest Ophthalmol Vis Sci 1990;.
104. Kwak HW, D'Amico DJ. Evaluation of the retinal toxicity and pharmacokinetics of dexamethasone after intravitreal injection. Arch Ophthalmol 1992;110: 259.
105. Diamond JG. Intraocular management of endophthalmitis: a systemic approach. Arch Ophthalmol 1981;99:96.
106. Rowsey JJ, Newson DL, Sexton DJ, et al. Endophthalmitis current approaches. Ophthalmology 1982;89:1055.
107. Peyman GA. Management of infectious endophthalmitis. Ophthalmology 1980;87:313.
108. Forster RK, Abbott RL, Gelender H. Management of infectious endophthalmitis. Ophthalmology 1980;87:313.
109. Olson JC, Flynn WH Jr, Forster RK, et al. Results in the treatment of postoperative endophthalmitis. Ophthalmology 1983;90:692.
110. Talley AR, D'Amico DJ, Talamo JH. The role of vitrectomy in the treatment of postoperative bacterial endophthalmitis. Arch Ophthalmol 1987;104/5:1699.

111. Forster RK. Endophthalmitis: diagnostic cultures and visual results. Arch Ophthalmol 1974;92:387.
112. Forster RK. Etiology and diagnosis of bacterial postoperative endophthalmitis. Ophthalmology 1978;85:320.
113. Allansmith MR, Anderson RP, Butterworth M. The meaning of preoperative cultures in ophthalmology. Trans Am Acad Ophthalmol Otolaryngol 1969;73:683.
114. Bohigian GM, Olk RJ. Factors associated with a poor visual result in endophthalmitis. Am J Ophthalmol 1986;101:332.
115. Donahue SP, Kowalski RP, Jewart BH, et al. Vitreous cultures in suspected endophthalmitis. Ophthalmology 1993;100:452.
116. Friberg TR. En bloc removal of inflammatory fibrocellular membranes from the iris surface in endophthalmitis. Arch Ophthalmol 1991;109:736.
117. Meisler DM, Zakov ZN, Bruner WE, et al. Endophthalmitis associated with sequestered intraocular *Propionibacterium acnes.* Am J Ophthalmol 1987;104:428.
118. Winward KE, Pflugfelder SC, Flynn HW Jr, et al. Postoperative *Propionibacterium* endophthalmitis: Treatment strategies and long-term results. Ophthalmology 1993;100:447.
119. Zambrano W, Flynn HW, Pflugfelder SC. Management options for *Propionibacterium acnes* endophthalmitis. Ophthalmology 1989;96:1100.
120. Brod RD, Flynn HW, Clarkson JG. Endogenous *Candida* endophthalmitis: management without intravenous amphotericin B. Ophthalmology 1990;97:666.
121. Williams DF, Meiler WF, Abrams GW, et al. Results and prognostic factors in penetrating ocular injuries with retained intraocular foreign bodies. Ophthalmology 1988;95:911.
122. Mieler WF, Ellis MK, Williams DF, et al. Retained intraocular foreign bodies and endophthalmitis. Ophthalmology 1990;97:1532.
123. Mieler WF, Glazer LC, Bennett SR, et al. Favorable outcome of traumatic endophthalmitis with associated retinal breaks or detachment. Can J Ophthalmol 1992;27:348.
124. Bauman WC, D'Amico DJ. Surgical techniques in diagnosis and management of suspected endophthalmitis. Int Ophthalmol Clin 1992;32:113.
125. Shaarawy A, Grand MG, Meredith TA, et al. Persistent infection after intravitreal antibimicrobial therapy. 1994 (in press).
126. Stern GA, Engel HM, Driebe WT. Recurrent postoperative endophthalmitis. Cornea 1990;9:102.
127. Nelsen PT, Marcus DA, Bovino JA. Retinal detachment following endophthalmitis. Ophthalmology 1985;92:1112.
128. Croxatto JO, Galentine P, Cupples HP, et al. Sympathetic ophthalmia after pars plana vitrectomy-lensectomy for endogenous bacterial endophthalmitis. Am J Ophthalmol 1981;91:342.
129. Forster RK, Zachary IG, Cottingham AJ Jr, et al. Further observations on the diagnosis, cause, and treatment of endophthalmitis. Am J Ophthalmol 1976;81:52.
130. Nobe JR, Gomez DR, Liggett P. Post-traumatic and postoperative endophthalmitis: a comparison of visual outcomes. Br J Ophthalmol 1987;71:614.
131. Mandelbaum S, Forster RK. Endophthalmitis associated with filtering blebs. Int Ophthalmol Clin 1987;27:107.
132. Mao LK, Flynn HW Jr, Miller D, et al. Endophthalmitis causes by streptococcal species. Arch Ophthalmol 1992;110:798.
133. Schemmer GB, Driebe WT. Post-traumatic *Bacillus cereus* endophthalmitis. Arch Ophthalmol 1987;105:342.
134. Laatikainen L, Tarkkanen A. Management of purulent postoperative endophthalmitis. Trans Ophthalmol Soc UK 1986;193:34.
135. Puliafito CA, Baker AS, Haaf J, et al. Infectious endophthalmitis: a review of 36 cases. Ophthalmology 1982;89:921.
136. Davey PG, Barza M, Stuart M. Dose response of experimental *Pseudomonas* endophthalmitis to ciprofloxacin, gentamicin, and imipenem: evidence for resistance to "late" treatment of infections. J Infect Dis 1987;155:518.

Ophthalmic Surgery Complications: Prevention and Management,
edited by Judie F. Charlton and George W. Weinstein.
J. B. Lippincott Company, Philadelphia © 1995.

19

Leonard Ferenz

Ethical Implications in the Practice of Ophthalmology

Ethics must be the concern of every ophthalmologist.
"Code of Ophthalmological Ethics," 1978, THE INTERNATIONAL ACADEMY OF OPHTHALMOLOGY

Competent ophthalmologic practice requires both moral and technical capacities.
"Information Statement," 1991, THE AMERICAN ACADEMY OF OPHTHALMOLOGY

The professional conduct of practitioners in the field of medicine has become the focus of sharply contested viewpoints regarding the moral responsibilities of health professionals. Some practices in the field of ophthalmology specifically have raised serious ethical concerns. Some physicians' questionable practice of performing cataract surgeries on patients whose need for it is marginal at best,[1] or of making false or misleading claims about procedures, such as radial keratotomy in advertisements,[2] are just two behaviors that many view as unethical. Other ethical matters that ophthalmology shares with medicine in general include, among others, respect for patient autonomy and human dignity, patient rights, questions of informed consent, obligations to third parties, and issues of justice in the distribution of limited health care resources.

The purpose of this chapter is to provide a general introduction to the role of ethics in medicine. It is not possible in the brief space here to explore the many ethical implications of medical practices, even if we limit ourselves to ophthalmic practices. Nor would it be possible to present and defend a comprehensive moral code of ethics in ophthalmology in this brief space. The primary task of this chapter, therefore, is to construct a more general and morally defensible framework that health care professionals, including ophthalmologists, can use to avoid and respond to the kinds of ethical problems likely to arise in their practices.

In this chapter, special attention is given to the Code of Ethics advanced by the American Academy of Ophthalmology (AAO). There are serious problems with this code that merit examination for two important reasons: first, because they are illustrative of problems of ethics in medicine generally; and second, because professionals licensed to practice ophthalmology in the United States are likely to join the academy and to be encouraged to accept the ethical guidelines offered in their Code of Ethics.[3]

Membership in the AAO is widespread with some 17,000 members and fellows. This figure exceeds the 1990 statistical figure of 16,703 ophthalmologists practicing in the United States, which was published by the American Medical Association in the 1992 publication *Physician Characteristics and Distribution in the U.S.* Therefore, newly licensed ophthalmologists will probably join the academy and consider the code of ethics.[3]

ROLE OF ETHICS IN MEDICINE

The AAO offers several of the many reasons why professionals might choose to act ethically in their practices. They suggest that ethical behavior in a profession such as ophthalmology is (1) professionally demanded, (2) personally elevating, (3) serves the best interests of patients, and (4) fulfills the sense of personal sacrifice that is characteristic of professional behavior in medicine.[4] The first two reasons offered are essentially grounded in self-interest, and the third and fourth in the interests of others. When we consider the interests of others before our own self-interest or give them equal weight with our own, we adopt what is generally regarded as the moral viewpoint. Reasons for ethical conduct that reflect this vantage point may be considered moral reasons. Thus, the academy, it would appear, is arguing for ethical behavior from the viewpoint of both self-interest and morality.

From the viewpoint of self-interest, ethical behavior in one's medical practice may indeed be prudent. For example, if persons tend to prefer doing business with those whom they regard as ethical in their business practices, then it would be prudent from the vantage point of economic self-interest (ie, it would be good business to appear ethical in one's business practices). Note, however, that it is important only that one be perceived by others as being ethical, not that one must truly be so.

Prudence might also instruct us to act ethically if we believe that our legal obligations coincide with, or are at least derived from, our ethical obligations. For example, if it were the case that the legal statutes in a given community and morality's demands were the same, then it would be prudent from the viewpoint of self-interest and compliance with the law to appear to conduct one's professional conduct ethically. As long as the demands of the law never exceed or conflict with the demands of morality, then ethical conduct could be a prudent way to avoid legal disputes and criminal liability. Ethical behavior in the effort to avoid malpractice suits would be an example of prudence in these circumstances. And, in fact, examples of this kind of prudential reasoning have appeared in journals advising members of the medical community on such nonclinical matters as how to avoid malpractice suits.[5]

From this viewpoint of self-interest and the law, however, it is not obvious why ethics should be the concern of every ophthalmologist. Indeed, it might be argued that an adequate understanding of legal requirements relating to medical practice is a sufficient warrant against both imprudent and illegal behavior. If this is the case, then it is probably the law that should be the concern of every ophthalmologist and not ethics.

There are objections to this kind of reasoning, however. From the viewpoint of self-interest, knowledge of the law alone is no guarantee against litigation and criminal liability. The right to refuse lifesaving treatment, for example, has become legally enforceable in the case of autonomous and informed refusals of treatment, though it has not always been.[6] The physician acting purely from beneficent motives to save a life during such transitional stages of the law may find himself or herself the object of personally damaging legal action. It is because of changes in the boundary between conduct that falls within the scope of the law and that which falls outside of it, that it may be prudent to look beyond the law for insurance against civil or criminal liability. If it is the case that precedents established in courts of law reflect ethical considerations not previously reflected in legal statutes, then it will, indeed, be prudent from the viewpoint of self-interest to be concerned with ethics as well as the law.

However, there is a deeper objection to the kind of reasoning that instructs us to be ethical for the sake of our own self-interest. That objection is simply that there would be no reason to behave ethically when we can get away with pretending to act ethically or when our own self-interests are better served by acting unethically. Thus, if we are to argue for ethical behavior in ophthalmic practices, our reasons must be moral reasons and not prudential ones serving self-interest.

The unique character of moral reasoning is that it forces us to consider the interests of others as equivalent and sometimes before our own self-interests. Indeed, the duties of morality are usually contrasted to the dictates of prudence and self-interest precisely because morality generally imposes obligations to promote the interests of others over one's own interests. Truth telling, for example, is a moral duty that imposes an obligation to tell the truth even though one's personal ends might be better served by lying. This does not mean that morality does not recognize duties to oneself; it does. However, the duties to oneself are generally second to the duties we have to others.

Moral reasoning in medicine especially is concerned with the duties that health professionals have toward others. In their highly instructive work on *Medical Ethics: The Moral Responsibilities of Physi-*

cians, Beauchamp and McCullough[7] suggest with others that moral principles and rules are designed to counteract the limited sympathies that individuals have for each other by directing them toward conduct that promotes the interests of others. In medicine, morality functions

> to keep things from going badly in the important interpersonal relationships intrinsic to medical practice by directing the physician to duties and virtues that promote the patient's best interests, rather than the physician's own personal interests.[7]

If this view is correct, then at least one important reason for ethical behavior in medicine is to practice those duties and virtues that promote the patient's best interests.

In many professions, and medicine especially, members of the profession are often regarded as having certain *role-specific duties* that define the special obligations that members of these professions have. We expect health care professionals, for example, to assume risks to their personal safety that we would not expect of persons generally, such as exposing themselves to the risk of infectious disease to help others in need of medical care. The duty to accept such risks is specific to the health profession; it is a special duty required of health professionals specifically.

The duty to promote the best interests of one's patients is also regarded as one of these, and sometimes the foremost of these, role-specific duties. Together, they are among the more compelling reasons for ethical behavior in a practice such as ophthalmology. Duty is not the only reason for ethical conduct, however, and it may not be the ultimate reason for it. In fact, the ultimate *reason* persons may be likely to choose to act ethically is not a reason at all but the *desire* to see good done and evil avoided.[8]

Beauchamp questions whether "it is even possible to adduce ultimate rational grounds in favor of morality" and that the "desire to see injustices rectified and human suffering reduced thus may be the deepest cause of our living moral lives."[8] The suggestion here is that it is the desire to live the moral life and not the persuasiveness of reasons that compel people to act ethically.

Although it might be a matter of great concern to some that persons choose to be ethical for the right reasons, we do not pursue that question here. It is enough that persons entering the health care profession have the desire to help others, and to do this even where it involves personal sacrifice and risk of personal injury. The purpose of our study of ethics in medicine, then, is not for the purpose of countering limited sympathies but rather for ensuring that these sympathies and good intentions are not misdirected.

Assuming, then, that we do want to be ethical in our practices, the question is how to go about it. In other words, how do we find out what the role-specific duties and moral responsibilities of health professionals are? The following are three possible options (though certainly not the only ones).

Subjective Approach to Personal Codes of Ethics

Members of many professions often think it is enough to act in a manner that they personally believe to be ethical for their conduct to be, in fact, morally correct. According to this approach, the moral responsibilities of health professionals are those recognized individually by each member of the profession. Awareness, sensitivity, and appeals to conscience, however, will not eliminate or resolve conflicts among persons equally concerned with acting ethically. The debate over abortion even among members of the health profession is a striking example of disagreement among persons—if not equally, at least enthusiastically—committed to doing what they believe is the right thing. Because of the extreme and often conflicting diversity of opinion in matters of morality, allowing each individual member of a profession to define his or her own personal code of ethics would almost certainly lead to as many different codes of ethics as there are differences of opinion. It is precisely because of disagreement at the level of personal opinion or personal intuition that the subjective approach to questions of morality is generally unacceptable.

Subscribing to Professional Codes of Ethics

Historically, health professionals have been held to a higher code of ethics, one that imposes more exacting moral obligations than those that are binding on society generally. The Hippocratic Oath is one such code.[9] Veatch provides a discussion of the Hippocratic and other Western and non-Western approaches to medical ethics.[10] The distinctive features of contemporary *professional codes of medical ethics* are (1) they are generally written by members of the profession or some specific discipline within the profession (such as ophthalmology) under the auspices of a particular institution or organization (such as the AAO); and (2) the profession itself (viz, the professional organization representing the profession) claims responsibility for adjudicating ethical disputes related to professional conduct.

Subscribing to a professional code of ethics appears to avoid at least one important criticism that we have of the subjective approach, namely, that many conflicting accounts of their moral responsibilities would arise if professionals were allowed, or encouraged, to establish their own personal codes of ethics. This alternative approach replaces the diverse and often conflicting judgments of individuals with the evaluative and normative judgments of a specific group of professionals, in this case ophthalmologists.

There are difficulties with this approach, however. Veatch[10] questions, for example, whether the "ethical and empirical judgment of doctors is a morally accurate one and whether it is in accord with the values of those outside the medical role." The concern here is that professional codes of ethics may not express a comprehensive or morally defensible viewpoint. It is possible that they might express such a view: however, there are reasons to doubt whether a segment of the population, even those closely involved with the kinds of issues that arise in their fields, are capable of constructing a medical code of ethics that reflects the moral sentiments and expectations of persons in general.

Universal Code of Medical Ethics

This third approach to matters of ethics in medicine is one that attempts to be as objective as possible, meaning not only that the perspective taken transcends the level of personal and professional opinion, but that the content of the code itself is universally accessible and verifiable. In other words, what we want is a code of ethics in medicine, and ophthalmology in particular, that is accessible to everyone and that can be confirmed by everyone.

Does such a code presently exist? In the field of ophthalmology, the answer must be "no," and it will become apparent why this is the case as we look more closely at professional codes of ethics and particularly the AAO's Code of Ethics in the following sections.

PROFESSIONAL CODES OF ETHICS

Acceptance of contemporary professional codes, such as the International Academy of Ophthalmology's (IAO's) or the AAO's Codes of Ethics, offers some distinct advantages to the practicing ophthalmologist. However, there are several criticisms of professional codes in general and the AAO's in particular. This section reviews both the merits and drawbacks of these codes.

Merits

One considerable advantage of professional codes in general is that they define what are considered within the profession to be the moral responsibilities of practitioners in the field. They do this by offering a specific set of principles and rules relating to what is regarded as ethical behavior in the profession. These guidelines also help to establish what we have called the role-specific duties of members of the professions.

An additional benefit provided specifically by the AAO is the periodic publication of advisory opinions on both clinical and nonclinical matters that pose ethical problems, such as marginally necessary or unnecessary surgery and misleading or deceptive advertising. The advisory opinions are intended to instruct the professional in the interpretation and application of the ethical guidelines presented in the AAO's Code of Ethics in these and similar real-life circumstances.

The AAO's Code of Ethics also stresses the importance of conformity to the requirements of our present legal system, insisting that "the Code is only permitted to represent standards within the law."[4] The idea here is that by confining the ethical guidelines offered in the code to standards established in the law, compliance with the code at least does not present the risk of violating the law. This is not to say that compliance with the code prevents physicians from breaking any laws pertaining to the practice of medicine but only that the guidelines themselves do not impose obligations that could lead to any apparent violations of the law. To this extent, the AAO's ethical guidelines are at least law abiding.

Professional codes in general may also be seen as promoting some uniformity in professional conduct and the manner in which ethical issues are addressed. For example, appointments to the AAO's Ethics Committee are made from among "respected ophthalmologists who will, to the extent practicable, assure that the Committee's composition is balanced as to relative age and experience and as to the emphasis of the appointees upon practice, education, research or other endeavors within ophthalmology."[3] If the evaluative judgments and opinions expressed by these committees are consistent with those we would expect of many, and perhaps most, other members of the profession, then the judgments made and guidelines offered are likely to lead to some uniformity in the professional conduct of members of the academy, which in the case of the AAO represents an overwhelming number of practicing ophthalmologists in this country. Not only might this lead to some uniformity in the way professionals treat ethical matters, but it might be seen as helping to establish a bond among professionals in the field.

Drawbacks and Criticisms

Criticisms and shortcomings of professional codes in general and the AAO's in particular are several, however. The most important ones are listed individually as follows.

Lack of Specificity and Problem-Solving Capability

Several commentators have observed that professional codes of ethics, including the AAO's, tend to be too general; therefore, they provide little guidance in specific circumstances and truly dilemmatic moral situations. Writing on ethical issues in ophthalmology, Weinstein and coauthors[11] argue that both the brevity and generality of a code of ethics, such as the AAO's "may make the principles contained in them difficult to apply in many situations." The authors suggest, for example, that "the prohibition against deceptive or misleading advertisements in the AAO Code may not help ophthalmologists decide whether particular advertisements they want to place violate the Code; they need to know specifically what kinds of statements are deceptive or misleading."[11]

General principles and rules, such as those contained in the AAO's Code of Ethics, also provide little guidance in situations presenting genuine moral dilemmas. For example, the preservation of life and the avoidance of pain and suffering are widely recognized values. It can be the case in the clinical setting, however, that these values will conflict (eg, when the preservation of life involves significant pain or suffering, such as in the treatment of cancer with chemotherapy). The dilemma occurs when these or other values are of equal importance or when two or more moral principles can be appealed to to justify opposing courses of action. In this example, both the preservation of life and the avoidance of pain are legitimate values that justify opposing course of action, treatment in the case of the former and nontreatment in the latter.

For the most part, medical practices presuppose the preeminence of the value of life and the overriding importance of the principle to preserve life. However, patients occasionally perceive this situation otherwise, such as when the avoidance of pain is valued more highly than the preservation of life or when religious convictions demand that certain medical procedures are avoided, even though this may eventuate in the loss of life (eg, refusals by Jehovah's Witnesses of lifesaving blood transfusions). In such instances, the principle of respecting the autonomy and personal integrity of individuals can conflict dramatically with the principle of preserving life. Weinstein[11] and coauthors again observe that "it is often the case that appealing to a code of ethics will not resolve an ophthalmologist's ethical concerns" precisely because codes of ethics do not and cannot decide how different values, such as the preservation of life and the avoidance of pain and suffering, are to be ranked in order of priority.

Narrowness of Scope and Lack of Moral Commitment

The IAO claims that "medical ethics cannot be otherwise than universal" and that "no restriction can be tolerated, if it is dictated by the doctor's religious, philosophic, sociological, political or linguistic convictions."[12] As noted earlier, however, the AAO's code of ethics confines itself to standards within the laws, apparently, of the United States, which are clearly not universal. Should we say, then, that the AAO's code of ethics lacks moral commitment?

The problem presented here is that of reconciling what may occasionally be the conflicting demands of the law with the demands of morality. A good example of this problem involves the proper management of medical information during the consent process for medical treatment. United States law has tended toward the position that any information relevant to the decision-making process for treatment in medicine should be made available to the patient. In the 1957 case *Salgo v Leland Stanford, Jr, University Board of Trustees,* for example, the court held that "A physician violates his duty to his patient and subjects himself to liability if he withholds any facts which are necessary to form the basis of an intelligent consent by the patient to the proposed danger."[13] Empiric evidence and the experience of many professionals in the medical setting, however, recognizes the potential harms, anxiety, frustration, and confusion that can arise when full disclosure of medically relevant information is made. If the law insists on full disclosure at all times, then health professionals who comply with the law may find themselves inflicting otherwise avoidable harms on their patients. In their discussion of the management of medical information, Beauchamp and McCullough[7] suggest that "the physician's commitment to the patient demands that he or she not abandon the patient to the mere formalities of contemporary legal requirements of informed consent."

Indeed, some would argue that when moral obligations exceed or conflict with one's legal obligations, one is morally bound to violate the law (eg, consider, the rationale behind civil disobedience). The IAO may be suggesting just that, for example, when it insists that ophthalmologists have "the moral obligation to cooperate in a militant manner with the private or public organizations whose objectives are to make medical care available to everyone."[12] In reality it is possible that the law could interfere with the ability to make such care available (eg, through the overregulation of pharmaceuticals and medical treatments, overly restrictive research protocols, and even public policies that hinder the professional from providing needed medical care to the children of negligent parents). In any of these cases, morality may indeed demand militant and possibly illegal behavior. The IAO seems to recognize this possibility.

The AAO, however, makes no such claims and might, therefore, be considered narrower in scope and intent. If legal standards and moral standards were identical, conformity to the dictates of the law could not be seen as morally inadequate. However, if morality does occasionally demand conduct that conflicts with or surpasses the demands of the law, then it may be argued that the AAO lacks moral commitment by insisting on standards that fall within the parameters of our present legal statutes.

Absence of Moral or Legal Authority

Still another criticism is that professional codes lack both moral and legal authority. They lack legal clout because organizations, such as the IAO or AAO, are not federal or state law enforcement agencies. Thus, the penalties they can levy against someone who violates the code are limited to such punitive measures as reprimands, publication of the transgressors name, and suspension or termination of membership in the academy, including the privileges such membership conveys.[3]

It can also be argued that these codes lack moral clout precisely because they are not grounded in universally accessible standards of morality. There are several ways in which this problem is manifest. First, discrepancies in the ethical demands of various professional codes directed at the same professional groups, such as those of the AAO and IAO, indicate that at least one and possibly both of these codes are not universal or objective, in the sense developed earlier. Thus, in the absence of some external standard or criteria, it is impossible to determine which of these competing codes of ethics is the morally correct code.

Second, the judgments of ethics committees made up exclusively or predominantly by members of the profession may not reflect the moral sentiments and expectations of persons generally. If they do not, these judgments are likely to carry very little weight with people outside of the profession. The concern here is that ethics committees comprised exclusively, or almost exclusively, of members of the profession are biased in favor of other members of the profession whose ethical conduct is in question. If we allow such committees to adjudicate ethical disputes relating to conduct within the profession, there are serious concerns about the impartiality and objectivity of the members of the committee. By analogy, we would have similar doubts about the impartiality and objectivity of a jury in a murder case made up exclusively of members of the defendant's family. Thus, only if the principles and rules themselves are grounded in universally accessible moral principles, and only if the moral integrity and objectivity of committee members is assured could we argue that the judgments of professional ethics committees carry any moral authority. We cannot know this without first knowing whether the principles themselves are universally accessible and verifiable.

Absence of a Justificatory Basis for the Code

The question of moral authority points toward a fundamental concern about the justificatory basis for professional codes of ethics in general. Are any of these codes grounded in universally accessible moral standards? Indeed, even though there are discrepancies between codes of ethics, this does not mean that none of them are grounded in such standards. The question we need to ask at this point is whether it just so happens that the ethical codes advanced by any professional organizations, in this case the AAO, are grounded in universally accessible and verifiable standards. If they are, then we would have a compelling reason for adopting the code. If they are not, we are as equally compelled to look elsewhere for moral guidance.

PRINCIPLE OF SERVING THE BEST INTERESTS OF THE PATIENT

The AAO asserts that it is the "exclusive goal" of the Code of Ethics to "insure that patients receive ophthalmological care that is in their best interest" and that "it is the duty of an ophthalmologist to place the patient's welfare and rights above all other considerations."[3,4] There are reasons for questioning, however, whether this goal is an appropriate first principle for ethical conduct in medicine. Our concerns can be grouped into two distinct areas: The first involves the interpretation of the patient's best interests. Are they the best interests of the patient according to the patient or according to the physician? Alternatively, are they the best interests as perceived by the patient or those established according to scientific or medical standards? How, in other words, are we to interpret what it means to serve the patient's best interests?

The second area of difficulty arises with the claim, here expressed as a principle of ethics, that the patient's welfare is the professional's *primary* consideration. This principle that "The best interests of the patient should come first," has a long tradition in medicine.[14] The AAO's version follows closely the World Medical Association's principle that "The health of my patient will be my first consideration."[14] However, many would argue that health professionals have other more important moral responsibilities that sometimes override their duties to patients.

In this section, only the problem of interpreting what is meant by serving the patient's best interests is discussed. Responsibilities to third parties and the relation between the principle of serving the patient's best interests and other important ethical principles are discussed later.

We begin by observing that there are two dominant interpretations of benefit used in contemporary medical practice to define the moral responsibilities of health professionals. They are the beneficence and autonomy models.

The *beneficence model* of moral responsibility in medicine interprets the best interests of the individual in terms of medicoorganic well-being. The foundation for the model is the moral *principle of beneficence*. In its most general form, this principle imposes a moral duty to benefit others. More specifically, it imposes a moral duty to promote the legitimate interests of others. Health is generally regarded as one of these legitimate interests; thus, the principle of beneficence may be seen as imposing obligations to prevent, remove, or alleviate conditions that threaten health.

One initial advantage of the model itself is that it provides an objective and scientifically determined basis for determining the best interests of the patient. Here "objective" is being used to describe standards of care that transcend the sometimes irregular and mistaken beliefs of care givers or patients. The standards that are represented are those that science and medicine establish. Thus, the best interests of the patient are interpreted from the more objective perspective that medicine and science take.

This perspective comports well with the traditional and generally prevailing views of medicine. The goal of medicine (though not necessarily the goal of persons practicing medicine) is to benefit the patient by providing health care that promotes the medical well-being of individuals. The Hippocratic formula, for example, instructs physicians to benefit patients according to their professional ability and judgment. Similarly, the goal in the beneficence model is to maximize the patient's medical well-being—meaning simply, that the caregiver should pursue that course of medical treatment that produces the greatest net benefit of medically related goods over medically related harms. In essence, then, the goals of both are similar; thus, the beneficence model can be seen as consistent with traditional medical practices.

The model also bypasses some of the problems associated with medical paternalism and the management of medical information. In moral philosophy, *paternalism* generally refers to acts that override an individual's autonomy, or personal freedom, to provide a benefit to that individual. An essential feature of paternalism is that the intervention is justified in terms of the benefit, or good, secured specifically for that individual (ie, by the intent to promote the individual's good). Medical paternalism, then, simply refers to paternalistic acts that promote the individual's medical well-being.

The situation that gives rise to instances of medical paternalism is when the goals of medicine and the goals of the individual patient conflict. A problem exists only if we acknowledge an obligation to respect the autonomously expressed goals of the patient. If we do acknowledge this obligation, then we need to be able to determine when someone's decisions or desires are autonomously expressed and whether there are limits to the demands of respect for autonomous choices—for example, whether there are other overriding moral obligations or whether there are limits to the kinds of decisions that must be respected, such as requests for exotic, expensive, or medically undesirable interventions.

These difficulties can be bypassed, however, if the goals of medicine are allowed to override the desires and preferences of the patient. By presupposing that the patient's medical well-being is a necessary good for that individual, the beneficence model bypasses some of the problems associated with medical paternalism by refusing to acknowledge the need to respect even autonomously expressed interests that do not comport with the goals of medicine. From this viewpoint, it is irrelevant whether the patient desires medical attention or whether the patient's personal conception of what is in his or her best interests is furthered through medical intervention.

Similarly, the beneficence model also bypasses some of the problems associated with the management of medical information. The moral obligation to tell the truth and legal requirements insisting on the full disclosure of medical information, for example, can lead to situations in which more harm may be done from a *medical viewpoint* than good promoted, again from the same view. We can bypass much of the debate about whether truth telling and full disclosure are overriding moral obligations by focusing exclusively on the patient's best medical interests. Disclosure is relevant here only to the extent that it promotes medical well-being.

Criticisms of the Beneficence Model

First, these last two features of the beneficence model that are merits from the viewpoint that medicine takes are extreme drawbacks from the view of personal autonomy. The demand for the respect of personal autonomy finds expression in the moral *principle of autonomy*, which imposes a moral duty not to interfere with an individual's autonomy. This includes respecting autonomous refusals of medical intervention. Thus, from the perspective of personal autonomy, medical paternalism is a problem precisely because paternalistic interventions by definition involve interference with personal freedoms. Likewise, the withholding of relevant medical information for reasons of beneficence is viewed from the perspective of autonomy as violating respect for personal autonomy because it denies persons access to information about themselves and their own well-being. From the viewpoint of personal autonomy, any information relevant to an informed decision-making process must be fully disclosed, whether or not that information might cause significant harm.

Second, within the province of medicine there is debate over the kinds of conditions that merit medical intervention. Some writers claim that not every physiologic condition that could be treated through medical intervention is a legitimate object of medical practices. For example, some physicians and philosophers argue that aging and conditions that are part of the aging process do not fall within the purview of medicine because they are *natural* or *species-typical* features of the human condition—terms that are meant to imply somehow that medicine should not try to alleviate the physiologic decrements associated with these kinds of processes. Others would argue that age-related conditions, such as age-related macular degeneration, are legitimate objects of medical intervention regardless of whether they are considered "normal" or "species-typical functional orientations." (The debate on the appropriateness of biomedical intervention into the aging process is lively and provocative. An overall review of the subject is provided by Ferenz[15] and Veatch.[15a])

A similar line of reasoning can be applied to the treatment of physiognomic deformities. If medicine does not recognize these as legitimate objects of medical intervention, then those who have these deformities might be forced to live with the condition or seek assistance from persons not in the medical field. MacGreggor[16] and others have argued persuasively for the appropriateness of treating physiognomic deformities as diseases and, therefore, legitimate objects of medical intervention. Still, however, we may not want to wait for a condition to be graced with the label "disease" before we use our medical resources to alleviate it.

It may be irrelevant to persons seeking medical treatment for conditions they disvalue, such as conditions associated with their general appearance or conditions associated with the aging process, that these conditions are regarded as deformities or diseases worthy of medical intervention. From the perspective of autonomy, any physiologic conditions disvalued by individuals will be regarded by them as legitimate objects of medical intervention. The beneficence model alone does reflect these considerations, which are the basis of many decisions to seek medical care.

Third, unproven procedures, those with unknown or uncertain risks, and others that promise little or no medical benefit may be denied to persons who would benefit from them psychologically or who are willing to undergo the procedure for the sake of medical knowledge. Indeed, much medical research could not be accomplished without the willingness of persons to be research subjects in trials that they know provide them no direct medical benefit.

Fourth, the numerous dimensions of life that contribute to overall well-being, such as physical, mental, economic, and social well-being, make it highly unlikely that anyone other than the individual would know what is in his or her best interests. Veatch argues persuasively that the beneficence model of serving the best interests of the patient is unrealistic precisely because health professionals cannot be expected to know how to maximize overall well-being among the many spheres of life that contribute to a person's good (Veatch RM, unpublished essay, July 1992). Thus, the perspective of medicine that the beneficence model takes is clearly too narrow to represent the best interests of an individual from the point of view of the individual's overall good.

Fifth, it may not be possible to conduct medical practices strictly according to scientifically established standards of due care because the legal parameters of due care may differ significantly. Legal standards of due care are often shaped through precedents established in the courtroom, where juries and judges may not always be guided by sound scientific judgment. If courtroom judgments are not identical to medical judgments, then health practitioners cannot be guided strictly by the beneficence model without running the risk of liability and litigation.

AUTONOMY MODEL OF MORAL RESPONSIBILITY

The autonomy model of benefit interprets the best interests of the patient in terms of the actual preferences and desires of the patient. According to this model, the health professional is obligated both to respect (ie, not interfere with) the patient's autonomous choices and further the patient's autonomously expressed interests in matters of care. The basis for the model is the principle of autonomy, which we noted earlier imposes a moral obligation to respect personal autonomy. As it stands, however, the principle of autonomy imposes only a negative injunction. That is, it requires that we *not* do something (viz, interfere with the autonomy, or personal freedom, of others). It does not require that we take positive steps to promote that freedom.

The patient–professional relationship, however, is one characterized by positive steps on the part of the professional (and sometimes the patient as well) to benefit the patient by promoting his or her best interests. The autonomy model interprets the benefits that are the objective of this relationship from the perspective of the patient and makes these the physician's primary concern.

However, the patient's perception of his or her own best interests becomes the primary concern of the physician only if the desires and preferences of the patient are autonomously expressed. That is, only if these desires are the patient's *own* desires, do they become the primary moral responsibility of the physician.

There may be a temptation to argue that the principle of autonomy and the autonomy model as well demand that any decisions expressed by persons should be respected. This would be an extreme misreading of the intent of the model, however. The autonomy model is designed to protect the autonomy of patients by requiring physicians to respect only those choices, desires, and preferences that are autonomous, not those that are nonautonomous. We do not protect autonomy by respecting nonautonomous decisions precisely because these decisions are foreign to the individual. In other words, such decisions are not the person's own decisions but rather the result of some internal or external constraints, such as emotional distress, disease, or the coercive influence of others. If we respect nonautonomous decisions (ie; decisions that are not self-determined), then we are respecting the controlling influence of some internal or external forces and not the individual's personal autonomy. We respect autonomy only when we respect decisions that are autonomous.

Recognizing that there is an obligation to respect autonomy, it becomes necessary to be able to discern autonomous from nonautonomous desires and preferences. We have associated autonomy with personal freedom and with some notion of the absence of internal and external constraints. The total absence of any constraining influences is impossible. However, we do presume that persons are capable of self-governance or self-determination—in other words, personal freedom—within the constraints that are a normal part of the human condition. Conditions that are *autonomy compromising* are those non-normal conditions, such as disease, that restrict an individual's ability to govern oneself or determine one's own life plan.

Many influences can adversely effect the kinds of choices and decisions people make. The influence of trauma, injury, physical or mental illness and disease, anxiety, drugs, mistaken beliefs about treatment, and the coercive influences of the clinical environment, medical personnel, family members, and others can all contribute to compromising an individual's ability to make decisions and express desires that are self-determined, or that are his or her own. This is not to say, however, that everyone acts or decides nonautonomously in the presence of these conditions. The same set of conditions that compromise one patient's decision-making capabilities may not compromise another's. For this reason, we cannot look to the presence of these autonomy-compromising conditions alone to determine whether the decisions or desires expressed under these or similar circumstances are autonomous.

Moreover, from the viewpoint of the autonomy model, it is also important to realize that what is at issue here is not whether a person or patient is autonomous, in the sense of possessing the freedom necessary to carry out and conduct a life plan. Under conditions necessitating medical attention, the autonomy of an individual is often substantially compromised. But this does not mean that the individual's ability to decide autonomously is compromised. What becomes important, then, is whether individual patients are *competent* within the health care setting to make autonomous decisions concerning their own medical care, not whether they are autonomous persons. If they are competent, then the decisions they make must be respected by the physician. If they are not, then we must consider these decisions and desires to be nonautonomous and, therefore, not binding upon the physician.

To many, the outstanding attraction of the autonomy model is this respect it shows for personal autonomy. By interpreting benefit in terms of the autonomously expressed preferences and desires of the patient, the autonomy model ensures that the health professional does not interfere with these autonomously expressed interests. Autonomous decisions to forego or suspend treatment must, therefore, be respected by the physician regardless of their outcomes. Similarly, the autonomy model requires that decisions concerning the management of medical information should be made in accordance with these autonomously expressed desires. If the patient desires autonomously full, partial, or even nondisclosure of relevant medical information, then it is the physician's moral responsibility to comply with these requests.

To a significant extent, the autonomy model also helps professionals avoid medical paternalism (in treatment decisions and in the management of medical information) by steering them away from some situations in which they might be tempted to substitute their own judgment for that of their patients. For example, some autonomously made decisions are clearly not in the patient's best medical interests, such as refusals of lifesaving blood transfusions by Jehovah's Witnesses patients. When they are not, the physician is tempted to substitute his or her judgment for that of the patient. For example, in a case involving total exsanguination after refusal of a blood transfusion by a Jehovah's Witness patient, Jewett laments that physician's efforts to prevent the needless loss of life should be frustrated by "intransigent adherence to a dogma inimical to life."[17] The autonomy model instructs the physician not to allow that to happen. According to the autonomy model, the physician's judgments must not be allowed to override the patient's decisions when these are autonomously made, regardless of whether these decisions are in the patient's best medical interests. Thus, the autonomy model avoids the more obvious cases of medical paternalism by requiring physicians to respect the patient's autonomous decisions concerning their own medical care.

Finally, when patients are incompetent to make decisions concerning their medical care, the autonomy model ceases to be the overriding model of moral responsibility. At that point, the beneficence model usually becomes the relevant model.

Criticisms

Difficulties in Determining Autonomy and Competence

There are serious practical and philosophical difficulties in determining precisely when a person or their decisions are autonomous or not autonomous. An entire range of behaviors describes the activities, desires, and decisions of persons that are regarded as autonomous. Somewhere outside of that range, individuals or the decisions they make become nonautonomous. The problem from both the philosophical and empirical viewpoint is in determining at what point individuals or their decisions become nonautonomous.

For the specific purposes of the autonomy model, the difficulty is in determining when patients are competent within the medical context to make decisions concerning their medical care. Thus, we need some criteria of competence. The problem, however, is that some amount of evaluative and normative judgment is inescapable in formulating such criteria, and this presents certain dangers. If approached from the view of medicine, the criteria selected will represent the evaluative and normative judgments of practitioners of medicine and are apt to be quite stringent. If approached from the general public's viewpoint, the criteria no doubt are much more liberal. The difficulty in determining what criteria should be used is the same difficulty that troubles the pursuit of ethical behavior in medicine and that is the problem of finding an ethical view that is objective and morally defensible. Once we can establish what that point of view entails, it should be possible to determine what criteria of competence are morally appropriate.

Limited Application

Another criticism of the autonomy model is that it applies only in the case of patients whose actual desires and preferences are autonomously expressed. The model itself says nothing about what other principles or models should take over when persons are no longer competent to make autonomous decisions.

Offensive and Excessive Desires and Preferences

Some autonomously expressed desires and decisions may seem excessive. They may involve exotic procedures of questionable or no medical value, or they may offend the sensibilities of the health professional or others, such as in the case of refusals to accept blood transfusions. When such requests violate the health professional's own moral sensibilities and more deeply cherished values, they pose a threat to the professional's own personal autonomy. In such cases, respect for the personal autonomy of the physician demands that the physician should be allowed to withdraw from the case, and the autonomy model appears still to require that the physician promote the patient's interests.

Undermines the Traditional Basis of the Patient–Professional Relationship

Some would argue that requiring health practitioners to respect the autonomous interests and preferences of individuals will undermine the traditional basis for the professional–patient relationship, a basis founded on beneficence.

In sum, the two models of moral responsibility discussed in this section represent two distinct interpretations of benefit. Occasionally, the best interests of the patient as viewed from the perspective of medicine conflict with the best interests as seen from the perspective of the individual patient. Without some way of establishing which, if either, of these interpretations is morally preferable, we cannot know which to adopt as a guiding principle of ethical conduct in medicine. By allowing the beneficence model to override interests in personal autonomy, we risk violating the personal integrity and dignity of individuals. Conversely, allowing the autonomy model always to override the beneficence model seriously jeopardizes many of the traditional values of medicine.

Moreover, as pointed out earlier, problems of interpretation are not the only concerns about the principle of serving the patient's best interests first. In addition to these problems are concerns about the moral responsibilities that health professionals have to persons outside of the professional–patient relationship (viz, to third parties). We turn now to these additional concerns.

OBLIGATIONS TO OTHERS AND THIRD-PARTY INTERESTS

The principle that "The best interests of the patient should come first," or "above all other considerations," is rejected by many writers in medical ethics. It is argued that health professionals have moral responsibilities to others that sometimes override the obligation to promote the best interests of their patients. This section looks briefly at several areas in which health professionals may have primary obligations to third parties and some of the reasons offered for them.

Obligations to Family and Guardians

Physicians treating children are sometimes faced with a serious dilemma when the best interests of the child are in conflict with the expressed interests of parents. For example, parents may request the withholding or discontinuance of lifesaving treatment in the case of seriously defective infants who have some chance at survival, even if only temporary, if aggressively treated. The beneficence model (not the principle of beneficence) demands aggressive care, whereas other considerations demand acquiescing to the parent's wishes.

One of these considerations is the widely accepted doctrine of parental rights. In cases such as those described, respect for these rights and the obligation to promote the best interests of the patient can pose a serious ethical dilemma. A similar dilemma also occurs if the principle of beneficence is seen as imposing a duty to promote the maximum amount of good over harm for all parties concerned. If, for example, the economic, emotional, and familial burdens of caring for a seriously ill child outweigh the good of promoting the child's best interests, then, according to some interpretations, the principle of beneficence would require removing or minimizing these burdens, for example, by allowing the child to die. The beneficence model, on the other hand, clearly imposes duties to promote the best medical interests of the child.

Obligations to Insurers and Third-Party Payers

Physicians working under contract as occupational physicians or in institutional settings, such as group practices, health clinics, or health maintenance organizations (HMOs), may have obligations to these parties that outweigh the interests of the patients they see in these settings. For example, members of HMOs generally agree to a package of benefits that include primary care by member physicians of the HMO. Depending on the benefits offered, however, some procedures, such as cosmetic or plastic surgery, may not be covered. Should a member of the plan ask their physician to perform a medically warranted (but not life threatening or handicapping) procedure not covered under the plan, there may be a serious conflict between the obligations of the physician to the HMO and to the patient.

As a member physician of the HMO, the physician has obligations to that organization. Conversely, according to the principle of placing the best interests of the patient first, the physician has an obligation to perform the requested procedure—on the basis of both the autonomy and beneficence models of benefit. The apparent ethical problem, however, is not really a problem of conflicting obligations but a question of the status of contracts. The physician has a contractual obligation to provide only those services offered under the plan. The patient, in subscribing to the plan, has also implicitly agreed to receive only those benefits covered. In essence, then, the patient has already expressed an interest in not receiving certain kinds of care. Thus, if we accept the moral legitimacy of the legal doctrine of contracts, then both the physician and the patient would be seen as having overriding moral obligations to honor their contracts. In this hypothetical situation, the patient may be seen as suffering what could be called buyer's remorse, but this change of mind would not materially effect the terms of the contract or the overriding obligation to honor them.

Obligations to Future Generations

There are several ways in which the interests of persons in the future can be affected by the conduct of health professionals in the present. In the management of limited health care resources, in the capacity as a research investigator, and as an educator of the next generation of caregivers, the health professional can have a profound impact on the quality of care available to future generations. This list is by no means exhaustive; however, in each instance, there is the potential for conflict between the interests of future persons and the present interests of the physician's patients. For example, to give physicians-in-training the experience they need as specialists in a particular area of medicine, it is necessary to give them an opportunity to perform delicate and sometimes extremely risky surgical or diagnostic procedures. Patients in such cases may be vehemently opposed to allowing the student to perform such procedures even under the direct supervision of their personal physician. Nevertheless, it is clear that the student must gain this experience to serve the interests of future generations of patients.

The ethical dilemma is in deciding whose interests are overriding. In the interest of justice and fairness, it might be claimed that today's patients owe future generations the opportunity to receive experienced care because they themselves are the beneficiaries of past patients who were likewise the teaching material of present physicians.

Obligations to Society and the State

Overriding obligations to society and the state are already part of the health professional's legal responsibilities. For example, physicians are required by law in most states to report bullet wounds to local law enforcement agencies. This violation of patient confidence is justified by the principle, expressed as a duty, to prevent harm from occurring to others. The reasoning here is that the public's interest and right to protect itself from persons whose activities may involve assault with a deadly weapon outweighs the physician's responsibility (grounded in respect for autonomy) to maintain patient confidentiality. The same principle could justify quarantining, mandatory inoculation programs, reporting carriers of communicable diseases, and other public health measures designed to promote public welfare and prevent harm to others. The ethical conflict present in each of these examples is the conflict between the health professional's obligation to serve the patient's interests and obligations to serve the public interest.

Not everyone, however, would argue that health professionals have a primary obligation to society or the state. From the traditional view of medicine, especially, primary obligations to the state would severely undermine the trust and patient confidence that is an important feature of the patient–professional relationship. There is a tremendous concern that routine violations of this trust to serve the purposes of the state would undermine the willingness of individuals to seek care and thus jeopardize the ability of physicians to treat those who need medical attention.

In the previous section, we observed numerous difficulties in the interpretation of the best interests of patients. In this section, we have considered several areas in which health care professionals may have primary moral obligations to parties other than their patients. Together, these difficulties present a considerable argument against professional codes of ethics that are designed foremost to promote the best interests of patients.

TOWARD AN ACCOUNT OF ETHICAL BEHAVIOR IN OPHTHALMOLOGY

To this point the discussion has focused mainly on the difficulties that exist in the interpretation of the moral responsibilities of health professionals. In this section, a more plausible and objective approach to the problem of ethics in medicine is discussed. The goal is to construct an ethical framework that helps the practicing ophthalmologist avoid and resolve ethical problems that typically arise in medical practice.

The first question we need to address in this section is how to write a code of medical ethics that meets the criteria of objectivity in ethics presented earlier in this chapter—that is, how do we construct an ethical system in medicine that is universally accessible and faithful to the moral sentiments and expectations of persons generally? As a practical matter, the formulation of such a code may seem an impossible task. Many would argue that disagreement in matters of morals is inescapable and that it would be impossible to arrive at any moral principles that persons would agree on in general.

The debate here, turns on the meaning of "in general." If this refers only to those moral sentiments and beliefs that are actually held in common, then the project would be prohibitive precisely because we cannot ask everyone their opinions on morality. Another possible interpretation of the phrase "in general" that deserves consideration is the interpretation referring to moral sentiments held by most individuals—giving it the meaning, then, "for the most part." The danger here, however, is of constructing a system of moral conduct that fails to represent or underrepresents the sentiments of others in the population. The literature on this subject has historically referred to the domination of majority-held beliefs as a "tyranny of the majority," which may not necessarily result in untoward consequences but presents the possibility of oppression and discrimination that many would argue should be avoided.

In consideration of these kinds of dangers, some writers have insisted that universal agreement is the only valid basis for an ethical system. The authority of ethical claims in public policy can only be established, according to one such account, if *all* persons can be presumed to agree to the ethical claims being made.[18] Thus, an actual consensus is not required but only the presumed agreement of all persons.

Universal agreement in matters of morality is highly unlikely, however, even if we limit agreement to that which is presumed to exist among rational persons only. The major criticism of this requirement is that the occasion of one dissenting voice either invalidates the ethical system or it must be dismissed as irrational or in some other way not relevant. This, of course, raises serious concerns about tailoring notions of rationality, or other criteria that are presumed relevant, to exclude those who do not, or would not, agree with the ethical claims being made.

The more plausible alternative to the above interpretations is one that gets its inspiration from social contract theory. The idea here is to interpret the moral sentiments and expectations of persons in general as those moral sentiments that are expressed in the terms agreed to in the social contract. If this is a plausible assumption, then it is this contract governing our cooperative social arrangements that we would look to for discovering the ethical guidelines and role-specific duties negotiated by members of a profession and the rest of society. This feature of the approach from social contract theory is what makes the ethical system upon which these social arrangements are based universally accessible. That is, we need only look to the structure and nature of our present cooperative social schemes in order to discover the ethical system upon which it is grounded.

In practice, however, we can only assume that the moral sentiments informing our cooperative social arrangements are those that would be agreed upon by individual contractors taking the moral point of view. Theoretically, if these are truly cooperative social schemes, then this may be a tenable assumption. If they are not, then the assumption is indefensible. As it turns out, any speculation about the nature of social contracts negotiated by persons taking the moral viewpoint (viz, the view that everyone's interests have equal weight) has to make assumptions about what these persons would agree to because we have no existing contracts of this kind to examine.

Robert Veatch develops this social contract approach in *A Theory of Medical Ethics*. He argues that the role-specific duties we identify with the medical profession

> cannot exist simply because a profession itself imposes them or alleges it alone possesses the ability to know what is ethical for professionals or patients. . . . If they are moral duties, . . . they must derive at least indirectly from the basic social contract.[10]

Veatch then goes on to describe what he calls a "triple-contract theory of medical ethics." According to this view, the content of the basic social contract will be

> what contractors taking the moral point of view . . . would invent or discover or have revealed to them as the basic ethical principles for society . . . a second contract, one between the society and a profession, can then spell out (again from the moral point of view) the special role-specific duties regarding interactions between lay people and professionals.[10]

The third level of contract would exist between individual lay persons and individual members of a profession, here spelling out the further terms of the relationship between professional and layperson. The result, as Veatch describes it, is a theory of medical ethics that is "accessible to all and applicable to all."[10]

If we accept this formulation as the most likely to yield an objective and morally defensible code of medical ethics, then the next question we need to ask is what the contract between society and health care professionals is likely to say. In other words, we want to know what the terms of these contracts are. Unfortunately, there is not enough space here to explore this question thoroughly. But the approach itself is one that merits considerable attention. We are much more likely to arrive at an ethic in medicine that is universally accessible and representative of the moral expectations of persons generally if we approach questions of ethics from the view of social contractors negotiating the rules that govern their cooperative social arrangements.

Because the construction of a complete ethical system for medical practices is beyond the scope of this chapter, the following guidelines are suggestions reflecting considerations touched on earlier that are likely to resurface in the contract between society and health professionals.

First, any acceptable formulation of medical ethics must incorporate the demands of all of society's moral principles (viz, autonomy, beneficence, the prevention of harm to others, and justice) as they relate to medical practice. Reliance on a single moral principle, no matter how intricately formulated, simply cannot capture all the moral responsibilities and values intrinsic to medicine. Exclusive use of the autonomy model, for example, does not provide guidance in the case of persons who are substantially nonautonomous, whereas the exclusive application of the beneficence model may result in failure to respect the personal autonomy of individual patients. In addition to the demands of the principles of beneficence and autonomy are the demands of justice and the prevention of harm to others, which can also be overriding in some cases. Consequently, a morally defensible code of medical ethics must incorporate all the demands generated by these principles with regard to the practice of medicine.

Second, it is important to recognize that all these principles that are integral to society's cooperative social arrangements, including the practice of medicine, are *prima facie* moral principles. The term *prima facie* (literally meaning "on first appearance") is used in moral philosophy to refer to moral principles that are always binding but that override other *prima facie* moral principles in certain circumstances. The *prima facie* principle of beneficence, for example, appears to be the guiding principle in clinical circumstances involving persons with substantially reduced autonomy. This is true, however, only on first appearance because a complete assessment of the moral implications of a given situation must consider the demands of all of morality's moral principles. The demands of justice, for example, may require allocations of limited health care resources that do not allow the physician to act fully in the patient's best medical interests. To the extent that each of these principles is *prima facie,* then, the professional must be aware in every individual case which principles apply and which are likely to be overriding according to the terms of the social contract.

Third, when patients are capable of autonomous decision making concerning their own medical care, the autonomy model should be the preferred model of moral responsibility for health professionals. The demands of the model include (1) noninterference with autonomous refusals of treatment, (2) efforts by the professional to use his or her professional skills to further the autonomously expressed interests of the patient, and (3) compliance with the patient's wishes regarding the management of relevant medical information. Thus, it is true that respect for autonomy requires both disclosure (truth telling) of information relevant to medical decision making (including economic and other nonclinical information) and confidentiality in the management of medical information; however, the autonomy model requires that both these derivative rules of the principle of autonomy should be practiced in accordance with the wishes of the competent patient—making these, then, also only *prima facie* rules.

The endorsement here of the overriding importance of autonomous decision making in the medical context reflects recent trends in court cases involving autonomous refusals of medical treatment. Through these decisions made in the courts, society appears to be endorsing the autonomy model of moral responsibility. It is debatable, however, whether paternalism in general is a widely acceptable principle of conduct in American society and whether these recent trends in the courts will continue.

The idea that physician, government, or others should override the autonomous interests of others for the explicit purpose of providing them a benefit (ie, for their own good), may be unpalatable to most Americans. Many would argue against this view, however, and there is ample evidence in the form of public safety requirements, such as seatbelt laws and helmet laws, that this view is incorrect. Indeed, it does appear that the public endorses some amount of paternalistic control of their personal liberties.

This tendency toward paternalism is also present in some of the criteria that have been suggested for determinations of competence among patients in the medical context. The criteria that are generally offered as reasons—presently in competition as the favored reasons—for considering a person incompetent to consent to or refuse medical interventions and therapies have been assembled from other sources by Beauchamp and McCullough.[7]

1. *Inability to decide.* This test asks only whether an individual can make a decision, not whether the decision is a good one.
2. *Inability to understand.* Does the person possess the basic cognitive abilities to understand and assess the risks, benefits, and alternatives to treatment discussed in decision-making contexts in medicine? This criterion does not test whether the individual possesses adequate information to decide but only whether they possess the cognitive ability to process the kind of information discussed generally in the health care setting.
3. *Inability to understand disclosed information.* This test asks whether the patient did in fact understand the information disclosed in a given circumstance, rather than whether the person is generally able to understand.
4. *Failure to give a reason.* That is, can the individual give a reason of any kind for the choice made?
5. *Failure to give a rational reason.* This test employs a minimal notion of rationality and insists only that there be some plausible connection between the reason and the choice.
6. *Failure to employ a risk–benefit calculus.* This test asks whether the individual has based their decision on a reasonable weighing of the potential risks and potential benefits already perceived by others as risks and benefits. The individual's subjective assessment of risks and benefits is not relevant.
7. *Inability to reach a reasonable decision.* This test demands that the decision arrived at is one that a reasonable person would make in similar circumstances.[7]

Note that the sixth and seventh conditions employ some notion of *reasonableness*, or what reasonable persons would decide, in order to establish whether someone is competent. If the decision is reasonable or if it reflects a reasonable balancing of what others already perceive to be potential harms and benefits, then the patient is competent to decide. Thus, the determination of whether someone is competent depends on what they decide. The purpose of such criteria are well-intentioned: they are designed to protect the incompetent patient from making harmful decisions.

The objection that must be raised here, however, is that proponents of criteria employing standards of reasonableness may be guilty of tailoring these criteria to justify paternalistic controls of behaviors and decisions that they simply find objectionable. Proponents of such a standard might argue, for example, that decisions that result in the needless loss of life, such as refusals of blood transfusions for religious reasons, indicate a choice or decision that is not autonomously made—that it is, in fact, the result of some form of coercion, such as a religiously coercive environment, or deeply seated psychological disturbances. The reason that the decision in this example is considered nonautonomous is because it results in what the proponent of the standard considers a needless loss of life. Implicit here, of course, is the idea that a needless loss of life is an unreasonable loss of life.

Indeed, it is in anticipation of such objectionable decisions and desires that philosophers such as Gerald Dworkin have argued for paternalism as part of a social insurance policy against what he calls "cognitive" and "evaluative delusions." Persons suffering these delusions act in a "nonrational fashion" by attaching "incorrect" weights to their values (the evaluative delusion) or by neglecting to act in accordance with their "actual" preferences and desires, i.e. with those preferences and desires that the individual has expressed or acted upon in the past (the cognitive delusion). Dworkin argues that people will agree to paternalistic controls, such as helmet laws, in order to protect themselves from irrational decisions resulting from these delusions.[19]

Criteria of rationality and reasonableness, however, are often seen as an attempt to smuggle in unjustified paternalistic controls over persons whose desires and preferences just happen to be out of the ordinary or in some other way objectionable. The danger that many writers see in standards of reasonableness and rationality is the attempt to control the behavior of persons whose decisions could result in harm to themselves. The point is, however, that even decisions that are harmful to oneself can be made autonomously and on the basis of eccentric or even absurd beliefs and ideas. Thus, if we are to avoid paternalism, criteria of reasonableness should pose a minimal constraint to considerations of competence and autonomous decision making.

Fourth, in those cases in which persons are substantially nonautonomous, (viz, when they are incompetent to make decisions concerning their own medical care), beneficence should be, prima facie, the guiding principle of moral responsibility. The working relationship between the autonomy model and the beneficence model will depend on the levels of competence possessed by patients. The general idea is that as competence decreases, the role of the beneficence model increases. The following guidelines borrow once again from Beauchamp and McCullough, although they have been condensed significantly and a fourth guideline has been added:

1. For patients with reversibly reduced autonomy, the patient's decisions should be given increasing weight, as demanded by an increased level of autonomy, as the patient improves.
2. In the case of persons whose autonomy cannot be restored, but a relevant and sufficiently complete set of the patient's values and beliefs can be reconstructed from prior autonomous determinations, such prior expression of the patient's autonomy should be respected.
3. If autonomy cannot be restored, and a value history cannot be obtained or reasonably constructed, or the patient may never have been autonomous, as in the case of the profoundly or severely retarded individual or a newborn infant, then the physician should look exclusively to the beneficence model.[7]
4. When in doubt, err on the side of beneficence. In other words, when the decisions of individuals cannot be considered autonomous, when there is reasonable doubt concerning the competence of the individual to make autonomous decisions, or in the absence of an explicit contractual arrangement in which an individual delegates his or her decision-making authority to their health provider, it is in keeping with traditional standards of care and, most probably, the expectations of society that health professionals would employ a beneficence-based model of moral responsibility.
5. From a practical view, respect for autonomy requires an interactive approach between professional and patient. Eraker and Politser[20] observe that "[a]s medical decisions become technically more complex and are associated with greater costs to the patient, physicians have been increasingly motivated to incorporate patient preferences in these critical decisions." The physician is expected to be in the best position to assess what course of treatment serves the patient's best medical interests and the competent patient (or guardian) is assumed best able to determine what serves his or her overall interests. Only together, therefore, are the professional and the patient likely to maximize the patient's overall best interests.

It would be unrealistic to suggest that the ethical requirements and responsibilities of physicians have been or could be adequately defined and defended in this brief chapter. The foregoing suggestions are made to assist the ophthalmologist in avoiding and resolving some of the more general ethical problems that are typical in the practice of medicine. The construction of a more comprehensive and morally defensible ethical system in medicine has been attempted by many writers whose works are well worth examining. However, there are no definitive and noncontroversial ethical guidelines that avert all ethical dispute in medicine. For this reason and because of the complexity of the task of caring for individuals whose needs and interests are diverse, the ophthalmologist should not expect, nor be expected, to pursue their practices without occasional ethical conflict. The best of intentions can meet with opposition. When ethical disputes do arise, therefore, it would be irresponsible of the health professional not to consult those who should be able to help resolve the conflict. This consultation includes but is not limited to the patient (or patient's guardian), someone adept in matters of ethics (such as an ethicist), and the physician's own deepest sense of compassion and commiseration with others.

References

1. Cataract surgery: fraud, waste, and abuse. Report of the House Select Committee on Aging, July 21, 1985.
2. Margo CE. Selling surgery. N Engl J Med 1986; 314:1575–1576.
3. American Academy of Ophthalmology. Code of Ethics, rev. San Francisco, American Academy of Ophthalmology, 1992:3,8.
4. American Academy of Ophthalmology. Ethics in ophthalmology: a practical guide. San Francisco, American Academy of Ophthalmology 1986:3,4,9.

5. So you think you know what's ethical. Medical Economics 1973;23:90–95.
6. President's Commission for the Study of Ethical Problems in Medicine and Biomedical and Behavioral Research. Deciding to forego life-sustaining treatment. Washington, DC, US Government Printing Office, 1983:244.
7. Beauchamp TL, McCullough LB. Medical ethics: the moral responsibilities of physicians. Englewood Cliffs, NJ, Prentice Hall, 1984:10,77,122–124.
8. Beauchamp TL. Philosophical ethics: an introduction to moral philosophy. New York, McGraw-Hill, 1982:303–335.
9. Jones WHS, trans. Hippocrates. Cambridge, MA, Harvard University Press, Loeb Classical Library, 1923.
10. Veatch RM. A theory of medical ethics. New York, Basic Books, 1981:15–75,106,127,138.
11. Weinstein BD, Weinstein GW, Burkard JL Jr. Ethical issues in ophthalmology. In: Tasman W, ed. Duane's Clinical ophthalmology, vol 5. Philadelphia, JB Lippincott, 1992:3.
12. International Academy of Ophthalmology. Code of Ophthalmological Ethics. Trans Ophthalmol Soc UK 1978:98:514.
13. *Salgo v Leland Stanford, Jr, University Board of Trustees,* 154 Cal App 2d 560, 578, 317 P2d 170. In: *Berkey v. Anderson,* App 82 Cal Rptr 67, 77.
14. World Medical Association. Declaration of Geneva. World Med Assoc Bull 1949;1:109.
15. Ferenz L. Social and ethical impacts of life extending technologies and interventions into the aging process. Washington, DC, Georgetown University, 1992. Dissertation.
15a. Veatch RM, ed. Life span: values and life-extending technologies. San Francisco, Harper & Row, 1979.
16. MacGreggor FC. After plastic surgery: adaptation and adjustment. New York, Praeger, 1979.
17. Jewett JF. Report from the Committee on Maternal Welfare: total exsanguination. N Engl J Med 1981;305:1218.
18. Engelhardt HT Jr. The foundations of bioethics. New York, Oxford University Press, 1986:39–49.
19. Dworkin G. Paternalism. The Monist 1972;56:79.
20. Eraker S, Politser P. How decisions are reached: physician and patient. Ann Intern Med 1982;97:262.

Bibliography

Beauchamp TL, Childress JF. Principles of biomedical ethics. New York, Oxford University Press, 1983.

President's Commission for the Study of Ethical Problems in Medicine and Biomedical and Behavioral Research. Securing access to health care, vol 1: report. Washington, DC, US Government Printing Office, 1983.

Veatch RM. The foundations of justice. New York, Oxford University Press, 1986.

Ophthalmic Surgery Complications: Prevention and Management,
edited by Judie F. Charlton and George W. Weinstein.
J. B. Lippincott Company, Philadelphia © 1995.

Robert R. Hobson
Donna Jo Wheeler
Judie F. Charlton

20

Biomedical Equipment Failure

Because of the variety of people handling operating room equipment and the need for reliability, most operating room equipment is designed to withstand more abuse than the standard office instruments. Power cables and controls are generally built with heavy duty switches, more stress connectors, better electrical contacts, extra ground connections and ground fault interrupters, moisture protection, and more readable controls. Frequently, isolation transformers are incorporated to disconnect the patient completely from the main electrical power source.

Naturally, all of these special requirements cause operating room equipment prices to be far above prices for clinical equipment. More stringent Occupational Safety and Health Administration regulations are providing greater protection but frequently require reengineering of specific items.

Despite all of these measures, operating room equipment does fail, often at inconvenient or critical times. More awareness on the part of the surgeon of how a piece of equipment works, and the reasons it might fail, helps reduce operating room time, surgical complications, repair costs, and frustration.

POWER FAILURE TO EQUIPMENT

Power failure to equipment frequently occurs when the unit is first turned on. The initial power surge can cause more electrical current drain than the fuse protector is designed to handle. Many pieces of equipment shut down or trip an equipment circuit breaker if the supply requirements are not within the tolerance range set by the manufacturer.

Variations in incoming line voltage can cause increased current demands from the equipment to the point that it shuts down to protect itself. Room electrical power circuit breakers trip less frequently since they are generally rated higher than the equipment circuit breakers. When equipment frequently shuts down, trips fuses, or requires repeated bulb changes, voltage variations may be occurring. Building maintenance shop personnel should be informed and a device attached to measure power line voltages continuously while equipment is being used. Installation of voltage regulators can often reduce the risk of shutdowns and damage to equipment.

When equipment power fails, potential sources of failure should be checked systematically (Table 20-1). First, check to see if any portion of the unit is functioning or a power indicator light is on. If some portion of the instrument has power, was a control setting on the unit changed that may have shut a portion of the unit down? If there is no indication of power to the unit, check to see if there is other equipment on the same electrical outlet working. If there is, one should try turning off the failed instrument's power switch and turning it on again. One should also check to see that the power plug has not been disconnected. Some units supply power to more than one piece of equipment or plug into the back of a larger piece of equipment. If electrical power strips are used, check the circuit breaker on the strip. Rooms with explosion proof electrical outlets often make it difficult to determine associated power lines.

If none of these measures reveals the source of the problem, one should look at all circuit breakers or fuses on the equipment. Back panels on most box-shaped instruments frequently have circuit breakers installed on them, often near the power cord. Some units have the circuit breakers built into the front on/off switch. When tripped, the switch lever usually

Table 20-1
Diagnostic Checklist: Equipment Power Failure

Is power going to any portion of the unit?
Is the electrical outlet working?
Has a control setting been changed?
Does turning the unit off and on again remedy the problem?
Is the power plug connected properly?
Is the circuit breaker on the electrical power strip tripped?
Are the circuit breakers and fuses on the unit functional?
Is the fuse the proper size and rating?

faces down. If the circuit breaker appears questionable, push the lever fully down, then up; one feels it click into position. Many operation microscopes have the fuses or circuit breakers mounted on the support column or base. Fuse holders usually unscrew or twist off at the cap. After removing them from the holder, one finds a small glass tube with a wire running through the center and metal contacts at each end[1] (Fig. 20-1*A*).

A blown fuse has a break near the center of the wire and frequently a burn mark on the glass (see Fig. 20-1*B*). The electrical current rating of the fuse is indicated on the side of the metal contact. One should make certain that the blown fuse is replaced with one of proper size and rating. Often the fuse's electrical current rating is printed on or next to the holder. If a fuse is replaced with one rated higher than the original, it could cause severe equipment damage. One rated lower requires often early replacement or blows when the equipment is turned on.

A push-type circuit breaker is often located on the microscope stand. It may serve not only as the circuit breaker but also as the on-off button. Also, it will frequently be illuminated. To reset the push type, one simply pushes the protruding button in and listens for a snap sound. If the button returns out, one should try turning off all switches on the equipment in question and resetting the breaker. If it resets, one needs to determine if a particular portion of the instrument is malfunctioning. This may be a portion for which another device may be substituted during the surgical procedure. To determine if a portion of the instrument is malfunctioning, turn on each switch in the sequence normally followed to start the instrument. When the breaker trips, this is an indication that the circuit to the malfunctioning portion is drawing more current than allowed, and possibly shorting. If the circuit involved contains a bulb, check that the correct bulb in the lamp housing is in place. If several attempts at identifying the problem are unsuccessful, one should call for service.

When replacing a part, make certain that the electrical power is off before removing the defective part.

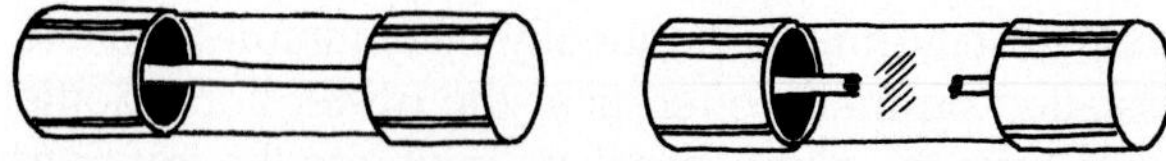

Figure 20-1. Fuses. (**A**) Normal glass cartridge fuse. (**b**) Burnt fuse.

MICROSCOPE PROBLEMS

No Light

It is disconcerting and potentially disastrous to lose the operating microscope light during an operation. The surgical team must be adept at diagnosing and treating this problem just as if it were an ocular problem (Table 20-2). If the fan and stand power indicator light are on, the lamp voltage is possibly set too low. If light is seen coming from the lamp housing, first check the intensity selector, then the fiberoptics bundle, if used, for a poor fiberoptics cable connection.[3]

If there is no light coming from the lamp housing, check the illumination lamp or bulb. If the microscope is fan cooled, one should listen for the fan. If the fan is audible, it is a good indication that this part of the microscope is receiving power. One should

Table 20-2
Diagnostic Checklist: Microscope Without Light

Is the microscope receiving power? (If not, see Table 20-1.)
Is the lamp voltage correct?
Is the bulb blown?
Is the voltage selector set correctly?
Is the fiber optics bundle connected properly?
Is the fan on? If not, there is probably no power going to this part of the unit.
Is there more than one light source available in the microscope?
Are the lamp house contacts pitted or corroded?
Are the circuit boards controlling the *x-y*, zoom, on focus, functional?
Are the lamp house electrical wires loose or broken?

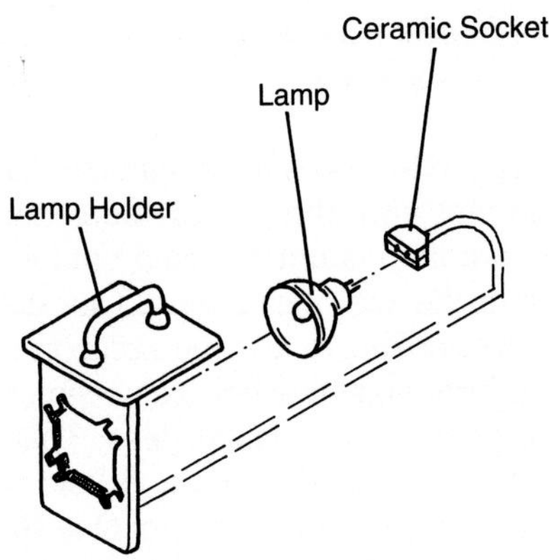

Figure 20-2. Common bulb and lamp housing.

replace the lamp or select a backup bulb from the bulb housing, if available (Fig. 20-2).

Some microscopes offer more than one light source. Often, each lamp has its own plug jack, on-off switch, and intensity regulator. If the microscope has a stand with a choice of plug jacks, the plug-in jack and the selector button on the stand are color coded. On older Zeiss microscopes, press the colored jack that matches the colored circle.[2] When replacing a bulb, one should check the lamp housing contacts for corrosion or pitting. If they show signs of corrosion, clean the contacts with a pencil eraser or contact electrical spray cleaner. One should file pitted areas with a fine file (eg, fingernail file) and have the contacts replaced as soon as possible; pitting continues if the contacts are not replaced, increasing the potential for overheating wires, poor illumination, and blown fuses.

When handling halogen bulbs, never touch the glass surface of the bulb; this can cause the bulb to age prematurely. If touched, clean the glass surface with alcohol before installing.[3]

If the fan and power indicator light are off, the microscope is probably not receiving power. Exchanging bulbs at this point would be premature. Instead, check the main power switch, electrical plug, and fuses or circuit breakers as described earlier. If none of these is the source of the problem, check the circuit board that controls the *x-y* positioner, zoom, focus, and lamps. If the circuit board has malfunctioned, contact the service company. Finish the operation with the room overhead operating lamp.

If the power indicator light is on, fuses or breakers are functional, and bulb replacement has no effect, one should check for a loose wire or connection. Move the lamp house wires to find a possible break in the wiring. Units with electrical connectors to the bulb can become loose and wires eventually break as a result of routine handling and movement of the microscope. Connectors can often be cleaned with electrical contact spray. Connectors with split pins that are loose can be spread and reinserted with slightly more force to assure good contact. If wires require frequent repair, try strapping the involved wires to the microscope arm or post. It is important to make certain that there is enough freedom in the wire to allow full swing of the microscope without causing undue stress on the wire.

Bulb Blows Frequently

There are several explanations for microscope bulbs blowing frequently. One is that the bulb is being used in overload rather than normal mode. Microscopes with intensity selectors are often left in the highest intensity position. Besides being potentially damaging to the patient's and surgeon's retinas, using the bulb at maximum intensity is hard on the electrical system and can cause more frequent fuse blowing or circuit breaker tripping, and burned bulb and housing contacts. Maximum intensity also increases the potential for the bulb to blow due to arcing within the housing contacts, and decreases the life of the bulb.

Bulbs also may need to be replaced frequently if the incorrect bulb is being used. Some lamp sockets hold bulbs rated for electrical currents different from the one required. If one replaces a bulb with one that has a lower current rating it requires a higher-intensity setting on the control panel to produce the same amount of light used before the original lamp expired. This causes premature aging of the new bulb because it is working at a higher voltage level than the original bulb. Often the filament is decentered in relation to the original bulb, requiring an additional increase in lamp intensity to compensate for light loss. Bulbs that have a higher electrical current rating could overheat the lamp housing and increase the need for fuse replacement. One should check the bulb's voltage and replace the bulb if necessary.

Bulbs may also blow as a result of arcing or pitting at the bulb contacts. Check the contacts for pitting, and clean or replace them as necessary. When replacing bulbs, one should make certain that the power is off. Bulbs should be turned off between uses; however, if the microscope is needed again in a few minutes, one should leave the bulb on. A bulb burns out prematurely if the filament is still hot when the bulb is turned on.

Zoom Malfunction

Another common problem is malfunction of the microscope's zoom feature. This might be the result of loose foot control connectors. The wiring connector should clip into its receptacle on the microscope stand. If it does not, clean the connector with contact cleaner and reinsert it. Also, trace the wires and connector looking for unsecured holders.

On connectors with small pins, one should clean them with an electrical contact spray cleaner, if available, and reinsert them. Also, it is important to look for wires that may have been pulled out of the connectors by mishandling. Foot switch wires are frequently pulled when moved across the floor. They have stress clamps yet still easily disconnect.

Assuming that the zoom setting is not in the extreme position and all other functions are working properly, fuse replacement or circuit breaker testing is generally the first step in attempting to correct zoom control problems. One should check the fuses or circuit breakers, and replace them if necessary.

On some units, a backup power supply is available. If the microscope has backup power, one should check to see whether it is on. When on, a light will blink indicating its availability. In this mode, none of the functions of the foot control are active, and a hand-actuated switch will have to be set. If the backup power is already on, turn it off and test the zoom function. Another possibility is that the zoom motor, gears, or foot switch may be jammed. Try pressing the foot pedal on different portions of the switch. If this fails, a service representative should be contacted. Many microscopes allow the use of manual zoom when the electric zoom jams.

Focus Malfunction

Most microscopes have a focus function that is analogous to the zoom function. Therefore, the same steps should be followed in diagnosing the problem. Naturally, if the electric focus does not function, the microscope can be moved up and down manually, or the patient's head level can be changed.

Assistant's Scope Not Axial to the Surgeon's View

It is frustrating to the assistant surgeon to have a field of view different from the primary surgeon. Unfortunately, this problem is not detected until everyone is scrubbed and the case has begun. One explanation frequently overlooked is that the surgeon's or assistant's scope front objective lens has been changed to a longer or shorter focal length lens. This naturally causes a different magnification and field which can appear to the viewer as malposition. One should simply replace the assistant's lens with one that matches the surgeon's.

Another possibility is that the assistant's scope is misaligned. Some assistant's scopes are externally mounted on dovetails that have positioning screws that become displaced from mishandling or movement (Fig. 20-3). If this becomes a problem during a surgical procedure, the surgeon should reduce magnification on the assistant's scope to create a wider field, which should include the area of the surgeon's field.

Internally mounted or beam-splitter–type assistant's scopes are usually not adjustable, but the mount can be checked to see if the assistant's scope was properly inserted before being tightened. The beam-splitter mount or the portion that attaches to the surgeon's scope could be loose. If moving the assistant's scope to the opposite side of the surgeon brings the assistant's scope into proper alignment, this is usually an indication that one of the surgeon's

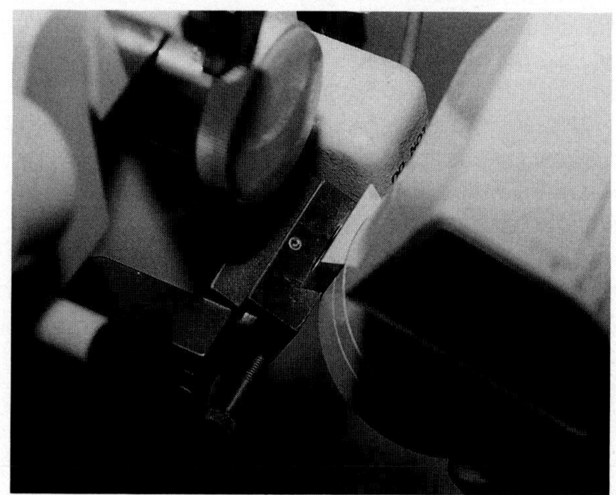

Figure 20-3. Dovetail microscope mount.

beam-splitter internal prisms is out of alignment. A microscope service representative will need to realign the prism. If both sides show malpositioning, the assistant's scope should be checked for possible damage or misalignment. This usually requires a service call.

X-Y Axis and Joy Stick Not Working Properly

Most microscopes allow the surgeon to move the microscope a few centimeters with a foot pedal control called the joy stick. In correlation with accepted mathematical standards, *x* movement gives horizontal or side-to-side movement while *y* gives front to rear movement. The *z* coordinate, which corresponds to vertical movement perpendicular to the surgical plane, is controlled by the focus mechanism.

If the *x-y* box is moving the microscope on its own, check the foot pedal protective cover and the joy stick. A plastic cover over the foot pedal can get twisted and pull on the joy stick, causing the *x-y* motor to run continuously.

If there is no movement of the *x-y* box, check the electrical connectors to the *x-y* box and the foot pedal. If the connectors are correct, one should check the fuse or circuit breaker. Some units have backup power which can be switched on when needed. When selected, the backup power disarms the foot switch function, and manual switching is required. The manual switches are located on the stand control panel.

If the *x-y* box moves, but will not center, the surgeon should check that the reference starting point is not too far to one side, limiting movement of the scope. One should look for a centering indicator and position the *x-y* axis at the indicator. The surgical field is centered while viewing it through the scope. On microscopes with a centering button, press the button and confirm that the scope is positioned in the center of its *x-y* box. The position of the patient's eye is adjusted manually while viewing it through the scope.

If the *x-y* control is centering with the joy stick, but there is difficulty controlling the direction of the movement of the scope, check the microscope *x-y* box orientation. Some microscopes can be turned and the *x-y* box left in a stationary position. During use this can cause the *x-y* box to be in a different respective position to the scope. Indicators on the *x-y* box should face the surgeon when properly oriented.

CAUTERY MALFUNCTION

Low Heat

Insufficient cautery heat leads to insufficient hemostasis, thus making subsequent surgical steps more difficult to perform. If the cautery unit is delivering insufficient heat, the surgeon should first check the controls and adjust them if appropriate. Also check to see if the tip is charred or loose. If charred, the tip is cleaned or replaced; if loose, the tip is adjusted or replaced. Loose connectors may also inhibit heat in the cautery tip. Both male and female connectors become loose after frequent use. Many plug-in connectors can be spread or cleaned to assure good contact. One should visually inspect and replace the cord if there is any sign of degradation indicated by broken insulation or frayed wires. When disconnecting the handle's power cord, the surgeon should hold the plug with one hand and the coagulator handle with the other. Separating the connectors by pulling on the cable can cause premature damage.

If the tip and connectors are in good condition, one should check for debris under the foot pedal. If there is no debris, the foot control pedal could be defective. For safety and reliability, the foot control pedal should be protected from water and debris by placing it in a small clear plastic bag, and tying the open end around the cable.

No Heat, and No Indicator Lights or Audio

If no heat, indicator lights, or audio are present, a problem with the power source is likely. It is important to check the power switch to be sure it is turned on and determine whether the power cord is unplugged or loose. One should also check the main power source for a tripped room circuit breaker as well as the instrument fuse or circuit breaker.

Power Indicator Is On, But No Heat

If the power indicator is on but the unit still produces no heat, check for a severely charred tip. Clean or replace the tip if appropriate. There could be loose connector contacts at the tip or handpiece wires. Both male and female connectors become loose after frequent use. Many plug-in connectors can be spread or cleaned to assure good contact. If the contacts are pitted, replace the tip or handpiece cable. Power with no heat might also be the result of a disconnected electrical connector or foot pedal. The surgeon should check these and reconnect if necessary. As mentioned earlier, the foot control pedal should be protected from water and debris by placing a small clear plastic bag over it and tying the open end around the cable.

IRRIGATION/ASPIRATION

Inadequate Irrigation

Problems with irrigation/aspiration can lead to multiple surgical complications such as a hypotonous eye, retained lens cortex, and prolonged surgical time. Inadequate irrigation may result if the irrigation bottle is too low or the irrigation line is kinked. It is helpful to check these and adjust the flow rate as necessary. Irrigation lines often become kinked if they are jammed between tables and instruments, if the system has been left on for a long period of time with the pinch valve keeping the tubing closed, or if the surgeon has wrapped the tubing around his or her forearm to have better control of the handpiece. Rarely does a tip clog at the irrigation end or a leak go unnoticed that will influence the flow rate. If the irrigation portion of the tip should clog, see the section on Inadequate Aspiration later. The only difference is that the irrigation line will be used in place of the aspiration line. If the aspiration is low, causing reduced irrigation, the surgeon should check for debris in the tip and reset the controls.

Bubbles in Irrigation Line

Every surgeon dreads the eye filling up with bubbles when performing a delicate maneuver. Bubbles in the irrigation line could have one of several causes. One should check the tubing to see if the irrigation line is properly primed and examine the tubing connections to determine if there is an air leak in the line. Another possibility is that the handpiece tip is leaking, possibly at the wound. It is important to check the wound site and the tightness of the tip. If the wound site is not leaking, one should remove the handpiece and check the tightness of the tip.

Irrigation Does Not Turn Off

If the irrigation does not turn off, the irrigation line might not be correctly aligned in the pinch valve. One should check the tubing position and place properly if necessary. Alternatively, the irrigation portions of the foot pedal could be sticking. The surgeon should check for debris or obstruction at the foot control as well as correct and test the pedal if appropriate.

Inadequate Aspiration

If the level of aspiration is inadequate, the aspiration setting may be incorrectly set. The surgeon should check the setting and reset if necessary. If the unit is a cassette type, the cassette that collects the fluid could be full. Many such models indicate on the front panel display that the cassette is full, and a sound is heard. Aspiration ceases until the cassette is replaced.

A clogged handpiece can also cause inadequate aspiration. It is important to remove and inspect the handpiece, and clear it if appropriate (Fig. 20-4). To clear the handpiece, the surgeon disconnects it from aspiration tubing and attaches a three-way stopcock. The two ends of the stopcock should be between the handpiece aspiration fitting and the aspiration tubing fitting. In the center port of the three-way stopcock, attach a 10-mL or larger syringe filled with balanced salt solution (BSS). The surgeon turns the stopcock valve to allow the syringe to flush BSS through the handpiece. It is helpful to push the syringe plunger, forcing fluid through the handpiece. The surgeon should not draw the flushing fluid back through the handpiece. When the syringe plunger resistance drops, the debris probably has been cleared. One should turn the stopcock to allow aspiration from the machine and insert the test chamber, if used, on the handpiece. The surgeon should fill the handpiece test chamber and test aspiration by seeing if the chamber will collapse. If a test chamber is not available, aspirate BSS from a sterile container. The surgeon should intermittently lift the tip out of the fluid to create bubbles in the aspiration line. The bubbles should move freely up the tubing.

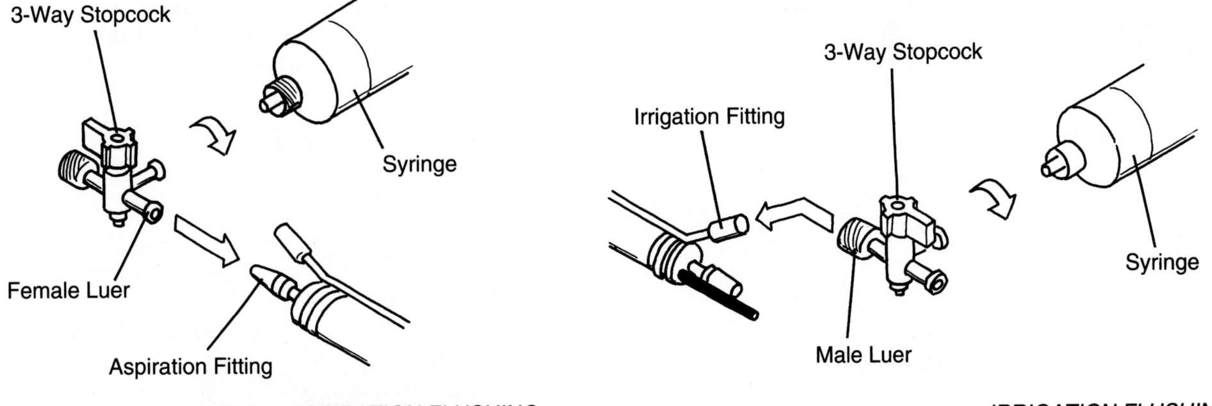

Figure 20-4. Handpiece flushing setup.

Tubing connectors might also be leaking. To test for leaks in tubing lines, one should remove the aspiration line from the handpiece, block the line with one's finger, and press the foot pedal for aspiration. The aspiration/vacuum meter should indicate high pressure. If the vacuum meter reads low, disconnect the tubing at the instrument and cover the vacuum fitting. Low vacuum indicates that the aspiration is set low or there is an internal vacuum problem. If the aspiration is not set low, service is needed.

Too Much Aspiration for Level of Irrigation

If the unit is delivering too much aspiration, one should first check to see if the maximum aspiration settings are too high. Reset the aspiration level and test. Irrigation could also be set too low. Check and adjust the irrigation settings or elevate the irrigation bottle height to equilibrate.

Setting Up Manual Irrigation/Aspiration

All ophthalmic surgeons should be skilled in manual irrigation/aspiration so that the operation may be completed despite equipment malfunction. If manual irrigation/aspiration is necessary, the surgeon first attaches a vented administration fluid set to an irrigating solution bottle for irrigation and anterior chamber maintenance. One should then push the output tubing of the administration set end into the tubing connector of an irrigation/aspiration cannula. Irrigation flow rate is controlled by adjusting the roller clamp supplied with the administration set. Attach a 5-mL syringe to the cannula's female Luer connector. The plunger of the syringe should be fully depressed to allow for maximum aspiration. The surgeon starts the irrigation flow, filling the tubing to release all bubbles from the system. It is important to leave the syringe plunger pushed in and the irrigation flow off until one is ready to start the procedure (Fig. 20-5).

Reflux Will Not Work

If the reflux does not work, the surgeon should check the aspiration port for debris and remove the handpiece from the eye. One should pinch the aspiration line approximately 2 feet above the connector and, while pinching, slide one's fingers down toward the handpiece. This should release any material obstructing the aspiration port. If a test chamber is available, the surgeon uses it to test the aspiration function. If the reflux mechanism still does not work, the surgeon simply pinches the irrigation tubing during the procedure to render a small burst of irrigation, which may be sufficient.

PHACOEMULSIFICATION

Phacoemulsification (phaco) is an elegant procedure and by nature is heavily reliant on the proper functioning of equipment. It is frustrating to make a small phacoemulsification incision only to learn that one must convert to a manual lens extraction because of equipment failure.

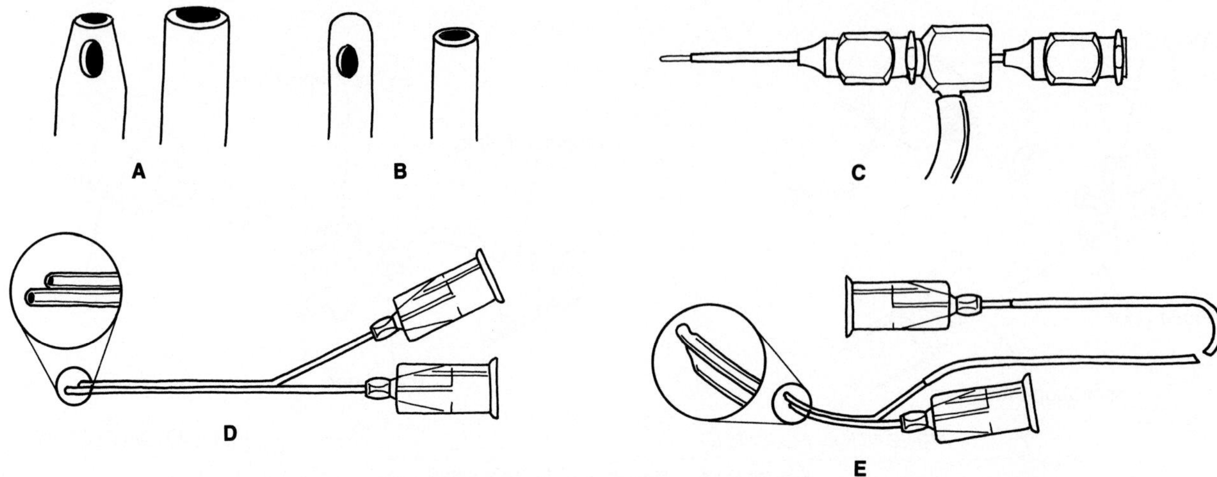

Figure 20-5. Manual irrigation/aspiration setups. (**A**) Irrigation cannulas. (**B**) Aspiration cannulas. (**C** through **E**) Irrigation and aspiration cannulas joined together.

Phaco Will Not Come On

Assuming that the irrigation/aspiration handpiece functions properly and that problems only occur when the phaco handpiece is connected, first check the handpiece electrical connections. Correct and retest the system. Electrically powered handpieces are usually powered by a cable with a connector that plugs into the side or front of the instrument. The surgeon should make certain that the connector plug is properly seated in the receptacle. If in doubt, remove and inspect the plug and reinsert it. If one does not hear power to the handpiece, install a backup handpiece. Hearing no power to the backup handpiece is an indication of control circuit failure. It is also important to check the handpiece tuning. Many models have either adjustable or automatic tuning, and do not run if not properly tuned. If your system has manual tuning, one should refer to the instruction booklet for tuning methods.

Too Little Phaco Power

If the phaco unit delivers too little power, the surgeon checks the instrument's power setting and adjusts it if necessary. It is helpful to examine the tip sleeve position and readjust as necessary. If the tip sleeve is too high, the port can be obstructed by the mouth of the incision pressing the sleeve against the tip. The surgeon also checks the phaco tip installation, and the tip itself (Fig. 20-6). Replacement of the tip is necessary if it is dull or bent; one must be certain to tighten and retest the handpiece.

Debris in the tip or handpiece might also interfere with power. If debris is present, the handpiece should be cleared. The surgeon should first disconnect the handpiece from the aspiration tubing and attach a three-way stopcock. The two ends of the stopcock should be between the handpiece aspiration fitting and the aspiration tubing fitting. On the center port of the three-way stopcock, attach a 10-mL or larger syringe filled with BSS. Turn the stopcock valve to allow the syringe to flush BSS through the handpiece. One should push the syringe plunger, forcing fluid through the handpiece without drawing the flushing fluid back through the handpiece. When the syringe plunger resistance drops, the debris probably has been cleared. The surgeon turns the stopcock to al-

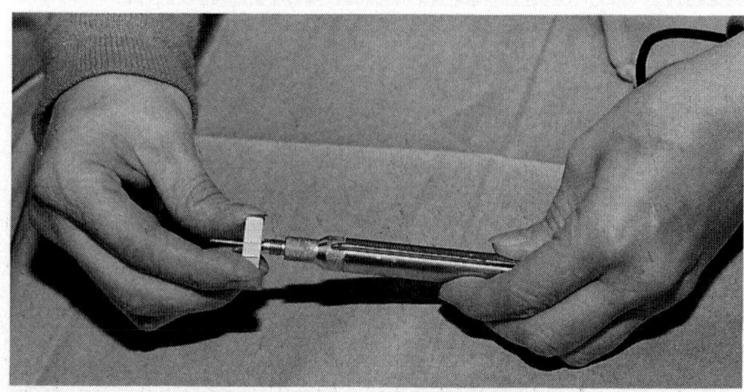

Figure 20-6. Phacoemulsification handpiece.

Table 20-3
Diagnostic Checklist: Too Little Phacoemulsification Power

Is the power set correctly?
Is the phacoemulsification tip sleeve position correct?
Is the phacoemulsification tip in good condition and has it been installed correctly?
Is there debris in the phaco tip or handpiece?
Is there adequate gas pressure going to the unit?
Is there an obstruction at the foot pedal?

low aspiration from the machine and insert the test chamber, if used, on the handpiece. One should then fill the handpiece chamber and test aspiration. If the irrigation line is in question, it is important to connect the stopcock to the irrigation line as described above. The stopcock port connectors are the reverse of when connecting to the aspiration lines (see Fig. 20-4).

Gas-driven units with low gas pressure can cause reduced phacoemulsification power. The gas tank or wall source driving the phaco unit should be checked. The gas may also be leaking through one of the lines or at the instrument.

Another source of power loss could be foot pedal obstruction. Look for debris around the foot pedal that might prevent the phaco pedal control from being fully depressed. Keep the foot controls clear of cables, tubing, surgical items and disposable needle and syringe caps, etc. For safety and reliability, the foot control pedal should be protected from water and debris by placing a small clear plastic bag over it and tying the open end around the cable. However, care must be taken to avoid twisting the plastic bag around the foot control, causing it to stick in a nonselected mode (Table 20-3).

Phaco Power Comes in Bursts

If the phaco power comes in bursts, several areas should be checked. The surgeon checks the phaco tip, and if it is loose, tightens it. One should also check the tip for obstructions and flush the handpiece if appropriate. It is also important to check the main control circuit for malfunction and recalibrate it if necessary. One must also check the foot pedal for debris, remove any debris, and retest the system.

Phaco Works, But Aspiration or Irrigation Not Working

If the phaco works but the aspiration or irrigation does not, the surgeon should check that the tubing and fittings are properly attached, and check fluid lines for kinked or pinched areas. One must also determine whether the handpiece tip is clogged and flush it if necessary. The surgeon checks the alignment of the handpiece tip sleeve. If the tip sleeve is too high, the port can be obstructed by the mouth of the incision pressing the sleeve against the tip. On cassette units, the cassette could be full. Empty the cassette and retest.

Another possible cause of aspiration or irrigation failure is electrical circuit malfunction. If recalibration is unsuccessful, service is needed.

VITRECTOMY

Problems with a vitrectomy unit can be related to the infusion port (inadequate flow or bubbles in the fluid line); the vitrector (guillotine action or aspiration); or the light pipe.

Infusion Port

If the infusion port is delivering inadequate flow, the surgeon checks the bottle of infusion fluid for adequate fluid level and bottle height. One should replace or adjust the level, and check the flow. The surgeon also evaluates whether the tubing stopcock is fully open, and whether the tubing is kinked, crushed, or twisted. It is important to check to be sure that the cannula has not disconnected from the infusion tubing, reducing eye pressure. If it has, the surgeon reconnects the cannula and carefully starts the flow.

Bubbles in the fluid line may also be a problem. Bubbles could result from inadequate priming. The surgeon should check the line for bubbles from the handpiece to the bottle. If bubbles are present, one must disconnect the irrigation line, checking that the drip chamber level is correct and running the fluid until all bubbles are out of the line. Bubbles might also be caused by vitreous in the port. If the presence of vitreous is suspected, the surgeon removes the handpiece and flushes the line with a fluid-filled syringe or clears the area around the infusion port with the vitrector while the infusion line is turned off. Again, it is important to check the flow.

If it is necessary, during an operation, to change from fluid to gas, the surgeon turns off the stopcock valve that controls the fluid line. One should turn on the gas and allow a few minutes for the gas to clear the line of fluid before proceeding.

Vitrector

If the guillotine action on a vitrector does not start, one checks to see if the tubing at the actuator end is pushed on too far, stopping the guillotine action. If it is, the surgeon slides the tubing back and restarts the unit (Fig. 20-7). If the actuator is jammed, one gently moves the actuator in a back-and-forth motion, and retest.

If the vitrector is providing inadequate aspiration, the aspiration canister may be full. The surgeon should also check all tubing connections, especially at the cassette, and tighten them if necessary.

If the surgeon has problems getting the reflux to work, he or she should check the port for debris. If debris is present, one removes the handpiece and pinches the aspiration line to release any material obstructing the aspiration port.

Light Pipe

The most common problem associated with the light pipe is lack of brightness. If this occurs, the illumination control might be set too low. Adjust it if appropriate. Debris on the light tip might also interfere with brightness. The surgeon removes the tip from the eye, cleans it, and views the light intensity. If it is correct, reinsert the tip and continue the procedure.

Another common problem is a burnt lamp. The surgeon removes the lamp and looks for dark spots on the glass, especially the part that faces the light pipe plug-in port. One then replaces the lamp. If the lamp is working, the fiberoptic bundle might be damaged. The surgeon unplugs the fiberoptic cable at the lamp housing, and views the light intensity. If the lamp intensity appears inadequate, one should remove the bulb and check for proper positioning, type, voltage, and wattage. If the output at the lamp housing port appears adequate, one must recheck the output at the fiberoptic cable tip. If the light output is inadequate, the surgeon should consider replacing the fiberoptic cable.

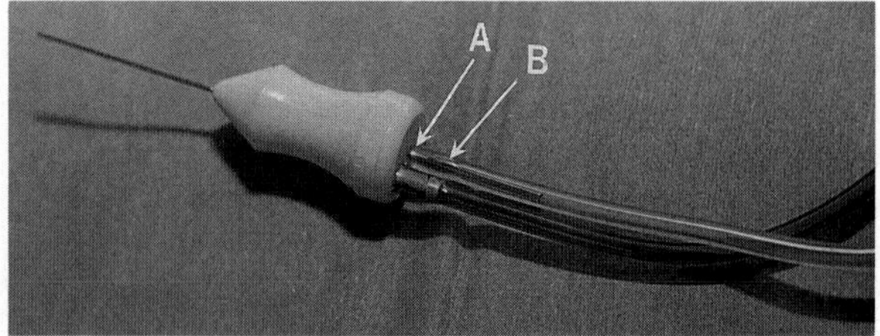

Figure 20-7. Vitrectomy handpiece with actuator end pushed on too far (**A**). Correct tubing position (**B**) is shown.

ENDOLASER

It is disconcerting to be peeling a macular membrane, find an inadvertent retinomy, and then learn that the endolaser is malfunctioning.

Unit Does Not Turn On

If the endolaser unit will not turn on, check the circuit breaker or fuse on the back of the unit. If the circuit breaker is not located on the back of the unit, the surgeon checks for other locations. If the circuit breaker cannot be found, it could be built into the on-off power switch. One should try pushing the power switch down and up again. Also check the room power line circuit breaker. If it is tripped, it is helpful to reset and restart the machine. Also, one should check to see if the power cable connector plug is loose. Power cable connectors rarely come loose, but they are often subjected to movements which cause bends and disrupt the connection. Tighten the connector, and restart the unit.

System Powers Up but Is Stuck in Standby Mode

If the system powers up but remains stuck in standby mode, the controls could be set incorrectly. One should check and reset the controls. Some systems require that the laser power and aiming beam controls be set at minimum before standby mode can be established.

Poor cable connections might also cause the system to remain in standby. Possibly the foot switch or fiberoptics probe is not connected properly. The surgeon should examine the foot switch connector for tightness and the probe for proper insertion. Often the "Stand-by" and "Treat" lamps are lit simultaneously.

A system might also revert to standby if the laser tube is overheating. One should let the system cool for 2 to 3 minutes and check the "Treat" lamp indicator.

An improper trigger signal to ignite the laser tube might also cause the system to stall. If this is suspected, the surgeon turns off the instrument for approximately 30 seconds and then restarts it. Most systems take approximately 45 seconds before the "Treat" light indicates readiness.[4]

The unit might be receiving inadequate power line voltage. Have in-house maintenance test the electrical supply during times when the system will not exit the standby mode. Generally, tolerances are set that do not permit the unit to ignite unless sufficient power requirements are met.

Extreme temperature might also be the source of the problem, especially in portable units. Often units that have recently been moved to a new area from outside the building require time to equilibrate. If the unit has been exposed to extreme temperatures, let the instrument run approximately 10 minutes before attempting to exit the standby mode.[4]

A disconnected "door switch interlock" also causes a unit to remain in standby. Some endolasers have a door closure shutdown connector in the rear of the unit. If the entrance door to the room is ajar, the system automatically shuts down. If this function is not being used, check the bypass shorting plug, located on the rear of the instrument, for tightness. It can be knocked loose or bent when moving the instrument for cleaning. This can cause the "Stand-by" and "Treat" lights to be on simultaneously.

Low Light Output, and Power Meter Reads Selected Level But Output Too Low

This problem may be caused by debris on the fiberoptic cable tip. The surgeon should check the light pipe tip, clean it, and reinsert it. Also check the main fiberoptic cable connections. The output from the fiberoptic cable can often be tested by placing the tip in front of the external output sensor, located on the face of the laser power unit, and setting the instrument in the test mode. If the output level from the cable reads low (although when surgically treating the internal output level reads correct), this is an indication that the optical filter in the instrument is dirty or discolored, or that the cable itself is damaged. Remember also that the external sensor is measuring light levels at the end of the cable, whereas the internal sensor is sensing light entering the cable.

CONTACT LENS WATER FOGGING AND WATER SPOTS

A contact lens obscured by fogging or water spots can become a problem during surgery. Inadequate visualization of the retina during critical steps of a procedure can induce unwanted surgical complications.

Fogging

If the adherent drape around the patient's eye is loose, the patient's breath may leak out to the surgical field. On intubated patients, pack the patient's nose with gauze sponges. If a local procedure is being performed, one should clean the skin around the nose with alcohol while carefully avoiding the eyes. It is important to allow the alcohol to dry and reapply the drape. Applying a skin prep can also help avoid loss of contact with the drape.

Water Spots on the Lens

Too much infusion fluid can cause water spots on a contact lens. If this becomes a problem, one must reduce the flow and wipe the lens. Wiping the lens with a cellulose sponge rather than a cotton-tipped applicator avoids adherence of cotton fibers to the lens. Water spots may also occur if a sclerotomy is too large, causing some of the irrigation fluid to be sprayed from the irrigation port onto the contact lens. If this is the case, the surgeon clamps the infusion line, wipes the surface of the lens with a sterile cotton ball, towel, or cellulose sponge, and restarts the irrigation solution. This procedure generally removes water spots. If it does not, one should rewet the surface of the lens and carefully wipe the lens dry.

CRYOTHERAPY

Cryotherapy (cryo) plays an instrumental role in treating peripheral retinal breaks. A malfunctioning cryotherapy unit can lead to a less than optimal surgical outcome.

Cannot Get Ice Formation

Failure to get ice formation with cryotherapy may result from the on-off valve being partially in the Off position, a closed gas cylinder valve, or cylinder pressure below 600 psi. If cylinder pressure is the problem, replace the gas cylinder. A newly replaced cylinder that is cold should be allowed to warm up to room temperature before use. The regulator pressure could also be set too low, or there could be moisture in the probe. A probe plug improperly engaged to the tank gasket could cause a leak.

Temperature Gauge Reading and Iceball Do Not Correlate

If the temperature gauge reading and the iceball do not correlate, the pyrometer may be out of calibration. Calibrate for the correct temperature. The pyrometer is usually calibrated with the probe connected to the unit and the system shut off. To calibrate the pyrometer more dynamically, submerge the probe tip in ice water and adjust the calibration screw, which is usually located on the front panel of the unit. To approximate the tip temperature, adjust the screw to 0°C.

If erroneous readings persist, replace the probe and retest the system for accuracy.

The problem could also be a defective thermocouple. One should replace the probe and retest the system for accuracy.

More Than the Cryo Tip Freezes

If more than the cryo tip freezes, the temperature is probably adjusted too high, or the pyrometer needs calibration. The plastic sleeve over the cryo tip may be torn and need to be replaced.

Temperature Not Registering on Console

If the temperature is not registering on the console, is an intraocular probe being used? Many intraocular probes are too small to contain a temperature-sensing thermocouple, and therefore the temperature gauge will not register. The unit may also have a bad probe temperature sensor, connector, or line. Try a replacement probe. If this does not correct the problem, then it is most likely in the temperature-sensing circuit or gauge.

CONCLUSION

Ophthalmic surgery is sophisticated and heavily reliant on technology. Equipment malfunctions can cause surgical complications with untoward patient outcome. At the least, equipment malfunctions cause surgical delays. The ophthalmic surgeon must be well versed in troubleshooting equipment problems. The responsibility to understand the equipment cannot be delegated to a nurse, technician, or other ancillary staff, because these persons are often not available for emergency off-hour cases. The authors hope that this chapter serves as a basic guide to troubleshooting unexpected equipment failures.

References

1. Grob B. Basic electronics. New York, McGraw-Hill, 1971:210–211.
2. Davidson J. Reference handbook of operating microscopes. Carl Zeiss Canada, 1987:135–136.
3. Hoerentz P. The operating microscope. V. Maintenance and cleaning. J Microsurg 1981;2:181–182.
4. HGM Operation manual. User maintenance and troubleshooting. HGM Utah:11-12.

Ophthalmic Surgery Complications: Prevention and Management,
edited by Judie F. Charlton and George W. Weinstein.
J. B. Lippincott Company, Philadelphia © 1995.

21 Legal Aspects

Jerome W. Bettman, Sr.

One of the unfortunate complications of surgery is a claim or suit against the surgeon. In the chapter on informed consent it was stated that the best prophylactic against a patient instituting legal action is the process of informed consent. The best defense is good documentation.

Almost everyone has heard that good records are of utmost importance, but few know why. There are three reasons:

1. The jury presumes that the facts are probably true because you took the time and trouble to write them;
2. The trial is years after the fact. By this time, the patient and the defendant frequently have different recollections of what occurred, but neither side truly remembers just what did happen. But the record was written at the time, and the jury knows this.
3. The jury is usually exposed to days or weeks of testimony during the trial. The testimony is frequently confusing and even benumbing, and most of it is forgotten before the jury deliberates, but the record is introduced into evidence and may be brought into the jury room where it can be looked at long after much else is forgotten.

There are essential precautions that should be taken. As indicated above, *never* alter a record in light of possible litigation. Although a record is frequently the most important instrument of defense, an altered record makes the case almost indefensible. The alterations indicate that you may not be trustworthy, and a jury will suspect that anything you say is untrue. Even the cleverest alterations can usually be detected. No matter how damning the record may be, never, never alter it.

Alteration in the record may be detected because the record had been copied previously for insurance purposes. In this situation the plaintiff's attorney can acquire the copy which shows the original unaltered record and a copy of the altered record, and the plaintiff has won the case. There are companies that specialize in detection of alterations. This method may be used if a copy of the original is not available.

The immediate question that frequently arises is what to do if a mistake is made while writing the record. Draw a line through the error, but allow the error to be visible.

The reason is that the record may have been copied in the interim. The copy may unexpectedly be in the possession of the plaintiff's attorney. If the correction is dated and initialed it is perfectly clear that it was not done to deceive, otherwise the inference of deception is used and this may be a great problem for the defense.

Records should be written at the time of occurrence. The following should be documented: any complications, mishaps or unusual occurrences; worries or concerns of the patient or family; instructions and warnings given to the patient at the time of discharge and date or advise regarding return visits; records of pertinent material from telephone calls. Avoid placing blame on others, the hospital, or economics.

There are other wise precautions regarding the record. Use the record for what it is intended—that is, a record of the patient's history, examination, and progress. Do not include personal remarks about the patient or other extraneous material. I was once associated with a doctor who would write "Stupid" on the record of a patient who might have been slow. There were frequently several exclamation points after "Stupid." Another associate wrote "S.C.", indicating "slow cerebrator." This was frequently followed by indications of the power, such as "S.C.^{3rd}," "S.C.^{9th}," or even "S.C.^{nth}." The power was frequently a more accurate indication of the doctor's indisposition than the patient's cerebration. Remember that any symbol on the record must be explained fully, under oath, during the deposition or the trial.

One should be just as careful concerning remarks on the patient's financial record. "Deadbeat" written on the record could give the jury the impression that the doctor is more interested in finances than the patient's welfare.

Information to be included in a medical record can be categorized as either essential or non essential. If the patient would be significantly endangered by failure to record the information (eg, the omission of a tonometry reading in a glaucoma patient), then it is *essential*, and must be recorded. Essential information is not usually extensive in quantity.

All other information is *nonessential;* although numerous nonessential readings and observations are commonly recorded in depth on an initial visit, such observations should not be recorded for follow-up visits unless they can be written every time the observations are made. If the handling of a particular case comes into question, the trier of fact is likely to presume that notations on the record are made on a consistent basis; thus if an observation that is made on every visit is recorded only on the patient's first two visits, for example, "fundus negative?", it might be assumed that the observation was made only on those two visits and was not made thereafter. If, on the other hand, the observation was never recorded on any follow-up visit, the trier of fact might be persuaded that the physician always makes the observation in such patients but customarily records only abnormal findings. Similarly, it is common practice for nurses to note when the doctor visits a hospitalized patient. If such a practice is evident from the records, and the nurse neglects to record a specific physician visit, the physician could have a difficult task proving the patient was seen unless a progress note was made on that occasion. Therefore, complete omission of nonessential information is preferable to inconsistent record-keeping practices.

Experienced attorneys have said, "If I can't defend the records, I can't defend the doctor."

There are four essential characteristics of a good record: completeness, objectivity, consistency, and accuracy. A poor record may encourage a plaintiff's attorney to pursue a case that seems otherwise defensible.

The length of time that records should be kept is a frequent subject of discussion. Although most states have a definite period after which the statute of limitations applies, the period varies in different states, and it is wise to consult an attorney or official in the given state. A caveat of which one should be aware is that the statute might begin to run *not* from the time the alleged substandard act occurred but from the time the patient should have been *aware* that the alleged substandard care caused the problem. This is frequently indefinite and may be subject to judgment of the court. Do not dispose of records until this period has elapsed. Consult your local medicolegal attorney.

If an irate patient telephones, it is wise to attempt to get him to come to the office so that the circumstances can be explained. This could forestall the suit. It should be made clear that there will be no charge for this visit. If the patient refuses to come, an explanation should be given over the telephone. Such an explanation must be delivered in a kind, patient, and lucid manner.

It is not as uncommon as one would expect that a patient who has instituted litigation will request the doctor he is suing to continue to care for him. The logic seems to be that "I really like you, I am just trying to get some money from the insurance company." The better judgment is to refuse to see the patient. At this point the patient is an adversary. The refusal should be done in a pleasant manner by stating that your attorney will not permit it. Some attorneys have advised that continuing to care for the litigating patient gives the doctor two advantages. One is that it is a demonstration of the patient's confidence in the doctor's ability if the matter should ever come to trial. The other reason is that it keeps the patient from going to another doctor who may be critical of the care. It is extremely unlikely that continued care will cause the patient to drop the suit, and the adversary position is very uncomfortable.

If the patient's attorney attempts to communicate with you, do not respond. The plaintiff's attorney knows what he wants and you don't. He may be most pleasant in requesting a report and add that you should send your full bill for this service. Report this to your attorney and let him or her handle it.

If the patient and his attorney decide to pursue the claim, it is important that the surgeon be aware of ensuing legal procedures and how to act during the course of development of the suit. The sequence of events are the interrogatories, the depositions, and the trial. Each is presented below.

THE INTERROGATORIES

The interrogatories are a series of questions sent by the opposing attorney on behalf of his/her client. They are a part of the discovery process and enable the attorney to obtain information to which he or she is entitled. The questions often seem shockingly searching and explicit. Examples of the questions that might be asked are: "Name every patient with this condition that you have ever treated and state the outcome"; "name every course in ophthalmology that you have ever attended"; "name every book and article related to this subject that you have ever read"; and "state in which way your handling of the case was substandard." There may be 200 questions.

Never attempt to answer them without your attorney's help. His responses might be: "This question violates physician–patient relationship"; "too numerous to list"; "irrelevant"; "see above"; and "see below."

Throughout the course of litigation always be completely open and honest with your own attorney. Always tell him everything, no matter how bad it sounds or how wrong you might have been. It is only by this open communication that the best defense can be formulated. One's own attorney is not going to divulge defects to the other side, but the other side may discover these defects, and you must enable your attorney to be prepared.

The physician who is being sued must work very closely with his attorney. No attorney can properly defend a doctor without a total effort on the doctor's part.

There is frequently a long period after the interrogatories before further overt developments occur. Either side may obtain advice from consultants during this period.

The next overt action is usually the deposition. The defendant, experts, the patient, and others such as nurses, hospital administrators, and other physicians may be deposed.

The deposition is so important that the entire chapter that follows is devoted to it, but before discussing the deposition or trial, it is necessary to be aware of the difference in philosophy between law and medicine and of the role of expert witnesses as well as consultants and defendants.

For all parties, the policy behind discovery is to prevent surprise at trial. The courts have determined that justice and judicial economy in the use of court facilities are best served by having both sides in litigation apprised of the facts, records, and witnesses the other may introduce at the time of trial. Statistically, many lawsuits, including medical malpractice cases, are dismissed or settled before trial because of information that has been developed during the discovery phase of the litigation. For example, an attorney representing the patient may advise his client to dismiss the case because he learns through discovery that the claimed injuries preceded the alleged acts of malpractice or because he believes that the physician is more convincing than the patient in testimony on whether informed consent was obtained before surgery or that the untoward result occurred in the presence of acceptable medical practice.

As the suit against the physician progresses, there will be depositions taken from the defendant, plaintiff, and potential witnesses. These procedures usually occur long after the interrogatories. After another long period the matter may come to trial, unless the case is dropped or settled. Before proceeding with a discussion of these developments, it is necessary for the physician, whether defendant or expert witness, to clearly understand the philosophical difference in focus between medicine and law.

Approximately 16,000 paid claims were reported to the National Practitioner Data Bank in its first year of existence. If one were to very conservatively estimate that there were at least that many that were dropped without payment and that there were only two experts on each side, we have a figure of 64,000 experts. There were probably many more. There are approximately 560,000 physicians in this country. Thus an average of one in eight physicians is called on each year. The actual number of experts required may be much greater.

PHILOSOPHY OF LAW AND MEDICINE

In these modern times, the majority of ophthalmologists will be involved in medicolegal suits, whether in the capacity of a defendant, an expert witness, or a consultant to an attorney.

In such actions, the philosophical concepts of the

law take precedence over those of medicine in terms of the aim of each profession with respect to a lawsuit. It is important for physicians who may be involved in medicolegal suits to understand the difference between these aims.

It is the aim of medicine to arrive at the "truth," which usually is the correct diagnosis, appropriate mechanism of action, realistic prognosis, and therapy. In medicine, an open discussion is frequent, either by consultation or presentation at grand rounds. All aspects of the case are discussed and everything is revealed. Physicians might expect medicolegal lawsuits to have similar aims, but they most certainly do not.

Lawsuits are not really intended to uncover the truth. Reduced to its essentials, a lawsuit is simply an extraordinary and complex mechanism for finally resolving a dispute, for reaching a decision. Attorneys are advocates for their clients and not primarily seekers of truth. Because society values some things more highly than truth and the proof necessary to arrive at the truth, the decision sought in a lawsuit must be reached in accordance with complex exclusionary rules of evidence and without the benefit of potentially determinative evidence which is inadmissible because it is protected by the constitutional privilege against self-incrimination, or by the privileges against disclosures of communications between a patient and his or her physician or a client and his or her lawyer.

Some physicians testifying as experts appear to believe that all aspects of a matter should be discussed openly, as one would in grand rounds. In the adversarial contest of a lawsuit, this openness can create serious difficulty, because the opposing side may intend to present a different or opposite viewpoint, irrespective of its appropriateness, and leave it to the court or a jury to determine where the "truth" lies between these differing viewpoints. An open discussion of all aspects of the case will create an unacceptable bias in favor of the other side because they will abide by the procedure that both sides should follow as stated in the following paragraph.

THE DEPOSITION

A witness or defendant should always respond to a question, whenever appropriate to do so, and always do so truthfully. The understandable temptation to respond with information other than or beyond that required in response to a specific question in order to "explain" something should be strenuously resisted. If a witness or defendant volunteers more information than necessary, a bias may be created in favor of the other side because the opposing attorney will present an adversarial position. Ordinarily, the answers of a witness or defendant should be as brief as possible, always consistent with a truthful response. Perhaps this will help to ensure, as nearly as possible, that the aim of a lawsuit to reach a decision will be based upon the truth.

It is probable that the importance of the deposition is underestimated by more people, except the attorneys, than any portion of the entire suit.

The physical structure of the deposition is reasonably simple. An attorney representing each of the interested parties is present, together with a certified court reporter. The reporter swears in the persons to be deposed so that the entire proceedings are conducted under oath. The reporter records every word and then has it typed. The transcription is submitted to the deposed for corrections and signature.

Anything said in the deposition can be read to the jury if there is a trial, and this is often years later. The deposition may determine the basis for a trial and whether or not there will be a trial. The deposition may take place in any mutually agreeable area: the attorney's office, the deponent's office or home, etc. The plaintiff's attorney often willingly comes to the physician's office. This enables him to gain an impression of the general milieu: what instrumentation and what books are present, and the impression of efficiency and economics.

There have been instances in which a reporter has recorded the name of every book and periodical in the doctor's office. These can then be checked to determine if they might be useful in evidence, especially if the plaintiff's attorney has not been able to get an expert witness to testify. The attorney can ask if the doctor relies on a publication to enable him to form an opinion. He might thus get the publication into evidence, and this could be very important.

The defense attorney sometimes has an additional reason for not wanting the deposition to be in the defendant doctor's office. The physician may have had little or no experience in testifying. He will eventually have to give testimony in the unfamiliar and relatively hostile environment of the courtroom. If his deposition is taken in the familiar and comfortable ambience of his own office, it will do less to prepare him for the courtroom experience than would having to give his deposition in the more hostile environment of the plaintiff's attorney's office. In this respect, the deposition may be used as a training experience.

The deposition is subject to a number of the same privileges as are also enforced in trial. Among these are the attorney-client privilege, the proceedings of committees of the organized medical staffs of hospitals, and the attorney's work product (that which counsel derives from his own consultants, or workup of the file based on skill and innovation). An important exception to privilege is that the patient-physician privilege is deemed waived when the patient files suit against the physician.

The purpose of the deposition is for the opposing attorney to gain information, and to provide the anlage for the deponent to contradict himself, if trial does ensue.

The attorney gains two types of information. The first is about the case: facts, weaknesses, general medical information, and what individuals or publications may have been consulted. He may ask almost anything. He can ask hundreds of questions, of which all but one may be irrelevant, but that one may make his case. The deposition may enable him to determine the weaknesses that may be exploited, and to prepare a defense against the strengths.

The attorney also gains information about the deponent and how he is likely to appear and act at the trial. As stated before, it may determine if there will be a trial. He may intentionally try to anger the deponent. Attorneys are pleased if the opposing witness is easily angered, or if he is snappish or rude, or if he is supercilious or arrogant. These characteristics may discredit the witness and create a very favorable environment for his opposition. The opposition is especially pleased if the deponent talks too much. Such mannerisms as rudeness, outbursts of temper, and garrulousness may cause the plaintiff's attorney to raise his estimate of the "payoff" from $200,000 to $400,000. On the contrary, the witness who is presentable, articulate, sincere, kindly, and honest but succinct is very discouraging to the opposition and may cause the plaintiff's attorney to drop the case or to settle for a trivial amount.

The attorney also evaluates personal appearance. Some individuals may be honest but look like liars, or the reverse. The witness who doesn't look others in the eye creates an unfavorable impression. Eye contact is an important aspect of communication.

Many attorneys use the deposition as a means of causing the witness to apparently or actually contradict himself during the trial. The more times a question is asked in a similar but somewhat altered manner and the more voluble a witness is, the greater is the chance that he will seem to contradict himself when asked similar material in trial. If a witness can be made to appear that he has given contradictory answers to questions asked in trial compared with his answers in deposition, credibility is lost.

When the attorney leaves the deposition he may dictate his impressions of how effective the witness might be on the stand and evaluate his case accordingly.

Proper and thorough preparation prior to the deposition is very important. One must know all details of the case history, including nurses' notes and results of laboratory tests and radiographs. If other questions or records have already been obtained, it is well to have reviewed them so that contradictions, or "traps," can be avoided. The doctor should know the names, actions, and possible complications of any drugs that were used. He should also know details of applicable surgical procedures, complications, and alternate procedures.

The doctor should meet with his attorney for a thorough discussion well in advance of the deposition. The attorney should be told everything good and bad about the case, and he should give advice on what might be asked in the deposition and what problems to anticipate. The witness or defendant should ask the attorney whether or not to read any literature or discuss the case with consultants. It is probable that he will be asked during the deposition what literature has been read and with whom he has discussed the case. Literature is considered hearsay and cannot be introduced into evidence unless someone cites it. One should therefore be cautious and consider whether it is advisable to risk introducing a given article into evidence as an exhibit by mentioning it. If the deponent says that he discussed the case with another expert, the latter may then be required to give a deposition. For these reasons, I neither read literature in preparation for the deposition, nor speak to others about the case without discussing the advisability with the attorney. A book that has become an exhibit can be carried into the jury room where the jury can read it long after they have forgotten what the witness has said.

Your attorney should review questions that might be asked. It is well to have him act as the devil's advocate. He should also tell you how to present your case most favorably. If you are a defendant, and your attorney will not spend a couple of hours preparing you well in advance of the deposition, you should consider getting another attorney.

The following guides are usually important when being deposed:

1. Always tell the truth and do not exaggerate or make statements that you cannot substantiate.
2. Do not volunteer any information unless your attorney has previously indicated that you should, and this is not usual. As previously mentioned, a point against you may make the case for the plaintiff's attorney; a point in your favor will give him the opportunity to prepare against it when it is introduced at the trial. I do not even amplify my training and credentials beyond an honest answer during the deposition. This is in marked contrast to my response during the trial.

   If a question can be answered honestly with a simple "Yes" or "No," say only that. Many witnesses have made serious mistakes by saying "Yes, but ...," and then adding a paragraph that does little but aid the opposition. Do not explain your thought processes in arriving at your answer.

   Your attorney may say, "Doctor, you have answered the question." Take the hint. The next step might be, "Doctor, will you please be quiet."

   Do not help the examiner by asking "Do you mean 'X' or do you mean 'Y'?" He will then ask both.

   The more you commit yourself, the more likely you are to contradict yourself in the deposition and in the trial. The defendant may set the standard of care for himself in the deposition, and this could be disastrous. He might even be called as the plaintiff's witness and have the unpleasant experience of being questioned by a hostile attorney immediately after mounting the witness stand.
3. Always wait for the entire question before answering. Wait five full seconds before you speak. This will enable your attorney to formulate objections and give you time to think. The last phrase may be important. It may contain a "hooker." If the question is a compound one, have it broken into its component parts before answering, otherwise your answer may imply something that you do not mean.
4. If you do not know an answer, say so. Don't guess. The court will accept opinions, but not guesses. Take all of the time that you wish to answer a question. The jury is not there to see how long you take. If the question is not clear, or you don't understand it, say so. Never hesitate to ask that the question be repeated.
5. I will almost never name any book or individual as *the* authority. If asked whether or not a given book or individual is the authority, I will answer that there are a number of authorities, which is nearly always true. If *one* is named as an authority, then all of the statements contained therein carry great weight, and some of these statements may be very damaging.
6. Usually, your personal notes are known as "work product" and are not disclosed to the opposition. However, if you use them to prepare yourself for the deposition, they may be acquired by the other side. Therefore, it is wise to be somewhat careful in writing your own notes. Do not write such things as "This might have been malpractice," or "I botched."

It is well for the expert to be aware of certain words or phrases of significance. These have been placed in groups.

1. *Words that the witness might say: "But" or "And."* What is said after either of these words may cause problems. The witness should be responsive to the question but should be concise and generally should not volunteer information. The more the witness says, the more likely that the testimony can be contradicted by others or by the witness in trial. Deviation from this policy should only be made after preliminary discussion with one's attorney.

"Inadvertent." A witness frequently uses this word to mean unavoidable. This is incorrect. The definition in Webster's Unabridged Dictionary is: not turning the mind to a matter; heedless; negligent; inattentive. This is rarely what the witness intends to convey. Don't use the word.

"I guess" or "I think" or "I speculate." Guesses and speculations are not permitted. It is proper to express an opinion. "In my opinion" is acceptable, but do not equivocate about that of which you are certain.

"Substandard" is equivalent to malpractice. Be certain that this is what you mean.

Do not characterize your own testimony. Phrases such as *"in all candor"* or *"honestly,"* or *"I am doing the best I can"* should not be used.

2. *Questions from the opposing attorney of which to be aware.*

"Who is an authority?" Take care in naming someone. That person's opinion will then prevail. There are many so-called authorities, but actually there is rarely an authority. It is best to specify that no person or book is authoritative or standard or classic in the sense that it sets the standard of practice.

"Is.....an acknowledged expert?" One might answer, "No, but he or she is a competent ophthalmologist and prominent in his or her field."

"Name an authoritative text or article." The remarks after "Who is an authority," above, apply here. One should also be aware that in most courts a text or article is considered "hearsay" and cannot be introduced in evidence unless the witness names it.

"Do you defer to .....?" If you do, that individual's opinion will prevail over yours.

"How often has this complication occurred in your hands?" If never, you might add that it does occur in the hands of other well-trained physicians (if this is the case) or, in trial, "I have been lucky." In deposition perhaps just say "never."

"I am almost finished, just one or two questions more." Be on guard. The attorney may save his most significant questions for the end when you don't expect them and are becoming relaxed and maybe less thoughtful.

"What do you charge for your testimony?" "I charge for my expertise and time, not for my testimony." But be open with the amount that you do charge.

3. *Statements from the attorney on your side. "Don't guess."* If you don't know do not hesitate to say so, or if you are uncertain say so, but don't guess. Never represent that you know something when you do not. A reasonable estimate is all right as long as you say it is just that.

"I object." Listen for any clue that might be coming. Your attorney may object because he actually does object to a question, but he might do it to give you time and have you rethink the answer, or to keep you out of trouble.

"But this is true, isn't it?" Listen to the attorney's implied suggestion, but don't be an advocate. Leave that role to the attorney.

4. *A few brief hints."Ordinary care"* is not necessarily what you or I would do, but what the hypothetical average person would do under the same circumstances. It is what at least *some* other good local physicians would have done.

"Is......acceptable practice?" It is if a minority of your reputable colleagues would have done the same thing under the same circumstances. Reputable simply means not disreputable.

This is not in my area of expertise." If this is the case do not hesitate to say so. It will keep you out of trouble and add to your credibility.

Do not permit an attorney to pressure you into giving percentages that indicate more precision than you know or mean to infer. One might say "I estimate that the incidence is less than 25%." The other attorney might then ask "Is it less than 15%? More than 10%?" etc. until you have been pressured into stating an incidence more exactly than you know. The other attorney might say at a later date that you testified that the incidence was between 10% and 15%, a fact that you do not know. I sometimes say that I do not play the numbers game.

The following is of special importance: Always tell the truth, respond to the question, but don't add anything unless it is necessary to be clear on an important issue in the case or unless it is agreed to in advance. Do not be an advocate. Do not permit an attorney to "put words in your mouth."

Look upon the deposition as a continuous cross-examination, which is essentially what it is. It is the other side's "show." If you leave the deposition feeling that you did not get a chance to tell your story, you were a great success. The other side failed.

After the deposition is transcribed, a copy should be sent to you for any corrections. Read it. If the case does come to court, re-read your deposition several times. This will be very helpful in avoiding contradictions which the opposing attorney would like to bring out.

After the deposition, each side may get experts. If you are a defendant, help your attorney with the selection of experts. They can make or break the case.

Approximately 80% of cases are settled after the deposition and before the trial. Attorneys usually prefer to settle because they then have some control over the outcome. They do not have this control if it is determined in trial.

THE TRIAL—WHETHER A DEFENDANT OR AN EXPERT

Careful preparation is an essential ingredient of a successful outcome in court.

It is naive not to recognize that a trial is a contest of

impressions. No matter how scientifically correct your testimony might be, it only weighs in the decision-making process if the jury believes it. Because of this, the physician-defendant and the expert witness must be aware of what is important in creating these impressions. In my opinion, a successful medical witness must be knowledgeable about the case and the subject, he must be honest, he must be discreet, and he must create the proper impression as will be discussed below.

To attain this end, extensive pre-trial conferences with the attorney are usually essential. In these conferences, the attorney should prepare the witness for the direct and the cross-examination. The good and bad aspects of the case must be discussed with complete candor. Every anticipated question and answer should be reviewed. Any inconsistencies in the record should be worked out. All important points brought out in all the depositions must be reviewed. The attorney must also instruct the witness on the salient points of the law. He should do more than this: he should instruct the witness in how to appear in court, how to dress, the proper demeanor, and to anticipate how the opposing attorney may act.

It is obvious that all of these things require time. The defendant must insist that his attorney spend hours with him, well in advance of the trial. These things cannot be done properly by meeting an hour before the trial is to take place. If the attorney does not devote the required time, the defendant should demand another attorney.

It is essential that the witness (defendant or expert) be completely familiar with the case record in its every aspect, including nurses' notes, laboratory tests, pathological specimens, and x-rays.

It is common practice that the average physician spends little time in reading the nurses' notes in the chart. The clinician frequently thinks that it is unfortunate that a trained nurse who has spent years in preparation for her vocation spends hours charting notes that no one looks at. Bear in mind that if litigation ensues, these notes become of great legal importance. They are a record of observations made at the time by a relatively impartial observer. One should look at nurses' notes and be sure of their accuracy.

THE TRIAL

The juror's decision is based largely on impressions, and the first impression of the witness is created when he qualifies himself as an expert. This occurs immediately after he is sworn in. No matter how correct one's testimony is, it only counts if the jury believes it. The credibility of the witness is first established by his qualification. These should be presented clearly, and as completely as one can without being too verbose or boring. This is not time for reluctance, but the qualifications should be presented in a somewhat humble manner, certainly not with arrogance. It can be helpful if one's attorney will say, "Doctor, I know that your natural modesty makes you reluctant to bring out all of your qualifications, but I must ask you to attempt to put this modesty aside for the moment." In my opinion, it is well for the attorney to ask occasional questions such as, "Please tell us about your teaching positions. Please tell us what you have published, what research you have done." In answer to each of these, the witness can and should amplify the subject, in a somewhat humble manner, but with due regard toward impressing the jury. The attorney who asks a question before *each* statement of the witness's accomplishments may sound as though he and the witness are in collusion, and this will not convey a good impression. At the other extreme, a witness who must expound on all his accomplishments without occasional intervening questions may sound too egotistical.

It is critical that the qualifications be brought out in the proper manner. If the witness is repeatedly asked leading questions regarding his accomplishments, it will avoid his appearing pompous.

The problem of the proper manner to bring out qualifications is particularly important when the defendant doctor is called as a witness by the plaintiff's attorney. This circumstance is not unusual. The plaintiff's attorney knows that the defendant's qualifications will come out, and he hopes that they will come out favorably. He hopes that the defendant will go on and on without being led. It is better for the qualifications to be kept simple at this time. The doctor's attorney can ask the appropriate questions to bring out any desirable qualifications when he questions him in the "cross-examination."

This entire procedure is done to impress the jury and hopefully make them feel that anything the witness says must be true. This can make or break the case. Actually, it is the judge who determines if the witness is a qualified expert.

The significance of the qualifying procedure is illustrated by my own experience in testifying in an alleged malpractice case. The opposing attorney knew me from other courtroom appearances. As soon as I was sworn in and was asked the first question about my qualifications, he jumped to his feet and said, "I will stipulate that the witness is qualified." He obviously did not want the jury to be told of my accomplishments. My attorney insisted that I be qualified, for obvious reasons. As my attorney led me, I went on at length in as modest a manner as possible about my academic positions, publications, research projects, etc., as I watched the pained facial expression of the opposing attorney. This is not an isolated instance.

It is amusing to recall an incident that involved Dr. Frederick Verhoff, the great Harvard ophthalmologist of the past generation, who was brilliant but sometimes irascible. While on the witness stand, he was asked who was the greatest authority on the subject. He answered simply, "I am." Afterward, a colleague questioned if that wasn't somewhat immodest. He said, "I had to say that, I was under oath." Few of us have that problem.

Assuming that the case will be decided by a jury, what is important in convincing a jury to return a verdict for the defendant physician? First, the physician and his attorney should have good credibility with the jury. Two key elements are involved here: trustworthiness and expertise. The jury has to believe that the attorney and the physician know what they are talking about and that they are being honest and candid. In addition, a high level of credibility is important for witnesses testifying in the physician's behalf. It is also important that the jury find the attorney and the physician likable. When a physician or his attorney appears obnoxious or arrogant, a jury will have greater psychological incentive to find against the physician in spite of a preponderance of evidence to the contrary.

It should be clear at this point that a physician cannot focus only on the medical testimony he intends to present. In many cases, the defendant physician will be portrayed by the plaintiff's attorney as having been grossly neglectful of the patient or too busy to be concerned with the patient's welfare. In attempting to decide whether these allegations are true, jurors will carefully watch the physician to see how he acts and whether he is the type of person that is being described by the plaintiff's attorney. In general, jurors who sit day after day listening to allegations about a physician naturally become curious about what he is really like. The time that the physician is on the witness stand often reveals little regarding his background, lifestyle, and character. In this context, simple matters such as the clothes he wears and the car he drives to court can be important. Jurors are drawn from the community and often carry prejudices and misconceptions; they may share the common prejudice that physicians make too much money. It is important that the physician not inflame this prejudice, if it exists, by his appearance. Modest, conservative clothing and the absence of a very expensive car and ostentatious jewelry may help in this regard. On the other hand, of course, the doctor should not dress to informally since this could suggest a lack of respect for the court or the legal system of which the jurors are a part. Everything that the physician does in the presence of the jurors, whether it is in the courtroom, in the hallways during the morning break, or at lunch in the courthouse cafeteria, can be important. The physician who appears at all times to be polite and well mannered will inevitably be regarded favorably by the jury when they adjourn to reach a verdict.

The qualifications of the witness are not the only things that are important in creating a desirable impression. The dress and attitude are likewise very significant. The jury expects the witness to dress and act like their image of a good doctor, which is usually derived from television. It is the image of a person whose dress is neat but not gaudy, who is kindly, wise and pleasant, who is never angry or arrogant, and who is helpful even to his opponents. This is the image the doctor on the witness stand should create.

The psychology of malpractice cases is very important. Usually a jury will vote for the defense and even forgive an error in judgment unless there are extenuating circumstances. Some of the factors that tip the scales in favor of the plaintiff are:

1. Arrogance of the physician
2. Lack of compassion for the patient
3. Altered records
4. Perjury (the jury may forgive a mistake, but not perjury)
5. Exorbitant fees
6. Refusal to admit a patient to the hospital
7. Discharging a patient too soon
8. Obvious lack of knowledge

The most effective witness is a doctor who has humility, compassion, and conveys the impression that he did the best he could.

When the weeks of testimony are over and the jury retires to their room for deliberations, they will have forgotten much, if not all, of what the witness has said, but they will have an impression of him. If this impression is favorable, if they think, "I would like to have him as my doctor," his side may win the verdict. If the pervading thought is "I wouldn't have him for my dog," the reverse is likely to be the case.

The attorney is under no such constraining image. His television personality is often portrayed as one who is tricky, argumentative, and is sometimes mean and angry. The jury expects and accepts these characteristics in an attorney, but not in a physician.

The witness will do well never to show anger, never to lose his temper, no matter how much the other attorney provokes him. Some attorneys deliberately attempt to provoke anger because it helps damage the image of the witness.

THE DIRECT EXAMINATION

After the witness has been qualified, the direct examination by the attorney on his side usually follows. Usually the questions and answers have been reviewed in advance, but not the precise terminology. The witness should listen carefully to every word of the question, and always wait for the complete question before answering.

During direct examination, one's attorney is usually 20 or 25 feet away in order to allow the jury to concentrate on the witness without being distracted by the attorney. The witness should look at the jury a reasonable portion of the time. Eye contact is important; it is the essence of credibility. Some jurors will later think, "Did he look me in the eye?" This may be the basis for their decision whether or not the witness is honest. An occasional friendly smile may be helpful.

My approach in talking to a jury is to treat them like a group of beginning medical students whom I really like. I attempt to teach them in the most lucid, patient, and comfortable manner that I can. I use scientific terminology but immediately explain it in simple lay language. The scientific terminology is important only for the record. In case of conflicting testimony by later witnesses, or an appeal of the case to another court, the record must show what you really mean. However, this is not meaningful to the jury, and they must be educated in simple terms. The witness should use diagrams whenever possible. In most instances, diagrams on large pieces of paper are preferable because they can be taken into the jury room, unlike a blackboard diagram which is erased soon after presentation.

As in the deposition, one should avoid overstatements and not say things that cannot be substantiated. It is well to avoid equivocation whenever possible. The court is not usually interested in the rare exception, guesses are not permitted. It is well to avoid, "I think," but the expert is entitled to his opinion, and it is well to say, "In my opinion ..." Always, always be honest. Do not permit the desire to win distort the truth.

The witness should discuss, in advance with his attorney, whether or not to amplify the answer to a question if it seems favorable. Generally it is not wise to do this during the direct examination, but amplification can be brought about during the re-direct, after the witness and the attorney have had an opportunity to discuss the question *(vide infra)*.

THE CROSS-EXAMINATION

The cross-examination questions by the opposing attorney are the next step. This is sometimes the type of performance that the jury has been conditioned by television to anticipate with interest.

The opposing attorney frequently comes very close to the witness stand during the questioning. He does this for two reasons. The jury's attention is diverted from the witness to the attorney, and he is better able to intimidate or anger the witness. Do not fall prey to these tactics. Look at the jury more often than at the attorney. Be kind to the attorney, smile at him. If he has difficulty with a word, help him in a kind, but not an arrogant, manner. It will figuratively kill him.

The attorney will attempt to demonstrate inconsistencies in what you have said on the stand or in your deposition, or in your statements compared with the testimony of other witnesses or what is in the written record. He may also attempt to develop uncertainty in your own mind. He will attempt to amplify minor inconsistencies to convince the jury that you are not worthy of belief.

In spite of the news media, the average layman still holds the physician in high esteem and does not expect mistakes and inconsistencies from him. The attorney will not usually say that the doctor is lying, but that he is busy and confused under the pressures of practice. If the doctor is the defendant witness, the attorney may say that this pressure of practice and confusion are unfortunate, *but* his client was injured by it and must be compensated.

You, the witness, *shall* listen carefully to the question and, as Shakespeare said, "Mark you his absolute 'Shall'." *(Coriolanus, Act III, Scene 1).* You shall always permit the attorney to finish the question before answering. Answers shall always be truthful but as brief as is consistent with the truth. As noted in the chapter on the deposition, the witness should not add phrases that are not required. Frequently, it is the "but" in "Yes, but" or "No, but" that gets the witness into difficulties.

The witness may be very tempted to add something that he considers favorable to his side. It is wise to avoid the temptation. During the recess the witness may ask his attorney to bring this out in the re-direct.

The witness must be sure that he understands the question. If he does not understand it, or does not hear every word, he should ask that it be repeated, no matter how long the question, or even if it has already been repeated. If the witness does not understand the question, he should say so. Do not answer a compound question. Break it into its component parts, or ask the attorney to do so. An affirmative or negative response to a compound question may include a response to one of the components that you do not mean.

If one of the attorneys objects, stop. If your attorney objects, he may be doing this for reasons based on the law, or he may be doing it because the witness is getting himself into difficulties, and he wants to give the witness a moment to think. Accordingly, if your attorney objects, think for a moment and evaluate your position and your answer.

It is common practice for the attorney, frequently the opposing attorney, to present a hypothetical case. This is done so that he can avoid establishing the legal background and face many objections from the other attorney with which he would probably be confronted. The hypothetical case generally corresponds in every detail to the actual patient involved in the litigation. It usually consists of many parts and may take several minutes to present. Listen very carefully to every part. It is not rare for the question to contain many portions that are obviously true but include one that is not. Consider the following example, "Doctor, I am going to ask you a hypothetical question. It is true, isn't it, that this three pound one ounce infant was born at approximately 33 weeks gestation, and that it was cyanotic and had a respiratory grunt, and the chest film showed a pneumothorax, and that it was given supplemental oxygen, and that at times the oxygen in the isolette was 70%, at times 40%, and at other times 32%, and that the accepted standard of practice is to maintain the oxygen level at or below 40%, and that this infant then developed a urinary infection and needed antimicrobial agents, which it received. This is true, isn't it doctor?" All but one of the phrases is true, and the witness may be lulled into nodding the affirmative and saying, "Yes, yes." The answer is "No!" because it is not below the standard of practice to exceed 40% oxygen if the status of the infant requires it. If the witness answers "yes," he has admitted that the practice was below standard, and thus was malpractice. If there is any doubt regarding any portion of the hypothetical presentation, request that it be repeated, even though it literally takes five minutes to do so. If one is still in doubt, have it repeated again. Do not fall into a trap. It is common practice that the expert witness will be asked what he is being paid. I answer truthfully. Sometimes, the question will be, "Doctor, you are being paid for your testimony, aren't you?" My answer is, "I am being paid for my time, knowledge, and ability, but not my testimony. My testimony is not for sale."

Occasionally, toward the end of the cross-examination or the deposition, the opposing attorney will say, "We are almost finished, excuse me for asking just one or two more questions, Doctor." Be careful; the attorney not infrequently saves his "best pitch," his most vital question, for this time, hoping that the witness is relaxed and off-guard.

THE IMPORTANCE OF THE RECESS

If the testimony has taken any significant length of time, the judge will declare a recess. Courts are usually in session for two or two and one-half hours in the morning or the afternoon. It is customary to have a recess during each period, which means that it is unusual for much more than an hour to elapse before the recess is declared. The recess is important. It provides an opportunity for the witness and his attorney to discuss what has transpired and what questions are likely to be presented after the recess. It is during this period that the witness who has felt that he would have liked to have added something to his testimony can suggest that his attorney ask the appropriate question after the recess. The attorney can also indicate to the witness the problems that have already arisen because of the answers and what might be done to correct the situation.

It is not wise for the witness to go right to the attorney at the start of the recess. The jury may think that the witness is being coached or unduly influenced by the attorney. It is preferable that the witness and the attorney agree in advance to meet in a more remote area, such as a washroom, and then they should be certain that no one is listening.

At the conclusion of the cross-examination there may be a re-direct examination, at which some of the problems noted above can be brought out. There may also be a re-cross examination.

Later in the trial, a witness may be brought back as a rebuttal witness. In this case, the questions that the attorney may ask are restricted to facts previously introduced into the trial, but the situation may otherwise be similar to the preceding.

On leaving the witness stand, it is desirable to avoid overt manifestation of great friendship for a defendant or another witness who might be in court because this could influence the jury.

The witness should avoid discussing the case with others after he has left the witness stand, just as he did before. The case may be declared a mistrial, or result in a "hung" jury, or be appealed, and remarks made even after leaving the stand might be regretted.

THE EXPERT WITNESS

If one is a defendant it is important that one helps the attorney in the selection of expert witnesses. They may make the difference between winning or losing.

The large number of suits means that many are called upon to be experts. It is important that one knows the role of the expert witness.

The function of an expert witness is to help define the standard of care as it pertains to the case under consideration and to render an opinion as to whether the care provided met this standard.

Legal standards of care are not necessarily what a majority do, but what a minority of acceptable ophthalmologists would do. The fact that the expert might not do it is not germane to his or her opinion.

Evaluating whether the care provided was substandard may be difficult. There are many gray areas and an expert witness should be cautious about stating that care was substandard because once this is indicated, the plaintiff's attorney will not desist.

The expert is not rushed and has the advantage of being able to evaluate all aspects of the case in retrospection. The treating physician did not have this advantage. Errors in judgment do not constitute substandard care. However, if care was indeed substandard the expert must say so and be willing to testify to it.

THE DISCOVERY PROCESS

It is essential that the expert be acquainted with certain fundamentals of giving a good deposition. These fundamentals were covered thoroughly earlier in this chapter. Review them if you are called to be an expert witness.

A CONTEST OF IMPRESSIONS

A trial is a contest of impressions. Juries are frequently faced by expert ophthalmologists on each side who give conflicting opinions. Expected to weigh one opinion against the other, juries must consider the relative qualifications and credibility of each expert and the basis for each opinion. Juries give great weight to the demeanor of witnesses and whether testimony is given in a logical, convincing manner.

An expert witness must meet certain ethical and legal requirements: expertise in the area of concern, honesty, impartiality, imperviousness to monetary considerations. Qualifications should be stated clearly but not arrogantly. The expert should dress and act conservatively, and speak to the jury as a kindly, helpful educator would speak to novices. Use both lay and scientific terminology. The former so the jury will understand it and the latter so the meaning is clear in the event of future disputes or retrials.

Listen carefully to the long hypothetical case that will be presented and attendant questions before answering. Do not agree unless you agree with every part of it. Do not hesitate to ask that it be repeated.

Never get angry or argue with an attorney. Be truthful. Do not exaggerate or amplify.

EXPERT FOR THE PLAINTIFF

Should an expert witness take cases for the plaintiff? There are several reasons why an expert who takes cases for the defendant also should accept them for the other side:

1. The vast majority of plaintiff's cases are without merit. An honest, knowledgeable expert can influence the plaintiff's attorney to drop these cases at an early stage, thereby saving time, money and emotional trauma.
2. It adds to one's credibility as an expert witness.
3. It is only fair that each side obtains good advice.
4. Dishonest witnesses are available if honest ones refuse.

SETTLING A CASE OUT OF COURT

Many physicians are reluctant to settle a case, especially if one feels that the care of the patient was not substandard. It is well not to be arbitrary about this, but many factors should be weighed. These include the following:

What impression on the jury is the appearance and testimony of the defendant, the experts for each side, and the plaintiff likely to make?

Is the trial to be held in an area from which a conservative or a liberal jury might be selected?

What are the consequences of settling?

Any payment must be reported to the National Practitioner Data Bank. In some states, payments over a certain amount must be reported to the state's medical board and payment over a larger amount may be investigated by them.

Index

Page numbers followed by "f" indicate figures; those followed by "t" indicate tabular material.

H

I

J

K

T

W